This book is dedicated to
Jerry Dolovich,
McMaster University,
Hamilton, Canada,
who has made so many
original and important
contributions to theoretical
and clinical allergy

Essential Allergy

NIELS MYGIND

Formerly Senior Lecturer, Otopathological Laboratory
Department of Otorhinolaryngology
Rigshospitalet, Copenhagen, Denmark

RONALD DAHL

Professor, Department of Lung Medicine
University of Århus
Kommunehospitalet, Århus, Denmark

SØREN PEDERSEN

Associate Professor, Department of Pediatrics
Kolding Hospital, Kolding, Denmark

KRISTIAN THESTRUP-PEDERSEN

Professor, Department of Dermatology
University of Århus
Marselisborg Hospital, Århus, Denmark

SECOND EDITION

Blackwell
Science

© 1986, 1996 by
Blackwell Science Ltd
Editorial Offices:
Osney Mead, Oxford OX2 0EL
25 John Street, London WC1N 2BL
23 Ainslie Place, Edinburgh EH3 6AJ
238 Main Street, Cambridge
   Massachusetts 02142, USA
54 University Street, Carlton
   Victoria 3053, Australia

Other Editorial Offices:
Arnette Blackwell SA
   1, rue de Lille, 75007 Paris
   France

Blackwell Wissenschafts-Verlag GmbH
   Kurfürstendamm 57
   10707 Berlin, Germany

   Feldgasse 13, A-1238 Wien
   Austria

First published 1986
Italian edition 1988
German edition 1989
Portuguese edition 1993
Second edition 1996

Set by Excel Typesetters, Hong Kong
Printed and bound in Italy
by G. Canale & C. SpA, Turin

DISTRIBUTORS

Marston Book Services Ltd
PO Box 87
Oxford OX2 0DT
(*Orders*: Tel: 01865 791155
         Fax: 01865 791927
         Telex: 837515)

North America
Blackwell Science, Inc.
238 Main Street
Cambridge, MA 02142
(*Orders*: Tel: 800 215-1000
               617 876-7000
         Fax: 617 492-5263)

Australia
Blackwell Science Pty Ltd
54 University Street
Carlton, Victoria 3053
(*Orders*: Tel: 03 9347-0300
         Fax: 03 9349-3016)

A catalogue record for this title
is available from the British Library

ISBN 0-632-03645-1 (BSL)
     0-86542-671-6
     (International Edition)

Library of Congress
Cataloging-in-Publication Data

Essential allergy / Niels Mygind . . .
[et al.]. — 2nd ed.
        p.   cm.
   Rev. ed.: Essential allergy /
   Niels Mygind. 1986.
   Includes bibliographical references
   and index.
   ISBN 0-632-03645-1
   1. Allergy.   I. Mygind, Niels.
II. Mygind, Niels.
Essential allergy.
   [DNLM: 1. Hypersensitivity.
   WD 300 E78 1995]
RC584.E85   1995
616.97 — dc20
DNLM/DLC
for Library of Congress   95-14201
                                              CIP

Contents

Preface

Essential Allergy is written for those who have just been appointed to a department dealing with allergic diseases. It will enable them to treat the patients, and to converse scientifically with the head of the department during tea break.

Essential Allergy is also intended for the interested medical student. Equipped with personal notes, the book may serve as a handbook and reference text. All physicians will be faced with allergic diseases during their career.

Essential refers to the most important tasks for a clinician, which are optimum patient care, exact diagnosis and treatment based on a cost–risk–benefit analysis.

The text describes both allergic and allergy-like diseases, and the term *allergy* in the title should, strictly speaking, be in inverted commas. The diseases, seen in an allergy clinic, are usually referred to as 'allergic diseases', but an allergic aetiology is only demonstrated in some of the patients, and non-allergic mechanisms are of importance even in genuine allergic states. Therefore, the diseases are described from a multifactorial, organ-related point of view.

Great effort has been made to ensure an easily readable text, and *Essential Allergy* consists of 110 short chapters with many illustrations (309 figures and 122 tables). You can quickly run through the book reading the 'key points' and the 'superheadings' to figures and tables.

The first edition was written by Niels Mygind. In the second edition, he covers rhinitis and the overall editing, Ronald Dahl and Søren Pedersen asthma, and Kristian Thestrup-Pedersen skin diseases.

Niels Mygind
Ronald Dahl
Søren Pedersen
Kristian Thestrup-Pedersen

Acknowledgements

We are grateful to a number of colleagues who have contributed with valuable help and comments to both the first and second edition of *Essential Allergy*: Louis A. Phillips, Carsten Bindslev-Jensen, T.J.H. Clark, Jens Korsgaard, Hans-Jørgen Malling, Ole Mejlsbo, Philip S. Norman, Minoru Okuda, Nils Svedmyr, Bent Weeke, John Widdicombe and Hugh Zacharia.

Abbreviations and Acronyms

APC	Antigen-presenting cell
ATP	Adenosine triphosphate
AU	Allergy unit
BAL	Bronchoalveolar lavage
b.d.	Twice daily
BU	Biological unit
C1–9	Complement components 1–9
CAM	Cell adhesion molecule
CD	Cluster of differentiation
C domain	Constant domain
CGRP	Calcitonin gene-related peptide
CNS	Central nervous system
COPD	Chronic obstructive pulmonary disease
DBPCFC	Double-blind, placebo-controlled food challenge
DPI	Dry-powder inhaler
ECP	Eosinophil cationic protein
ELAM-1	Endothelial leucocyte adhesion molecule 1
ELISA	Enzyme-linked immunosorbent assay
EDN	Eosinophil-derived neurotoxin
EPO	Eosinophil peroxydase
EPX	Eosinophil protein X
ESR	Erythrocyte sedimentation rate
Fab	Fragment antigen binding
Fc	Fragment crystallizable
FcϵR1	High-affinity receptor for IgE
FcϵR2	Low-affinity receptor for IgE
FEIA	Fluorescence immunosorbent assay
FEV_1	Forced expiratory volume in 1 second
FVC	Forced vital capacity
GALT	Gut-associated lymphoid tissue
GM-CSF	Granulocyte-macrophage colony-stimulating factor
GP	Guinea-pig or general practitioner
H chain	Heavy chain
HIV	Human immunodeficiency virus
HLA	Human leucocyte antigen
HML-1	Human mucosal lymphocyte receptor 1

HPA	Hypothalamic–pituitary–adrenal
ICAM-1	Intercellular adhesion molecule 1
IFN	Interferon
IgE	Immunoglobulin E
IL	Interleukin
IU	International unit
kDa	Kilodalton
kPa	Kilopascal
L chain	Light chain
LFA	Leucocyte function-associated antigen
LT	Leukotriene
Mac	Macrophage antigen
MALT	Mucosa-associated lymphoid tissue
MC_{TC}	Mast cell containing chymase and tryptase (connective tissue mast cell)
MC_T	Mast cell containing tryptase (mucosal mast cell)
MBP	Major basic protein
MDI	Metered-dose inhaler
MHC	Major histocompatibility complex
NANC	Non-adrenergic non-cholinergic
NEP	Neutral endopeptidase
NPY	Neuropeptide Y
NK	Neurokinin
NKA	Neurokinin A
o.d.	Once daily
$Paco_2$	Arterial blood gas tension of CO_2
PAF	Platelet activating factor
Pao_2	Arterial blood gas tension of O_2
PEEP	Positive end-expiratory pressure
PEP	Positive expiratory pressure
PCA	Passive cutaneous anaphylaxis
PC_{20}	Provoking concentration (of histamine), which reduces lung function 20%
PD_{20}	Provoking dose (of histamine), which reduces lung function 20%
PG	Prostaglandin
PGD	Prostaglandin D

PGE	Prostaglandin E
PGF	Prostaglandin F
PNU	Protein nitrogen unit
PRIST	Paper radioimmunosorbent test
PRN	*Pro re nata*. Latin for: accordingly as circumstances may require. When a drug is used on an as-needed basis
RANTES	Regulated upon activation, normal T cell expressed and secreted
RAST	Radioallergosorbent test
RIA	Radioimmunoassay
RIST	Radioimmunosorbent test
RV	Residual volume
Sao_2	Arterial blood gas saturation of O_2

SP	Substance P
SLE	Systemic lupus erythematosus
Tc cell	T cytotoxic cell
TCR	T-cell receptor
TDI	Toluene diisocyanate
Th cell	T helper cell
t.i.d.	Three times daily
TNF	Tumour necrosis factor
TXA	Thromboxane A
VCAM-1	Vascular cell adhesion molecule 1
VC	Vital capacity
V domain	Variable domain
VIP	Vasoactive intestinal polypeptide
VLA	Very late antigen

Part 1 Basic Mechanisms

1.1 History of allergy
From reagin to IgE

Key points
- It was not until the middle of the last century that the diseases, which we now call atopic allergic diseases, were recognized as entities.
- In 1873, Charles Blackley showed beyond any doubt that hay fever is caused by pollen.
- Richet and Portier demonstrated that repeated injections of jelly fish toxin into a dog, instead of providing protection, caused its death.
- They used the term anaphylaxis to describe this, the opposite of protection (prophylaxis).
- von Pirquet noted that under some conditions, humans, instead of developing immunity, had an increase in reactivity: this he called allergy.
- Arthus showed that non-toxic substances, such as horse serum, can, after repeated injections, cause tissue injury and necrosis (Arthus' reaction).
- Coca and Cooke proposed the term 'atopy' for those clinical forms of allergy, manifest by hay fever and asthma.
- Prausnitz and Küstner showed that atopic allergic sensitivity can be passively transferred from one individual to another by a serum factor, which they called reagin.
- It was not until 1967 that it was shown by Ishizaka and Ishizaka and by Johansson and Bennich that reagin belongs to a new immunoglobulin class, IgE.
- Allergy then became part of the exact discipline, clinical immunology.

A London doctor with summer catarrh

John Bostock (Fig. 1.1.1), speaking to the Royal Medical Society of London in 1819, described his own 'periodical affection of the eyes and chest', which he called *Catarrhus aestivus* or 'summer catarrh'. This condition also acquired the popular name of '*hay fever*', 'since the idea has generally prevailed, that it is produced by the effluvium from new hay'. Later Bostock reported a survey of the disease but was able to find only 28 cases in all England.

Another sneezing doctor

Half a century later, Charles Blackley of Manchester (Fig. 1.1.2) established beyond any doubt that pollens

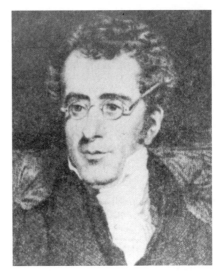

Fig. 1.1.1. John Bostock (1773–1846) described *Catarrhus aestivus* or hay fever. From Cohen SG, Samter M, eds. *Excerpts From Classics in Allergy* 2nd ed. Providence: OceanSide Publications, 1992: 1–211.

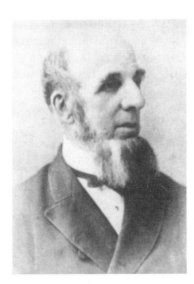

Fig. 1.1.2. Charles Blackley (1820–1900), a British allergy pioneer, who described the cause of hay fever. From Cohen SG, Samter M, eds. *Excerpts From Classics in Allergy* 2nd ed. Providence: OceanSide Publications, 1992: 1–211.

play an important role in the causation of hay fever. As a sufferer of the disease, he sampled pollens, and rubbed them into a scratch on his arm, which elicited a reaction. He also provoked conjunctivitis, rhinitis and asthma.

By microscopy of sticky slides, he counted pollen in the air and showed a correlation between the count and his symptoms. He attached sticky glass slides to the string of a kite and found pollens 500m above ground level. This discovery he took to be the explanation as to why he also suffered from hay fever in the city of Manchester.

Following the publication of his book, *Experimental Researches on the Causes and Nature of Catarrhus Aestivus* (London: Baillière Tindall, 1873), Blackley received a letter from Charles Darwin who stated: 'I have read two-thirds of the book with much interest . . .'. He wisely suggested that Blackley should investigate the differences that might be inherent in pollens transferred by the wind and those which were transferred by insects.

Description of other diseases

Hay fever was not the only entity described in the nineteenth century; *vasomotor rhinitis* (non-infectious perennial rhinitis) dates back to 1881 (Herzog), and *Quincke oedema (angioedema)* was described by the German, Dr Heinrich Quincke (Fig. 1.1.3). Although it was demonstrated that these diseases, and *bronchial asthma*, could in some cases be caused by exposure to foreign substances not damaging *per se*, the mechanisms behind the symptoms were not elucidated until the beginning of this century.

The unexpected death of a dog

In 1901, the French scientist Charles Richet (Fig. 1.1.4) and Paul Portier (Fig. 1.1.5) went on a Mediterranean cruise with Prince Albert of Monaco. He suggested that they study the poisonous jellyfish, the Portuguese man-of-war, the sting of which is extremely painful. After his return to Paris, Richet tried to make dogs immune to the poison. He used the method of the Greek King Mithradates (132–63 BC) who took repeated small doses of poison in order to make himself resistant to food that was poisoned by his enemies. One of the test-subjects was a 'fine big dog by the name of Neptunus'. Twenty-two days after the first injection, he was given a second one, this time one-tenth of a fatal dose. To Richet's astonishment, the animal became extremely ill and died within minutes.

As the phenomenon was considered to be the opposite of *prophylaxis*, which means protection, it was called *anaphylaxis*. Although Richet's interpretation of the experiment was wrong—he thought that a natural resistance against the toxic substance had been broken down—the concept of anaphylaxis proved to be very useful in the future study of allergy. The term, anaphylaxis, is still used for severe systemic allergic reactions.

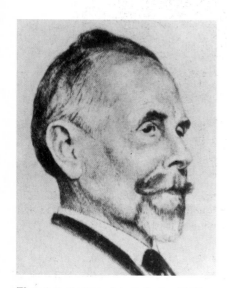

Fig. 1.1.3. Heinrich Quincke (1842–1922) gave his name to the disease, Quincke oedema (angioedema). From Cohen SG, Samter M, eds. *Excerpts From Classics in Allergy* 2nd ed. Providence: OceanSide Publications, 1992: 1–211.

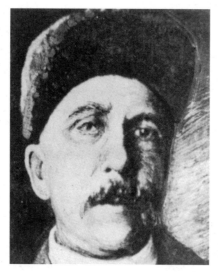

Fig. 1.1.4. Charles Richet (1850–1935) who, together with another French scientist, Paul Portier (see Fig. 1.1.5), described anaphylaxis. From Cohen SG, Samter M, eds. *Excerpts From Classics in Allergy* 2nd ed. Providence: OceanSide Publications, 1992: 1–211.

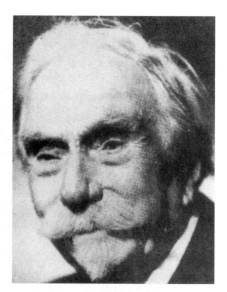

Fig. 1.1.5. Paul Portier (1866–1962). From Cohen SG, Samter M, eds. *Excerpts From Classics in Allergy* 2nd ed. Providence: OceanSide Publications, 1992: 1–211.

A few years later, it was suggested that hay fever (Wolff-Eisner, 1906) and asthma (Meltzer, 1910) were 'human anaphylaxis'. Richet, who was a multitalented scientist, was awarded the Nobel Prize in 1919.

Injury from non-toxic substances

In the year following Richet's experiment, Maurice Arthus (Fig. 1.1.6) showed that anaphylactic reactions can be triggered by substances that are not in themselves toxic. Arthus injected horse serum into rabbits without causing any reaction the first time. When he repeated the injection after a few weeks he observed a strong reaction, the tissue becoming inflamed and, in some cases, necrotic. This local anaphylactic reaction became known as the *Arthus' reaction*.

Derivation of the word 'allergy'

Two paediatricians, the Austrian Clemens von Pirquet (Fig. 1.1.7) and the Hungarian-born Bela Shick (Fig. 1.1.8), reported, in 1905, that children who were given repeated injections of horse streptococcal antitoxin serum sometimes developed fever, swollen glands and nettle rash, *serum sickness*. von Pirquet, in an article in the *Münchener Mediziniche Wochenschrift* in 1906, proposed

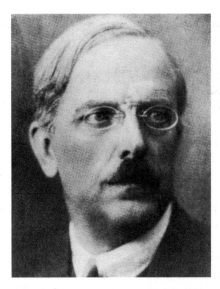

Fig. 1.1.7. Clemens von Pirquet (1874–1924) coined the word 'allergy', and, together with Bela Shick (see Fig. 1.1.8), described serum sickness. From Cohen SG, Samter M, eds. *Excerpts From Classics in Allergy* 2nd ed. Providence: OceanSide Publications, 1992: 1–211.

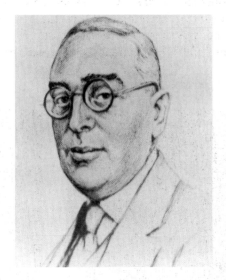

Fig. 1.1.8. Bela Shick (1877–1967). From Cohen SG, Samter M, eds. *Excerpts From Classics in Allergy* 2nd ed. Providence: OceanSide Publications, 1992: 1–211.

the term *allergy* for the concept of changed reactivity. He put together the Greek words '*allos*', meaning different or changed, and '*ergos*', meaning work or action.

Derivation of the word 'atopy'

The American researchers Cooke and Coca (Figs 1.1.9–10), in 1923, proposed the term *atopy* for those clinical forms of allergy, manifest by hay fever

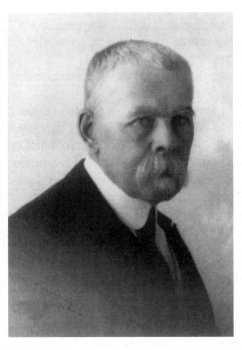

Fig. 1.1.6. Nicholas-Maurice Arthus (1862–1945). From Cohen SG, Samter M, eds. *Excerpts From Classics in Allergy* 2nd ed. Providence: OceanSide Publications, 1992: 1–211.

and asthma, in which 'the individuals as a group possess a peculiar capacity to become sensitive to certain proteins to which their environment and habits of life frequently expose them'. Thus, an *inherited predisposition* to become sensitized is a characteristic feature of atopy. Later, another characteristic was added, the presence of 'reagin' and a positive skin test to allergen.

A dramatic horse-ride in Central Park

In 1919, Dr Maximillian Ramirez of New York reported an unusual case of asthma in the *Journal of the American Medical Association*. He was consulted by a man who had developed an asthma attack for the first time in a horse-drawn carriage in Central Park. A fortnight earlier, this patient had had a blood transfusion, and Dr Ramirez found out that the blood donor was an asthmatic with a positive skin test to horse dander. This was the first observation indicating that asthma can be mediated by a serum factor.

Prausnitz and Küstner

That allergy can be transferred by serum was confirmed in 1921 by Dr Prausnitz (Fig. 1.1.11) in his classical experiment. Serum from the fish-allergic Küstner (Fig. 1.1.12) was injected into Prausnitz's arm. The next day, Prausnitz was injected with fish extract in the same place and, for the first time in his life, he exhibited a positive skin reaction. The serum factor responsible for the *Prausnitz–Küstner reaction* was named *reagin* by Coca and Cooke.

Reagin and immunoglobulin

It later became clear that reagin was associated with antibody, but compared with antibody against micro-organisms, the reaginic antibody had some distinctive features. First, it could not be demonstrated in serum by the usual precipitation reactions. Second, it was heat labile. Third, it had a peculiar ability to become fixed to the skin for prolonged periods and to elicit a wheal (oedema) and flare (erythema) reaction.

When the different immunoglobulin classes were later identified, attempts were made to relate reaginic antibody to one of these classes. However, it soon became obvious that reagin was associated with neither IgG, IgM, IgA nor with IgD.

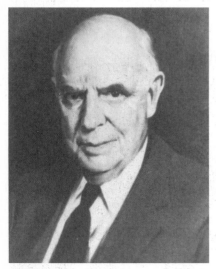

Fig. 1.1.9. Robert A. Cooke (1880–1960), an American allergy pioneer, who, together with A.F. Coca (see Fig. 1.1.10), first used the term 'atopy', and also, together with M.E. Loveless, described blocking antibody. From Cohen SG, Samter M, eds. *Excerpts From Classics in Allergy* 2nd ed. Providence: OceanSide Publications, 1992: 1–211.

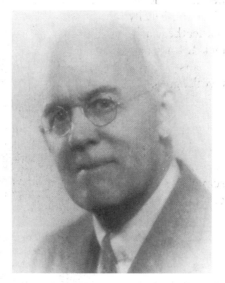

Fig. 1.1.10. Arthur Fernandez Coca (1875–1959). From Cohen SG, Samter M, eds. *Excerpts From Classics in Allergy* 2nd ed. Providence: OceanSide Publications, 1992: 1–211.

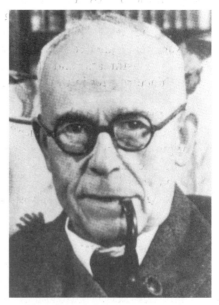

Fig. 1.1.11. Carl Prausnitz (1876–1963) who, together with Heinz Küstner, first reported on passive transfer of allergy. From Cohen SG, Samter M, eds. *Excerpts From Classics in Allergy* 2nd ed. Providence: OceanSide Publications, 1992: 1–211.

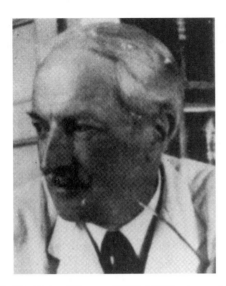

Fig. 1.1.12. Heinz Küstner (1897–1963) who, aside from being the subject with allergy in the Prausnitz–Küstner reaction, was professor of obstetrics and gynaecology. From Cohen SG, Samter M, eds. *Excerpts From Classics in Allergy* 2nd ed. Providence: OceanSide Publications, 1992: 1–211.

The ugly duckling –

While other fields of immunology were rapidly developing in the 1950s and 1960s, the discipline of allergy remained the ugly duckling. The empirically founded practice of injecting extracts of feather cushions, vacuum cleaner contents and chicken soup into the skin of asthmatic and rhinitis patients did not inspire much respect in the allergists' colleagues.

– becomes a swan

The situation changed dramatically in 1967. Due to the original observations (described below) the ugly duckling became a swan and allergy is now a highly respected member of the exact discipline, clinical immunology. The metamorphosis took place when *reagin became IgE.*

Logic and genius

The husband and wife team, Ishizaka and Ishizaka (Fig. 1.1.13), working in Denver, Colorado, isolated a reagin-rich serum fraction from a person with extreme allergy to ragweed pollen (Fig. 1.1.14). A Prausnitz–Küstner (PK) reaction demonstrated the reaginic content of the serum, which was used to raise antibodies (antiserum) in rabbits. Human IgG, IgM, IgA and IgD were added to the antiserum to precipitate anti-IgG, IgM, IgA and IgD antibodies. The supernatant should then be empty of the

known immunoglobulin classes, but it still produced a positive PK reaction. The addition of the original reagin-rich serum to the 'empty' supernatant produced a small precipitate and the new supernatant thus obtained was devoid of skin-sensitizing activity. Furthermore, the precipitate bound isotope tagged ragweed allergen, indicating that it had antibody activity.

The Ishizakas had thus produced evidence that reaginic antibody belongs to a previously undiscovered immunoglobulin class, which they named *gamma E globulin.*

Luck and genius

Working at the same time as the Ishizakas but independently of them, S.G.O. Johansson (Fig. 1.1.15) and Hans Bennich (Fig. 1.1.16) in Uppsala, Sweden, obtained a myeloma protein, which differed from the known immunoglobulin classes. They called the new immunoglobulin *IgND* after the initials of the patient.

Using a very sensitive radioimmunoassay, they demonstrated the presence of small amounts of IgND in normal serum and of increased levels in allergic patients. These observations led to the conclusion that reagin belongs to this new immunoglobulin class.

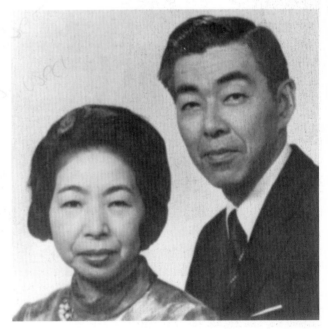

Fig. 1.1.13. Teruko and Kimishige Ishizaka who first described IgE. From Avenberg KM, Harper DS, Larsson BL. *Footnotes on Allergy* Uppsala: Pharmacia, 1980: 1–103.

Original experiment to identify IgE

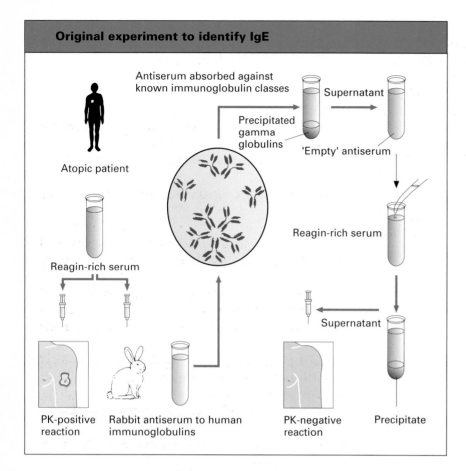

Atopic patient

Antiserum absorbed against known immunoglobulin classes

Precipitated gamma globulins

'Empty' antiserum

Supernatant

Reagin-rich serum

Reagin-rich serum

Supernatant

PK-positive reaction

Rabbit antiserum to human immunoglobulins

PK-negative reaction

Precipitate

Fig. 1.1.14. This scheme outlines the experiments that led to the conclusion that reaginic antibodies belong to a distinct immunoglobulin class, IgE. Refer to text for interpretation. From Ishizaka K. The identification and significance of gamma E. In: Dixon FJ, Fisher DW, eds. *The Biology of Immunologic Diseases*. Sunderland: Sinauer Associated Inc., 1983: 13–23.

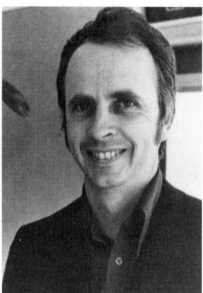

Fig. 1.1.15. S. Gunnar O. Johansson who, together with Hans Bennich (see Fig. 1.1.16), described IgE independently of the Ishizakas and who also developed radioimmunoassays for its determination. From Avenberg KM, Harper DS, Larsson BL. *Footnotes on Allergy* Uppsala: Pharmacia, 1980: 1–103.

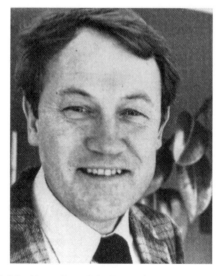

Fig. 1.1.16. Hans Bennich. From Avenberg KM, Harper DS, Larsson BL. *Footnotes on Allergy* Uppsala: Pharmacia, 1980: 1–103.

IgE

When the two teams met in 1968, it became clear that they had studied the same immunoglobulin class, which they agreed to call *immunoglobulin E (IgE)*. It is now established that this immunoglobulin class is the carrier of the biological features of reaginic antibody.

Discovery

Discovery is seeing what everybody has seen, and thinking what nobody has thought.

Claude Bernard

1.2 The immune system
A brief introduction

Key points

- The immune system is able to distinguish between self and non-self macromolecules.
- The system consists of lymphocytes and antibody molecules.
- An immune response is characterized by specificity towards the antigen.
- Lymphocytes are classified into T and B cells.
- They become stimulated when antigen is presented to them in a processed form by antigen-presenting cells.
- Stimulation of T cells results in the formation of sensitized lymphocytes, which secrete a series of active substances, cytokines (a cell-mediated immune response).
- When B cells are stimulated, they are transformed into plasma cells, which synthesize antibody (a humoral immune response).
- T lymphocytes, as helper cells, control the immune response.
- Antigen-specific memory is a key property of the immune system.
- An immune response can lead to immune protection or to immune disease: allergic and autoimmune disease.

Basic knowledge of the immune system is a prerequisite for a full understanding of allergic diseases. Immunologists have in recent years made considerable progress in the study of the immune system. Of particular importance for allergists are the description of the receptor for IgE, the regulation of IgE synthesis, and the characterization of lymphocyte receptors and cytokines. Molecular biologists have now cloned the genes' encoding for most of these proteins and mediators and have defined their amino acid sequence.

Self and non-self

The first of three fundamental properties of the immune system is its ability to *distinguish between 'self' and 'non-self'*, that is, between macromolecules that are products of the individual's own genes and those that are not.

Some 10^{12} *lymphocytes* and 10^{20} *antibody molecules* constantly patrol the body checking every cell and molecule in order to detect non-self structures and eliminate them, a function called *immunological surveillance*.

Specificity for antigen

Specificity is the second key attribute of the immune system. When a non-self protein macromolecule penetrates the organism, it can act as an *antigen* and stimulate the immune system exclusively towards that molecule or towards a part of it, an *epitope*.

The foreign proteins are phagocytized by *antigen-presenting cells*, which belong to the macrophage/monocyte/dendritic cell system. These cells are present in every surface tissue of the body.

The patrolling lymphocytes can recognize as many as 10^7 antigens, but each cell is only able to recognize a few. When an antigen binds to a lymphocyte, which has specificity for one of its epitopes, the antigen-stimulated lymphocyte is activated; it proliferates and starts a production of identical offspring cells, all with the same antigen specificity, *clonal proliferation*. This antigen-driven selection of cells is called *clonal selection* (Fig. 1.2.1). As humans, fortunately, do not encounter every thinkable antigen, it follows that many lymphocytes ('virgin cells') grow old and die without ever having met their respective antigen and becoming stimulated by it.

T and B lymphocytes

The lymphocyte is 'the conductor of the immunological orchestra', and, as such, is the most important cell in the immune system. This revelation is recent; only 3 decades ago the same cell was described in a textbook of pathology as 'a phlegmatic spectator of inflammatory reactions'.

All lymphocytes develop from a common lymphoid precursor cell in the bone marrow, from where they will migrate to the peripheral lymphatic tissues. There are two main groups: B and T cells.

T lymphocytes (thymus-dependent lymphocytes) need a period of maturation in the thymus, where they express their T-cell receptor and other surface markers of differentiation (see later).

The other major cell type, the *B lymphocytes*, develop fully in the bone marrow and migrate directly to the peripheral tissues (Fig. 1.2.2).

Antigen stimulation of lymphocytes

Lymphocytes that have not been in contact with their antigen are called 'naïve cells' or 'virgin cells'.

When *B lymphocytes* are stimulated by antigen, they multiply and are transformed into *plasma cells*,

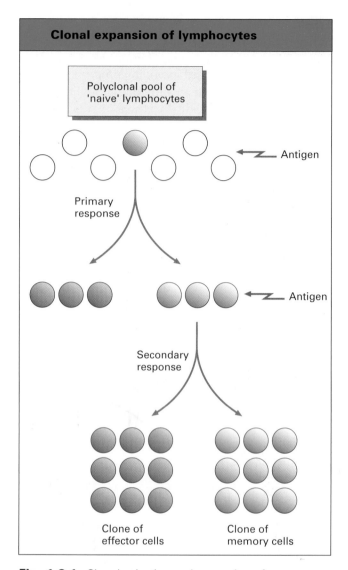

Fig. 1.2.1. Clonal selection and expansion of lymphocytes. Lymphocytes with different specificity for antigen form a pool of 'naïve' or 'virgin' lymphocytes. Following stimulation by antigen only those cells with specificity for that particular antigen proliferate and form clones of identical cells, which may either function as effector cells or as memory cells. When memory cells are again stimulated by the antigen, the secondary response will be faster and more vigorous than the primary response.

which commence synthesis of *antibody* against the antigen in question (Fig. 1.2.2).

Antigen stimulation of *T lymphocytes* causes them to proliferate and differentiate into *activated T cells*. Some of these act as T helper cells (CD4+ subsets; see later), while others develop into *cytotoxic cells* or effector cells (CD8+ subsets), which can destroy antigen-containing cells. Activated T cells also produce

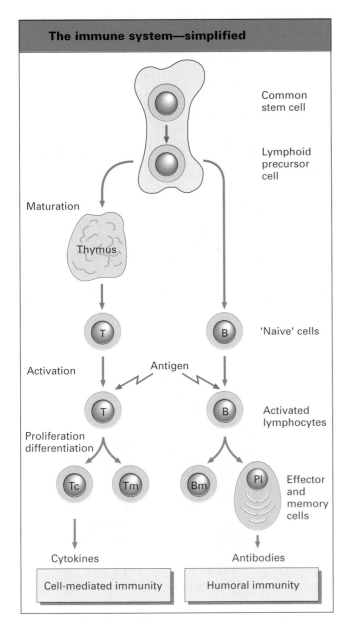

The immune system—simplified

- Common stem cell
- Lymphoid precursor cell
- Maturation
- Thymus
- 'Naive' cells
- Activation
- Antigen
- Activated lymphocytes
- Proliferation differentiation
- Effector and memory cells
- Cytokines
- Antibodies
- Cell-mediated immunity
- Humoral immunity

Fig. 1.2.2. Simplified presentation of the immune system. The two lymphocyte subsets, T and B cells, are both derived from precursor cells in the bone marrow. Maturation in the thymus is only needed for the T cells. Antigen stimulation activates the cells, which proliferate and differentiate into memory cells (Tm, Bm) and effector cells. The T cell line operates by effector or cytotoxic T cells (Tc) and the production of cytokines, while the B cell line operates by the formation of antibodies. Cell-mediated immunity (left arm) and humoral immunity (right arm) are exemplified by the tuberculin reaction and hay fever, respectively.

and release a series of biologically active proteins, *cytokines*.

There is now overwhelming evidence that T cells and cytokines play an important role both in IgE synthesis and in recruiting and activating inflammatory cells in the IgE-mediated allergic reaction.

Historically, immunologists have distinguished between two types of immune responses. 1, A *humoral immune response* (right arm in Fig. 1.2.2), which is dependent on B cells, plasma cells and antibodies. This type of immunity can be transferred passively to another individual by plasma. 2, A *cell-mediated or cellular immune response* (left arm in Fig. 1.2.2), which is dependent on T cells and cytokines. This type of immunity needs cells for passive transfer.

However, both immune responses do require cells and humoral factors. This distinction is therefore more didactic than real. More precise names are *B-cell mediated immune response* and *T-effector cell mediated immune response* (see Chapter 1.6).

T helper and T cytotoxic cells

The T cell orchestrates all types of immune responses, and can, as a *T helper cell* (belonging to the CD4+ subset), stimulate B cells and facilitate their transformation into plasma cells. Earlier, both T helper and T suppressor cells were described, but it is doubtful whether suppressor cells exist as a separate subset.

The T cell is also an effector cell and it can, as a *T cytotoxic cell* (belonging to the CD8+ subset), kill antigen-containing cells by direct contact and by release of cytokines.

Immunological memory

When the body is re-exposed to an antigen, the *secondary immune response* is faster and stronger than was the *primary response* (Fig. 1.2.1). This *immunological memory*, which is the third key attribute of the immune system, is due to *memory cells*, which are antigen-stimulated T and B lymphocytes that can circulate in blood and lymph for years.

Immunological memory provides the basis for vaccination and protection against infection, but it also means that an allergic sensitization may be life-long.

Immune protection and immune disease

A teleological distinction between *immune protection* (against infection) and *immune disease* (allergy and autoimmune disease) is useful for clinical practice. However, it is difficult to say with certainty whether an immune response will be beneficial or harmful for the body. It can therefore be argued that it is theoretically more correct, in all cases, to use the term *hypersensitivity*, indicating a specifically increased response of the body depending upon a reaction between antigen and antibody or sensitized lymphocytes leading to symptoms for the host.

Definition of allergy

In this book, the term *allergy* is used in the same sense as in clinical work, that is, when a substance, which is not harmful in itself, causes an immune response and a reaction that gives rise to symptoms and disease in a few predisposed individuals only. Thus, allergy is an immune reaction that apparently causes nothing but misery. Most of the allergy discussed in this book is *IgE-mediated allergy*. An antigen that induces an IgE response is traditionally called an *allergen*.

You and molecular biology?
To be conscious that you are ignorant of the facts is a great step to knowledge.

Benjamin Disraeli

1.3 Type I–IV hypersensitivity reactions
A useful over-simplification

Key points
- Antigen stimulation of the immune system results in an integrated immune response involving both antibodies and sensitized lymphocytes.
- Nevertheless, the simplified classification of Gell and Coombs into four distinct types is convenient.
- The Type I reaction depends on an interaction between antigen and IgE antibody attached to mast cells. T cells and eosinophils are also activated.
- Symptoms of a Type I reaction occur immediately and are caused by histamine and other chemical mediators.
- Type II is a cytotoxic reaction between cell-bound antigen and circulating IgG or IgM antibody.
- Type III is an immune complex reaction between circulating antigen and IgG antibody. It can result in vasculitis.
- Type I–III are humoral immune responses.
- Type IV is a cellular immune response mediated by sensitized lymphocytes; these react with antigen-containing cells and via the release of cytokines.

Allergic or hypersensitivity reactions have been classified in different ways. 1, They can be based on a *humoral or cellular* immune reponse. 2, If symptoms occur within minutes following antigen exposure, it can be called an *immediate reaction*; if symptoms start after hours, it is a *late reaction*, and after days, it is a *delayed reaction*. 3, According to Gell and Coombs, the hypersensitivity reactions can be classified as *Type I–IV*, which tends to follow known clinical disease patterns. Considering the extreme complexity of the immune system, this can be at most a useful over-simplification. Generally, different types of reactions act in concert.

Type I–IgE-mediated reaction
When allergen reacts with IgE attached to the surface of a mast cell, the cell degranulates and liberates *chemical mediators* (Fig. 1.3.1). Symptoms occur within minutes, and a Type I reaction is, therefore, an *immediate reaction*. This reaction is followed by eosinophilia and chronic inflammation, which are

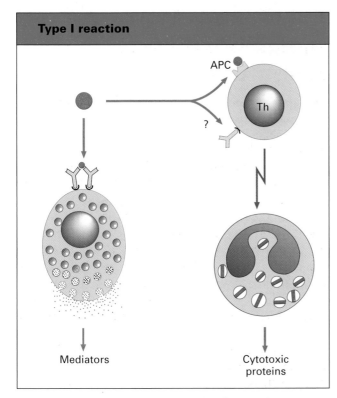

Fig. 1.3.1. *Type I reaction.* Antigen interaction with IgE, bound to high-affinity receptors on mast cells, causes release of histamine and other biochemical mediators. Antigen also stimulates T helper cells via antigen-presenting cells (APC) and possibly by interaction with IgE bound to low affinity receptors on the T cells. The result is activation of eosinophils, which secrete cytotoxic proteins.

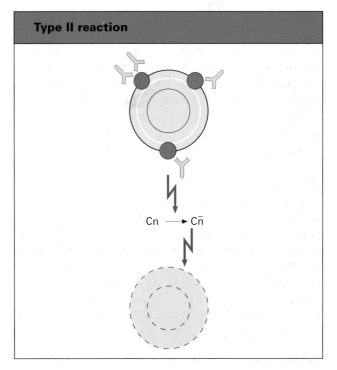

Fig. 1.3.2. *Type II reaction.* Interaction between cell-bound antigen, for example on an erythrocyte, and IgG antibody causes cell damage by activation of the complement cascade (Cn).

caused, at least in part, by T cell secretion of cytokines. *Allergic rhinitis and asthma*, most cases of anaphylactic shock, some cases of urticaria and of angioedema are based on Type I allergic reactions. Type I reactions occur commonly among patients with *atopic dermatitis*.

Type II – cytotoxic reaction

The antigen is localized to the cell membrane (Fig. 1.3.2). It is either a molecule synthesized by the cell (e.g. blood type antigen) or a foreign molecule (e.g. a drug) attached to the cell. The cell membrane is damaged by the interaction between *cell-bound antigen* and *circulating IgG antibody* (or IgM). Activation of the *complement cascade* results in *lysis of the cell*. *Transfusion reactions*, drug-induced *haemolytic anaemia*, thrombocytopenia, and agranulocytosis are examples of Type II reactions.

Type III – immune complex reaction

Complexes are formed between *circulating antigen* and specific antibody, especially of the *IgG* class (Fig. 1.3.3). The *complement cascade* is activated, causing local infiltration by *neutrophils*, which, in turn, release tissue-damaging lysosomal enzymes.

Antibody and antigen often interact perivascularly, resulting in *vasculitis*. Experimentally, this is known from the *Arthus' reaction*, which is a necrotizing vasculitis in the skin, induced by local injection of antigen in a sensitized animal. Immune complex vasculitis in the skin can occur in a series of clinical conditions, such as serum sickness, autoimmune diseases (systemic lupus erythematosus, rheumatoid arthritis), drug reactions and infections. Henoch–Schönlein purpura is an allergic vasculitis on an infectious basis.

Type III reactions cause symptoms 4–6 hours after antigen exposure, a *late reaction*. Note that the late bronchial response to inhaled allergen (e.g. pollens or mites) is not Type III reactions, but inflammatory consequences of a Type I reaction (see later).

Type III reaction

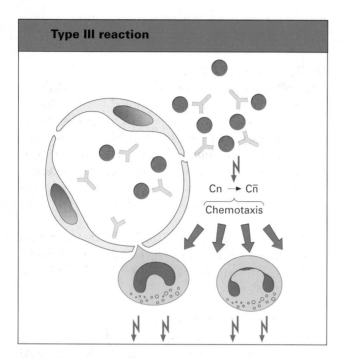

Fig. 1.3.3. *Type III reaction.* Immune complexes of antigen and IgG antibody activate complement and attract neutrophils, which release tissue damaging lysosomal enzymes. As Type III reactions often occur in the perivascular tissue, they result in vasculitis.

Type IV reaction

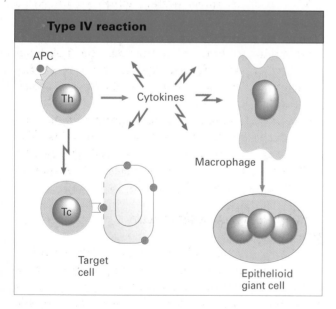

Fig. 1.3.4. *Type IV reaction.* Antigen presentation for a T helper cell results in the formation of cytokines, and in stimulation of T cytotoxic cells. These cells kill target cells containing the antigen, for example a virus. Cytokines attract and activate macrophages, which can transform into epithelioid giant cells.

Type IV – cellular immune reaction

This *cell-mediated immune reaction* is the classical *delayed type hypersensitivity* in which symptoms appear 24–48 hours after antigen exposure. The T lymphocyte has receptors in its cell membrane, which, in the same specific way as antibody, are able to recognize and react with the antigen (Fig. 1.3.4). When the antigen is part of a cell, for example a virus infected cell, the immune reaction between cytotoxic T cells and the target cell results in lysis of the target cell. The *sensitized T lymphocytes* also act by liberating *cytokines*, which mobilize non-sensitized cells to fight the antigen, causing inflammation, tissue damage, and formation of epithelioid and giant cells. Delayed type hypersensitivity often occurs as a result of persistent microbial infection. A well known example of a Type IV reaction is the *Mantoux reaction* to tuberculin. In contrast to the neutrophilic infiltrative response in Type III reactions, the cell infiltrate is dominated by lymphocytes, monocytes, macrophages and, eventually, epithelioid cells. Allergic *contact eczema* is another example of a Type IV reaction.

The term allergy
It seems likely that the term allergy would itself have been dropped long since had it not been for the strong general feeling that a word so beautiful must mean something.

David Harley
Modern Practice of Dermatology

1.4 Antigen processing and presentation
— by macrophages and dendritic cells

Key points
- T cells will not recognize antigen in solution; they need to have it presented by antigen-presenting cells (APCs).
- Macrophages and dendritic cells are APCs.
- APCs have major histocompatibility complex (MHC) class II molecules on their surface.
- APCs pick up antigen and break it down into peptide fragments.
- The simultaneous presentation of processed antigen and MHC class II molecules is necessary for T cells to recognize the antigen.

A T lymphocyte cannot recognize an antigen in solution, for example in plasma or in tissue fluid. It needs to be processed by another type of cell and presented for the T cell.

Antigen-presenting cells
Antigen-presenting cells (APCs) belong to the monocyte/macrophage system and the dendritic cell/Langerhans' cell system. These cells originate from the same stem cell in the bone marrow (Fig. 1.4.1). Characteristically, APCs bear *class II MHC molecules*, necessary for antigen presentation.

Macrophages/monocytes
Cells of the macrophage/monocyte lineage populate all parts of the body including connective tissue, airways and alveoli (Fig. 1.4.1). In any inflamed tissue, they will become activated and increase their expression of MHC class II molecules.

Dendritic cells
Dendritic cells, as interdigitating cells, are found in the lymph nodes and spleen. As Langerhans' cells in the skin, they make up about 2% of all epidermal cells. Such cells have recently been described in the human airway epithelium.

When the dendritic cells have picked up their antigen, for example in the skin, they travel to the lymph node, where T cells, having specificity for the same

antigen, can be selected from the recirculating pool of cells (Fig. 1.4.1).

MHC molecules
The *major histocompatibility complex* (MHC), consisting of a group of glycoprotein molecules on the cell surface, is an important recognition structure in the immune system. The MHC in humans is also called the *human leucocyte antigen (HLA) system*, well known from transplantation medicine. These molecules play an important role in the immune system's discrimination between 'self' and 'non-self'.

MHC (HLA) molecules can be divided into two major classes: class I molecules (HLA-A, HLA-B and HLA-C), and class II molecules (HLA-DR, HLA-DQ and HLA-DP).

Class I and class II effects
T cells can only respond to antigen when it is presented by cells expressing MHC class I or II molecules.

MHC class I molecules are present on the surface of all nucleated cells. It can present *endogenous antigen* for *T cytotoxic cells*. In this way, virus-infected cells and cells containing autoantibodies are recognized and eliminated.

MHC class II molecules are expressed on APCs (macrophages only in the activated form) and on B cells. However, induced expression can occur in a large number of cells, when they become stimulated by a cytokine. As described above, class II molecules are necessary for the presentation of *exogenous antigen* for *T helper cells*.

The class II molecules form a groove on the cell surface into which the processed antigen fits. The simultaneous presentation of processed antigen and MHC class II molecules is necessary for T cells to recognize the antigen (Fig. 1.4.2).

Antigen processing and presentation
Antigens are large molecules with a complex three-dimensional structure. They are not presented whole to the T cell but have to undergo processing in an APC, where they are broken down into peptide fragments, which, bound to MHC class II molecules, are transported to the cell surface (Fig. 1.4.2). This membrane-bound complex is now ready for antigen presentation, that is, interaction with the *T-cell recep-*

tor on a cell having specificity for this particular antigen (see Chapter 1.5).

The cell-to-cell contacts in the immune system, between APCs and T cells (and between T and B cells) is enforced by a number of *adhesion molecules*, which hold the cells together as long as 'communication' goes on (see Chapter 1.10). They are especially important for stimulation of naïve T cells.

A MHC class II molecule is able to bind to a large number of antigens, but the binding affinity for different antigens or epitopes varies. Thus, the antigen-

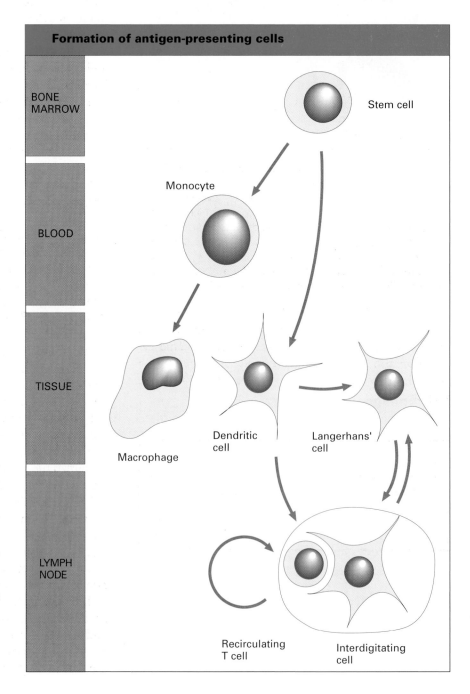

Formation of antigen-presenting cells

BONE MARROW

BLOOD

TISSUE

LYMPH NODE

Stem cell

Monocyte

Macrophage

Dendritic cell

Langerhans' cell

Recirculating T cell

Interdigitating cell

Fig. 1.4.1. Development and circulation of APCs. The two systems, the macrophage/monocyte and the dendritic cell/Langerhans' cell systems, form a functional unit, but are composed of cells that in various tissues and functional situations express a large number of different receptors, by which they can be identified. When Langerhans' cells have picked up antigen, they travel to regional lymph nodes, where they, among the large number of recirculating T cells, can select and stimulate cells with the right antigen specificity.

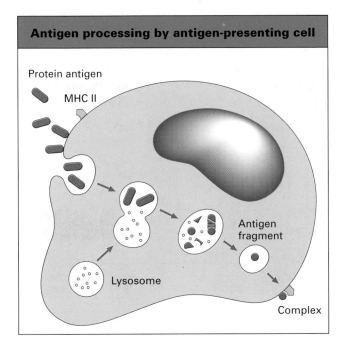

Antigen processing by antigen-presenting cell

Protein antigen

MHC II

Antigen fragment

Lysosome

Complex

Fig. 1.4.2. Model for APC (macrophage) handling of an antigen in solution. The antigen adheres to the cell membrane and is taken up by endocytosis. Lysosomal enzymes break down the protein molecule (which may be composed of hundreds of amino acids) into short peptide chains (consisting of about 20 amino acids). The antigen fragment becomes bound to MHC class II molecules and this complex is transported to the cell membrane, where it is ready for specific interaction with a T cell.

icity of a foreign protein molecule will depend upon the affinity of its epitopes for the class II molecules. A single amino acid change can profoundly alter both the affinity and the ability to induce an immune response.

Go on reading
If you do not understand a particular word in a piece of technical writing, ignore it. The piece will make perfect sense without it.

Arthur Bloch
Murphy's Law Book

1.5 Antigen recognition
—by T cells and by immunoglobulins

Key points
- Cell membrane receptors are necessary for specific recognition of the antigen by T and B lymphocytes.
- On T cells, the structure is called the T-cell antigen receptor (TCR)
- On B cells, the receptor is a modified antibody molecule.
- The membrane-bound receptors are glycoproteins and many of them have now been defined in molecular terms.
- The membrane receptors have specificity for other proteins (counter-structures or ligands).
- Each receptor is given a cluster of differentiation (CD) number, which is also used for identification of the cells.
- For example, T helper cells are named $CD4^+$ cells because they have a CD4 receptor.

The first step in the immune response is the APCs' handling of the antigen. The next step, stimulation of T lymphocytes and the formation of antibodies, is antigen specific and requires antigen recognition. It is effectuated by cell membrane receptors, which are described briefly below.

Membrane receptors
Membrane-bound receptors are the 'senses of the cell', through which it communicates with the environment. The receptors are glycoproteins. They consist of an extracellular region, which reacts with antigen or epitope, a short part that anchors the receptor in the cell membrane, and a cytoplasmic part, through which the receptor transmits signals into the cell (Fig. 1.5.1).

Like all proteins, receptors are folded into a three-dimensional structure. It is this structure that can be recognized by other proteins (counter-structures or ligands), which bind to the receptor because of complementarity of shape and the electric charge of adjacent amino acids.

The membrane receptors that form the basis for the specific recognition of antigens are expressed by T and B lymphocytes. On T cells, the structure is called the *T-cell antigen receptor*, and the B cell structure is a modified form of *immunoglobulin* anchored in the

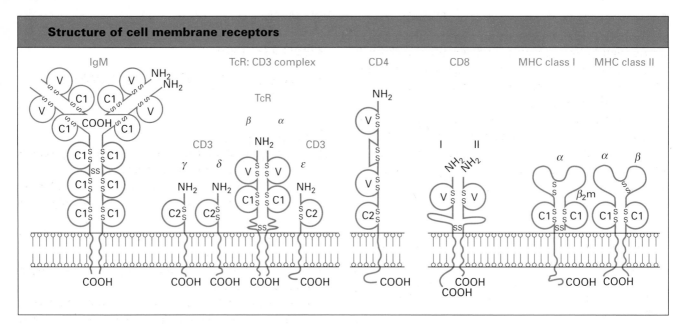

Structure of cell membrane receptors

Fig. 1.5.1. Models for some molecules in the immunoglobulin superfamily. The circles represent immunoglobulin domains. Membrane IgM has, like IgE, five heavy-chain domains. TCR–CD3 is the T-cell receptor with the accessory proteins CD3. MHC, major histocompatibility complex. Modified from Williams AF. *Immunol Today* 1987; **8**: 298.

Cluster of differentiation markers

Marker	Distribution	Function
CD3	T cell	Part of T-cell receptor complex
CD4	T helper cell	Class II MHC interaction, HIV receptor
CD8	T cytotoxic/effector cell	Class I MHC interaction
CD20	B cell	
CD25	T cell	Marker for IL-2 receptor, shows activation of T cell

Table 1.5.1. Examples of human CD markers. IL, interleukin. A full and updated list of the CD antigens is described in Schlossman SFL, Boumsell W, Gilks JM, *et al. Leucocyte Typing* V: *White Cell Differentiation Antigens* Oxford: Oxford University Press, 1994

cell membrane. The clusters of differentiation (CD) markers (described below) perform an important task in antigen recognition together with the T-cell receptor.

CD markers

Following the description in the late 1960s of the two major subsets of lymphocytes, T and B cells, the identification of lymphocyte surface markers by monoclonal antibodies has now allowed the identification of a large number of lymphocyte subsets. These membrane proteins are referred to as *clusters of differentiation (CD) markers*, and cells containing a marker, for example the T-lymphocyte marker CD3, are named CD3+ cells.

The CD markers, widely used to identify and name lymphocyte subsets, also play important roles in cell biology, for example in antigen recognition (CD3) and HIV infection (CD4) (Table 1.5.1).

The T-cell antigen receptor

The *T-cell antigen receptor* (TCR) consists of an α- and β-chain, which are responsible for antigen recognition. The TCR is at the cell surface associated with three short polypeptide chains, called CD3, which are involved in signal transduction to the cell nucleus. This *TCR–CD3 complex* (Fig. 1.5.1) is the structure that can recognize processed antigen.

CD4 markers, present on T helper cells, determine binding to MHC class II molecules in APCs. CD8 markers, present on T cytotoxic cells, determine binding to MHC class I molecules in other cell types.

Immunoglobulins and the B-cell antigen receptor

Immunoglobulins are glycoproteins produced by B cells and plasma cells. The antigen specificity depends upon recognition structures in the variable or V region of the molecule.

The molecules occur as free *circulating immunoglobulins*, which reach all parts of the body, including the surface of mucous membranes, and as *membrane immunoglobulins*, bound to the surface of B cells, which recognize antigen by these surface molecules.

Make it easy
To take something difficult and make it easy—that is difficult. To take something easy and make it difficult—that is easy.

Soya

1.6 Lymphocyte responses
—and the cytokine network

Key points
- As 'hormones of the immune system' cytokines control cell-to-cell communication
- The lymphocyte response to antigen (stimulation, proliferation and activation) is controlled by cytokines.
- Cytokines are proteins with a molecular weight of 10 000–50 000 kDa.
- They are produced by lymphocytes, macrophages and some other cells.
- Cytokines are sequenced at the amino acid level and most genes encoding these proteins have now been cloned.
- Cytokines act as haemopoietic growth factors, they have a regulatory role in the immune system and pro-inflammatory effects.
- Antigen stimulation of virgin T cells and their cloned expansion and differentiation requires antigen presentation by APCs and co-signals from interleukins IL-1 and IL-2.
- Antigen stimulation of B cells occurs via T cells, but B cells can also be stimulated directly by antigen interaction with their immunoglobulin receptors.
- There are two types of T helper cells: Th1 and Th2.
- Th1 cells are stimulated by microbial antigens.
- Th2 cells are stimulated by parasites and allergens.
- The two systems, by their release of cytokines, are mutually suppressive.
- Th2 cells produce IL-3, IL-4, IL-5 and granulocyte-macrophage colony-stimulating factor (GM-CSF), cytokines of considerable importance in allergic inflammation.

Cytokines

Antigen stimulation of lymphocytes and their subsequent activation, proliferation and differentiation is controlled by *cytokines*. They are small soluble proteins produced by one cell that alter the behaviour or properties of another cell.

Terminology

A number of cytokines are referred to as *interleukins* (IL-1 to IL-15, at present). The numeration relates to their discovery, not their importance. Other cytokines are named *granulocyte-macrophage colony-stimulating factor* (GM-CSF), *interferons* (IFN) and *tumour necrosis factor* (TNF).

Role in cell-to-cell communication

In a functional immune system, a network of cells must coordinate their activities, as in the nervous system. This cell-to-cell communication is effected by the cytokines.

Cytokines are proteins with a molecular weight of 10 000–50 000 kDa. They are synthesized by lymphocytes and by a series of other cell types (macrophages, mast cells, epithelial cells, etc.). In popular terms, cytokines act as 'hormones of the immune system', but, in contrast to real hormones, they usually act in the microenvironment of an inflamed tissue.

A series of cytokine molecules work in collaboration, providing the *cytokine network* fundamental to every function of the immune response and inflammation. In popular terms, each cytokine is a single 'word' in the 'sentence' of instruction given to the cell.

Cytokines are effective at very low concentrations because they bind to high-affinity cytokine receptors on the cell surface (not described further in this text).

Cytokines have now been sequenced at the amino acid level and most of the genes encoding these proteins have been cloned. Cytokines have recently become crucial to the understanding of the mechanisms underlying allergic diseases.

Table 1.6.1. Characteristics of some cytokines of importance for allergic reactions and disease. * Proliferation and differentiation. † Cells of the Th1 subset. ‡ Cells of the Th2 subset

Cytokines		
Cytokine	**Principal cell source**	**Primary type of activity**
IL-1	Macrophages	T and B cells* Pro-inflammatory: fever and synthesis of acute-phase proteins
IL-2	T cells†	T (and B) cells*
IL-3	T cells†‡	Haemopoietic stem cells* and progenitors* to all myeloid cell lines including eosinophils, basophils and mast cells
IL-4	T cells‡	B-cells* Promotes IgE class switch
IL-5	T cells‡	Eosinophils* and prolongation of their survival
IL-6	Macrophages Fibroblasts T cells	B cells* Pro-inflammatory: synthesis of acute-phase proteins
IFNγ	T cells†	Inhibition of viral replication Macrophage activation Inhibition of IgE class switch
GM-CSF	T cells†‡ Epithelium Endothelium Fibroblasts	Haemopoiteic stem cells* Activates mature granulocytes

Cytokine effects

Most cytokines are multifunctional (Table 1.6.1). *Haemopoietic growth factors* can stimulate the proliferation and differentiation of lymphoid and myeloid stem cells in the bone marrow and of circulating progenitor cells (see Chapter 1.10). Cytokines have a major *regulatory role in the immune system*; importantly, they affect T cell orchestration of the immune response. Some cytokines (e.g. IL-1, IL-6, IL-8, TNF) have *pro-inflammatory effects*, attracting non-sensitized lymphocytes, macrophages and granulocytes to the site of the specific immune reaction, which thereby becomes amplified. Other cytokines (e.g. IL-2) have an effect on T cells, whereas some (e.g. IFNγ, TNF, IL-10) have *cytotoxic or inhibitory effects* suggesting a role in killing bacteria and virus-infected cells and in dampening pro-inflammatory cytokine release (IL-10).

IL-1 is synthesized by many cells but most abundantly by macrophages in response to cell damage, infection or antigen (Table 1.6.1). It *stimulates T and B cells* and induces inflammatory responses. It induces *fever* and, in the liver, the production of *acute-phase proteins*. Virtually all cells in the body have receptors for IL-1 and can respond to it.

IL-2 is produced by T cells, chiefly by CD4+ cells. It is the most powerful *growth factor and activator of T cells* (all types); it also acts on B cells to induce growth and differentiation.

IL-3 stimulates the growth of all precursors of all the *haemopoietic lineages*, including *eosinophils, basophils and mast cells*.

IL-4 acts on B cells to induce activation and differentiation, thus increasing the production of immunoglobulin. IL-4 plays an important role in allergic disease, as it induces IgE isotype switch and *IgE production*.

IL-5 is, like IL-3 and IL-4, produced mainly by T cells. It is chiefly a growth and differentiation factor for eosinophils. It also prolongs their survival and is, at least in part, responsible for the *eosinophilia* in allergic and parasitic diseases.

IL-6 is produced by many cells, including T cells, and macrophages. It is particularly important in inducing B cells to differentiate into antibody-forming plasma cells. In the liver, it stimulates the production of *acute-phase proteins*.

IFNγ is produced by activated T cells. It has *anti-viral activity*, activates macrophages and regulates the function of APCs. It inhibits stimulation of Th2 cells (see later) and *inhibits IgE synthesis*.

GM-CSF is synthesized by many cells. It stimulates growth and differentiation of the *haemopoietic stem cell* and activates mature granulocytes.

TNF has pro-inflammatory and cytotoxic effects.

Cytokine-forming cells

Cytokines are not exclusively produced by lymphocytes and monocytes/macrophages. Other cell types have similar capacity. Eosinophils, for example, produce GM-CSF, and mast cells have recently been shown to produce IL-4. In the tissues, stromal cells, such as epithelial cells and fibroblasts, can produce chemotactic cytokines of significance for the local accumulation of inflammatory cells.

Lymphocyte response to antigen

T-effector cell mediated immune response

Antigen-induced activation of a naïve T helper cell requires antigen presentation by physical contact with an APC, as well as IL-1, produced by the APC (Fig. 1.6.1).

The activation of the T cell results in the synthesis of IL-2 and expression of receptors for IL-2, which is necessary for the growth, cloned expansion and differentiation to T cells.

The end result is a clone of antigen-specific activated T cells (IL-2 receptor-positive), which can act as cytotoxic cells.

When the antigen exposure ends, the T cells will gradually stop the production of IL-2, loose their IL-2 receptors and become resting cells, acting as memory cells.

The number of committed antigen-specific T cells initially stimulated in this manner is limited. Pro-inflammatory cytokines have the important task of attracting and activating non-committed T cells as well as a broad range of other inflammatory cells (Fig. 1.6.2). Without this amplification system many immune responses would not be successful in eliminating the antigen.

B-cell mediated immune response

Naïve B cells can, by their membrane immunoglobulin, recognize and react with antigen and become activated (T-cell independent response). Most antigens, however, require T cell collaboration in order to induce B cell proliferation and differentiation (T-cell dependent response).

When processed antigen is presented to the T cell by an APC, the activated T cell conveys the antigen-specific message, in a MHC class II restricted way, to a B cell, having the same antigen specificity. Thus, T-cell receptor and antigen on the T cell react with class II molecules and membrane immunoglobulin on

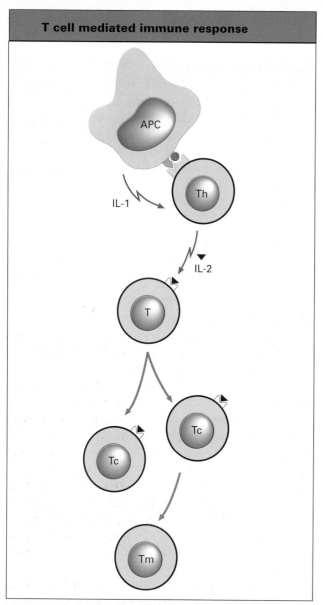

Fig. 1.6.1. Immune response mediated by T effector cells. A T helper cell is stimulated by antigen and by IL-1 from an APC. The activated T cell expresses IL-2 receptors and starts synthesizing this cytokine. Cell proliferation results in a clone of cytotoxic T effector cells and T memory cells.

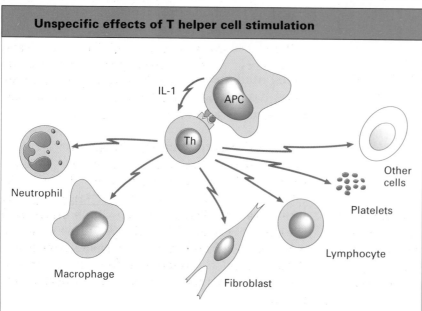

Fig. 1.6.2. The antigen-specific stimulation of a T helper cell results in the release of a series of pro-inflammatory cytokines, which, in an unspecific way, recruits a series of cells to the site of inflammation.

B cell mediated immune response

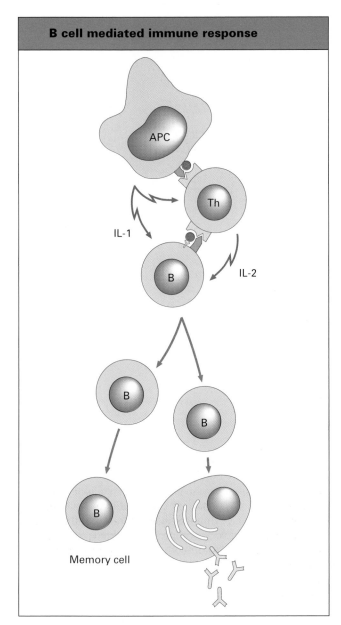

Fig. 1.6.3. Immune response mediated by B cells. The interaction between the APC and the T helper cell is the same as in Fig. 1.6.1. Antigen-specific stimulation of the B cell requires interaction between the T helper cell (T-cell receptor and antigen) and the B cell (immunoglobulin and class II molecule), as well as IL-1 and IL-2.

Cytokine profiles of Th1 and Th2 cells

Cytokine	Th1	Th2
IL-2	+	−
IFNγ	+	−
IL-4	−	+
IL-5	−	+
IL-3	+	+
GM-CSF	+	+

Table 1.6.2. Cytokines produced by Th1 and Th2 clones

Th1 and Th2 cells

Studies in recent years have identified two functional subsets of T helper cells, Th1 and Th2 cells, characterized by their cytokine profiles.

Whether a naïve T cell, a Th0 cell, develops towards a Th1 or a Th2 cell depends on: 1, the patient's genetic background and atopic predisposition; 2, the way, perhaps, the antigen is presented for the immune system (route, amount, timing and adjuvance); and 3, the nature of the antigen. Antigens from viruses, bacteria and, in particular, mycobacteria preferably stimulate Th1 cells by the effect of IL-12 produced by macrophages. Helminth antigens and allergens, on the other hand, preferably stimulate Th2 cells by the effect of IL-4 (from T cells? from mast cells?).

Activation of *Th1 cells* causes the release of *IL-2 and INFγ*, while *Th2 cells* respond with synthesis of *IL-4 and IL-5* (IL-10 and IL-13). Both cell types produce IL-3 and GM-CSF (Table 1.6.2).

While the cytokine profile of Th1 cells leads, predominantly, to delayed-type hypersensitivity (IFNγ), that of Th2 cells intitiates the synthesis of IgE (IL-4). Interestingly, stimulation of Th1 cells inhibits the Th2 system, and vice versa (Fig. 1.6.4).

Th2 cytokines and allergic inflammation

The cytokines produced by activated, allergen-specific Th2 lymphocytes are involved in: 1, the IgE synthesis (IL-4); and 2, the triggering and maintenance of allergic inflammation in tissues. IL-3 favours the growth, differentiation and activation of mast cells. IL-3 and IL-5 promote the growth and differentiation of eosinophils from bone marrow precursors and prolong eosinophil survival in the tissue.

the B cell (Fig. 1.6.3). The B cell becomes stimulated by this direct contact, by secretion of IL-1 from the APC and IL-2 from the T cell. The B cell proliferates by clonal expansion and differentiates, helped by IL-6, into antibody-producing cells, including plasma cells.

Th1 and Th2 pathways

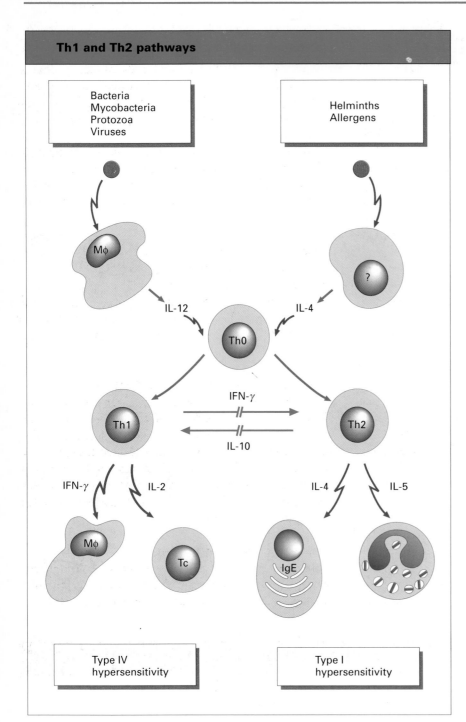

Bacteria
Mycobacteria
Protozoa
Viruses

Helminths
Allergens

Mφ

?

IL-12

IL-4

Th0

IFN-γ

IL-10

Th1

Th2

IFN-γ

IL-2

IL-4

IL-5

Mφ

Tc

IgE

Type IV
hypersensitivity

Type I
hypersensitivity

Fig. 1.6.4. Stimulation with different types of antigen of 'naive' or 'virgin' Th0 cells results in the formation of one of two functional Th lymphocyte subsets with different cytokine profile. Antigens, derived from micro-organisms, stimulate Th1 cells by the release of IL-12 from macrophages, while allergens stimulate Th2 cells by IL-4. Stimulation of Th1 cells results in a cell-mediated, delayed-type hypersensitivity (a Type IV reaction), while Th2 cells are responsible for humoral immunity and IgE-mediated allergy (a Type I reaction). The two systems are mutually repressive.

True in medicine also
There is nothing permanent, except change.
Heraclitus, 513 BC

1.7 Immunoglobulins
The smallest tool in the world

Key points

- The basic monomer immunoglobulin molecule is composed of two heavy chains and two light chains.
- Immunoglobulins are sub-divided into five classes: IgG, IgA, IgM, IgD and IgE.
- IgG is the major immunoglobulin class in plasma. It combats micro-organisms by activation of the complement chain, and it plays a role as blocking antibody in allergy to Hymenoptera venoms.
- IgA, as secretory IgA, is the dominant immunoglobulin in mucous membranes. It is actively transported through the epithelium and functions as an antiseptic surface paint.
- IgM, as a large molecule (pentamer), is mainly intravascular.
- IgD serves, as does IgM, as a surface marker of virgin B cells.

The immunoglobulin classes

Human immunoglobulins belong to five classes or isotypes: *IgG, IgA, IgM, IgD and IgE*, listed in order of their decreasing plasma concentration. IgE, most important for allergy, is present in very small amounts (Fig. 1.7.1).

Immunoglobulin structure

Heavy and light chains

Immunoglobulins are glycoproteins synthesized by B cells and plasma cells. They have a symmetric four-chain structure composed of *two heavy (H) and two light (L) chains* joined together by disulphide bonds (Fig. 1.7.2). There are five kinds of heavy chains, named by the Greek letter equivalent to their class name: gamma γ, alpha α, mu μ, delta δ, and epsilon ε. There are two light-chain types, called kappa κ and lambda λ.

In addition to the inter-chain disulphide bridges, there are intra-chain bonds dividing the chain into *domains* (Fig. 1.7.3). These represent symmetrical 'homology regions', each with about 110 amino acids.

The *variable or V domains* form the antigen-binding sites, and display an immense diversity of heterogeneity, matching that of the foreign molecules in our environment. The *constant or C domains* have a constant amino acid sequence for any one heavy or light chain. There are two C domains in light chains, four in γ, α and δ, and five in μ and ε heavy chains.

Monomers, dimers and pentamers

IgG, IgD and IgE are present as *monomers* (i.e. two heavy and two light chains). While most IgA in serum is a monomer, it is found as a *dimer* in secretions. The dimer consists of two monomers linked together by a *J chain* (Fig. 1.7.4), which combines with *secretory component* in the glandular epithelium. IgM, which is a *pentamer*, also has J chains as receptors for secretory component.

Bivalency – a key attribute

Based on experimental enzyme degradation of the immunoglobulin molecule (at the hinge region), the globulin can be described as consisting of two *Fab*

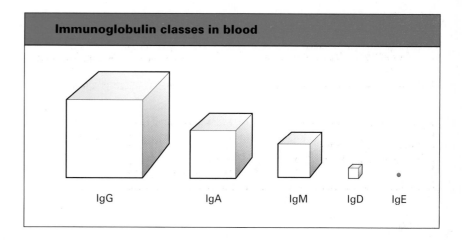

Fig. 1.7.1. Relative amounts of the five immunoglobulin classes in normal serum. It was impossible to make the IgE cube small enough (IgG, 12 mg/ml; IgA, 2 mg/ml; IgM, 1 mg/ml; IgD, 30 μg/ml; IgE, 50 ng/ml).

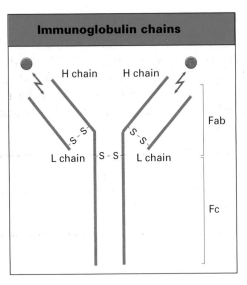

Fig. 1.7.2. The Y-shaped monomer immunoglobulin molecule consists of two identical heavy chains and two identical light chains. The two Fab (fragment, antigen-binding) fragments are responsible for antigen binding, while the Fc (fragment, crystallizable) fragment is necessary for binding to cell surfaces.

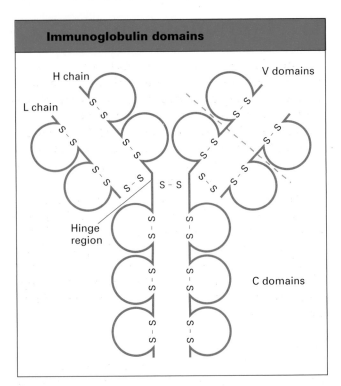

Fig. 1.7.3. Secondary structure of immunoglobulin molecule consisiting of domains of varying (V) and constant (C) amino acid sequence.

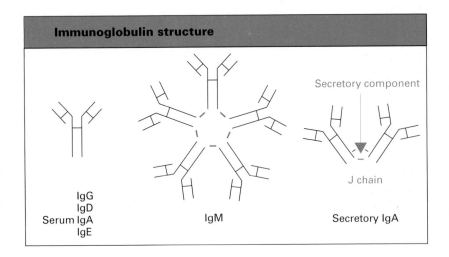

Fig. 1.7.4. Structure of immunoglobulins showing monomer, pentamer and dimer.

fragments (fragment, antigen-binding) and one *Fc fragment* (fragment, crystallizable).

Each Fab fragment has one site that can bind to antigen. Thus, each single monomer has *two antigen-binding sites*, which allows the antibody to form a bridge between two antigen molecules. *Bridge formation* between two IgE molecules is necessary for degranulation of mast cells.

The Fc fragment is necessary for cell binding (Fig. 1.7.2). Receptors in the cell membrane, which can bind immunoglobulin, are therefore called Fc-receptors (e.g. the receptor for IgE is FcεR).

IgG

IgG is the immunoglobulin that is *quantitatively dominant in the blood*. It is the only immunoglobulin class that crosses the placental barrier, conveying antibodies to a series of viruses and bacteria to the fetus.

When IgG binds to micro-organisms, the organisms are assailed by activation of the complement cascade. The cascade consists of a number of plasma proteins, each with enzymatic properties.

In general, IgG does not have the ability to bind to mast cells, but one of the four subclasses (IgG4) has a low binding affinity. It can, in animals, act as *short-term sensitizing antibody*, but it is dubious as to whether it plays any role in humans. In atopic allergic disease, IgG plays a role as *blocking antibody*, developing during immunotherapy with Hymenoptera venom (see Chapter 13.3). IgG antibody, in addition to causing complement activation, also plays a role in allergic bronchopulmonary aspergillosis, extrinsic allergic alveolitis and some allergic drug reactions.

IgA

As *secretory IgA* (Fig. 1.7.4), IgA is the quantitatively dominant immunoglobulin in *external secretions*, and in the entire body.

Secretory IgA covers the mucosal surface as an '*antiseptic paint*' and protects the body against intruding micro-organisms by inhibition of their attachment to the mucosal surface.

An important feature of this *first line of defence* is that the immune reaction takes place on the surface of the body, and secretory IgA does not activate complement. When the intruder has overcome this system, a *second line of defence*, the IgG and IgM systems in the mucous membrane, are stimulated. As these antibodies employ complement, inflammation will be the result.

Possibly, secretory IgA can prevent the penetration of the mucous membrane by non-self macromolecules. It was formerly believed that IgA could prevent the formation of IgE antibody and the development of allergy.

IgM

IgM is mainly intravascular due to its size (1 million kDa) (Fig. 1.7.4). Its principal function is agglutination of particles and molecules. It participates in some adverse reactions to drugs.

IgD

IgD and IgM serve as surface markers on naïve B cells, before they are switched to, for example, IgE production.

IgE

IgE is a *minor immunoglobulin class* in that it normally comprises less than 0.001% of the total circulating immunoglobulin. Even allergic patients have low levels, averaging 2–10 times the normal. Nevertheless, it is of paramount importance for atopic allergy.

> **A problem with a multiauthor book**
> Two or more people getting together to write something is like three people getting together to make a baby.
> Evelyn Waugh

1.8 Immunoglobulin E
—and receptors for IgE

Key points
- IgE is produced by plasma cells in the airway, gastro-intestinal tract and regional lymph nodes.
- It comprises less than 0.001% of circulating immunoglobulin.
- The IgE molecule binds to mast cell receptors for long periods.
- Isotype switching of B lymphocytes to IgE+ cells and IgE production can be induced by IL-4 and inhibited by IFNγ.
- High-affinity receptors for IgE, FcεR1, are present on mast cells and basophils.
- There are low-affinity receptors, FcεR2, on other cells (T cells, eosinophils and APCs) but their role is uncertain.
- The amino acid sequence of the IgE molecule and the receptors for IgE have now been characterized.

The IgE molecule
Injection of IgE antibody can sensitize the skin to allergen, a property first demonstrated in the Prausnitz–Küstner experiment. It is now well established that the *skin-sensitizing* ability of IgE antibody is due to its binding to mast cells. While IgE sensitizes the skin for 2–4 weeks, its plasma half-life is only 2–4 days.

While the antigen-binding properties of IgE are connected to the Fab fragments, the Fc fragment determines the capacity for binding to the IgE receptor and fixation to mast cells and basophils (see Fig. 1.7.2).

Like other immunoglobulins, IgE has two heavy chains (ε-chains) and two light chains, organized into globular domains. Having five domains in its heavy chain, IgE is slightly larger than IgG, which has only four domains (molecular weight of IgE is 190000 kDa and of IgG is 150000 kDa).

The gene encoding for the human ε-chain has now been cloned, and the IgE molecule characterized in detail. Apparently, the amino acid sequence of the ε-chain may not make meaningful reading to the clinician (Table 1.8.1). However, the fact that molecular biologists have now sequenced IgE, the IgE receptor and a series of other molecules of importance for allergy implies a fascinating possibility for new therapeutic modalities, for example with synthetic peptide fragments, which block reactive sites in the allergic reaction.

IgE synthesis and regulation

Genetic control
The familial inheritance of atopic diseases suggests that *genetic factors* regulate IgE biosynthesis. Some genetic loci seem to control the level of total IgE, others the immune recognition of specific allergens and the subsequent formation of IgE antibody. However, the genes that encode for IgE antibody synthesis and predispose to atopic allergy have not been identified.

Allergen exposure
The synthesis of IgE antibody is *stimulated by allergen exposure*, for example in the pollen season. However, antibody synthesis persists for long periods in spite of allergen avoidance. If that were not the case, IgE antibody, having a plasma half-life of only 2–4 days, would be undetectable a few weeks after the pollen season.

Amino acid sequence of the ε-chain in IgE

QTQLVQSGAEVRKPGASVRVSCKASQYTFIDSYIHWIRQAPGHGLEWVGWINPN
SGGTNYAPRFQGRVTMTRDASFSTAYMDLRSLRSDDSAVFYCAKADPFWSDYY
NFDYSYTLDVWGQGTTVTVSS) (ASTQSPSVFPLTRCCKNIDSNATSVTLGCLAT
GYFPEPVMVTCDTGSLNGTTMTLPATTLTLSGHYATISLLTVSGAWAKQMFTCR
VAHTPSSTDWVDNKTFS) (VCSRDFTPPTVKILQSSCDGGGHFPPTIQLLCLVSGY
TPGTINITWLEDDQVMDVDLSTASTTQEGELASTQSELTLSQKHWLSDRTYTSQV
TYQGHTFEDSTKKSA) (DSNPRVGSAYLSRPSPFDLFIRKSPTITCLVVDLAPSKGT
VNLTWSRASGKPVNHSTRKEEKQRNGTLTVTSTLPVGTRDWIEGETYQCRVTHP
HLPRALMRSTTKTS) (GPRAAPEVYAFATPEWPGSRDKRTLACLIQNFMPEDISV
QWLHNEVQLPDARHSTTQPRRKTKGSGFFVFSRLEVTRAEWEQKDEFICRAVHEA
ASPSQTVQRAVSVNPGK

Table 1.8.1. Amino acid sequence in the ε-chain. From Peng C. *J Immunol* 1992; **148**: 129–36

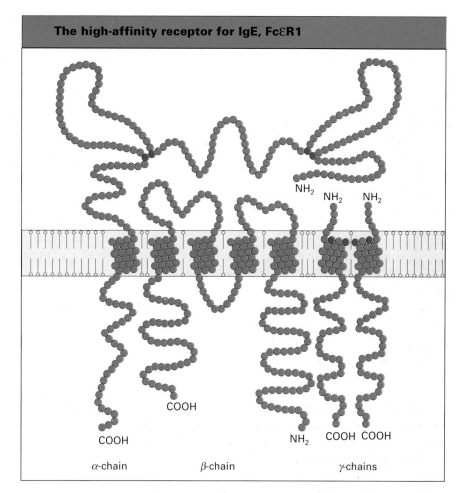

The high-affinity receptor for IgE, FcεR1

NH₂   NH₂   NH₂

COOH

COOH

NH₂   COOH COOH

α-chain   β-chain   γ-chains

Fig. 1.8.1. The model for the high-affinity receptor for IgE, FcεR1. It contains four transmembrane polypeptide chains with IgE-binding function contained within the α-chain, which has two immunoglobulin-like domains projecting out of the cell. While it is the extracellular part of the receptor that binds to IgE, it is the transmembrane and cytoplasmic parts that are necessary for signal transduction to the cell and release of mediators. From Holgate ST, Church MK. *Allergy.* London: Gower Medical Publishing, 1993: 1–250.

Site of production

IgE-producing cells are distributed primarily in lymphoid tissue adjacent to the *respiratory and gastro-intestinal tract*. Thus, IgE antibody is synthesized near the site of antigen encounter, but it is eventually *distributed throughout the whole body*. In contrast to dimer IgA, it is *not actively transported* through the epithelium.

Isotype class switch to IgE

While a lymphocyte cannot change its specificity for antigen, a B cell can, at an early stage, change its immunoglobulin class or isotype. Thus, it is the C domains that change while the V domains, responsible for antigen specificity, remain the same.

Immature B cells synthesize μ and δ heavy chains and have membrane-bound IgM and IgD on the cell surface. Antigen stimulation can result in isotype switching to any of the five immunoglobulin classes. Switching to IgE requires two signals: one from a T

helper cell with the same antigen specificity, and the other from IL-4. Both these signals can be supplied by a Th2 cell.

IFNγ, produced by Th1 cells, can antagonize the IL-4-induced switch to IgE⁺ B cells. The ratio between activated Th2 and Th1 cells and the balance between IL-4 and IFNγ seems a critical mechanism in IgE regulation.

Receptors for IgE

High-affinity receptors

High-affinity receptors for IgE, *FcεR1*, are present on *mast cells and basophils*, and their number is increased in atopic subjects with high levels of plasma IgE. Recently, FcεR1 receptors have also been described on Langerhans' cells.

FcεR1 consists of four transmembrane polypeptide chains (one α-, one β- and two γ-chains). The IgE-binding function is contained within the α-chain (Fig. 1.8.1). This chain belongs to the immunoglobulin superfamily. It has two immunoglobulin-like do-mains that project out of the cell.

The four-chain structure of the high-affinity recep-tor has been characterized, the receptor has been cloned and the binding site on the IgE molecule identified. It may, therefore, be possible in the future, at least in theory, to block the allergic reaction in one of two ways: 1, by IgE fragments, which can inhibit the interaction between IgE and FcεR1; or 2, by extracellular fragment of FcεR1, which can react with circulating IgE and block its cell binding sites.

Low-affinity receptors

A number of inflammatory cells, including *lympho-cytes, eosinophils, macrophages, Langerhans' cells and platelets*, also have receptors for IgE in the cell membrane. Their expression is enhanced by acti-vation of the cells. These receptors, *FcεR2*, have low binding affinity and the potential to be preferentially activated by IgE immune complexes. Their role in mediating reactions dependent upon monomer IgE is therefore debatable at present.

Fact, idea, proof
A fact in itself is nothing. It is valuable only for the idea attached to it, or for the proof which it furnishes.
Claude Bernard

1.9 Mast cells, basophils
—and chemical mediators

Key points
- Mast cells and basophils are the primary initiating cells of IgE-mediated allergic reactions.
- Progenitors of mast cells are formed in the bone marrow under the influence of GM-CSF and IL-3.
- There are two types of mast cells: connective tissue mast cells (MC_{TC}) and mucosal mast cells (MC_T).
- There is an accumulation of MC_T cells in tissues experiencing allergic reactions.
- High-affinity membrane receptors for IgE are unique to mast cells and basophils.
- They act as amplifiers of the allergen-IgE interac-tion by release of biochemically active mediators.
- Chemical mediators are either stored in the gran-ules or newly synthesized in the cell membrane.
- Histamine is a preformed mediator, which is of considerable importance in conjunctivitis, rhinitis and urticaria.
- It stimulates nervous irritant receptors, contracts smooth muscle and increases vascular permeability.
- The newly synthesized, membrane-derived me-diators, prostaglandin D_2 (PGD_2), leukotriene (LTC_4) and platelet activating factor (PAF), are probably relatively more important in asthma.
- The prostaglandins are generated from arachidonic acid by the enzyme cyclo-oxygenase, and the leukotrienes are products of lipoxygenase.
- Mast cells, but not basophils, also release enzymes (tryptase and chymase).
- The cell reactivity is modulated by a series of drugs, hormones, chemical mediators and neuro-transmitters.
- Mediator release can also occur after challenge with a series of non-specific stimuli.

Mast cells and basophils are the primary mediator cells of IgE-mediated allergic reactions. They are very important for the expression of symptoms in allergic rhinitis and urticaria. Their role for asthma and atopic dermatitis seems far less significant.

Cellular characteristics

Mast cells
Mast cells are found in the loose connective tissue of all organs, except the brain. They lie along blood

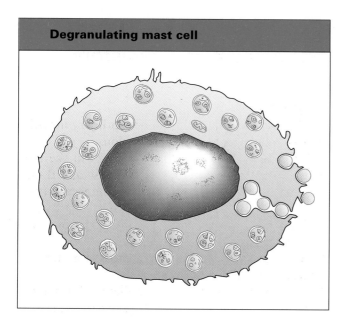

Degranulating mast cell

Fig. 1.9.1. Human mast cell with secretory granules, showing the characteristic laminar structure. Degranulation is indicated on the right of the cell. Fusion of the perigranular and the cell membranes forms a complicated labyrinth of channels, which are geographically within the confines of the cell, but communicating freely with the extracellular fluid. Granules need not be extruded from the cell to release mediators to the extracellular fluid.

vessels and are predominant in the skin, airways and gastro-intestinal tract.

The mast cell contains *granules*, which are of uniform size and stain metachromatically with toluidine blue. They are bounded by a thin *perigranular membrane*, which surrounds some laminar structures consisting of *whorls and scrolls* (Fig. 1.9.1). When the cell is activated, the perigranular and the cell membranes fuse, and, as the mediators are released, the laminar structure of the granules is replaced by loose flocculent material (Figs 1.9.2–3).

Heterogeneity of mast cells

Mast cells can be divided into two subpopulations by morphological, cytochemical and functional criteria. *Connective tissue mast cells* and *mucosal mast cells* were first described, in the rat, by their staining characteristics and sensitivity to formaldehyde fixation. More recently, the development of monoclonal antibodies to enzymes of human mast cells (MCs) has allowed an identification of MC_{TC}, which contains *tryptase and chymase*, and MC_T, which contains *tryptase only*. MC_{TC} correspond to connective tissue mast cells, and MC_T to mucosal mast cells.

The ratio between MC_{TC} and MC_T vary between tissues and between normal condition and disease. While the MC_{TC} predominates in the skin, the MC_T is prevalent in the lungs and the gastro-intestinal mucosa. In allergic reactions, it is the MC_T that migrate into the epithelium of the nose and bronchi (Table 1.9.1).

Basophil leucocytes

The basophil differs structurally from the mast cell by having a bilobar nucleus, and fewer granules, which are of unequal size. It acts as a 'circulating mast cell', which mediates systemic allergic reactions. In addition, basophils migrate to the tissues and participate in local allergic reactions. This commonly occurs in allergic contact eczema, and probably in IgE-mediated allergic airways disease.

Haemopoietic development

Mast cells

Stem cell differentiation into mast cell progenitors takes place in the bone marrow under the influence of the pluripotent haemopoietic growth factors, GM-CSF and IL-3 (Fig. 1.9.4). The precursor cells are released into the blood and migrate into the tissue where they develop into mature mast cells. Whether it

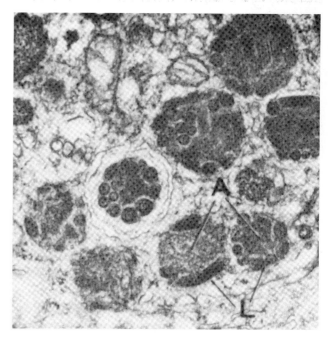

Fig. 1.9.2. Portion of mast cell from healthy nasal mucosa. Each granule consists of an amorphous core (A) and a laminar peripheral zone (L) with whorls and scrolls.

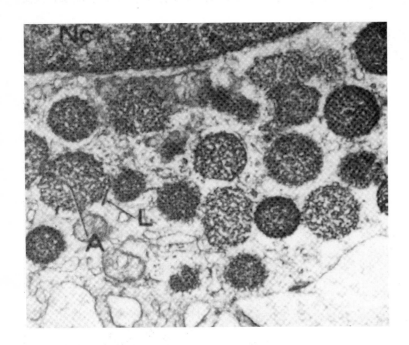

Fig. 1.9.3. Portion of mast cell from a nasal polyp. The granules consist of a loose flocculent material (A), while the peripheral lamellar material (L) is mostly absent, suggesting release of chemical mediators. Transmission electron micrograph ($\times 30\,000$). From Cauna N, Hinderer KH, Manzetti GW, Swanson EW. Fine structure of nasal polyps. *Ann Otol Rhinol Laryngol* 1972; **81**: 41–58.

Distribution of mast cell subsets		
	MC_{TC}	**MC_T**
Skin	+++	–
Intestine		
Mucosa	–	+++
Submucosa	++	+
Conjunctiva	++	+
Nose		
Epithelium	–	+++
Lamina propria	++	+
Lungs		
Epithelium	+	++
Alveoli	–	+++

Table 1.9.1. Tissue distribution of mast cell subsets based on tryptase and chymase immunocytochemical staining (–, <10%; +, 10–50%; ++, 50–90%; +++, >90%)

will be MC_{TC} or MC_T depends on factors, especially cytokines, in the local microenvironment. There is evidence that the MC_T, in contrast to the MC_{TC}, is dependent on T-cell products. There is a predominance of MC_T in areas of inflammation with heavy T cell infiltration.

Basophils

The development of the haemopoietic stem cell into a myeloid progenitor cell is stimulated by GM-CSF and IL-3. There is a common progenitor cell for basophils and eosinophils. IL-5 is a specific growth and differentiation factor for these two leucocyte types (Fig. 1.9.4).

Receptors for IgE

As described earlier, mast cells and basophils have *high-affinity receptors* for IgE, *FcεR1*. The extremely high binding constant and the *long residence time* for IgE permits the cell to concentrate IgE antibody. Without this mechanism, it would seem that the very low level of plasma IgE and the short half-life would make this trace immunoglobulin ineffectual and of negligible importance.

Degranulation

Factors causing degranulation

In allergic diseases, *allergen* causes degranulation by interaction with IgE antibody bound to the FcεR1 receptor. Degranulation can also occur in non-allergic asthma, rhinitis and urticaria, but the nature of the trigger mechanism is unknown.

Anti-IgE antibody, raised in immunized animals, will release mediators from human mast cells, and this experimental model has been used to study the release mechanisms.

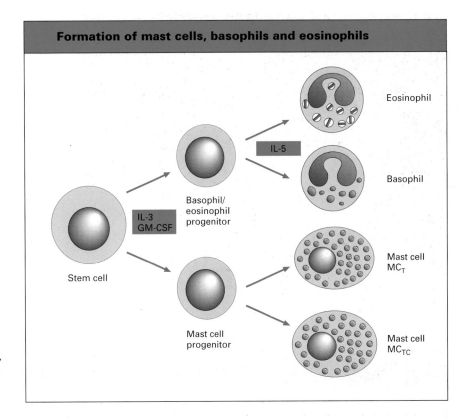

Fig. 1.9.4. The haemopoietic differentiation of allergic effector cells, including mast cells, basophils and eosinophils, mediated by growth factors.

Recently, *autoantibodies* to the FcRε1 receptor have been identified as a cause of mast cell degranulation and skin symptoms in a few cases of severe chronic urticaria.

Histamine-releasing factor is a cytokine produced by activated T cells and macrophages. Its exact role in disease remains to be established.

Non-immunological factors can cause degranulation. The list is long and includes mechanical and thermal trauma, venoms, anaphylatoxin (C3a and C5a) produced by activation of the complement cascade, cytokines, lysosomal enzymes, drugs (such as plasma expanders, muscle relaxants and morphine), organic iodide compounds (used as radiocontrast media), and agents that result in calcium influx into the cell.

Mechanism of degranulation

Degranulation of mast cells and basophils is an *active secretory process* requiring energy and calcium. The process starts on the cell surface with allergen *bridging* between two IgE molecules attached to FcεR1 receptors (Figs 1.9.5–6). This, in turn, *activates enzymes*, which re-orientate the phospholipids in the cell membrane. The calcium gates open, and an *influx of extracellular calcium* takes place. This has two main results. 1, Calcium activates microtubules resulting in a flowing together of perigranular and cell membranes with release of *preformed, granule-associated mediators* (e.g. histamine) (Fig. 1.9.5). Histamine liberation takes place by *ion exchange* with Na^+. 2, Calcium, via enzyme activation and arachidonic acid synthesis, induces the release of *newly synthesized, membrane-associated mediators* (e.g. prostaglandins and leukotrienes) (Fig. 1.9.6).

Chemical mediators

Mast cells and basophils have a similar content of mediators, but there are differences. The lipid mediators, but not histamine, are also synthesized by other cell types (e.g. eosinophils) (Table 1.9.1). Recent data have shown that mast cells can also synthesize and release cytokines (IL-3, IL-4, IL-5 and IL-6).

Each mediator has many effects in the tissue, and the role of individual mediators in the pathophysiology of allergic disease, for example asthma, is not yet clear (Table 1.9.2).

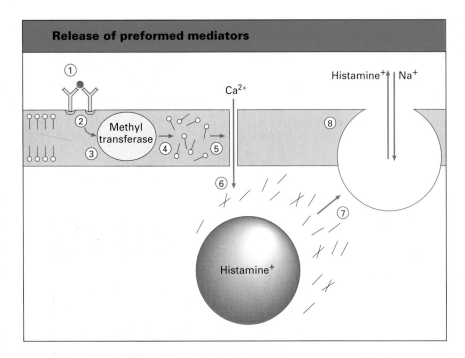

Release of preformed mediators

Fig. 1.9.5. IgE-dependent release of histamine from a mast cell: 1, antigen−IgE interaction on the cell surface; 2, cross-linking of adjacent IgE receptors; 3, activation of membrane-associated enzyme; 4, re-orientation of membrane phospholipids; 5, opening of calcium gates and influx of calcium; 6, activation of perigranular microtubules; 7, fusion between perigranular and cell membranes; and 8, histamine, as a cation is finally released by ion exchange with Na^+.

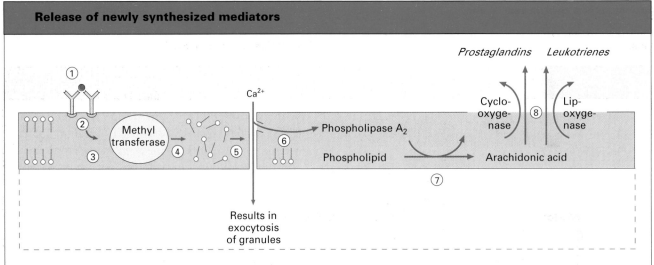

Release of newly synthesized mediators

Fig. 1.9.6. IgE-induced synthesis and release of arachidonic acid metabolites: 1–5, as described in Fig. 1.9.5; 6, calcium activation of phospholipase A_2; 7, metabolism of phospholipid to arachidonic acid; and 8, metabolism of arachidonic acid via either the cyclo-oxygenase or the lipoxygenase pathway.

Histamine

Histamine (Fig. 1.9.7) is formed from the amino acid, *histidine* by the action of *histidine decarboxylase*. Its role in allergic rhinitis and urticaria is well established but its normal function is not known.

Histamine-induced symptoms are elicited within a few minutes by stimulation of nervous irritant receptors, contraction of smooth muscles and an increase in vascular permeability.

In the *skin*, histamine induces the typical pruritic wheal-and-flare reaction. It causes itching, hypersecretion and blockage in the *nose*. *Bronchial* histamine inhalation results in cough and smooth muscle contraction leading to bronchoconstriction. Hypersecretion of gastric acid, cramp and diarrhoea are histamine effects in the *gastro-intestinal tract*. High plasma levels can cause *anaphylaxis*.

Cell sources of lipid mediators

	LTC$_4$	LTB$_4$	PAF	PGD$_2$
Mast cells	++	+/−	++	++
Basophils	+	+/−	−	−
Eosinophils	++	−	++	−
Neutrophils	−	++	++	−
Monocytes	−	++	++	−
Platelets	−	−	++	−

Table 1.9.2. Principal cell sources of lipid mediators in humans

Histamine

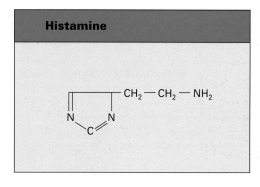

Fig. 1.9.7. Histamine.

Arachidonic acid

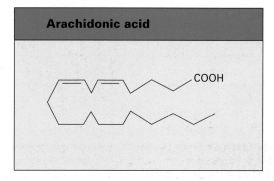

Fig. 1.9.8. Arachidonic acid.

Fig. 1.9.9. (*Below*.) Lipoxygenase and cyclo-oxygenase pathways for the synthesis of arachidonic acid metabolites.

Arachidonic acid metabolites

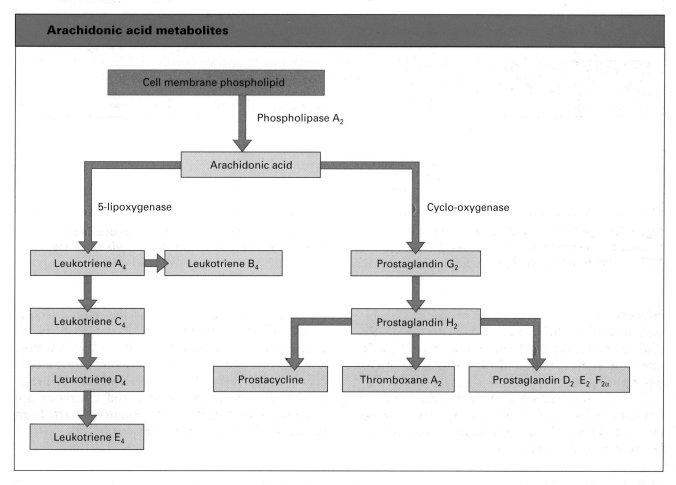

Effects of mediators					
	Bronchoconstriction	**Airway secretion**	**Microvascular leakage**	**Chemotaxis**	**Bronchial hyper-responsiveness**
Histamine	+	+	+	–	–
PGD_2, $PGF_{2\alpha}$	++	+	?	?	+
PGE_2	–	+	–	+	–
TXA_2	++	?	–	±	+
LTB_4	–	–	±	++	±
LTC_4	++	++	++	?	±
PAF	++	+	++	++	++
Bradykinin	+	+	++	–	–

Table 1.9.3. Effects of inflammatory mediators implicated in asthma. From Barnes PJ. Pathophysiology of allergic inflammation. In: Middleton E, Reed CE, Ellis EF, Adkinson NF, Yunginger JW, Busse WW, eds. *Allergy. Principles and Practice* 2nd ed. St Louis: The CV Mosby Company, 1993: 243–301

Arachidonic acid metabolites

Bridging of FcεR1 receptors, and the subsequent calcium influx, activates the membrane-associated enzyme, *phospholipase A_2*. This enzyme transforms phospholipid to arachidonic acid (Fig. 1.9.8), which is rapidly metabolized by either of the two enzymes, *cyclo-oxygenase* and *lipoxygenase* (Fig. 1.9.9).

Cyclo-oxygenase products

Pertubation of the cell membrane of almost all nucleated cells induces the generation of one or more of the cyclo-oxygenase products: *prostaglandins* (PGD_2, PGE_2 and $PGF_{2\alpha}$) and thromboxane A_2 (TXA_2). The specific product formed varies widely between cell types. Human mast cells generate *PGD_2 and TXA_2*, which contract smooth muscle; TXA_2 also activates blood platelets (Table 1.9.3).

Lipoxygenase products

Leukotrienes are lipoxygenase products (Fig. 1.9.6). Mast cells are rich in lipoxygenase, and, when they become activated, they synthesize the *sulphidoleukotrienes*, LTC_4, LTD_4 and LTE_4 (formerly called slow-reacting substance or SRS-A). These leukotrienes are potent mediators, producing smooth muscle contraction, mucus secretion and increased vascular permeability. Mast cells (and neutrophils) also produce LTB_4, which is chemotactic for neutrophils and eosinophils.

Platelet activating factor

PAF was first identified in rabbits and subsequently in humans. It aggregates platelets and activates their release of serotonin. It also contracts bronchial smooth muscle, increases vascular permeability and induces airway hyper-responsiveness.

Serotonin

In allergic disease, serotonin may be *released from platelets* by the mast cell products, PAF and TXA_2. It stimulates sensory nerves and increases vascular permeability. About 90% of the body's serotonin (5-hydroxytryptamine) is located in the gastro-intestinal tract. Mast cells in animals, but not in humans, contain serotonin.

Enzymatic mediators

A variety of enzymes (inflammatory proteases) have been identified in mast cells and basophils. Some of these, such as *kallikrein*, contributes to inflammation by the formation of *bradykinin*, which has a number of inflammatory properties: 1, it contracts bronchial smooth muscle; 2, it dilates blood vessels; 3, it increases vascular permeability; and 4, it causes pain, redness and oedema of the skin. The role of other enzymes, such as tryptase and chymase, is largely unknown. However, they are released during degranulation, and tryptase can be detected in the skin during urticaria, in nasal lavage fluid following allergen challenge and in plasma during anaphylaxis.

Oh, Histamine!
You give asthmatics wheezes,
pollinosis patients sneezes,
you smooth muscle
stimulating Histamine.

Though obscure as yet,
the fact is you're involved
in anaphylaxis—you
capillary poison, Histamine.

We've extracted you
and weighed you,
by the living gut assayed you,
you decarboxylated son of Histidine.

Carl A Dragstedt
Northwestern University
Medical School, 1947

1.10 Eosinophils
—and adhesion molecules

Key points
• The eosinophil leucocyte is a pro-inflammatory cell, which contributes to allergic inflammation.
• The eosinophil can be identified by its biloped nucleus and cytoplasmic granules, which stain bright red with eosin.
• Each granule contains a typical crystalline structure.
• The cell is biochemically characterized by its content of cytotoxic proteins (eosinophil cationic protein (ECP), eosinophil-derived neurotoxin (EDN), eosinophil peroxydase (EPO) and major basic protein (MBP)).
• These proteins contribute to tissue damage, for example epithelial shedding in asthma.
• The eosinophil is formed in the bone marrow under the control of cytokine growth factors (GM-CSF, IL-3 and IL-5).
• It leaves the circulation when adhesion molecules are activated.
• Cellular adhesion molecules, on leucocytes and endothelial cells, play a very important role in physical cell-to-cell contact.
• These proteins and their ligands hold two cells together as long as it is necessary for their 'communication'.
• Adhesion molecules are grouped into the immunoglobulin superfamily, the integrins and the selectins.
• Cytokines, in inflamed areas, up-regulate adhesion molecules, and passing leucocytes become 'sticky'.
• A freely circulating eosinophil becomes attached to endothelial cells, rolls slowly along them, flattens (selectins) and migrates between the cells (intercellular adhesion molecule-1 (ICAM-1) and vascular cell adhesion molecule-1 (VCAM-1)).
• It passes through the extracellular matrix (very late antigen-1 (VLA-1)) by directed migration towards chemotactic factors (RANTES?).
• In the tissue, the eosinophil becomes activated and secretes its cytotoxic proteins and also other mediators.
• The local survival of eosinophils is considerably prolonged during allergic inflammation (GM-CSF, IL-3 and IL-5).

• Thus, simple eosinophilia has become very complicated.

Having first described the mast cell, Paul Erlich, in 1879, named a new leucocyte, eosinophil, after Eos, the Greek goddess of dawn. The cell stains bright red with the acidic dye, eosin.

Only a few decades ago, the eosinophil leucocyte was referred to as 'the cell of beauty and mystery'. Today, we know that the cell contributes to allergic inflammation; it releases cytotoxic proteins and causes cell damage.

Structure

The eosinophil is easily identified in the light microscope by a bilobed nucleus and by 100–200 bright red *granules* in the cytoplasm. In the electron microscope, the granules have a crystalline-like core surrounded by a less electron-dense matrix (Fig. 1.10.1).

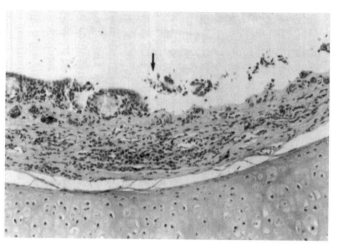

Fig. 1.10.2. Damage to the surface epithelium of the guinea-pig trachea after a single injection of ECP.

Eosinophil proteins and mediators

Granule proteins

The granules are made up of eosinophil-specific proteins. *Major basic protein (MBP)* is in the core; *eosinophil cationic protein (ECP), eosinophil protein X (EPX)*, also called *eosinophil-derived neurotoxin (EDN)*, and *eosinophil peroxydase (EPO)* are present in the matrix (Fig. 1.10.1).

All these basic proteins are toxic to mammalian cells, including airway epithelium (Fig. 1.10.2). They are also toxic for helminthic parasites, supporting the idea that the teleological role for eosinophils is to protect against parasitic infections. ECP and EDN are potent neurotoxins.

Lipid mediators

In addition to the cytotoxic proteins, eosinophils secrete some of the arachidonic acid metabolites or lipid mediators, described in Chapter 1.9.

PAF, produced both by eosinophils and by mast cells, possibly plays a role in the bronchial hyper-responsiveness, associated with allergic eosinophil inflammation. It is a potent chemotactic factor for eosinophils and neutrophils, and, under certain conditions, it can activate the eosinophil cell. So far, however, therapeutic trials with PAF-antagonists in asthma have been disappointing.

Activated eosinophils produce appreciable amounts of LTC_4, LTD_4 and LTE_4; they also generate PGE_2, TXA_2 and *cytokines* (e.g. GM-CSF).

Eosinophil receptors

Like all leucocytes, eosinophils express a *large num-*

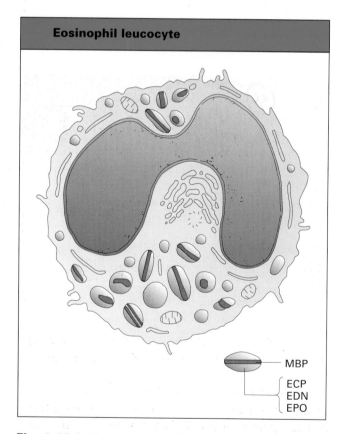

Eosinophil leucocyte

MBP

ECP
EDN
EPO

Fig. 1.10.1. Eosinophil leucocyte with bilobed nucleus and eosinophil granules with crystaloids. Localization of cytotoxic proteins in granule matrix and crystalloid.

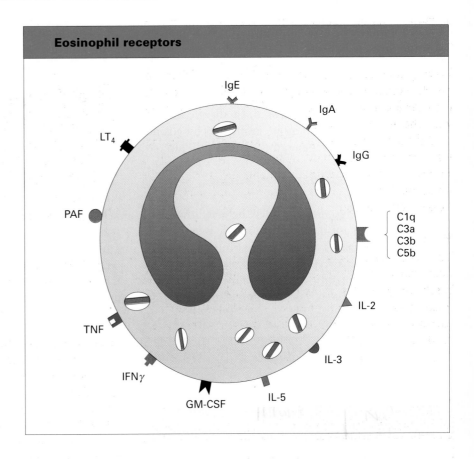

Fig. 1.10.3. Cell receptors on the eosinophil leucocyte for immunoglobulins, complement, cytokines and mediators.

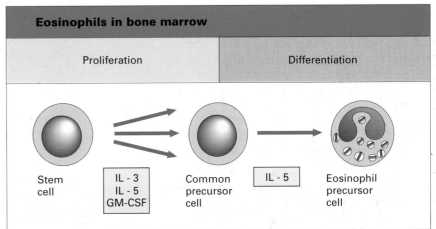

Fig. 1.10.4. A simplified model of the life and function of the eosinophil leucocyte is presented in Figs 1.10.4–1.10.6. Proliferation and differentiation takes place in the bone marrow, where the cell lives 4–5 days.

ber of membrane receptors (Fig. 1.10.3). These include Fc receptors, receptors for complement, adhesion receptors (see below), and receptors for soluble mediators and cytokines.

The low-affinity receptor for IgE, *FcεR2*, not operative on resting eosinophils, is expressed on activated cells. The FcεR2 receptor reacts with IgE and participates in the effector function of eosinophils against parasite larvae. Its role in allergic inflammation is less clear, as the receptor combines with aggregated IgE, and not with monomer IgE.

Formation and differentiation

Eosinophils, like other leucocytes, differentiate from haematopoietic stem cells *in the bone marrow* under the control of cytokine growth factors, *GM-CSF, IL-3 and IL-5* (Fig. 1.10.4), all of which can be produced by Th2 cells.

Eosinophils have a transit time in the bone marrow of some days, a half-life in the blood of less than 1 day, and live the rest of their life, a few days, in the tissues. Normally, the gut appears to be the most heavily populated site. Few cells are present in the airways, and none in normal skin. In allergic disease, however, many organs may be infiltrated by eosinophils, and their kinetics may be significantly altered.

Eosinophil recruitment and accumulation

Not many years ago, it was widely believed that mast cell release of an eosinophil chemotactic factor (ECF-A) was the cause of tissue eosinophilia in allergy. Unfortunately, this hypothesis was too simple to be correct, and we must now realize that the mechanism behind eosinophilia is *very complex* and *not fully understood*.

Factors of importance for tissue eosinophilia
Haemopoietic stem cell growth factors
Haemopoietic precursor cell differentiation factors
Cellular adhesion molecules
Chemotactic factors
Cell activation factors
Cell survival factors
Molecules that up-regulate various types of cell receptors

Table 1.10.1. The accumulation of eosinophils at the site of an allergic reaction depends upon a series of factors

The accumulation of eosinophils at the site of an allergic reaction depends upon a series of factors (Table 1.10.1). Further discussion of this topic necessitates a brief introduction to one of the 'hot topics' in modern allergy research, that is, adhesion molecules.

Adhesion molecules

Role in cell-to-cell contact and communication

To act effectively, leucocytes must be able to circulate as free, non-adherent cells in the blood, and, as adherent cells, to stick to the endothelium and migrate through the tissues. A number of intercellular adhesion molecules, on both leucocytes and endothelial cells, are operative in this process.

Adhesion molecules are *membrane-bound proteins*, which can be thought of in terms of *receptors* and their specific counterparts or *ligands*. It is their function to hold two cells together as long as it is necessary for their 'communication'.

Adhesion molecules are not exclusively expressed on *leucocytes* and *endothelial cells*, they are also, for example, expressed on *epithelial cells*. They are operative in many types of cell-to-cell communication. An important example is their holding together of *APCs/T helper cells* and *T helper cells/B cells* during the immune response. A detailed description of these activities is beyond the scope of this book.

Superfamilies

The adhesion molecules are grouped into three gene superfamilies. 1, The *selectin family*, with E-selectin (or ELAM) and P-selectin expressed on endothelial

Adhesion molecules		
Superfamily	**Receptor on endothelial cells**	**Ligand on leucocytes**
Selectin	P-selectin E-selectin	Lewis X Lewis X
Immunoglobulin	ICAM-1 and -2 VCAM-1	LFA-1 (β_2-integrin) VLA-4* (β_1-integrin)
Integrin	β_1-, β_2-, β_3-integrins	Collagen Laminin Fibronectin

Table 1.10.2. Examples of adhesion molecules, described as receptors on endothelial cells and their specific counter-structures or ligands on leucocytes. ICAM, intercellular adhesion molecule; VCAM, vascular cell adhesion molecule. LFA, lymphocyte function-associated antigen; VLA: very late antigen. *Except neutrophils.

cells and L-selectin on leucocytes (Table 1.10.2). They are involved in the early phase of leucocyte–endothelial cell interaction (Fig. 1.10.5). 2, The *immunoglobulin supergene family*, including intercellular adhesion molecules, ICAM-1, and ICAM-2, and vascular cell adhesion molecule-1 (VCAM-1), all of which are expressed on vascular endothelium. Compared to the selectins, their expression is delayed and prolonged. 3, The *integrin family* (β_1-, β_2-, β_3-integrins) comprises lymphocyte function–associated antigen-1 (LFA-1), expressed on all leucocytes, and very late antigen-4 (VLA-4), expressed on eosinophils and lymphocytes. Integrins are both involved in leucocyte–endothelial cell adhesion and in cell-matrix adhesion (Fig. 1.10.6).

As cell membrane receptors, the adhesion molecules are also given a number in the CD nomenclature (from 1 to 130+ and impossible to remember). Apart from the superfamilies, described above, there are several newly recognized CD molecules that are important in T–B cell interactions. An example is CD40 and CD40 ligand, which is intensively studied at present. A defective CD40 gene in T cells leads to failure of B cells to undergo immunoglobulin class switching and to immunodeficiency syndromes.

Receptor up-regulation

In inflamed areas, the endothelial cells become 'sticky' for the circulating leucocytes because inflammatory mediators and *cytokines up-regulate* the ex-pression of the *adhesion molecules* and their respective ligands (Fig. 1.10.6).

Transmigration

In order to make adhesion molecules operative in leucocyte trans-endothelial migration, where attachment to endothelial cells is followed by detachment, a temporary adjustment of function and up-regulation is required (Fig. 1.10.6). Initially, the leucocyte becomes *attached* to the endothelial wall and *rolls slowly* along it. It then comes to a halt, *flattens* and starts to *migrate* through the junction between endothelial cells (diapedesis). It then dissolves the basement membrane and migrates into lamina propria, where it interacts with proteins of the extracellular matrix (collagen, laminin, fibronectin). These proteins also have adhesion molecules attached.

In short, selectins are responsible for leucocyte attachment to the endothelium, the immunoglobulin superfamily (ICAM-1, ICAM-2 and VCAM-1) for flattening and diapedesis, and integrins (VLA-1 to VLA-6) for passage through the extracellular matrix.

Allergen-induced eosinophilia

Cytokines, released during an inflammatory reaction, up-regulate adhesion molecules on endothelilal cells in the local microvasculature. IL-1, IFNγ and TNFα up-regulate ICAM-1 and E-selectin. They interact with ligands expressed on all leucocytes, and the cellular infiltration will be dominated by neutrophils.

IL-4 up-regulates VCAM-1, which interacts with

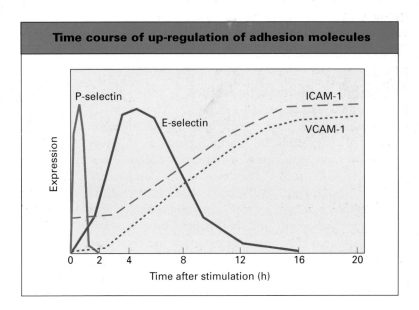

Fig. 1.10.5. Time course of cytokine-induced up-regulation of leucocyte–endothelial cell adhesion molecules. From Gundel RH, Wegner CD, Letts ALG. Leuococyte–endothelial adhesion. In: Busse WW, Holgate ST, eds. *Asthma and Rhinitis*. Oxford: Blackwell Science, 1995: 752–63.

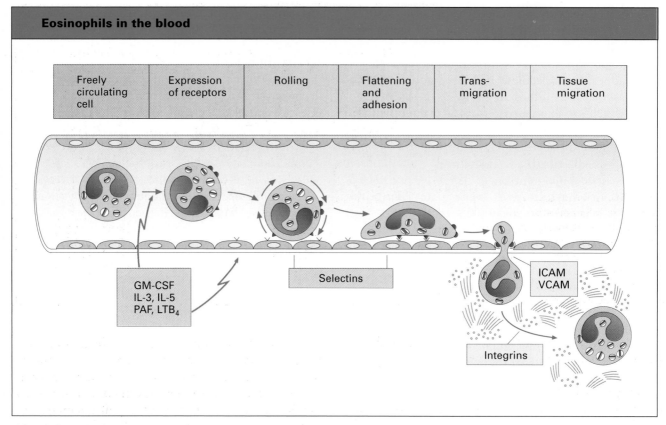

Fig. 1.10.6. In inflamed microvasculature, adhesion molecules are expressed on eosinophils and endothelial cells. The sticky eosinophil rolls, stops, flattens and migrates through the blood vessel and the tissue, a process controlled by sequential up- and down-regulation of a series of adhesion molecules. Eosinophils circulate in the blood for less than 1 day.

VLA-4, expressed on eosinophils and lymphocytes, but not on neutrophils. An up-regulation of VCAM-1, which occurs in vasculature following allergen challenge, will therefore produce an infiltrate in which the eosinophil predominates.

Local tissue eosinophilia

Eosinophil chemotactic factors

Eosinophils can respond to stimuli by chemokinesis (non-directional movement) and by chemotaxis (directed migration to a site across a stimulus concentration gradient). *In vitro* studies have ascribed *eosinotactic activity* to many compounds (Table 1.10.3; Fig. 1.10.7), but a chemotactic factor, or chemoattractant, which, *in vivo*, exclusively attracts eosinophils and not neutrophils, has yet to be isolated. However, recent data indicate that a substance, called RANTES (a chemotactic peptide related to IL-8 and released by T cells), is chemotactic for eosinophils, but not for neutrophils. At present, it

Eosinophil chemoattractants	
	Known major cell source
PAF	Eosinophils, neutrophils, macrophages, basophils and endothelial cells
LTB$_4$	Mast cells
IL-3	T cells
IL-5	T cells
GM-CSF	T cells and epithelial cells
RANTES	T cells
C5a	Activation of the complement cascade

Table 1.10.3. Molecules with a positive chemotactic activity on eosinophils

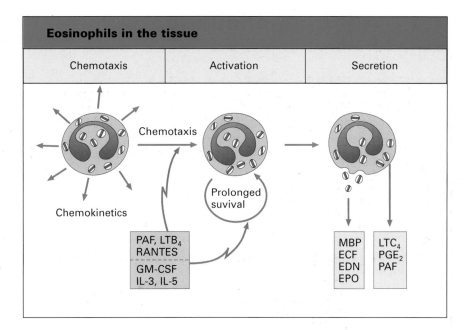

Fig. 1.10.7. Eosinophils are attracted to inflamed areas by chemotactic substances; they become activated and secrete their cytotoxic proteins and mediators. Normally they live 2–5 days in the tissue, but the period can be prolonged to some weeks during inflammation.

is not known whether RANTES is released in diseased human airways and skin.

Eosinophil survival

When eosinophils are cultured in the presence of GM-CSF, IL-3 and IL-5, their *survival is prolonged* by up to several weeks. These cytokines, released by Th2 cells during the allergic reaction, may, in part, be responsible for eosinophil accumulation by prolonging the persistence of cells in the tissue.

Eosinophil activation and secretion

Many of the substances chemotactic for eosinophils (GM-CSF, IL-3, IL-5, PAF and LTB$_4$) can also activate the cells, as judged by increased surface receptor expression and enhanced secretion. The role of these molecules for eosinophil activation and secretion *in vivo*, however, is not clear.

Eosinophils, like mast cells, *release preformed granule-associated molecules* (basic proteins) and *newly synthesized membrane-derived mediators*. They release their granule components by exocytosis, individual granules fusing with the plasma membrane.

Activated eosinophils lose some of their granule material during secretion, and they are referred to as *hypodense cells* in contrast to normodense cells.

Demonstration of cell activation

Activated cells can be identified in the tissue by staining with a monoclonal antibody, *EG2*, which is spe-

cific for ECP in activated cells (ECP changes its antigen specificity during cell activation). As an immunoassay exists for *ECP*, it can be measured in plasma and body fluid. These methods make it possible to identify and quantitate the eosinophil inflammatory reaction both in research and in clinical practice (see Chapter 4.4).

> **Short text is best**
> I have only made this letter rather long because I have not had time to make it shorter.
>
> Blaise Pascal

> **Why read this book?**
> Read not to contradict and confute, nor to believe and take for granted, nor to find talk and discourse, but to weigh and consider.
>
> Francis Bacon

1.11 Allergen challenge
Early and late responses

Key points
• An allergen challenge is used as a simple and simplified model for studying the pathophysiology of allergic diseases.
• The allergen challenge is followed by an early and a late response.
• During the early response, there is evidence of mast cell degranulation and plasma exudation.
• During the late response, which follows after 4–6 hours, there is T cell activation, up-regulation of adhesion molecules and accumulation of eosinophils.
• In the skin, the early response consists of the wheal-and-flare reaction, inhibited by H_1 antihistamines.
• In the bronchi, the early response is caused by smooth muscle contraction, prevented and reversed by inhaled beta$_2$ agonists.
• In the nose, the early response consists of sneezing, watery rhinorrhoea and blockage, which H_1 antihistamines inhibit to a high, a moderate and a poor degree, respectively.
• In the eye, the early symptoms, itching and redness, are effectively inhibited by H_1 antihistamines.
• A late response often develops when the allergen challenge is severe and when the tissue is inflamed before challenge.

• Glucocorticoids very efficiently block the development of late responses in all tissues.
• In the skin, a late response consists of a diffusely demarcated induration.
• In the bronchi, the late and the early responses typically form a biphasic curve.
• In the nose, the late response, consisting of intermittent sneezing and persistent blockage, is poorly defined in time and without the typically biphasic pattern.

Although it is more than a hundred years since Charles Blackley artificially introduced allergen into the skin and airways, it is only during the last 2–3 decades that allergen challenge has been widely used for studying the pathophysiology of asthma and rhinitis.

When using *artificial challenge* as a model for disease, it should be noted that a single challenge with a large allergen dosage in the laboratory differs fundamentally from *natural exposure* to minute amounts of allergen inhaled by 15 000 breaths a day. Thus, the description below of an allergic reaction, composed of an early and a late response (Figs 1.11.1–2), is a simplified model, which mainly serves a didactic purpose. In chronic disease with continuous allergen exposure, the condition at a given point of time will constitute the sum of accumulated early and late responses.

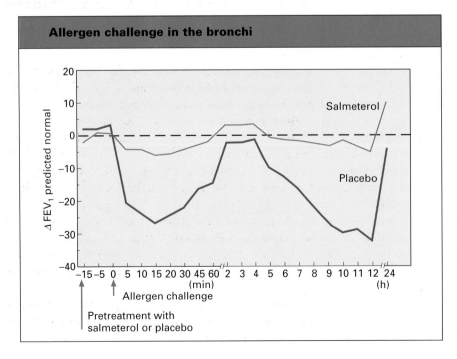

Allergen challenge in the bronchi

Fig. 1.11.1. Allergen inhalation challenge can cause an isolated early response, but it often results in a dual early and late response, showing a typical biphasic curve. In this study, both early and late responses were effectively inhibited by the inhalation of a long-acting beta$_2$ agonist (salmeterol 50 µg) (upper curve), as compared with placebo (lower curve). From Pedersen B, Dahl R, Larsen BB, Venge P. The effect of salmeterol on the early- and late-phase reaction to bronchial challenge. *Allergy* 1993; **48**: 377–82.

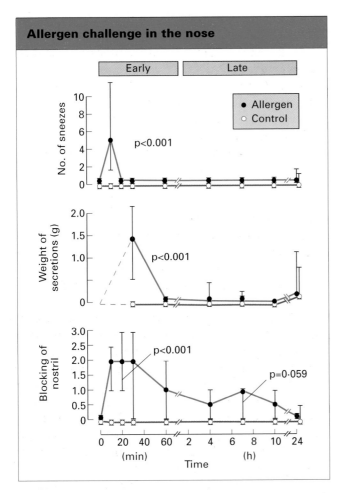

Fig. 1.11.2. Allergen challenge in the nose is dominated by the early response, consisting of marked sneezing, rhinorrhoea and nasal blockage. It is followed by a late response consisting of a few scattered sneezes and partial blockage without a typical biphasic time curve. From Durham SR. Allergic inflammation. *Pediatr Allergy* 1993; **4** (suppl 4): 7–10.

Early response

The early response to an allergen challenge starts within minutes, and symptoms and signs have usually resolved within 1 hour. In all tissues challenged, there is morphologic and biochemical evidence of *mast cell degranulation* and of plasma exudation. The early response can be modified by pretreatment with drugs as shown in Table 1.11.1.

It is during the early response that processes, which initiate the late response, such as up-regulation of adhesion molecules, take place (Fig. 1.11.3).

Skin

The early response in the skin is characterized by

itching and a *wheal-and-flare* reaction. Both itching and the wheal reaction can be almost completely blocked by an H_1 antihistamine. This indicates that the itching is caused by *histamine* acting on nervous H_1 receptors. Similarly, the wheal reaction is due to histamine stimulation of vascular H_1 receptors, which results in plasma extravasation and oedema formation. The flare (erythema) reaction is only partly inhibited by H_1 antihistamines. It is caused by histamine stimulation of vascular H_1 and H_2 receptors and also of other mediators. An *axon reflex* also contributes to vasodilation and erythema. This reflex is mediated by substance P, and, experimentally, it can be inhibited by pretreatment with capsaicin, which depletes the sensory nerves for substance P.

Bronchi

The complete prevention and reversal of all symptoms and signs of asthma by a *beta₂ bronchodilator inhaler* suggests that the early bronchoconstriction is due to *smooth muscle contraction* rather than oedema formation. Antagonists of histamine and of arachidonic acid metabolites have partial effects, showing some contribution by histamine, sulphidoleukotrienes (LTC_4, LTD_4, LTE_4) and prostaglandins. However, their added effects cannot completely block the response, indicating a role played by some unopposed bronchoconstrictor substances.

The allergen-induced early response can be imitated by inhalation of histamine, sulphidoleukotrienes, prostaglandins and PAF.

Nose

Allergen challenge results, within 1–2 minutes, in *sneezing* followed, with some minutes' delay, by *rhinorrhoea* and *blockage* (Fig. 1.11.2).

Biopsy studies have shown that mast cell degranulation occurs predominantly in the superficial layer of the mucous membrane. Release of mast cell derived mediators (histamine, tryptase, prostaglandin D_2 and leukotrienes) can be detected in nasal lavage fluid (Fig. 1.11.4).

Kinins, albumin and other plasma components are also increased in nasal lavage fluid, indicating increased vascular leakage and plasma exudation, more pronounced in the early than in the late nasal response.

Histamine, but not the other putative mediators, can imitate the entire early response with its intense itching, sneezing, rhinorrhoea and blockage.

Drug effect on early responses					
	H$_1$ antihistamine	**Beta$_2$ agonist**	**Oral steroids**	**Topical steroids**	**Cromoglycate**
Skin					
Itching	+++	+	–	+	–
Wheal	+++	+	–	+	–
Flare	++	+	–	+	–
Bronchi					
Bronchocon-striction	+	+++*	+	++	++
Nose					
Sneezing	+++	+*	–	++	++
Rhinorrhoea	++	+	–	++	++
Blockage	+	+	–	++	++
Eye					
Itching	+++	?	–**	?	++
Redness	+++	?	–**	?	++

Table 1.11.1. Effect of pretreatment with various drugs on the early response to allergen challenge (–, 0–10%; +, 10–40%; ++, 40–70%; +++, 70–100%). *Topical application. **Treatment for 3 days

While an H$_1$ antihistamine is highly effective on itching and sneezing, and moderately so on rhinorrhoea, it can only slightly inhibit nasal blockage. This indicates that blockage is mediated, predominantly, by other substances. Pretreatment with topical glucocorticoids has some effect on the early response, but the mode of action is not clear.

Eye

Itching and *conjunctival redness* can be almost completely inhibited by *H$_1$ antihistamines* indicating that *histamine* is the most important mediator.

Studies of tears have shown increased levels of mast cell derived mediators (tryptase and PGD$_2$) after allergen challenge. Conjunctival scrapings have shown an up-regulation of epithelial adhesion molecules (ICAM-1), starting during the early response (Fig. 1.11.3).

Late response

When a large dosage of allergen is used for challenge, the early response is often followed by a late response. This typically begins after 2–4 hours, is maximal between 6–12 hours and has usually ended within 24–48 hours (Figs 1.11.1–2).

It was formerly believed that the late response was caused by a Type III allergic reaction. However, strong evidence against this hypothesis has been pro-

vided by Dolovich and coworkers in Canada, who showed a late dermal response to the injection of anti-IgE antibody. Thus, the late response is a direct consequence of the IgE-mediated reaction.

There is morphological and biochemical evidence of: 1, *T cell* activation; 2, up-regulation of adhesion molecules (initiated earlier); and 3, *eosinophil* accumulation, activation and secretion.

Although there is little doubt that the eosinophil, with its content of cytotoxic proteins, is very important in the late response, other inflammatory cells (lymphocytes, neutrophils, macrophages, monocytes, platelets, Langerhans' cells and basophils) and stationary cells (epithelial cells and fibroblasts) may all contribute with release of mediators and cytokines. No single mediator has been implicated in the generation of the late response. The combined effect of a series of molecules in the 'mediator soup' certainly can cause a multitude of effects. The precise role played by each of these mediators and cells has yet to be defined.

The high efficacy of *glucocorticoids* in inhibiting the late response (Table 1.11.2) is compatible with a T-cell induced inflammatory reaction as lymphocytes are very sensitive to steroids.

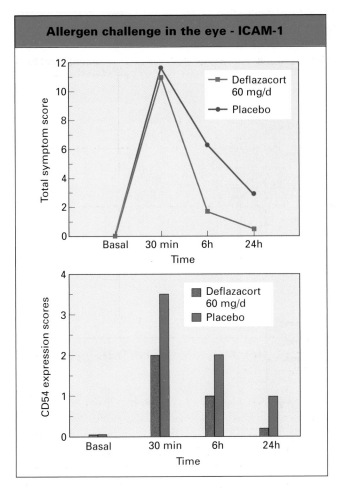

Allergen challenge in the eye - ICAM-1

(top graph) Total symptom score vs Time (Basal, 30 min, 6h, 24h)
— ■ Deflazacort 60 mg/d
— ● Placebo

(bottom graph) CD54 expression scores vs Time (Basal, 30 min, 6h, 24h)
■ Deflazacort 60 mg/d
■ Placebo

Fig. 1.11.3. Allergen challenge of the eye results in an early response with sneezing and redness, and, in severe cases, redness and discomfort continues during a late phase. Conjunctival scrapings showed a clear up-regulation of epithelial adhesion molecules (ICAM-1 or CD54). It was, like the late symptom response, inhibited by pretreatment for 3 days with an oral steroid (Deflazacort 60 mg/day). From Ciprandi G, Buscaglia S, Pesce GP, Iudice A, Bagnasco M, Caconica GW. Deflazacort protects against late-phase but not early-phase reactions induced by the allergen-specific conjunctival provocation test. *Allergy* 1993; **48**: 421–30.

Skin

The late cutaneous response is a *diffusely demarcated induration* without the characteristic itching of the wheal-and-flare reaction.

Histologically, it is characterized by oedema and by increased numbers of *eosinophils* and *T helper lymphocytes* having a cytokine profile of Th2 cells (Fig. 1.11.5).

While histamine induces only an early response, the injection of mast cell degranulating compounds (anti-IgE, codeine and PAF) can elicit both an early and a late response.

Bronchi

A severe challenge, especially of already inflamed airways with eosinophilia, usually results in a dual symptom response with the early and the late responses forming a typical *biphasic curve* (Figs 1.11.1–2).

The late response is associated with an increase in bronchial responsiveness (see next chapter), often with exaggerated airflow variation and asthma for some days. There is strong evidence that the late response is a better *model for chronic asthma disease* than the early response.

The late symptoms are more severe and protracted than the early bronchoconstriction. They can be completely abolished by pretreatment with *glucocorticoids*, and inhaled beta$_2$ bronchodilators are also effective.

While the level of histamine and its metabolites in lavage fluid, plasma and urine are raised during the early response, they are unchanged during the late response. This suggests that the role of mast cell or basophil degranulation is of little importance during the late inflammatory response.

Studies of *lymphocytes* and of lymphocyte subsets in bronchoalveolar lavage (BAL) and biopsies have failed to find an increase in number. However, a recent study of BAL, using a sensitive flow cytometry method, has shown a significant increase in the number of activated CD4$^+$ T cells 24 hours after allergen challenge. These cells had the cytokine profile of Th2 cells. Thus, allergen challenge results in *local activation of Th2 cells* in the bronchi.

Examination of ECP in BAL fluid and of EG2$^+$ eosinophils in bronchial biopsies have shown signs of *eosinophil activation and degranulation* as early as 3 hours after challenge, and the number of cells is maximal after 24 hours.

The eosinophilia is related to the magnitude of the late response, the degree of T cell activation and the level of cytokine expression. Although this finding does not prove a causal association, it supports the concept that the eosinophil contributes to the late asthmatic response.

Cell infiltration during the late response is dependant on *adhesion molecules*. Bronchial allergen challenge studies have shown that an increase occurs in ICAM-1 and E-selectin in endothelial cells at 5–6 hours, and in VCAM-1 at 24 hours following the

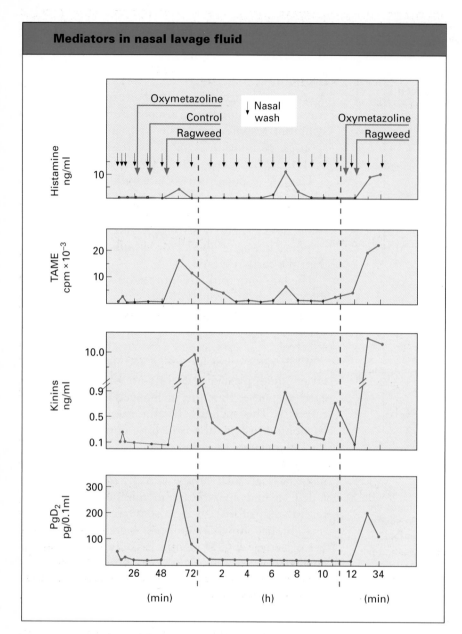

Fig. 1.11.4. Mediators in nasal lavage fluid during early, late and rechallenge responses of allergic subject to nasal challenge with ragweed extract. From Naclerio RM, Proud D, Togias AG, *et al.* Inflammatory mediators in late antigen-induced rhinitis. *N Engl J Med* 1985; **313**: 65–70.

Drug effect on late responses

	H₁ antihistamine	Beta₂ agonist	Steroids	Cromoglycate
Skin	+	−	+++	−
Bronchi	+	+/+++*	+++	++
Nose	+	−	+++	++

Table 1.11.2. Effect of pretreatment with various drugs on the late response to allergen challenge (−, 0–10%; +, 10–40%; ++, 40–70%; +++, 70–100%). *+ for inhaled short-acting drugs; +++ for inhaled long-acting drugs

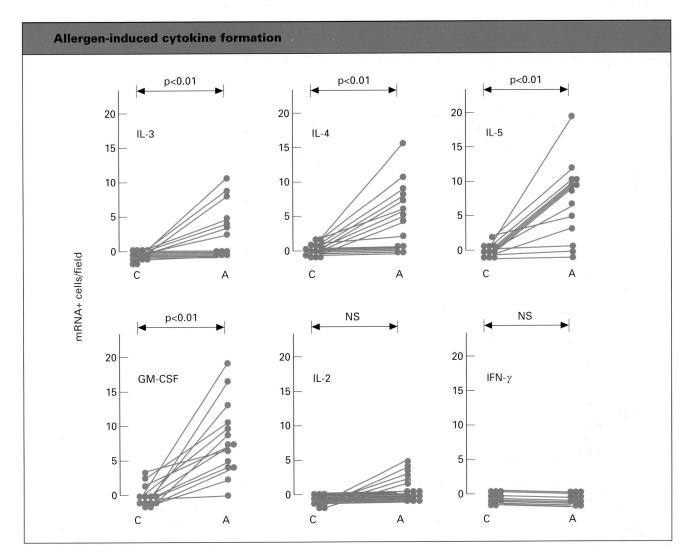

Allergen-induced cytokine formation

Fig. 1.11.5. *In situ* hybridization of allergen-induced late cutaneous responses (A). When compared to control sites (C), significant increases in IL-3, IL-4, IL-5 and GM-CSF, but not IL-2 and IFNγ, were observed. From Kay AB, Sun Ying, Varney V, *et al.* Messenger RNA expression of the cytokine gene cluster, IL-3, IL-4, IL-5 and GM-CSF in allergen-induced late-phase cutaneous reactions in atopic subjects. *J Exp Med* 1992; **173**: 775–8.

challenge. This up-regulation in the airway microvasculature is comparable to findings in the skin and conjunctiva at similar time points.

Nose

The early attack of sneezing and hypersecretion can be severe (25 sneezes and 1ml of secretion), it is followed by minor bouts of sneezing and discharge for the rest of the day. While nasal blockage is worst during the first hour, some stuffiness remains for the rest of the day (Fig. 1.11.2). Unlike the late response in the bronchi, the late response in the nose is less severe than the early response, more *variable in time* and *not strictly biphasic*.

Some hours after the challenge, there is a local *influx of metachromatic cells* to the epithelial surface (mast cells of the mucosal type, MC_T, and probably some basophils). There is a marked *influx of eosinophils*, and a striking increase in the concentration of *ECP in lavage fluid*. This shows that the eosinophils migrate to the epithelium and release their proteins.

In biopsies, taken 24 hours after challenge, there is an increased number of *activated T helper cells* (IL-2 receptor positive or CD25[+] cells), and of cells expressing messenger ribonucleic acid (mRNA) for IL-4 and IL-5 (Th2 cells), but not IL-2 and IFNγ (Th1 cells).

A positive correlation between numbers of activated eosinophils (EG2[+]) and mRNA for IL-5 supports the notion that the eosinophilia is IL-5 induced.

Eye

There is histological evidence of a late response with *eosinophilia* in conjunctival scraping 6 hours after challenge. This response is subclinical unless the challenge is very heavy. When a late symptom response follows allergen challenge, it consists of persistent redness and ocular discomfort without a quiescent symptom-free period (Fig. 1.11.3).

A late response
Sickness comes on horseback and departs on foot.
Dutch proverb

1.12 Allergic inflammation
—in the skin, bronchi, nose and eye

Key points
* In atopic dermatitis, there is an increased number of Th2 cells, eosinophils, mast cells and Langerhans' cells.
* In asthma, there is eosinophil inflammation in severe cases and in mild disease.
* In allergic and non-allergic asthma, the number of epithelial mast cells, of the MC_T type, is increased and they show signs of degranulation.
* In asthma, an increased number of Th2 cells are activated and secrete IL-5 of importance for eosinophil accumulation. The reaction is blocked by steroids.
* In asthma, there is an up-regulation of ICAM-1 in vasculature and also in surface epithelium.
* Epithelial shedding occurs in severe asthma but, even in mild cases, there is damage of the surface epithelium.
* In the allergic nose, there is an increased number of Langerhans' cells, eosinophils and mast cells of the MC_T type in the epithelium, and an enhanced expression of adhesion molecules (ICAM-1 and VCAM-1).
* In the eye, allergic inflammation is more pronounced in vernal kerato-conjunctivitis than in allergic conjunctivitis.
* In vernal kerato-conjunctivitis, mast cells of the MC_{TC} dominate, and there is an increased number of CD4[+] T cells of the Th2 type.
* A tissue-driven cytokine production may explain the allergen-induced, self-perpetuating inflammation, which causes chronic disease.

Atopic dermatitis
The lesion of atopic dermatitis is characterized by a *lymphocyte infiltrate* dominated by CD4[+] cells, up to 10% *eosinophils*, and an increased number of *mast cells* and of *Langerhans' cells*. It has features in common with an allergic contact dermatitis reaction, which represents delayed-type hypersensitivity. This has been studied in atopic dermatitis patients, who have a patch test with mite antigen performed and develop a cutaneous reaction, which clinically is fully

compatible with a Type IV skin reaction. Cloning of T lymphocytes from such skin reactions show a predominant Th2 cytokine profile.

Asthma

It has long been recognized that, in fatal asthma, there is bronchial inflammation, characterized by massive intraluminal plugging with mucus containing sheets of epithelial cells and huge numbers of eosinophils. More recently, bronchoscopy studies, with lavage and biopsy, have provided evidence of *inflammation even in clinically mild asthma.*

Mast cells and mediators

There is an *increased number of epithelial mast cells* in both allergic and non-allergic asthma. They have the staining characteristics of mucosal mast cells, MC_T, and show ultrastructural signs of degranulation; a feature confirmed by increase of histamine, PGD_2 and tryptase in lavage fluid (Fig. 1.12.1).

The marginal effect of H_1 antihistamines in clinical asthma indicates, however, that the mast cell derived mediator, histamine, does not play a major role in chronic asthma.

T cells and cytokines

In asthma, study of cells recovered by lavage and in bronchial biopsy material, have shown an increased number of activated Th2 cells, which express IL-3, IL-4, IL-5 and GM-CSF.

In a recent study from The National Heart and Lung Institute in London, there was an increased number of activated T cells (CD4[+] and CD25[+]) in the peripheral blood in patients who required peroral glucocorticoids for exacerbation of asthma. They also had detectable plasma IL-5 and an increased eosinophil count. All parameters were normalized by the glucocorticoid therapy. These observations are consistent with the hypotheses that exacerbations of asthma are associated with activation of memory cells, of the Th2 type, which secrete IL-5 and induce eosinophilia.

Adhesion molecules

A more recent study has reported *up-regulation of ICAM-1* expression in the *vasculature* of bronchial biopsies from patients with non-allergic asthma.

Interestingly, an increased expression of ICAM-1 is found in *airway epithelium* from asthmatics as compared with normals. It is possible that eosinophil-mediated damage of the surface epithelium is

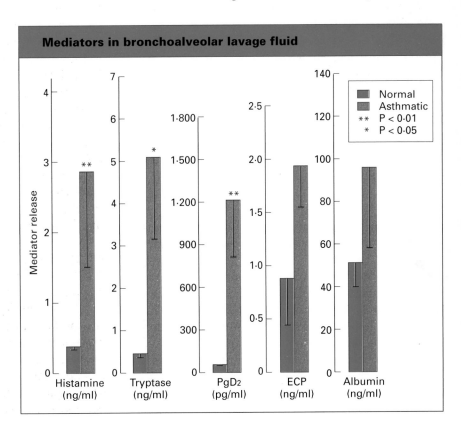

Fig. 1.12.1. Mediator concentrations in bronchoalveolar lavage fluid in matched normal and asthmatic subjects. From Holgate S. Mediator and cytokine mechanisms in asthma. *Thorax* 1993; **48**: 103–9.

facilitated by binding between epithelial receptor (ICAM-1) and eosinophil ligand (LFA-1).

Eosinophils and basic proteins

The eosinophil is found in increased number in the full thickness of the airway wall, and there is bronchial *eosinophilia* even in mild cases of asthma. Like mast cells, eosinophils in the bronchial wall have the ultrastructural features of degranulation, and their secretion of basic proteins is shown by lavage studies (Fig. 1.12.1).

Surface epithelium

Epithelial sloughing is seen in bronchi of patients who have died in status asthmaticus (Fig. 1.12.2). A series of recent studies have shown signs of *epithelial damage* even in mild asthma. There is an increased number of opened, tight junctions and widened intercellular spaces. The number of ciliated cells is reduced. It is of considerable clinical significance that treatment with topical glucocorticoids reduces the number of eosinophils, and other infiltrating cells (Fig. 1.12.3), and tends to normalize the epithelial changes.

It is now a widely accepted hypothesis that eosinophil-induced damage of the bronchial epithelium is a major cause of airway hyper-responsiveness (Figs 1.12.4–5; see next chapter).

Other structural changes

Chronic asthma is associated with a series of changes in the bronchial tissue: 1, basement membrane thickening; 2, tissue fibrosis; 3, smooth muscle hyperplasia; and 4, glandular hyperplasia. These changes may be responsible for the partial irreversibility of airway obstruction, which often occurs when chronic asthma has persisted for decades.

Allergic rhinitis

The number of *Langerhans' cells* in the nasal epithelium is increased by allergen exposure, experimental as well as natural. The number is reduced by topical treatment with glucocorticoids.

The numbers of progenitors of eosinophils and basophils are elevated in the peripheral blood of patients with allergic rhinitis, and asthma, and these cells fluctuate inversely with symptoms.

There is an increase of *mast cells of the* MC_T *type* in the epithelium and of total and *activated eosinophils* in the epithelium and lamina propria. Although there is an increased level of eosinophil

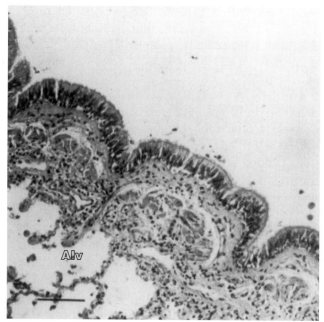

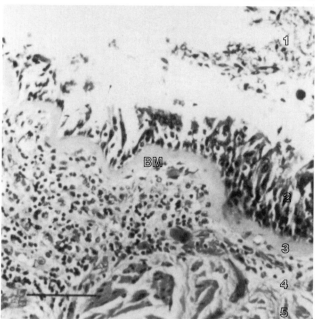

Fig. 1.12.2. Bronchial mucous membrane in a normal subject (× 160) (upper part) and in a patient who died from severe asthma (× 500) (lower part). The latter demonstrates: 1, cellular exudate in the airway lumen; 2, the fragility and sloughing of surface epithelium; 3, the thickened and prominent basement membrane; 4, marked cellular infiltrate; and 5, hypertrophy of bronchial smooth muscle. From Barnes PJ. Pathophysiology of allergic inflammation. In: Middleton E, Reed CE, Ellis EF, Adkinson NF, Yunginger JW, Busse WW, eds. *Allergy. Principles and Practice* 2nd ed. St Louis: The CV Mosby Company, 1993: 243–301.

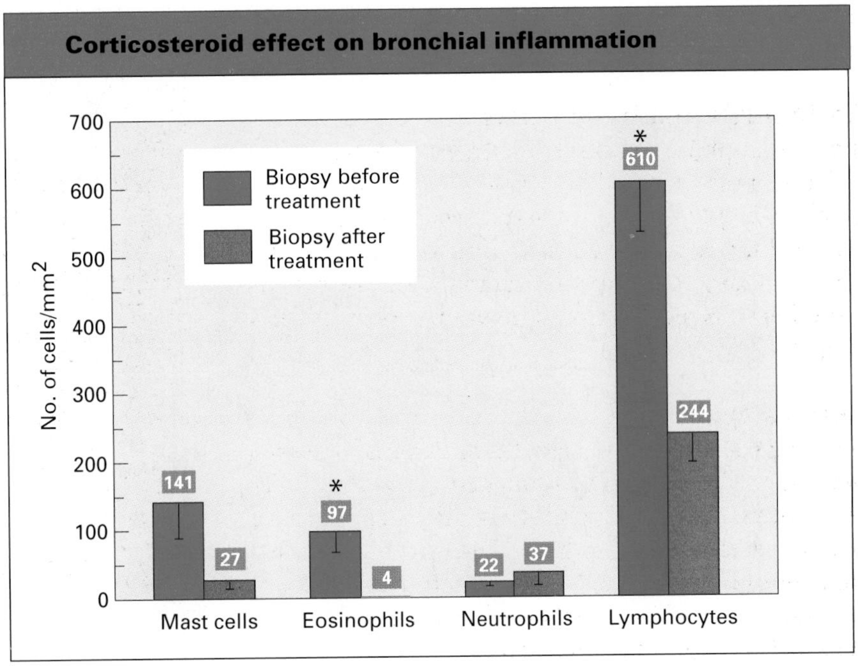

Fig. 1.12.3. Number of infiltrating cells in the bronchial epithelium of 14 asthmatic patients before and after treatment for 3 months with the inhaled steroid, budesonide. The number of eosinophils and lymphocytes decreased significantly (*$p < 0.05$). From Laitinen LA, Laitinen A, Haathela T. A comparative study of the effects of an inhaled corticosteroid, budesonide, and a β_2-agonist, terbutaline, on airway inflammation in newly diagnosed asthma. *J Allergy Clin Immunol* 1992; **90**: 32–42.

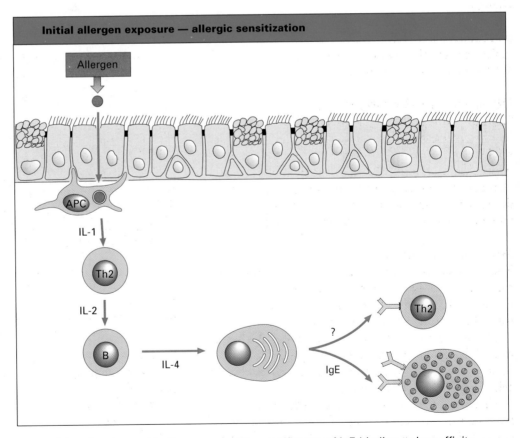

Fig. 1.12.4. Simplified summary of the allergic sensitization process. The significance of IgE binding to low-affinity receptors on T cells is unknown.

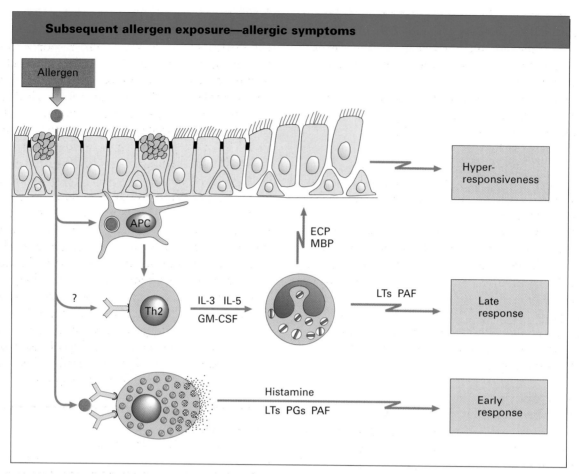

Fig. 1.12.5. Simplified summary of the allergic reaction. It is uncertain whether antigen stimulation of Th2 cells always takes place through APCs or whether it also can occur by interaction with IgE bound to low-affinity receptors.

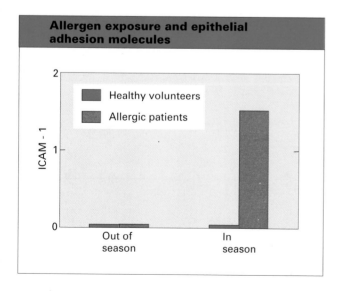

Fig. 1.12.6. ICAM-1 expression on nasal epithelial cells increases during the *Parietaria judaica* pollen season in sensitized patients (*n* = 10) and not in healthy volunteers (*n* = 10). From Ciprandi G, Prontzto C, Ricca V, Bagnasco M, Canonica GW. Evidence of intercellular adhesion molecule-1 expressed on nasal epithelial cells in acute rhinoconjunctivitis caused by pollen exposure. *J Allergy Clin Immunol* 1994; **99**: 738–46.

cytotoxic proteins in nasal secretion and lavage fluid, a series of histological studies have failed to show any morphological damage to the surface epithelium in the nose after natural and experimental allergen exposure.

Immunohistochemical investigation of nasal vasculature in seasonal allergic rhinitis have identified *enhanced expression of VCAM-1* and also in perennial allergic rhinitis of ICAM-1.

Adhesion molecules on *epithelial cells* may also be up-regulated during inflammatory reactions contributing to the accumulation of inflammatory cells in airway secretions (Fig. 1.12.6).

A study of seasonal allergic rhinitis has failed to reproduce the change in T-cell numbers seen after allergen challenge. This indicates that inflammation is more pronounced following artificial than natural exposure to allergen.

The significant effect of H_1 *antihistamines*, even in chronic perennial allergic rhinitis, shows that histamine plays an important role in the nose − in contrast to the bronchi.

Allergic conjunctivitis and vernal kerato-conjunctivitis

The number of mast cells is increased in allergic conjunctivitis and in vernal kerato-conjunctivitis in particular. Although there is an increased number of mast cells of the MC_T type in vernal kerato-conjunctivitis, the MC_{TC} *cells dominate* (80–100%) over MC_T at all locations. This is at variance with the relative occurrence of these cells in the airways.

Mast cell derived tryptase is detectable in tears in vernal kerato-conjunctivitis but not in allergic conjunctivitis.

The local *eosinophil infiltration* is more pronounced in vernal kerato-conjunctivitis, both allergic and non-allergic, than in allergic conjunctivitis. The same applies to the concentrations of ECP in conjunctival lavage fluid.

The major histological feature differentiating *vernal kerato-conjunctivitis* from seasonal and perennial allergic conjunctivitis is the *large number of T cells*, particularly of the CD4+ type, in the stroma of vernal kerato-conjunctivitis. T cell clones have been produced from conjunctival biopsies, having the cytokine profile of *Th2 cells*.

In summary, the changes in seasonal and perennial allergic conjunctivitis is far less dramatic than in vernal kerato-conjunctivitis, and, on examination, inflammation appears to be mild.

Self-perpetuating allergic inflammation

An allergen challenge with a late response can cause asthma symptoms for days and even weeks. The asthma disease can continue for prolonged periods after complete avoidance of allergens, which is demonstrated by occupational asthma due to the red-cedar tree (see Chapter 3.6). The pathophysiological basis for this phenomenon may be an allergen-induced, self-perpetuating inflammatory reaction.

As described earlier, a series of cells in the allergic inflammation can synthesize and release haemopoietic and pro-inflammatory cytokines, having an effect on circulating progenitor cells to mast cells and eosinophils, as well as on the mature cells. The local cytokine production in the inflamed tissue may provide a positive feedback loop for allergic tissue responses. Thus, a local, *tissue-driven cytokine response* may explain the *chronicity and self-perpetuation of the pathology* of such conditions as atopic dermatitis, asthma and nasal polyposis. Accordingly, these conditions may then be considered expressions of an ongoing cytokine over-production.

Clinical trials needed
Each physician thinks his pills best.

German proverb

1.13 Hyper-responsiveness
A consequence of inflammation?

Key points

- Non-specific hyper-responsiveness to stimuli is a characteristic of allergic disease.
- Bronchial hyper-responsiveness is a constant feature of chronic asthma.
- Asthma patients, therefore, bronchoconstrict in response to non-specific stimuli, such as exercise, cold air and irritants.
- Allergen exposure can induce hyper-responsiveness and symptoms for prolonged periods of time.
- This is probably due to eosinophil accumulation, release of cytotoxic proteins and epithelial damage.
- The eosinophil inflammation and the hyper-responsiveness can, in part, be normalized by glucocorticosteroids.
- However, this hypothesis does not explain all features of airway hyper-responsiveness, and steroid therapy does not completely normalize the responsiveness.
- There is clinical evidence that patients with rhinitis show increased responsiveness to non-specific stimuli, but testing is not clinically useful.
- Patients with chronic urticaria and patients with atopic dermatitis have a considerably reduced threshold for itching following non-specific physical and chemical stimulation.

It is characteristic of allergic diseases that a series of non-specific physical and chemical stimuli, causing little or no reaction in normal subjects, result in sneezing, coughing, wheezing, itching and scratching. This abnormal responsiveness, of great clinical importance, is best studied in asthma, and bronchial hyper-responsiveness is the main subject of this chapter.

Bronchial hyper-responsiveness

Bronchial responsiveness is defined as the degree to which airways constrict in response to non-sensitizing physical or chemical stimuli. It can be measured by *inhalation challenge with histamine* or methacholine. In asthma, there is an increase both in the ease with which airways narrow and in the magnitude of the airway constriction (Fig. 1.13.1).

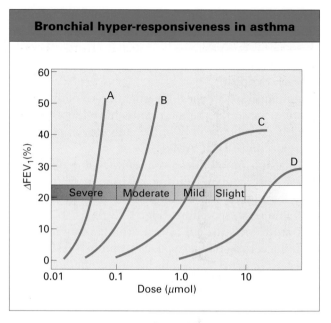

Bronchial hyper-responsiveness in asthma

Fig. 1.13.1. Dose–response curves to inhaled histamine or methacholine. Severe asthma (A) is characterized by a shift to the left of the curve (increased sensitivity), and an elevation of the maximal response with a loss of the plateau (excessive narrowing), as compared to a normal subject (D). The response is measured as the change in forced expiratory volume in 1 second (FEV_1), and the result is usually given as the dosage causing a 20% reduction in FEV_1 (see Chapter 9.11). From Woolcock AJ, Salome CM, Yan K. The shape of the dose–response curve in asthmatic and normal subjects. *Am Rev Respir Dis* 1984; **130**: 72–5.

—in asthma definition and diagnosis

Although not synonymous with asthma, bronchial hyper-responsiveness, or hyper-reactivity, is *a constant feature of chronic asthma* and has become part of recent definitions of the disease. In selected patients, a histamine inhalation test is used as an adjunct to establish the diagnosis and for assessment of the disease severity.

Episodic or persistent asthma

Although patients with episodic or seasonal allergic asthma have airways that narrow excessively in response to allergen, they may have normal responsiveness to histamine. Patients with chronic persistent asthma, on the other hand, have hyper-responsiveness as a consistent feature of the disease. Clinically, this is important, as asthma subjects get symptoms from exposures to non-specific stimuli (i.e. exercise, inhalation of cold air and irritant gases).

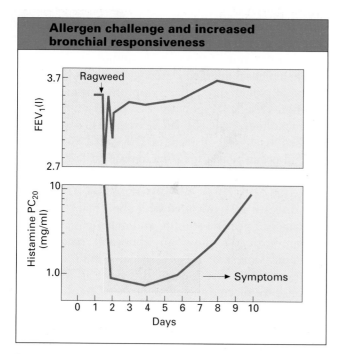

Fig. 1.13.2. An allergen inhalation challenge, provoking a late bronchial response, induces an increased bronchial responsiveness to histamine, associated with symptoms provoked by non-specific stimuli. From Cockroft DW. Mechanism of perennial allergic asthma. *Lancet* 1983; **2**: 253–6.

Transient or persistent hyper-responsiveness

Patients with chronic asthma have a relatively stable degree of airway hyper-responsiveness. Superimposed on this persistent 'baseline responsiveness', transient increases develop following exposure to a number of 'inducers', which are allergens, low-molecular weight chemical sensitizers, noxious gases, such as ozone and sulphur dioxide, and viral respiratory tract infections.

Allergen is an important 'inducer', and there is convincing evidence that both artificial challenge and natural exposure is associated with an increase in non-specific responsiveness (Fig. 1.13.2). When the exposure stops, it can take weeks or months before the reactivity returns to its former level. It has recently been realized that, in some cases of occupational asthma, hyper-responsiveness and disease may continue indefinitely in spite of complete avoidance of the offending substance. Obviously, exposure to allergen, or to low-molecular weight occupational sensitizers, creates a vicious circle (Fig. 1.13.3) and may result in a self-perpetuating inflammatory reaction.

Eosinophil inflammation

The observation that even individuals with mild asthma can have airway inflammation has recently been emphasized. Asthma is now considered primarily as an inflammatory disease with broncho-constriction, and symptoms as secondary features to bronchial hyper-responsiveness.

There are data to link airway responsiveness to inflammation, at least the transient form induced by allergens and by other 'inducers'. Studies have shown a correlation between the degree of airway hyper-responsiveness and the numbers of mast cells and eosinophils in the bronchi (Fig. 1.13.4).

It is our present working hypothesis that airway hyper-responsiveness is mainly due to release of cytotoxic proteins from eosinophils, which cause epithelial damage and the exposure of sensory nerve endings to irritants.

Effect of steroids

In support of the above hypothesis is the findings that glucocorticoid treatment, especially when inhaled over prolonged periods, has the following effects. 1, In allergen challenge, it inhibits influx of eosinophils

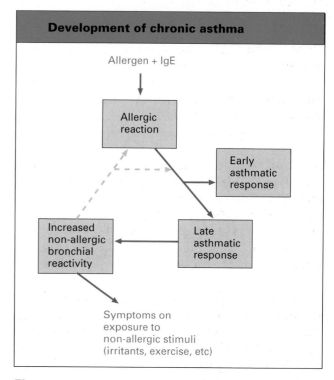

Fig. 1.13.3. Diagram of hypothesis explaining development and maintenance of perennial allergic asthma. From Cockroft DW. Mechanism of perennial allergic asthma. *Lancet* 1983; **2**: 253–6.

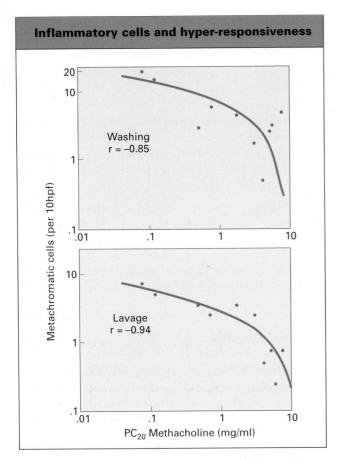

Inflammatory cells and hyper-responsiveness

Fig. 1.13.4. Positive correlation of the number of inflammatory cells in bronchial lavage fluid and the degree of methacholine airway hyper-responsiveness in mild asthmatic subjects. From Kirby JC. Bronchoalveolar cell profiles in asthmatic and non-asthmatic subjects. *Am Rev Respir Dis* 1987; **136**: 379–85.

and the late response. 2, In clinical asthma, it reduces bronchial eosinophilia and epithelial damage. 3, In chronic asthma, it decreases airway hyper-responsiveness and symptoms.

It must be emphasized, however, that this hypothesis does not explain all features of airway hyper-responsiveness and that even long-term steroid therapy is unable to normalize the responsiveness, except in a few mild cases.

Nasal hyper-responsiveness

In patients with rhinitis, symptoms are provoked by exposure to a series of non-specific stimuli (e.g. cold air, dust and fumes), which suggests hyper-responsiveness of the nasal mucosa. This can be demonstrated by a nasal challenge with histamine (sneezing, hypersecretion and blockage) or methacholine (hypersecretion only). However, these tests cannot

separate a normal and a diseased population as efficiently as an inhalation test in asthma. Their usage is, at present, confined to research studies.

When a nasal allergen challenge is repeated, within hours or some days, the symptom response, and the non-specific responsiveness to histamine and methacholine, will be increased. This allergen-induced hyper-responsiveness, also called 'priming of the end organ', lasts for some days or a few weeks.

Cutaneous hyper-responsiveness

Skin diseases are associated with abnormal reactivity, especially to pruritic stimuli, and many patients with chronic urticaria show an abnormal reaction to mechanical stress or other physical stimuli.

Patients with atopic dermatitis have an abnormal response to injected metacholine (see Chapter 6.3).

Books and patients
To study the phenomenon of disease without books is to sail an uncharted sea, while to study books without patients is not to go to sea at all.

William Osler

Further reading

Books

AVENBERG KM, HARPER DS, LARSSON BL. *Footnotes on Allergy* Uppsala: Pharmacia, 1980: 1–103.

BARNES PJ, RODGER IW, THOMSON NC, eds. *Asthma. Basic Mechanisms and Clinical Management* 2nd ed. London: Academic Press, 1992: 1–782.

BUSSE WW, HOLGATE ST, eds. *Asthma and Rhinitis* Oxford: Blackwell Science, 1995: 1–1488.

COHEN SG, SAMTER M. *Excerpts from Classics in Allergy* Providence: OceanSide Publications, 1992: 1–211.

GODARD P, BOUSQUET J, MICHEL FB, eds. *Advances in Allergology and Clinical Immunology* Carnforth: The Pantheon Publishing Group, 1992: 1–696.

HOLGATE ST, CHURCH MK. *Allergy* London: Gower Medical Publishing, 1993: 1–250.

JANEWAY CA, TRAVERS P. *Immunobiology. The Immune System in Health and Disease* London: Current Biology Ltd, 1994: 1–12.48.

KAY AB, ed. *Eosinophils, Allergy and Asthma* Oxford: Blackwell Scientific Publications, 1990: 1–163.

KLEIN J. *Immunology* Oxford: Blackwell Scientific Publications, 1990: 1–508.

PAGE CP, GARDINER PJ, eds. *Airway Hyperresponsiveness: Is It Really Important for Asthma?* Oxford: Blackwell Scientific Publications, 1993: 1–344.

ROITT I. *Essential Immunology* 7th ed. Oxford: Blackwell Scientific Publications, 1991: 1–356.

WARDLAW AJ. *Asthma* Oxford: Bios Scientific Publishers, 1993: 1–195.

Articles

ADAMS DH, SHAW S. Leucocyte–endothelial interactions and regulation of leucocyte migration. *Lancet* 1994; **343**: 831–6.

BARNES PJ. Inflammatory activities. *Nature* 1991; **349**: 284–5.

BENTLEY AM, JACOBSON MR, CUMBERWORTH V, *et al*. Immunohistology of the nasal mucosa in seasonal allergic rhinitis: increases in activated eosinophils and epithelial mast cells. *J Allergy Clin Immunol* 1992; **89**: 877–83.

BOCHNER BS, SCHLEIMER RP. The role of adhesion molecules in human eosinophil and basophil recruitment. *J Allergy Clin Immunol* 1994; **94**: 427–38.

BROIDE DH, GLEICH GJ, CUOMO AJ, *et al*. Evidence of ongoing mast cell and eosinophil degranulation in symptomatic asthma airways. *J Allergy Clin Immunol* 1991; **88**: 637–48.

CANONICA GW, BUSCAGLIA S, PESCE G, BAGNASCO M. Adhesion molecules in allergic inflammation: recent insights into their functional role. *Allergy* 1994; **49**: 135–41.

GORRIGAN CJ, HACZKU A, GEMOU-ENGESAETH S, *et al*. T-lymphocyte activation in asthma is accompanied by increased serum concentration of interleukin-5. *Am Rev Respir Dis* 1993; **147**: 540–7.

CORRIGAN CJ, KAY AB. T cells and eosinophils in the pathogenesis of asthma. *Immunol Today* 1992; **13**: 501–7.

DEL PRETE G. Human Th1 and Th2 lymphocytes: their role in the pathophysiology of atopy. *Allergy* 1992; **47**: 450–5.

DURHAM SR. Allergic inflammation. *Pediatr Allergy Immunol* 1993; **4**(suppl 4): 7–12.

FREW AJ, O'HEHIR R. What can we learn from studies of lymphocytes present in allergic sites? *J Allergy Clin Immunol* 1992; **89**: 783–8.

GEHA RS. Regulation of IgE synthesis in humans. *J Allergy Clin Immunol* 1992; **90**: 143–50.

GIBSON PG, ALLEN CJ, YANG JP, *et al*. Intraepithelial mast cells in allergic and nonallergic asthma. *Am Rev Respir Dis* 1993; **148**: 80–6.

GLEICH GJ. The eosinophil and bronchial asthma: current understanding. *J Allergy Clin Immunol* 1990; **85**: 422–36.

GORDON JR, BURD PR, GALLI SJ. Mast cells as a source of multifunctional cytokines. *Immunol Today* 1990; **11**: 458–63.

GREWE M, GYUFKO K, SCHÖPF E, KRUTMAN J. Lesional expression of interferon-γ in atopic eczema. *Lancet* 1994; **343**: 25–6.

GUNDEL RH, LETTS LG, GLEICH GJ. Human eosinophil major basic protein induces airway constriction and airway hyperresponsiveness in primates. *J Clin Invest* 1991; **87**: 1470.

HANSEL TT, WALKER C. The migration of eosinophils into the sputum of asthmatics: the role of adhesion molecules. *Clin Exp Allergy* 1992; **22**: 345–56.

HOLGATE ST. Mediator and cytokine mechanisms in asthma. *Thorax* 1993; **48**: 103–9.

HOLGATE ST, CHURCH MK. The mast cells. *Br Med Bull* 1992; **48**: 40–50.

KAMEYOSHI Y, DORSCHNER A, MALLET AI, CHRISTOPHERS E, SCHRODER J-M. Cytokine RANTES released by thrombin stimulated platelets is a potent attractant for human eosinophils. *J Exp Med* 1992; **176**: 587–92.

KAY AB. Asthma and inflammation. *J Allergy Clin Immunol* 1991; **87**: 895–910.

LAITINEN LA, LAITINEN A, HAAHTELA T. A comparative study of the effects of an inhaled corticosteroid, budesonide, and a β$_2$ agonist, terbutaline, on airway inflammation in newly diagnosed asthma: a randomized, double-blind, parallel-group controlled trial. *J Allergy Clin Immunol* 1992; **90**: 32–42.

LEE TH, LANE SJ. The role of macrophages in the mechanisms of airway inflammation in asthma. *Am Rev Respir Dis* 1992; **145**: S27–S30.

LOSEWICZ S, WELLS C, GOMEZ E, *et al*. Morphological integrity of the bronchial epithelium in mild asthmatics. *Thorax* 1990; **45**: 12–15.

LUI MC, BLEEKER ER, LICHTENSTEIN LM, *et al*. Evidence for elevated levels of histamine, prostaglandin D$_2$ and other bronchoconstricting prostaglandins in the airways of subjects with mild asthma. *Am Rev Respir Dis* 1990; **142**: 126–32.

MAGGI E, PARRONCHI P, MANETTI R, *et al*. Reciprocal regulatory effects of IFN-γ and IL-4 on the *in vitro* development of human Th1 and Th2 clones. *J Immunol* 1992; **148**: 2142–7.

MARKERT ML. Molecular biology and allergy: current status and future prospects. *Pediatr Allergy Immunol* 1992; **3**: 49–60.

METZER H. The receptor with high affinity for IgE. *Immunol Rev* 1992; **125**: 37–48.

MONTEFORT S, HERBERT CA, ROBINSON C, HOLGATE ST. The bronchial epithelium as a target for inflammatory attack in asthma. *Clin Exp Allergy* 1992; **22**: 511–20.

MONTEFORT S, HOLGATE ST, HOWARTH PH. Leucocyte–endothelial adhesion molecules and their role in bronchial asthma and allergic rhinitis. *J Respir Cell Mol Biol* 1992; **7**: 393–401.

OHASHI Y, MOTOJIMA S, FUKUDA T, MAKINO S. Airway hyperresponsiveness, increased intracellular spaces of bronchial epithelium, and increased infiltration of eosinophils and lymphocytes in bronchial mucosa in asthma. *Am Rev Respir Dis* 1992; **145**: 1469–76.

O'HEHIR RE, GARMAN RD, GREENSTEIN JL, LAMB JR. The specificity and T cell regulation of responsiveness to allergens. *Ann Rev Immunol* 1991; **9**: 76–95.

RICCI M, ROSSI O, BERTONI M, MATTUCI A. The importance of Th2-like cells in the pathogenesis of airway allergic inflammation. *Clin Exp Allergy* 1993; **23**: 360–9.

ROBINSON DS. Interleukin-5, eosinophils and bronchial hyperreactivity. *Clin Exp Allergy* 1993; **23**: 1–3.

ROBINSON DS, DURHAM SR, KAY AB. Cytokines in asthma. *Thorax* 1993; **48**: 845–53.

ROBINSON D, HAMID Q, BENTLEY A, *et al*. Activation of CD4+ T cells, increased Th2-type cytokine mRNA expression, and eosinophil recruitment in bronchoalveolar lavage after allergen challenge in patients with atopic asthma. *J Allergy Clin Immunol* 1993; **92**: 313–24.

RODGERS JR, RICH RR. Molecular biology and immunology: an introduction. *J Allergy Clin Immunol* 1991; **88**: 535–51.

ROMAGNANI S. Human Th1 and Th2 subsets: doubt no more. *Immunol Today* 1991; **12**: 256–7.

ROMAGNANI S. Induction of Th1 and Th2 responses: a key role for the 'natural' immune response? *Immunol Today* 1992; **13**: 379–81.

SCOTT P. IL-12: initiation cytokine for cell-mediated immunity. *Science* 1993; **260**: 496–7.

SPRINGER TA. Adhesion receptors of the immune system. *Nature* 1990; **346**: 425–34.

VENGE P. The eosinophil granulocyte in allergic inflammation. *Allergy* 1993; **4**(suppl 4): 19–24.

WALKER C, VIRCHOW J-C, BRUIJNZEEL PLB, BLASER K. T cell subsets and their soluble products regulate eosinophilia in allergic and non-allergic asthma. *J Immunol* 1991; **146**: 1829–35.

WEGNER CD, GUNDEL RH, REILLY P, *et al*. Intercellular adhesion molecule-1 (ICAM-1) in the pathogenesis of asthma. *Science* 1990; **247**: 456–9.

WELLER PF. Immunobiology of eosinophils. *N Engl J Med* 1991; **324**: 1110–16.

ZIMMERMAN GA, PRESCOTT SM, McINTYRE T. Endothelial interactions with granulocytes: tethering and signalling molecules. *Immunol Today* 1992; **13**: 93–100.

Part 2 Diseases and Epidemiology

2.1 Atopic diseases
Atopic dermatitis, allergic rhinitis and asthma

Key points
- Atopy refers to an inherited predisposition to produce IgE antibody.
- Atopic subjects respond with persistent production of IgE antibody on exposure to minute amounts of inhaled allergen.
- The atopic status of a person can be determined by skin testing with a battery of common aero-allergens.
- The most important atopic diseases are atopic dermatitis, allergic rhinitis and asthma.
- Allergic rhinitis and asthma are IgE-mediated atopic, allergic diseases.
- Atopic dermatitis is an IgE-associated atopic disease, for symptoms are not, or only to a minor degree, caused by allergen exposure.
- Highly atopic patients develop atopic dermatitis, allergic rhinitis and asthma, and easily become sensitized to new allergens.
- People with a low degree of atopy merely develop hay fever, and this is by far the most frequent.

Definitions
Atopy refers to a hereditary predisposition to produce IgE antibody. When *atopic subjects* are exposed to the minute amounts of allergen in ambient air, they respond with a persistent production of IgE antibody. The *atopic status* of a person can be determined by skin testing with a battery of common aero-allergens (e.g. mite, cat and pollen). The most important *atopic diseases* are atopic dermatitis, allergic rhinitis and asthma.

While allergic rhinitis and asthma are *IgE-mediated* diseases, atopic dermatitis is, in most cases, merely *IgE-associated*. In other words, allergic rhinitis and asthma are *atopic and allergic diseases* in which symptoms are the result of allergen exposure, while atopic dermatitis is an *atopic disease but not an allergic disease*, for symptoms are not, or only to a minor degree, caused by allergen exposure. It is confusing that an atopic disease can be both allergic and non-allergic. When atopic dermatitis is called 'allergic' by laymen the results are many futile attempts to find the offending allergenic substance.

A patient with a high degree of atopy
The patient has parents with atopic disease. Atopic dermatitis starts within the first year of life and may be aggravated by food allergy. After some bouts of 'wheezy bronchitis' the patient develops attacks of asthma not preceded by infection. The asthma becomes chronic and is accompanied by allergic rhinitis and multiple positive skin tests.

In adolescence, the eczema may improve, but the skin is still dry and vulnerable. The asthma usually continues and drugs are needed on a daily basis.

This patient has a high atopic status; he or she is an 'allergy machine' who easily becomes sensitized upon exposure to new potent allergens. Allergy, disease and medication constitute a life-long burden.

A patient with a low degree of atopy
A typical example is a young man of non-atopic parents, who develops a positive skin test to grass pollen and suffers from rhino-conjunctivitis in the pollen season. Treatment is easy and the symptoms improve in middle age.

This patient has a low atopic status. His risk of further sensitization and the development of other atopic manifestations is only slightly increased. Fortunately, this example is by far the most frequent.

A specialist in allergy
An expert is one who knows more and more about less and less.

Nicholas M Butler

2.2 Non-atopic diseases
Urticaria, nasal polyps and non-allergic asthma

Key points
- Atopic allergy is the cause of perennial rhinitis and asthma in 90% of children and 30% of adults.
- Chronic urticaria and nasal polyposis are, as a rule, non-allergic.
- Intolerance to acetylsalicylic acid can cause profuse rhinorrhoea, violent asthma, urticaria, angioedema, shock and death.
- It is a non-immunological reaction to all cyclo-oxygenase inhibitors, that is, acetylsalicylic acid and other non-steroidal, anti-inflammatory drugs (NSAIDs).
- The so-called ASA triad consists of intolerance to *Acetylsalicylic* acid, nasal polyps/hyperplastic *Sinusitis* and non-allergic *Asthma*.
- Acetylsalicylic acid and NSAIDs act as inhibitors of cyclo-oxygenase and block the formation of prostaglandins.
- NSAID intolerance occurs in about 20% of adults with rhinitis, nasal polyps and non-allergic asthma.
- It usually develops in middle-aged patients.
- Patients with non-allergic rhinitis often develop nasal polyps and hyperplastic sinusitis.
- Nasal symptoms usually precede bronchial asthma, which may again precede manifest intolerance to NSAIDs.
- While acute urticaria is usually allergic, chronic urticaria is non-allergic.
- The diagnosis of NSAID intolerance is based on the history and oral provocation testing.
- A provocation test with acetylsalicylic acid, which is potentially dangerous, is performed as a titration, starting with a low dose.
- In patients with NSAID intolerance, avoidance must be strict and life-long.

Allergic and allergy-like disease
In childhood, 90% of patients suffering from rhinitis and asthma are allergic, as compared with only 30% in adults. Thus, many patients with diseases discussed in this book are not allergic. The diseases are 'allergy-like', as their histopathology and clinical presentation are similar to that of atopic allergic diseases, but the aetiology is unknown.

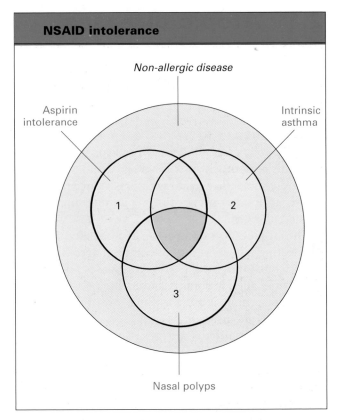

Fig. 2.2.1. The ASA triad only accounts for a minor part of the non-allergic asthma/rhinitis cases, but it has a central position in the comprehension of this entity.

The ASA triad
Sensitivity to acetylsalicylic acid is more frequent in 'allergy-like' than in allergic disease. Typically, it is part of the so-called ASA triad which consists of: 1, *intolerance to Acetylsalicylic acid*; 2, *nasal polyps/hyperplastic Sinusitis*; and 3, *non-allergic Asthma* (intrinsic or idiopathic asthma). Only a minority of patients with 'allergy-like' disease have the ASA triad fully expressed; each of the components can occur alone or in combinations (Fig. 2.2.1).

Intolerance to acetylsalicylic acid – Aspirin intolerance
Acetylsalicylic acid was first marketed in 1899 as Aspirin. A few years after its introduction, angioedema and generalized urticaria were reported as adverse reactions. Soon, added to the list, were profuse rhinorrhoea, violent asthma, shock and death.

The term intolerance is used instead of allergy, as the adverse effect is *not based on an immune reaction*. Aspirin-intolerant patients invariably react to

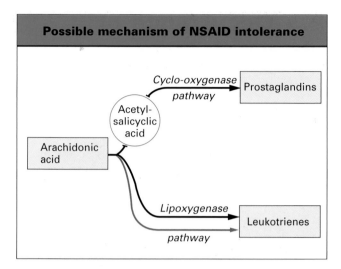

Fig. 2.2.2. Acetylsalicylic acid inhibition of the cyclo-oxygenase pathway may increase the formation of lipoxygenase products. This mechanism is possibly responsible for NSAID-induced symptoms.

indomethacin and other non-steroidal, anti-inflammatory drugs (NSAIDs), which are chemically different. It follows that the term, *NSAID intolerance* is more correct than Aspirin intolerance, which, however, is widely used.

Pathogenesis

Arachidonic acid is generated in the cell membrane by immunological and non-immunological stimuli (see Chapter 1.8). Its metabolism to prostaglandins is blocked by acetylsalicylic acid and NSAIDs, which act by *inhibiting the enzyme, cyclo-oxygenase*. In theory, more arachidonic acid is then available for the synthesis of lipoxygenase products, the leukotrienes and thromboxanes. It is possible, but not proven, that an increased quantity of these inflammatory substances accounts for the adverse reaction to acetylsalicylic acid (Fig. 2.2.2).

Dyes and preservatives

A few NSAID-intolerant people also react to the ingestion of *tartrazine* and other dyes and preservatives (see Chapter 5.2).

Prevalence

The prevalence of NSAID intolerance appears to be 2–4% among patients visiting an allergic clinic, but it varies considerably between subgroups. About 20% of all adults with rhinitis, nasal polyps and non-allergic asthma are NSAID intolerant. The highest prevalence rate is found among patients with severe disease.

Age

NSAID intolerance is rare in children and the full expression of the ASA triad usually develops in *middle-aged patients*.

Non-allergic rhinitis, nasal polyps and hyperplastic sinusitis

Typically, the nasal symptoms initially present as non-allergic or vasomotor rhinitis with intermittent, profuse nasal hypersecretion. The rhinorrhoea is followed, after some years, by chronic blockage that is increasingly less responsive to vasoconstrictors. The sense of smell disappears and nasal polyps are seen at rhinoscopy. The mucous membrane of the paranasal sinuses is hyperplastic and the sinus X-ray abnormal.

Non-allergic asthma

Nasal symptoms usually precede bronchial asthma, which may again precede manifest intolerance to NSAID. Non-allergic asthma often becomes chronic severe and *requires corticosteroid therapy*.

Chronic urticaria and angioedema

While acute urticaria is usually allergic, the reverse is the case with chronic disease. Urticaria and/or angioedema may be the only manifestation of NSAID intolerance or it may occur in association with rhinitis/polyps/sinusitis and asthma. Urticaria can initially present only after ingestion of a NSAID, but often persists even after the drug is discontinued. Laryngeal oedema following ingestion of NSAIDs can be a threat to life.

Diagnosis

History

A correct diagnosis is important as exposure can have serious consequences. The diagnosis of intolerance is based on the history and oral provocation testing as there is no reliable laboratory test.

Provocation test

Challenge with acetylsalicylic acid is a *potentially dangerous procedure*, and it should only be carried out in hospital with the patient under close observation. The patient must be symptom-free or at least in a stable phase. The provocation is performed as a titration, starting with a low dose (1–10 mg). A provocation test should not be performed in a patient with a clear-cut positive history.

Management

Avoidance must be strict and life-long. NSAID-intolerant patients are warned not to take any preparations containing acetylsalicylic acid, indomethacin or other cyclo-oxygenase inhibitors. Most patients tolerate salicylic acid and paracetamol. Steroids and morphine are the only anti-inflammatory and analgesic drugs that are completely safe in patients who have had a life-threatening reaction to acetylsalicylic acid.

Avoidance of acetylsalicylic acid and NSAIDs will not improve the basic disease. Neither will a diet without dyes and preservatives cure the patient, but some exacerbations may be avoided in a few patients.

The goal for writing
Everything should be made as simple as possible, but not one bit simpler.

Albert Einstein

2.3 Occurrence of atopic diseases
– and natural history

Key points
• A positive skin test to aero-allergens occurs in 20–30% of the total population.
• About 15–20% of the population develop an atopic disease.
• The prevalence rate is highest between 15 and 30 years of age.
• The accumulative prevalence rate of atopic dermatitis is 10–15%.
• The debut of atopic dermatitis is early: 50% within the first year and 90% by 3 years.
• The symptoms usually improve and often disappear (80%) during childhood, but they relapse in 10–20%.
• The symptoms usually improve (90%) and often disappear (50%) in adolescence.
• Children with atopic dermatitis usually develop asthma or allergic rhinitis (60–70%).
• Allergic rhinitis is a frequent disease but the usually reported figures of 10–20% include mild cases.
• In most countries, pollens are the main cause of allergic rhinitis.
• Hay fever usually develops in childhood or adolescence, and the symptoms invariably improve in middle age.
• The prevalence rate of asthma is 5–10% and it is the most common chronic disease in children in the western world.
• Allergy to aero-allergens is an important predisposing factor for the development of asthma in childhood.
• While 90% of children with asthma are allergic, this is the case in only 30% of those with adult-onset asthma.
• Asthma improves in adolescence in 50% of the cases, predominantly the mild ones, but it returns in 30%.
• In severe chronic asthma, irreversible airway obstruction may develop.

Reported prevalence rates of atopic dermatitis, allergic rhinitis and asthma *vary considerably*, which may be explained, in part, by differences in the selection of a study population, criteria used for diagnosis

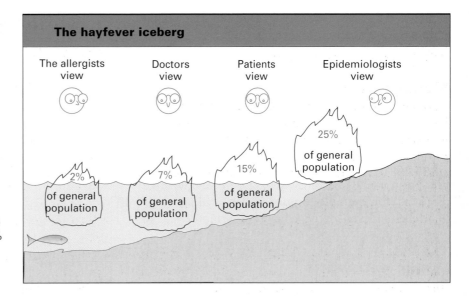

Fig. 2.3.1. The problem of defining allergic rhinitis is illustrated in a study of medical students. While 25% had a positive skin test to pollen, 15% suffered from rhinitis symptoms, 7% received pharmacotherapy, and 2% were treated with immunotherapy.

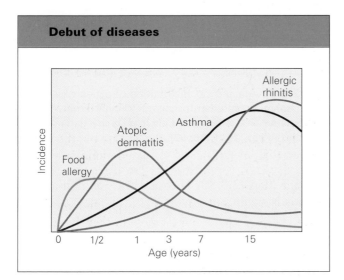

Fig. 2.3.2. Approximate incidence (first appearance of symptoms) of various atopic diseases in relation to age.

and definition of the disease. It can be difficult to make an unequivocal diagnosis, and, in all cases, to make a clear distinction between, for example, asthma and chronic obstructive bronchitis (see Chapter 9.13). The manifestation of a disease can range from minimal to severe symptoms and a reported prevalence rate depends upon an arbitrary distinction made between a normal and a diseased state as, for example, in allergic rhinitis (Fig. 2.3.1).

Reported prevalence figures also depend upon whether accumulated or point prevalence rates are given, as spontaneous cure can occur. The age of the population studied is of importance as the various diseases characteristically start at different ages (Fig. 2.3.2).

Positive skin test

A *positive skin test* to aero-allergens occurs in *20–30%* of the total population (Table 2.3.1). Thus, atopy with the original meaning 'strange or unusual' is usual, and it is curious that 75% of a population never become sensitized.

Some skin test positive subjects never get symptoms, others only have insignificant symptoms and about *15–20%* of the total population will develop an *atopic disease* (mild cases included). The highest prevalence rate is reached at *15–30 years of age*. While a positive skin test strongly correlates with the

Prevalence of disease	
Positive skin test	20–30%
Atopic dermatitis	10–15%
Urticaria	10–20%*
Allergic rhinitis	10–20%
Non-allergic rhinitis	2–4%
Asthma	5–10%

Table 2.3.1. Accumulated prevalence rates for atopic allergic diseases and non-allergic allergy-like diseases. Estimates based on recent publications from industrialized western countries. *Single episodes included

occurrence of atopic disease in children and young adults, the association weakens beyond the age of 35 years.

A positive skin test is an indicator of *predisposition to further sensitization*. A single positive test implies a low risk and multiple positive tests imply a high risk. A pollen-allergic subject more often becomes sensitized to other pollens than to animal protein and vice versa.

Once developed, a positive skin test *does not disappear* but it usually becomes weaker with age. Positive reactions, for example to grass pollen, will continue to be elicited, even after the hay fever symptoms have ceased.

Atopic dermatitis

The reported accumulative prevalence rates (have and have had) vary with *10–15%* as a reasonable average figure. The *debut is early*: 50% of the cases have developed before the age of 1 year and 90% before the age of 3 years. The more serious the severity, the earlier the start.

The symptoms *usually improve* and *often disappear* (80%) in adolescence. Predictive for a chronic course, persisting into adult life, are in order of importance: 1, widespread severe eczema; 2, associated allergic rhinitis/asthma; 3, a family history of atopic dermatitis; and 4, early start of the symptoms.

Even patients who have complete clinical remission in childhood or adolescence have a considerably increased risk of later development of hand eczema (see Chapter 6.4).

Children who develop atopic dermatitis usually have a family history of atopic disease (60–70%). As many as 60–70% of these children will develop asthma (20–40%) or allergic rhinitis (50–60%), often delayed by some years.

Allergic rhinitis

Allergic rhinitis is a frequent disease but the usually reported figures of *15–20%* includes mild cases not seen by a doctor (Fig. 2.3.1). In most countries, pollens are the main cause of allergic rhinitis. Non-allergic rhinitis is less frequent, affecting about 2–4%, but the figures are uncertain due to poor diagnostic criteria. The frequency of nasal polyps may be 1% or less.

Hay fever usually develops in childhood or adolescence, the symptoms remain stationary for 2–3 decades, after which they will invariably *improve considerably* in middle age and almost disappear in

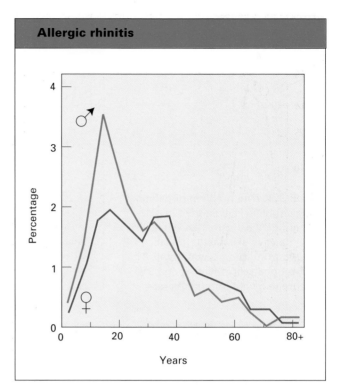

Fig. 2.3.3. Age and sex distribution of patients visiting their general practitioner for allergic rhinitis. From Weeke ER, Pedersen PA. Allergic rhinitis in a Danish general practice. *Allergy* 1981; **36**: 375–9.

old age (Fig. 2.3.3). The outcome of non-allergic rhinitis is significantly worse.

Asthma

The prevalence rates of asthma reported from western Europe and the USA are *5–10%*. This makes asthma the most common chronic disease in children in the western world.

Allergy to aero-allergens is an important predisposing factor for the development of asthma, but only in childhood. While 90% of children with asthma are allergic, this is the case in only 30% of those with adult-onset asthma.

It was formerly believed that childhood asthma was a self-limiting disorder, which would improve spontaneously in adolescence. This seems to be an over-simplification, which only applies to children with mild, episodic symptoms. Overall, asthma *improves in adolescence* in 50% of the cases, but it *often returns* (in 30%), and allergy is then of less importance. The age-related curve for asthma occurrence is biphasic (Fig. 2.3.4), in distinction from that of allergic rhinitis. The reason for this later recurrence of

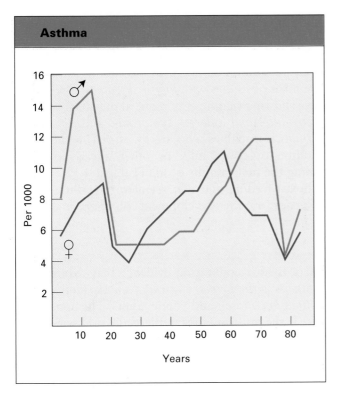

Asthma

Fig. 2.3.4. Age and sex distribution of patients visiting their general practitioner for asthma. From Weeke ER, Pedersen PA. Allergic rhinitis in a Danish general practice. *Allergy* 1981; **36**: 375–9.

the bronchial, in contrast to the nasal, symptoms is unknown.

In some cases of severe chronic asthma, *irreversible airway obstruction develops* and the prognosis is dubious due to steadily decreasing lung function.

The problem of prognosis
Prediction is difficult – especially about the future.
Robert Storm Petersen

2.4 Development of atopic diseases
Predisposing factors

Key points
- The development of atopic allergic disease depends on genetic predisposition, allergen exposure and, possibly, adjuvant factors.
- A child inherits a predisposition for atopic disease in general, for involvement of certain organs and for the severity of the disease.
- The risk for the child is doubled when one parent is atopic and quadrupled when both are atopic.
- There is a male predominance of atopic diseases in childhood, which disappears with age.
- Early exposure of high-risk babies to cow's milk increases the risk of gastro-intestinal symptoms and atopic dermatitis.
- Children exposed to high levels of mite antigen have a five- to 10-fold increased risk of asthma.
- Patients born in the months immediately before a pollen season have an increased risk of developing pollen allergy.
- Adjuvants (e.g. air pollution) are believed to facilitate the sensitization process, but their role remains speculative.
- Parenteral smoking is an important factor in the occurrence of wheezing in infants and children.
- The hypothesis that diesel exhaust increases the frequency of hay fever is poorly supported.
- The role of early infection with respiratory syncytial virus in the development of asthma remains unsettled.
- There is a slightly higher prevalence of atopic diseases in urban than in rural areas.
- Western style of living is associated with a high prevalence of atopic disease.

Simplified, the development of atopic allergic disease depends upon: 1, the *genetic predisposition*; 2, *exposure to allergens* in food and air; and, possibly, 3, exposure to *adjuvants*, which may facilitate the sensitization process. The role of adjuvants, however, remains speculative, and their nature and mode of action are badly defined.

Genetic factors
The importance of genetic factors can be exemplified

by a reported concordance rate for atopic dermatitis of 86% in monozygotic and only 21% in dizygotic twins. The mode of inheritance is probably polygenic and complex. It is far from being elucidated, although a group in Oxford recently has incriminated a gene on the long arm of chromosome 11.

A child inherits a predisposition for: 1, *atopic disease in general*; 2, involvement of *certain organs*; and 3, *severity* of the disease. A child of parents with severe eczema and asthma is therefore at greater risk than a child of parents with simple hay fever.

The child's risk of developing an atopic disease is increased by a factor of two if one of the parents is atopic and by a factor of four if both parents have an atopic disease.

Sex

Studies of the prevalence of asthma and hay fever in children have usually shown a *male predominance*, which *disappears with age* (see Figs 2.3.3–4).

Exposure to food allergens

There is increasing evidence that an early introduction of potential allergens in infant feeding is associated with an increased risk of atopic disease. This may not be surprising, as mother's milk is the natural food for babies and cow's milk for cattle.

The risk of early introduction of cow's milk and other potential food allergens has been illustrated by a number of studies with *high-risk babies*. The results have shown a significantly reduced prevalence rate of *gastro-intestinal allergy symptoms* and of *atopic dermatitis* in babies who are *breast-fed*, without the addition of cow's milk or other allergenic foods during the first months of life (Table 2.4.1).

Breast-feeding and diet seem to have little or no influence on the development of *allergic airways disease*.

Exposure to aero-allergens

There is now convincing evidence that exposure to allergens is *the primary cause of the development of asthma in children* and young adults. The house dust mite is the most important allergen world wide, and, for example, in the UK, 80% of asthmatic children are sensitized to mites.

There is a *clear dose–response relationship* between the prevalence of sensitization to mites and the degree of exposure during infancy. Children, who have been exposed to high levels of mite antigen (>100 mites or 10 µg *Dermatophagoides pteronyssinus* I/g dust) have *a five- to 10-fold increased risk* of mite sensitization and asthma. To put this risk in perspective the risk of developing lung cancer is increased by a factor of 10–20 in cigarette smokers.

When house dust mite exposure is the dominant cause of asthma, one can expect a higher prevalence of the disease in areas of high mite exposure. Indeed, the prevalence of asthma is higher in children born in Marseille, at sea level, than in Briacon in the French Alps (high altitude, dry air and therefore no mites). There are also significant differences in adult asthma in these two locations (2.4% compared to 4.1%).

Another example is reported from Papua New Guinea, where changed sleeping habits with the introduction of blankets, which became heavily infested with mites, was followed by a dramatic increase in the prevalence of asthma (by a factor of 40).

Interestingly, there is a good correlation not only between a child's exposure to mites and its risk of developing asthma but also *atopic dermatitis*.

An increasing number of studies suggest that allergens, derived from cats, cockroaches and fungi, are

Preventive programme and disease			
	With preventive programme	**Without programme**	***p* value**
Atopic dermatitis	14%	31%	<0.01
Vomiting/ diarrhoea	5%	20%	<0.01
Colic	9%	24%	<0.01
Cow's milk allergy	5%	20%	<0.01

Table 2.4.1. Occurrence of atopic dermatitis and food allergy at age 18 months in high-risk infants with and without preventive programme, consisting of breast-feeding and/or hypoallergenic formula combined with avoidance of solid foods during the first 6 months of life. From Halken S, Høst A, Hansen LG, Østerballe O. Effect of an allergy prevention programme on incidence of atopic symptoms in infancy. *Allergy* 1992; **47**: 545–53

capable of increasing the prevalence of allergy and asthma, although their overall importance is secondary to that of mites.

The therapeutic implications of these studies are that *allergen avoidance regimens could prevent the onset of asthma* in a considerable number of susceptible infants.

Month of birth

The first few months of life, when the immune system is immature, appear to be a vulnerable period with increased risk of sensitization in both the gastrointestinal tract and the airways. Evidence for the latter is nicely presented by a number of studies that relate month of birth and subsequent sensitization to pollen. Patients born in the months immediately before a pollen season have twice the risk of developing pollen allergy compared with their friends born immediately after the season. As the symptoms of hay fever usually do not develop until an age of 5–15 years, it is theoretically interesting that stimulation of the immune system during the first months of life apparently can influence the development of a disease years later.

Adjuvants

Epidemiological studies have shown a positive correlation between the occurrence of wheezy illness in children, and parental smoking, indoor gas heating and outdoor air pollution. While these factors may induce wheezing in asthmatics, it is dubious, however, whether they can facilitate the sensitization process.

Parenteral smoking

Evidence that this is an important factor for the occurrence of wheezing in infants and children is provided by a series of studies. In, for example, a study from Boston of unselected children aged 5–9 years, persistent wheeze occurred in 1.9% of children from households where neither parents smoked, 6.9% of children from households with one parent currently smoking and 11.8% of children from households in which both parents were currently smoking.

Air pollution

While it is easy to demonstrate the association between passive cigarette smoking and respiratory illness in infancy, it is less easy to define the contribution of other air pollutants to the morbidity of atopic disease.

Pollinosis and air pollution	
Exposure to pollen and air pollution	**Prevalence of pollinosis**
Along roads lined with cedar trees	13.2%
Area with less cedar trees but heavy traffic	9.6%
Cedar forest with little traffic	5.1%
Area with few cedar trees and little traffic	1.7%

Table 2.4.2. Prevalence of Japanese cedar pollinosis in the Nikko area. From Miyamoto T. Increased prevalence of pollen allergy in Japan. In: Godard P, Bousquet J, Michel FB, eds. *Advances in Allergology and Clinical Immunology* Carnforth: The Panthenon Publishing Group, 1992: 343–7

There is circumstantial evidence from laboratory experiments and from epidemiological studies to indicate that air pollution, in particular diesel exhaust, may be associated with an increase in sensitization to aero-allergens. Special support comes from a study in Japan, where a higher frequency of cedar pollinosis was reported in areas with heavy traffic than in those with light traffic (Table 2.4.2). However, exact measurements of air pollution and of pollen counts were lacking in that study.

An excellent epidemiological study from Germany has failed to show a positive correlation between air pollution, as such, and occurrence of atopic diseases. In a comparison between Leipzig (in the former East Germany) and Munich (in the former West Germany), there was a significantly greater prevalence of hay fever in Munich, in spite of a much higher degree of pollution in Leipzig (Table 2.4.3).

Early airway infection

Gastro-intestinal infections increase the frequency of cow's milk protein intolerance in early childhood. The relationship between respiratory infections and the development of respiratory allergy is less clear. There is some dispute as to whether respiratory syncytial virus infections in infancy merely increase respiratory symptoms or contribute to the actual development of allergy. Indeed, the former is more likely to be the case.

Air pollution and disease			
	Leipzig	Munich	*p* value
Sulphur dioxide (μg/m³)	203.8	10.7	
Particulate matters (μg/m³)	133.5	51.1	
Asthma	7.3	9.3	NS
Bronchitis	30.9	15.9	<0.01
Hay fever	2.4	8.6	<0.01
Atopic dermatitis	13.0	13.9	NS

Table 2.4.3. Prevalence of respiratory and allergic disorders among 9- to 11-year-old children in two German cities with different levels of air pollution. From von Mutius E, Fritzsch C, Weiland SK, Röll G, Magnussen H. Prevalence of asthma and allergic disorders among children in united Germany: a descriptive comparison. *Br Med J* 1992; **305**: 1395–9

Allergy in city and countryside		
	Allergic rhinitis	**Asthma**
Countryside	6.5%	2.5%
Town	8.5%	2.7%
Stockholm	10.1%	3.3%

Table 2.4.4. Prevalence of allergic rhinitis and asthma in rural and urban areas in Sweden. From Åberg N. Asthma and allergic rhinitis in Swedish conscripts. *Clin Exp Allergy* 1989; **19**: 59–63

Rural and urban areas

A series of epidemiological studies have shown a higher prevalence of childhood asthma, allergic rhinitis and atopic dermatitis in urban than in rural areas, with a ratio of about 2:1 (Table 2.4.4). It is a common, but poorly substantiated, belief that the influence of air pollution, acting as 'adjuvant', is the explanation of this finding.

Western style of living

The prevalence of atopic disease apparently increases when people move to industrialized countries, chang-ing from native to a western lifestyle and living conditions. A well-known example is West Indians who move to Britain. A more recent and striking example is from Polynesia, where the prevalence of atopic dermatitis and allergic rhinitis in Tokelauan islanders were found to be 0.1% and 13.7% compared with 8.5% and 28.3% in their peers who had moved to New Zealand.

> **Modern allergy prevention**
> Some million years of practical experience and about 70 years of medical research have made it probable that mother's milk is suitable food for babies.
> Mikael Rode

2.5 Increasing prevalence of atopic diseases
The cause is unknown

Key points
- The prevalence of atopic dermatitis, allergic rhinitis and asthma has increased in western countries since World War II.
- There are a number of possible causes but none are satisfactory.
- Increased awareness of allergic diseases may be part of the explanation.
- Reduced breast-feeding in modern society may explain some of the increase in atopic dermatitis.
- In Northern Europe, new energy-saving homes with little ventilation and high humidity have caused an increased number of mites and allergies.
- In Japan, the number of cedar trees and the prevalence of cedar pollen allergy have increased considerably since World War II.
- Otherwise, the quantity of aero-allergens has not increased in general.
- The evidence of a role for air pollution as an adjuvant in allergic sensitization is merely circumstantial.
- Infections may, by the production of IL-12 and IFNγ, inhibit Th2 cell activation, synthesis of IgE and development of allergy.

Evidence
Epidemiological studies in many western countries have consistently shown increasing prevalence rates of atopic dermatitis, allergic rhinitis and asthma since World War II.

A study from Great Britain reported an increase of the cumulative prevalence of *atopic dermatitis* from 5.1% for children born in 1946, to 12.2% in children born in 1970, and similar results were obtained in Denmark (Fig. 2.5.1).

While John Bostock, in 1819, was able to find 28 cases of *hay fever* in all England, a similar number of patients are now seen by a single general practitioner. More scientific evidence for the increase in allergic rhinitis is available (Table 2.5.1).

In the USA, the prevalence of *asthma* among 6- to 11-year-old children increased from 4.8 to 7.6% between the first (1971–74) and second (1976–80) National Health Survey.

Possible causes
Although an *increased awareness* of allergic diseases may have had some influence on studies based on patient questionnaires, the reported increase in prevalence rates, as for example shown by skin testing, cannot exclusively be explained on this basis.

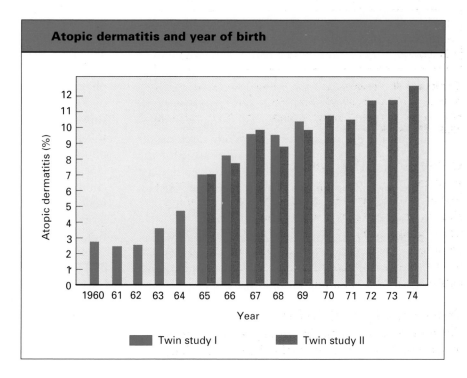

Fig. 2.5.1. The cumulative incidence rates for atopic dermatitis in children (0–7 years) according to year of birth. From Schultz Larsen F, Hanifin JM. Secular change in the occurrence of atopic dermatitis. *Acta Derm Venereol (Stockh)* 1992; (suppl 176): 7–12.

Increasing prevalence of disease			
	1971	1981	*p* value
Allergic rhinitis	4.4%	8.4%	<0.01
Asthma	1.9%	2.8%	<0.01

Table 2.5.1. Prevalence of allergic rhinitis and asthma in 112 000 Swedish conscripts. From Åberg N. Asthma and allergic rhinitis in Swedish conscripts. *Clin Exp Allergy* 1989; **19**: 59–63

Change in genetic factors cannot occur over a few decades so the explanation of the increase in atopic disease must therefore be sought in *environmental factors*.

The reduced practice of *breast-feeding* in modern society and early introduction of cow's milk may explain some of the increase seen in atopic dermatitis.

There is no indication that the quantity of *aeroallergens* has increased in general. In certain microenvironments, however, an *increased mite exposure* may be associated with an increased frequency of allergic rhinitis and asthma. As mentioned, this can occur when native people change their sleeping habits by the use of blankets. In Scandinavian countries, mite allergy has increased as buildings have become better insulated with less air changes, higher humidity and, consequently, greater mite infestation.

In a few areas, the increased prevalence of allergic rhinitis can be explained by an increase of airborne *pollens*, as, for example, in Japan, where the number of cedar trees has increased considerably since World War II.

While *air pollution* undoubtedly contributes to asthma morbidity, the evidence of a role for 'adjuvants' in allergic sensitization is merely circumstantial. We have to admit that the main reason for the increasing prevalence of atopic disease over the last decades remains *unknown*. This is highly unsatisfactory and needs to be addressed.

A sign of health?

A dietary compromised population frequently develops chronic recurrent infections, which easily become invasive, for example mastoiditis following acute otitis media. Allergic diseases, on the other hand, are rare.

An affluent western population, getting adequate food, proteins, vitamins and minerals, has a low fre-

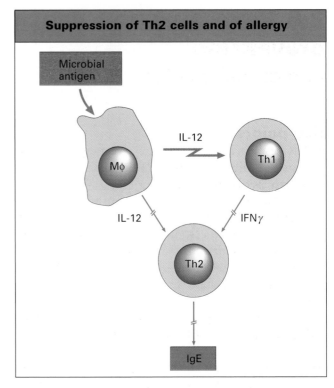

Fig. 2.5.2. Possible explanation of a Yin–Yang relationship between chronic recurrent infection and atopic allergy. Microbial stimulation of macrophages and development of Th1 clones may suppress Th2 cells by IL-12 and IFNγ production.

quency of severe invasive infections, but the prevalence of atopic diseases is high.

A possible theoretical explanation of this apparent Yin–Yang relationship between infection and allergy has emerged. Microbial antigens stimulate macrophages to release IL-12, which induces the expansion of Th1 cell clones. Th2 cells, and IgE synthesis, are suppressed by macrophage-produced IL-12 and by IFNγ produced by Th1 cells (Fig. 2.5.2). If this hypothesis is correct, then the two green strings of purulent secretion, obligatory beneath the noses of children living under poor socioeconomic conditions, may yield protection against the development of allergy. If allergy is a sign of wealth and health, prevention will be difficult.

> Increasing prevalence of allergists
> It is not the number of diseases and patients that has grown, but the number of doctors able to study the diseases.
>
> Anton Chekhov

2.6 Prediction and prevention
In high-risk babies

Key points
- Advice of prevention programmes is given to the parents of a high-risk baby (fetus).
- A high-risk baby has both parents with atopic disease or one with severe disease.
- A prevention programme consists of breast-feeding, and avoidance of food allergens, aero-allergens and passive smoking (Table 2.6.1).
- Smoking parents are told that their habit will double the risk of development of a wheezy illness in their child.
- Even the best avoidance programme can only reduce and not eliminate the risk of atopic disease.

Atopic diseases are chronic disorders with a high morbidity and their prevalence is increasing. As environmental factors have a major impact on the development, manifestation and severity of atopic diseases, their prevention may be possible by environmental control. This could have far greater impact on the disease than conventional approaches to treatment.

Prevention programmes consist of combined avoidance of food and aero-allergens as described below. Changing exposure to air pollution and respiratory viruses is a difficult practice and the effect is uncertain. Similarly, advice about the month of birth is not given.

Identify high-risk babies
Allergen avoidance trials and dietary intervention have only shown convincing results in high-risk infants. Stringent prevention programmes, which are expensive and easily cause significant disturbances in family life, are only advised in selected high-risk babies, comprising about 5% of all newborns.

In investigational studies, an elevated level of cord blood IgE has shown a positive correlation to the later development of atopic disease, but the precision of this test is too poor for it to be useful in clinical medicine.

In daily routine, the identification of high-risk babies is based exclusively on the family history, that is, *both parents with atopic disease* or *one with severe manifestations*.

Time period for intervention
As described in Chapter 2.3, the first months of life are most important for allergic sensitization, and prevention programmes are usually advised for at least 4–6 months.

Table 2.6.1. Prevention programme recommended for high-risk babies

Prevention in high-risk babies
Breast-feeding, at least for 4–6 months, but preferably as long as possible
Avoidance of cow's milk in the maternity unit before breast-feeding is started ('the hidden bottle')
Hypo-allergenic formula as a substitute for breast-feeding when this is needed for nutrition during the first 4–6 months
Complete avoidance of cow's milk during the first 4–6 months
Late and step-wise introduction of solid food
Preferably, avoid highly allergenic food in the first year (fish, nuts, chocolate, citrus fruits, tomatoes and strawberries)
No smoking in the home
No furred pets in the home
Mite avoidance programme in the child's bedroom before birth

Preventive diet

Mother's diet

Maternal avoidance of potent food allergens during pregnancy has no proven effect on the development of diseases in the child and it is not recommended.

Protein molecules in the food can be absorbed unchanged, reach the baby with the milk and cause sensitization, but the risk is very small. It is difficult for lactating mothers to diet for there is a risk of malnutrition of the mother and reduced nutrition and weight gain in the baby. Therefore, maternal dieting during lactation *cannot be recommended* as a preventive measure.

Strict breast-feeding

Studies have shown that breast-feeding provides protection against the development of atopic dermatitis and food allergy (Table 2.3.2), although it is not clear whether it prevents disease or merely delays the onset of problems.

Strict breast-feeding for 4–6 months and delayed introduction of solid food is recommended for high-risk babies (Table 2.4.1). When necessary, breast milk can be supplemented by a hypo-allergenic formula, which, however, is expensive, and it can be difficult strictly to follow this programme for practical and economical reasons. Single administrations of cow's milk given to crying babies, by maternity personnel or grandmothers, must be discouraged. Considerable support for the mother at this time is mandatory.

Avoidance of aero-allergens

The intervention programme is best started before the child is born. In arranging the bedroom, all effort should be made to render it as clean and 'mite-hostile' as possible (see Chapter 3.4). As mentioned earlier, a heavily mite-infested bedroom increases the risk of asthma with a factor similar to the one with which cigarette smoking increases the risk for lung cancer.

Furred pets should not be in the home; they should be removed months before birth as allergen can remain in the furniture for prolonged periods.

Avoidance of smoking

There should be no exposure to tobacco smoke in the home both ante-natally and post-natally. Smoking parents should be told that their habit will more than double the risk of development of a wheezy illness in their child.

Information to parents

Parents with a high-risk baby are usually motivated to intervention programmes. They will become very disappointed when the infant, in spite of their effort, develops an atopic disease. It is therefore prudent to inform them beforehand that even the best programme can only reduce but not eliminate the risk.

Prevention preferable
An ounce of prevention is worth a pound of cure.
Old English proverb

Further reading

ARSHAD SH, MATTHEWS S, GANT C, HIDE DW. Effect of allergen avoidance on development of allergic disorders in infancy. *Lancet* 1992; **339**: 1493–7.

BJÖRKSTÉN B. Risk factors in early childhood for the development of atopic diseases. *Allergy* 1994; **49**: 400–7.

BLUMENTHAL M, BLUMENTHAL M, BOUSQUET J, BURNEY P. Evidence for an increase in atopic disease and possible causes. *Clin Exp Allergy* 1993; **23**: 484–92.

BURROWS B, MARTINEZ FD, HALONEN M, BARBEE RA, CLINE MG. Association of asthma with serum IgE levels and skin test reactivity to allergens. *N Engl J Med* 1989; **320**: 271–7.

BUSINCO L, DREBORG S, EINARSSON T, *et al*. Hydrolysed cow's milk formulae. Allergenicity and use in treatment and prevention. An ESPACI position paper. *Pediatr Allergy Immunol* 1993; **4**: 101–11.

CHARPIN D, BIRNBAUM J, HADDI E, *et al*. Altitude and allergy to house-dust mites: a paradigm of the influence of environmental exposure on allergic sensitization. *Am Rev Respir Dis* 1991; **143**: 983–6.

DOWSE GK, TURNER KJ, STEWARTH GA, ALPERS MP, WOOLCOCK AJ. The association between *Dermatophagoides* mites and the increasing prevalence of asthma in village communities within the Papua New Guinea highland. *J Allergy Clin Immunol* 1985; **75**: 75–83.

GERGEN PJ, MULALLY DI, EYANS R. National survey of prevalence of asthma among children in the United States. *Pediatrics* 1988; **81**: 1–7.

HALKEN S, HØST A, HANSEN LG, ØSTERBALLE O. Effect of an allergy prevention programme on incidence of atopic symptoms in infancy. A prospective study of 159 high-risk infants. *Allergy* 1992; **47**: 545–53.

HOLT PG, McMENAMIN C, NELSON D. Primary sensitisation to inhalant allergens during infancy. *Pediatr Allergy Immunol* 1990; **1**: 3–13.

KORSGAARD J. Mite asthma and residency. A case-control study on the impact of exposure to housedust mites in dwellings. *Am Rev Respir Dis* 1983; **128**: 231–5.

LARSEN FS. Atopic dermatitis: a genetic–epidemiologic study in a population-based twin sample. *J Am Acad Dermatol* 1993; **28**: 719–23.

LARSEN FS, HANIFIN JM. Secular change in the occurrence of atopic dermatitis. *Acta Derm Venereol (Stockh)* 1992; (suppl 176): 7–12.

LAU-SCHADENDORF S, WAHN U. Exposure to indoor allergens and development of allergy. *Pediatr Allergy Immunol* 1991; **2**: 63–9.

NELSON HS. The natural history of asthma. *Ann Allergy* 1991; **66**: 196–203.

SAVAL P, FUGLSANG G, MADSEN C, ØSTERBALLE O. Prevalence of atopic disease among Danish school children. *Pediatr Allergy Immunol* 1993; **4**: 117–22.

SEARS MR. Epidemiology. In: Barnes PJ, Rodger IW, Thomson NC, eds. *Asthma. Basic Mechanisms and Clinical Management* 2nd ed. London: Academic Press, 1992: 1–19.

SPORIK R, CHAPMAN MD, PLATTS-MILLS TRAE. House dust mite exposure as a cause of asthma. *Clin Exp Allergy* 1992; **22**: 897–906.

SPORIK R, HOLGATE ST, PLATTS-MILLS TAE, DOGSWELL JJ. Exposure to house-dust mite allergen (*Der p* I) and the development of asthma in childhood. A prospective study. *N Engl J Med* 1990; **323**: 502–7.

TAYLOR B, WADSWORTH J, WADSWORTH M, PECKHAM C. Changes in the reported prevalence of childhood eczema since the 1939–1945 war. *Lancet* 1984; **2**: 1255–8.

VON MUTIUS E, FRITZSCH C, WEILAND SK, RÖLL G, MAGNUSSEN H. Prevalence of asthma and allergic disorders among children in united Germany: a descriptive comparison. *Br Med J* 1992; **305**: 1395–9.

WAITE DA, EYLES EF, TONKIN SL, O'DONNALL TV. Asthma prevalence in Tokelaun children in two environments. *Clin Allergy* 1980; **10**: 71–5.

WEISS ST, TAGER IB, SPEIZER FE, ROSNER B. Persistent wheeze. *Am Rev Respir Dis* 1980; **122**: 697–707.

WICKMAN M, NORDVALL SL, PERSHAGEN G. Risk factors in early childhood for sensitization to airborne allergens. *Pediatr Allergy Immunol* 1992; **3**: 128–33.

ZEIGER RS, HELLER S, MELLON MH, *et al*. Genetic and environmental factors affecting the development of atopy though age 4 in children of atopic parents: a prospective randomized study of food allergen avoidance. *Pediatr Allergy Immunol* 1992; **3**: 110–27.

Part 3 Allergen Sources

3.1 Allergens
Characteristics and determination

Key points
- Allergens are antigens that initiate and elicit an IgE-mediated Type I allergic reaction.
- Analysis of allergen extracts has revealed a large number of antigens, both major and minor.
- The important major allergens represent only about 1% of the crude allergen source material.
- An allergenic molecule consists of a number of epitopes (antigenic determinants), which are polypeptide pieces.
- Techniques are now available for sequencing the amino acids and for epitope mapping.
- Patients vary in their response both to different allergens and to different epitopes in the same allergen molecule
- This variation in responsiveness is genetically determined and depends upon the MHC class II molecules.
- B and T lymphocytes, in the individual patient, react with different epitopes in the same allergen molecule.
- The B-cell epitopes are dependent on the three-dimensional configuration of the protein molecule.
- The T-cell epitopes consist of short segments of the protein molecule.
- Similarities in amino acid sequences, sequence homology, between different protein antigens result in cross-reactivity.
- It can be clinically informative to quantitate environmental allergens.
- Airborne pollens can be determined by a pollen trap, for example, a Burkard sampler.
- Counting of mites in dust from a vacuum cleaner is used for research work.
- Airborne mould spores, sedimented and allowed to grow on culture plates, are quantitated by colony counting.
- Immunochemical methods can be used clinically to quantitate mite and animal allergens in the environment.

We are all exposed to the numerous antigens present in the environment. However, under natural conditions of exposure only genetically predisposed persons, about 10–20% of the population, become allergic to some of these antigens. Antigens that initiate and elicit an IgE-mediated Type I allergic reaction are called *allergens*. Immunochemically, the term refers to a pure compound, but clinically it is often used for the source of allergenic molecules, such as pollens, animal proteins and mites. Water extraction from these materials will give a complex mixture of molecules, an *allergen extract*.

Physico-chemical characteristics
An increasing number of allergenic molecules have been purified, cloned and characterized with regard to amino acid sequence. They are all *proteins* or glycoproteins with a molecular weight of *5–50 kDa*. The lower limit is determined by the degree of molecular complexity required for immunogenicity, the upper limit by the ability to penetrate a mucous membrane. Otherwise, there are *no physico-chemical differences* between allergens and other protein antigens to explain their ability to elicit an IgE response. No common feature in the amino acid sequences of allergens has been noted. Thus, allergens are *functionally characterized antigens*.

Analysis of allergen extracts have revealed a *large number of antigen molecules* (Fig. 3.1.1) (about 20 for animal proteins, 40 for pollens and mites, and 60 for moulds). Some of these antigens are not allergenic, others only sensitize a few patients (minor allergens) and some, *major allergens*, evoke an IgE response in most patients. There are between one and four major allergens in an allergen extract, and they represent *only a small proportion* of the crude source material (about 1% of the total weight). In the last decades, major allergens have been identified and characterized in pollens, from grass and trees, mites, moulds and the common animal species (Table 3.1.1).

One allergen molecule consists of a number of *epitopes* (antigenic determinants), which are polypeptide pieces with a specific amino acid sequence. Techniques are now available for sequencing the amino acids and for epitope mapping.

Individual patients vary not only in their responses to different allergens but also in their responses to different epitopes of the same allergen molecule. This variation in responsiveness is genetically determined. A patient's sensitivity to an allergen depends upon his or her histocompatibility gene products (MHC class II molecules), which combine with processed antigen in the antigen-presenting cells.

In the individual patient, it is not the same epitopes

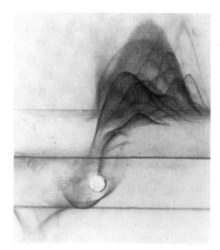 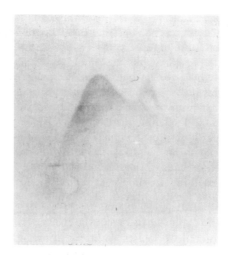

Fig. 3.1.1. Crossed immunoelectrophoresis (left), depicting the considerable number of antigen molecules in ragweed pollen. Crossed radioimmunoelectrophoresis (right), where first patient serum and second radioactively labelled anti-IgE are added, shows that, in this particular patient, only a few of the antigens act as allergens. From Løwenstein H. Quantitative immunoelectrophoretic methods as a tool for the analysis and isolation of allergens. *Progr Allergy* 1978; **25**: 1–62.

of the allergen molecule that react with B cells and with T cells. There are B-cell epitopes and T-cell epitopes.

The membrane antibody molecules on the B cells can recognize and combine with the full allergen molecule. The three-dimensional configuration of this protein molecule determines the specificity of the *B-cell epitope*, which combines with the B cell.

A T cell is not able to recognize and bind a full protein antigen. *T-cell epitopes* consist of short linear segments of the protein molecule (about eight to 15 amino acids). T-cell epitopes of several allergens have been studied and attempts made to use them in immunotherapy (see Chapter 10.3).

Different protein antigens may have some similarities in amino acid sequences, *sequence homology*, which may or may not result in partial immunological identity or *cross-reactivity* (e.g. between different grasses).

The chemical configuration of an antigen and its antibody-binding activities are influenced by denaturation, for example enzymatic degradation in the gastro-intestinal tract, and physico-chemical processes during the manufacture of allergen extracts.

Determination and quantification

It can be *clinically useful* to quantitate environmental allergens for evaluating the significance of an allergic sensitization, prescribing adequate medication, and judging the consistency of an allergen elimination programme.

Morphological methods

Pollens

The simplest and most inexpensive way to sample pollen is to use a *gravitational method* (Fig. 3.1.2). A greased slide is exposed for 24 hours in a shelter and the number of pollen grains per square centimeter of slide are counted. This sampler (Durham) does not give direct measurement of pollens in the air because variations in wind velocity influence the number of grains falling on the slide. Small particles are largely underestimated.

Volumetric methods are better indicators of particle prevalence as they reduce the size-dependent bias and give quantitative and comparable data. In the *rotating arm impactor*, an adhesive-coated stick is whirled in a circular path through the air (Fig. 3.1.3) while *suction samplers* (Burkard) aspirate air at fixed rates into flow channels with sharp bends (Fig. 3.1.4).

Mites

The number of mites in dust from a vacuum cleaner (treated with lactic acid and stained with lignin pink) can be counted in a stereo microscope and the type of mite can be identified. This is a time-comsuming specialist task only employed *for research* work.

Table 3.1.1. Some important and well-characterized major allergens with complete sequence data. They are named by the first three letters of the genus (*italics*), the first letter of the species name (*italics*) and a roman numeral

Some important and well-characterized allergens		
Common name	**Latin name**	**Major allergens**
Pollens		
Birch	*Betula verrucosa*	*Bet v* I–II
Japanese cedar	*Cryptomeria japonica*	*Cry j* I–II
Bermuda grass	*Cynodon dactylon*	*Cyn d* I
Bluegrass	*Poa pratensis*	*Poa p* I, V, IX
Orchard grass	*Dactylis glomerata*	*Dac g* I, V
Ryegrass	*Lolium perenne*	*Lol p* I–V
Timothy grass	*Phleum pratense*	*Phl p* I, IV–VI
Mugwort	*Artemisia vulgaris*	*Art v* I–III
Olive	*Olea europaea*	*Ole e* I–II
Parietaria	*Parietaria judaica*	*Par j* I
Ragweed, short	*Ambrosia artemisiifolia*	*Amb a* I–VII
Ragweed, giant	*Ambrosia trifida*	*Amb t* V
Moulds	*Alternaria alternata*	*Alt a* I
	Aspergillus fumigatus	*Asp f* I
	Cladosporium herbarum	*Cla h* I–II
House dust mites *Dermatophagoides*	*D. pteronyssinus*	*Der p* I–II
	D. farinae	*Der f* I–III
	D. microceras	*Der m* I
Inhalant insect allergens		
Cockroach, American	*Periplaneta americana*	*Per a* I
Cockroach, German	*Periplaneta germanica*	*Per g* I–II
Midges	*Chironomus thummi thummi*	*Chi t* I
Mammals		
Cat	*Felix domesticus*	*Fel d* I
Dog	*Canis familiaris*	*Can f* I
Domestic cattle	*Bos domesticus*	*Bos d* I–III
Horse	*Equus callabus*	*Equ c* I–III
Mouse	*Mus musculus*	*Mus m* I–II
Rat	*Rattus norvegicus*	*Rat n* IA–B
Stinging insects		
Honey bee	*Apis melifera*	*Api m* I–IV, VI
Yellow jacket	*Vespula germanica*	*Ves g* I, II, V
Wasp	*Polistes annularis*	*Pol a* I, II, V
Imported fire ant	*Solenopsis invicta*	*Sol i* I–IV
Foods		
Cod	*Gadus callarias*	*Gad c* I
Egg white, chicken	*Gallus domesticus*	*Gal d* I–III

Gravitational pollen sampler

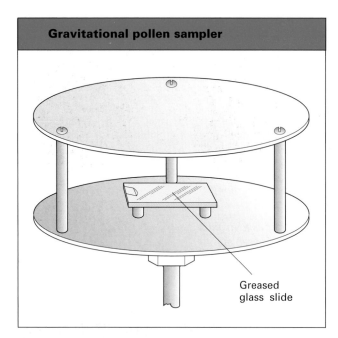

Fig. 3.1.2. Durham pollen sampler, which uses the gravitational method.

Moulds

Culture plates are placed inside houses for sampling of airborne spores, sedimented during a 20-minute period and then allowed to grow under optimal conditions for later microscopic identification and quantification (colony counting) (Fig. 3.1.5). The quantity of indoor mould spores generally reflects the outdoor concentration but sampling from single rooms can disclose local mould growth.

Immunochemical methods

Allergen sources can be identified and quantified by immunochemical methods (enzyme-linked immunosorbent assays (ELISAs), radioimmunoassays (RIAs) and radioallergosorbent test (RAST) inhibition). The patient provides some grams of vacuum cleaner dust for the laboratory where the allergenic molecules are extracted. Assays, using monoclonal antibodies, are

Fig. 3.1.4. (*opposite.*) A suction sampler deposits particles at bends in its internal flow system. This device has especially high efficacy for small particles, which readily enter the trap from a moving airstream. From Solomon WR. Common pollen and fungus allergens. In: Bierman CW, Pearlman DS, eds. *Allergic Diseases from Infancy to Adulthood* 2nd ed. Philadelphia: WB Saunders Company, 1988: 141–64.

Rotating arm pollen sampler

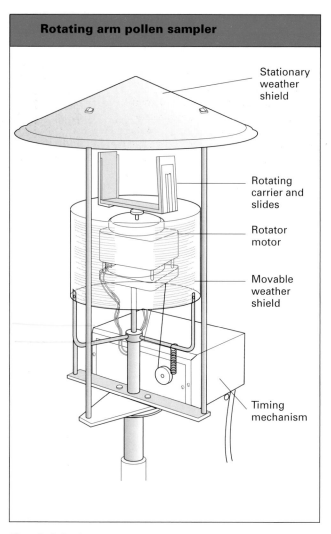

Fig. 3.1.3. A rotating arm impactor (Ogden), which is a quantitative pollen sampler.

Volumetric pollen sampler

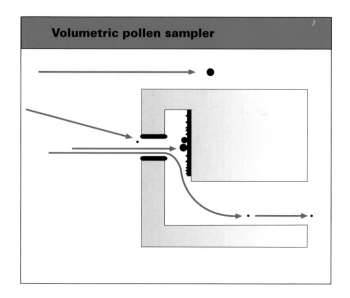

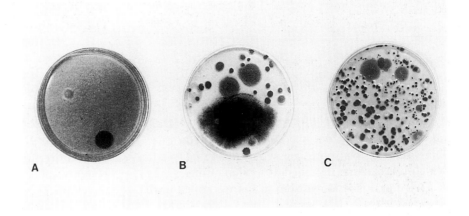

Fig. 3.1.5. Petri dishes with agar and antibiotics exposed for 20 minutes to indoor air. Mould growth from single sedimented spores at 26°C are counted after 1 week. 'A' is typical for January and 'B' for August (Northern hemisphere); 'C' is from a room with local mould growth. From Gravesen S. Fungi as a cause of allergic disease. *Allergy* 1979; **34**: 135–54.

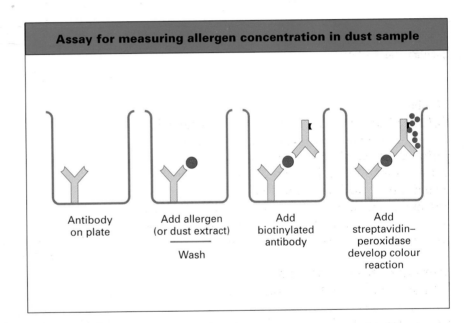

Fig. 3.1.6. Principles of monoclonal ELISA assay for measuring allergen concentration in dust samples.

extremely sensitive and are technically straightforward (Fig. 3.1.6). Assay results on several hundred samples can be obtained in a few days and these assays are ideal for routine use or for epidemiological surveys.

Diagnosis = disease
One of the most common diseases is the diagnosis.
                                                    Karl Kraus

Psychological sense
It is much more important to know what sort of patient has a disease than what sort of disease a patient has.
                                                    William Osler

3.2 Pollen
The most common cause of allergy

Key points
• Insect-pollinated plants produce few pollen grains and only close contact will result in allergy.
• Most dangerous are the wind-pollinated plants, which release huge numbers of pollen grains.
• Pollen grains, 15–50 µm in size, are trapped in the upper airways.
• Allergens, released from pollen in dew and rain drops as small dust particles, can reach the bronchi and cause asthma.
• There are three major groups: tree, grass and weed pollen, with seasons in spring, summer and autumn, respectively.
• Birch is important and it cross-reacts with hazel and alder.
• Oak, elm, plane and olive trees are also of significance.
• Japanese cedar is the most frequent cause of hay fever in Japan.
• Grass is, world wide, the most common cause of pollinosis.
• There is extensive cross-reactivity between most grass species (timothy, rye grass, orchard grass, etc.).
• Bermuda grass does not cross-react with the above species.
• The grass pollen count is low on cold, rainy days and high on hot, dry days.
• Ragweed is a significant source of morbidity in North America.
• Ragweed is prominent on spoil heaps, at construction sites, along roads and, in particular, in grain fields.
• Consequently, cultivated areas (the Mid-west in the USA) pose the greatest risk to ragweed-sensitive subjects.
• Mugwort and parietaria are weeds of some significance in Europe.

A pollen grain is the male sexual cell essential for reproduction of seed plants. It is released from one plant and transferred to another by insects or by wind.

Insect-pollinated plants produce few, heavy pollen grains designed to stick to the legs of insects. The plants have colourful flowers to attract the distribu-tors of their pollen. Only close contact with insect-pollinated plants, for example chrysanthemum in a market garden, will result in allergy.

The *wind-pollinated* plants, having no colourful flowers, release huge amounts of pollen grains. They are the most dangerous plants for allergic subjects.

Structure of pollen grains
Wind-borne pollen grains are 15–50 µm in size and roughly spherical in shape. They consist of an outer envelope, exine, a middle cellulose-rich layer, intine, and an inner protoplast containing the genetic material. The exine is a tough impervious structure used in geology for determination of the age of sediments. It is prominently sculptured, bears a number of apertures (Fig. 3.2.1) and stains readily with dyes (fuchsine). Pollens from different trees and weeds can be identified under the microscope (Fig. 3.2.2) but it is not possible to distinguish between different grasses.

Tree pollens

Deciduous trees
Many deciduous trees are allergen producers. Pollination usually takes place in the *spring* and is of short duration. The pollen count can be high (Fig. 3.2.3)

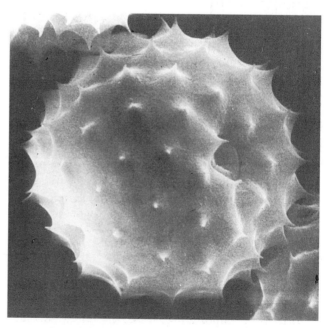

Fig. 3.2.1. Scanning electron micrograph of a pollen grain of the giant ragweed plant (× 12 000).

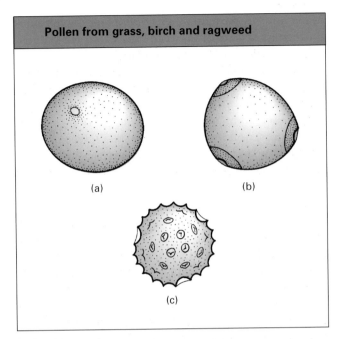

Pollen from grass, birch and ragweed

Fig. 3.2.2. Pollen from: (a) grass (30μm, one aperture); (b) birch tree (25μm, three apertures); (c) ragweed (20μm, three apertures).

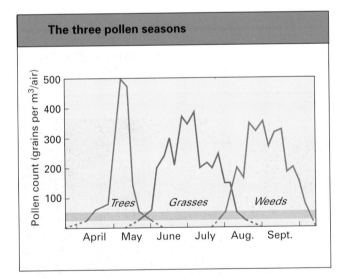

The three pollen seasons

Fig. 3.2.3. Example of pollen count with: a tree season in the spring; a grass season in the summer; and a weed (ragweed) season in the early autumn. Most patients develop symptoms when the pollen count reaches 25–50 grains/m².

and symptoms severe in patients living in an area with many trees.

Birch is an important cause of allergy in northern parts of Europe, Asia and North America. There is considerable immunological cross-reactivity between birch and other members of the birch family, hazel and alder.

Oak, elm and *plane trees* give symptoms in a limited number of subjects while beech and chestnut are not causes of morbidity. The *olive tree* is a major cause of pollen allergy in the Mediterranean countries.

Conifers

Japanese cedar is the most frequent cause of hay fever in Japan (season: February–April). In the USA, *mountain cedar* (Texas season: late fall–late winter) and cypresses are of some significance.

Pine trees produce immense quantities of pollen. Rarely do they cause hay fever, although they are often accused of doing so by patients who associate their symptoms with the yellow film of pine pollen visible on forest lakes.

Grass pollen

Species

On a world wide scale, the grasses are clearly the most common cause of pollinosis. There is *extensive cross-reactivity* between most grass species (timothy, rye grass, orchard grass, blue grass, red top grass, sweet vernal grass, and meadow grass), so the number of extracts necessary for diagnosis and treatment can be limited to one or a few. *Bermuda grass*, Bahia grass and Johnson grass, which are important allergen sources in some subtropical regions, belong to another family and do *not cross-react* with the above species.

Pollination

The considerable amounts of pollen released from *wild and cultivated grass* (hay) are carried several miles by the wind and can reach the victim even in the centre of a city.

The start of the pollen season is correlated to the *soil temperature*. In the Northern hemisphere, it is later in the north than in the south (important for the planning of summer holidays).

The amount of pollen in the air closely relates to the weather. Pollen counts are low on cold, rainy days and high on *hot, dry days*. *Wind conditions* have a profound effect on pollen release and distribution.

Pollens are only *liberated during the day*. Grains, released in the morning, are carried high into the air by noon, only to descend again late in the afternoon (Fig. 3.2.4). The highest pollen count occurs in the

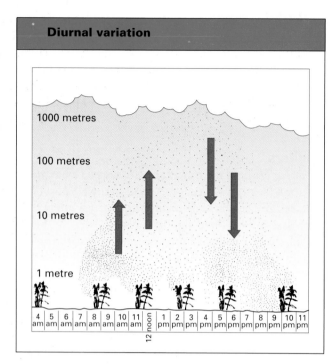

Diurnal variation

1000 metres

100 metres

10 metres

1 metre

4am 5am 6am 7am 8am 9am 10am 11am 12 noon 1pm 2pm 3pm 4pm 5pm 6pm 7pm 8pm 9pm 10pm 11pm

Fig. 3.2.4. Pollen, released in the morning is carried high into the air around the middle of the day, to descend again late in the afternoon, often several miles away.

morning and in the late afternoon. The diurnal variation is delayed by distance from the source plants, reflecting transport time.

Weed pollen

Species

Among weeds, *ragweeds* (ambrosia) hold a leading position as they are the most significant source of morbidity in North America where six cross-reacting species are widely distributed. These plants are very rare in the Old World where only *mugwort*, with little success, tries to keep up with its American relative. *Parietaria* is a common weed and an important allergen source around the Mediterranean basin. It flowers and releases pollen almost all year round.

Pollination

Recurring *disturbance of soil and plant cover* is essential to the success of the ragweeds for they compete poorly with perennial species in undisturbed areas. Natural disturbance is provided by running water so ragweeds grow on sand-bars and flood plains. Man's activities are more important; ragweeds are therefore prominent on spoil heaps, at construction sites, along

roads and, in particular, *in grain fields*, which have the highest density of ragweed growth. Consequently, cultivated areas (the Mid-west in the USA) pose the greatest risk to ragweed-sensitive subjects.

The ragweed plants shed pollen in *late summer–early autumn* (August–September), depending on locality and climate. Diminishing *length of day* stimulates maturation and, as a result, the ragweed season occurs later in more southerly areas (in contrast to grass pollen). The daily fluctuation in pollen level in the air is largely influenced by the same factors as the grass pollen level.

Pollens and asthma

Pollen grains, as large particles, are *trapped in the upper airways* and only reach the bronchi in minute amounts. Nevertheless, a fair proportion of pollen-allergic patients experience asthma in the season. This is probably because they are exposed to pollen allergen in particles much smaller than intact pollen grains. Pollen grains, in contact with rain or dew, will rapidly *release allergen molecules to water*. They will later, as *small dust particles*, become airborne, and be inhaled and deposited in the lower airways.

> **Allergic allergists**
> Every physician almost has his favourite disease.
> Henry Fielding, 1707–54

3.3 Microfungi
Spores as a cause of allergy

Key points
• Microfungi (moulds) are microscopic plants that depend on plant or animal material for nourishment.
• A high relative humidity is essential for growth.
• Moulds produce vast numbers of small spores (2–5 µm), which become airborne.
• Common mould species are *Cladosporium, Alternaria, Aspergillus, Penicillium* and *Mucor*.
• The frequency of mould allergy is uncertain and varies in published reports; it is higher in children than in adults.
• Wet weather favours mould growth, and sunny, windy weather favours spore release, while snow reduces both considerably.
• In warm, humid climates, fungi are present in vast quantities all the year round.
• In temperate zones, spore counts are highest during late summer.
• Indoor exposure largely depends upon humidity.
• Mould growth can be immense in badly constructed houses ('sick house syndrome').
• Moulds can efficiently be disseminated in a building when they grow in a humidifier of an air-conditioning system.
• Occupational exposure can occur during manufacture of bread, cheese, beer and wine.
• In recent years, the use of moulds has been extended to include antibiotic, enzyme and steroid manufacture.
• Inhalation of small numbers of mould spores can evoke an IgE response and asthma.
• Massive exposure to saprophytic moulds growing in the airway can evoke an IgE and an IgG response in bronchopulmonary aspergillosis.
• The inhalation of large amounts of mould antigen in organic dust can cause an IgG response and extrinsic allergic alveolitis.

Microfungi (moulds) are microscopic plants lacking chlorophyll. They cannot synthesize starches from carbon dioxide and water. They must *depend on plant or animal material* for nourishment. Moulds are *ubiquitous* and play an important ecological role converting waste organic matter to humus. They are commonly saprophytic on dead matter, parasitic on plants and occasionally invasive in humans.

A *high relative humidity* is essential for growth, and most species favour a temperature above 10°C. Moulds survive unfavourable conditions by producing vast numbers of *spores*, which outnumber the pollen grains in the air. While the large pollen grains (20–30 µm) mainly cause conjunctivitis and rhinitis, the major symptom of allergy to the small mould spores (2–5 µm) is asthma.

Species
Cladosporium, Alternaria, Aspergillus, Penicillium and Mucor (Figs 3.3.1–4) are the most important causes of mould allergy. The frequency of allergy to inhaled mould spores varies in published reports (Table 3.3.1); it is higher in children than in adults.

Outdoor exposure
Wet weather favours mould growth, and sunny, windy weather favours spore release, while snow reduces both considerably. In warm, humid climates, fungi are present in vast quantities all the year round. In temperate zones, spore counts for *Cladosporium* and *Alternaria* are highest during *late summer*. The count will be high in areas of decaying plant material but the spores may be wind borne for many kilometres.

Indoor exposure
The spore count indoors is usually lower than that outdoors. Indoor spores are derived from outside and from internal growth foci. Nutritional sources are abundant (Table 3.3.2), as moulds have enzymes that can split cellulose, starch and organic material. *Humidity*, however, is the determining factor for growth, which can be immense in badly constructed houses ('sick house syndrome'). Moulds can efficiently be disseminated in a building when they grow in a humidifier of an air-conditioning system. The sites of maximum growth can be determined by placing culture plates in various parts of the house (see Fig. 3.1.5).

Cross-reactivity
Very little cross-reactivity exists between genera but is common between species belonging to the same genus. Each mould organism produces several different allergenic molecules, which may or may not cross-react.

Fortunately, patients who are allergic to the drug penicillin do not develop asthma from inhalation of

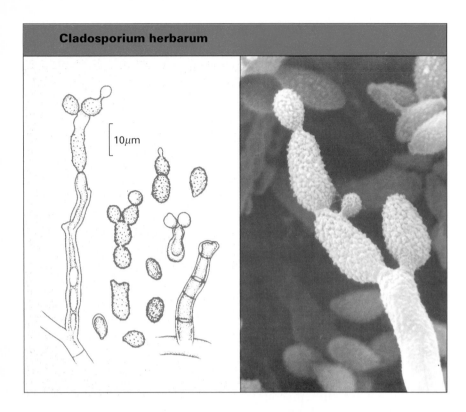

Cladosporium herbarum

10μm

Fig. 3.3.1. *Cladosporium herbarum.* Line drawings from Samson RA, Hoekstra ES, van Oorschot CAN, eds. *Introduction to Food-borne Fungi* Delft: Institute of the Royal Netherlands Academy of Arts and Sciences, 1981: 1–247. Scanning electron micrographs from Gravesen S, Frisvad JC, Samson RA. *Microfungi* Copenhagen: Munksgaard, 1994: 1–168.

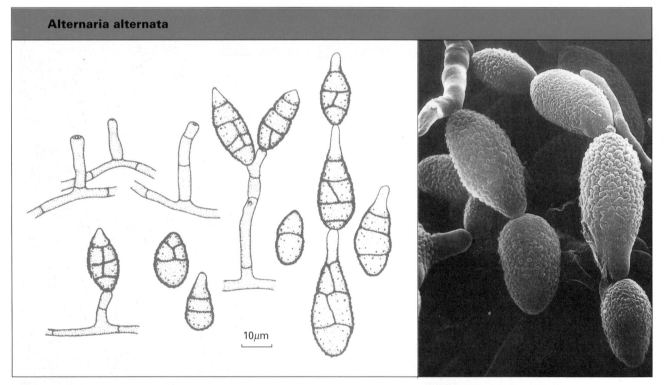

Alternaria alternata

10μm

Fig. 3.3.2. *Alternaria alternata.* Line drawings from Samson RA, Hoekstra ES, van Oorschot CAN, eds. *Introduction to Food-borne Fungi* Delft: Institute of the Royal Netherlands Academy of Arts and Sciences, 1981: 1–247. Scanning electron micrographs from Gravesen S, Frisvad JC, Samson RA. *Microfungi* Copenhagen: Munksgaard, 1994: 1–168.

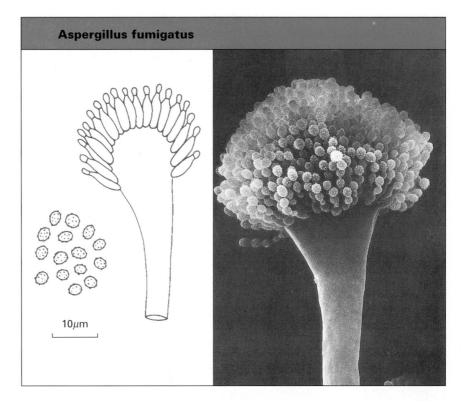

Fig. 3.3.3. *Aspergillus fumigatus.*
Line drawings from Samson RA,
Hoekstra ES, van Oorschot CAN, eds.
Introduction to Food-borne Fungi
Delft: Institute of the Royal
Netherlands Academy of Arts and
Sciences, 1981: 1–247. Scanning
electron micrographs from Gravesen
S, Frisvad JC, Samson RA. *Microfungi*
Copenhagen: Munksgaard, 1994:
1–168.

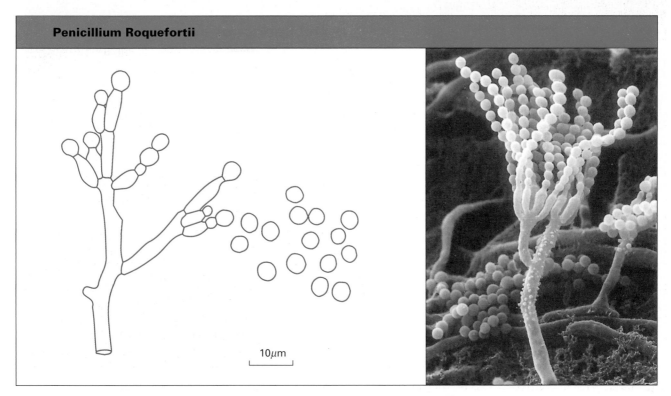

Fig. 3.3.4. *Penicillium Roquefortii.* Line drawings from
Samson RA, Hoekstra ES, van Oorschot CAN, eds.
Introduction to Food-borne Fungi Delft: Institute of the
Royal Netherlands Academy of Arts and Sciences, 1981:

1–247. Scanning electron micrographs from Gravesen S,
Frisvad JC, Samson RA. *Microfungi* Copenhagen:
Munksgaard, 1994: 1–168.

The diagnosis of mould allergy is difficult
Mould spores are ubiquitous, indoors and outdoors
Growth foci are, as a rule, invisible
There are hundreds of different species
Each mould organism produces many different allergenic molecules
The relative content of mycelium, spores and enzymes depends on the growth conditions
Some species fail to grow on laboratory media
Skin reactions to mould extracts are not always convincingly positive
Skin test, RAST and bronchial provocation test correlate poorly
Some of the saprophytic moulds can occasionally be invasive pathogens
Moulds can elicit different immune responses and different diseases

Table 3.3.1. Reasons why the diagnosis of mould allergy is difficult and the importance of this allergy controversial

Sources of mould spores
Outdoor sources
Rotting leaves (forest, compost heap and greenhouse)
Grass, hay, straw, grain and flour (lawn cutting, harvesting, and work in barns, mills and bakeries)
Dust storms (refloating spores)
Indoor sources
Summer cottages, closed part of the year
Damp cellars
Bathrooms with insufficient ventilation
Wallpaper on cold walls
Window frames, where condensation is prominent
Moist textile materials
Stored food (even at 5°C)
Artificial humidifiers

Table 3.3.2. Common sources of mould spores

Penicillium spores, but there is a theoretical risk from eating Roquefort (Fig. 3.3.4) and blue cheese.

Occupational exposure

Microfungi have been used throughout history for the manufacture of bread, cheese, beer and wine. In recent years, this use has been extended to include antibiotic, enzyme and steroid manufacture. The production of purified mould extracts carries a risk of occupational allergy, necessitating great care during manufacture.

Allergic responses

The inhalation of small amounts of allergen in mould spores in the ambient air can evoke an *IgE response* and cause *asthma* in atopic individuals. Massive exposure to antigens from saprophytic moulds growing in the airway can evoke an *IgE and an IgG response* in *bronchopulmonary aspergillosis*. The inhalation of large amounts of mould antigen in organic dust can also cause an *IgG response* in non-atopic persons, *extrinsic allergic alveolitis*.

> **For research in mould allergy?**
> If anyone of you, dear friends, should be the owner of a pair of mouldy shoes, I would like to have them. I need them for something which I am working on in my laboratory.
>
> Alexander Fleming, 1928

3.4 House dust mites
– and cockroaches

Key points
- House dust mites are the most important indoor allergen source.
- *Dermatophagoides pteronyssinus* and *D. farinae*, showing strong cross-reactivity, are the most important species.
- House dust mites can find all their requirements, that is, food, high humidity and temperature, in the human bed.
- They are vulnerable to desiccation and die when the relative humidity in the surrounding air is below 55%.
- There are many mites in bedding and mattresses and also in stuffed furnitures and carpets.
- Mites are frequent in warm, humid areas, and rare in dry areas and at high altitudes.
- In airtight, energy-efficient homes, the reduced ventilation leads to increased indoor humidity and mite levels.
- Mite allergens, as large faeces particles, are only airborne for short periods following vacuum cleaning and making the bed.
- Major exposure takes place at night when heads are close to mite-infested material.
- Exposure to 100 mites/gram of dust is associated with an increased risk of sensitization.
- Exposure to 500 mites/gram increases the risk of episodes of asthma.
- Storage mites, requiring very high humidity, are common in granaries, warehouses, food and farm stores.
- They are more frequent than house dust mites in tropical dwellings.
- Storage mites do not cross-react with the *Dermatophagoides* species.
- Cockroaches are important indoor allergens in urban dwellings, especially in lower socioeconomic communities.

Studies from most parts of the world have shown the presence of large numbers of mites in house dust, and the dust mites are, on a world wide basis, the most ubiquitous and important indoor allergen source.

House dust mites

From dust to mite
Pioneer allergists at the beginning of this century noted that the symptoms in some asthma and rhinitis patients were related to exposure to house dust and feather pillows. They made aqueous extracts of vacuum cleaner content and feather pillows for skin testing and injection therapy.

House dust is a heterogeneous hotchpotch of substances (Fig. 3.4.1). It contains animal proteins (cat and dog), which, in some patients, accounts for a

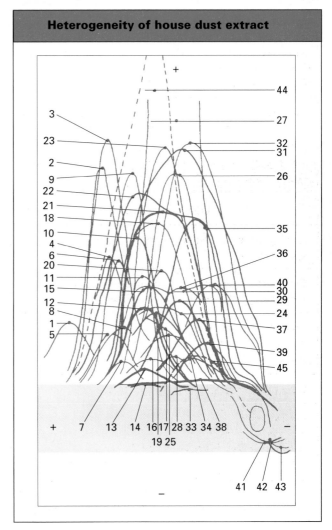

Heterogeneity of house dust extract

Fig. 3.4.1. Line drawing of crossed immunoelectrophoresis showing the heterogeneity of a house dust extract. Each precipitation line represents one antigen. From Carlsen SD, Weeke B, Løwenstein H. Analysis of antigens in a commercial house dust extract by means of quantitative immunoelectrophoresis. *Allergy* 1979; **34**: 155–65.

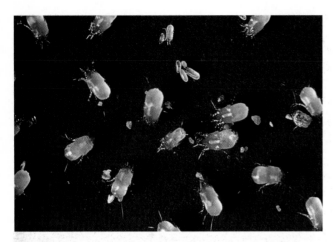

Fig. 3.4.2. House dust mites seen alive in a stereo microscope. By courtesy of Matthew J. Colloff, Scottish Parasite Diagnostic Laboratory, Stobhill Hospital, Glasgow, Scotland.

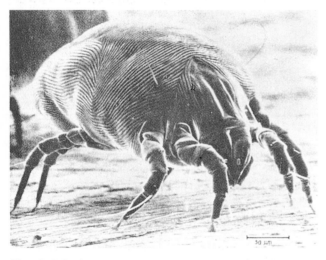

Fig. 3.4.3. Scanning electron micrograph of the house dust mite, *Dermatophagoides farinae*. From Wharton CW. Mite and commercial extracts of house dust. *Science* 1970; **167**: 1382–5.

positive skin test to house dust extract. In 1964, Voorhorst, Spieksma and coworkers in Holland showed that a mite, *Dermatophagoides pteronyssinus (Der p)* (Figs 3.4.2–3), is the chief cause of *'house dust allergy'*. *'Feather allergy'* is also caused by contamination with *D. pteronyssinus*, which, in Greek, means 'the skin-eating feather mite'. Thus,

the state of art has improved considerably in recent decades.

Types of mites

Two major species, *D. pteronyssinus* and *D. farinae*, are, world wide, the most important causes of dust mite allergy. Other species, such as *D. microceras* and *Euroglyphus maynei*, may also be important in more limited geographical regions. They are all close to each other from an allergenic point of view, and the major allergens of the *Dermatophagoides* species are very similar in structure, sharing a >90% amino acid sequence homology, and are strongly cross-reacting.

Growth in culture

House dust mites can grow in culture, where they, for example, *feed from human skin scales*. They have a temperature and humidity optimum for proliferation of 25°C and 75% relative humidity (acceptable ranges 17–32°C and 55–80% relative humidity).

Mite anatomy and requirements

The mites are too small to have lungs and therefore respire through the skin. Their thin skin permits the exchange of oxygen and carbon dioxide, and water vapour easily evaporates from their surface. As they feed from dry skin scales and other debris, they are *vulnerable to desiccation* and die when the relative humidity in the surrounding air is below 55%. Although it is common practice to measure ambient humidity, it is the humidity within their living places (mattresses, bedding, carpets and sofas) that is relevant.

As food is abundant (one person sheds 0.5–1 gram of skin scales per day, which is enough to feed thousands of mites for months) and their temperature preference is equal to our preferred indoor temperature, *air humidity* becomes the most important environmental factor determining the size of a mite population.

'Bed companions'

As humans spend roughly one-third of their time in bed and evaporate about 500 ml water while there, the mites have found an ecological niche in this micro-climate where they live their whole life: they forage, excrete faeces, make love, lay eggs and die there. These activities are only noted by allergic persons as the mites (0.3 mm) are hardly noticeable to the naked eye. Predominantly, the *faeces pellets* (Fig.

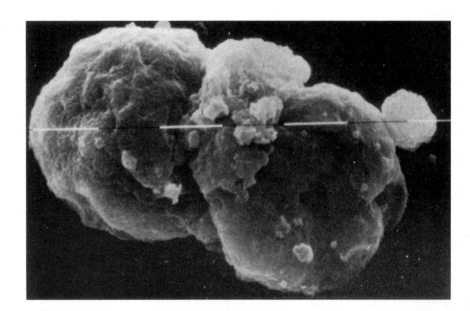

Fig. 3.4.4. Mite faeces are a major source of house dust allergens. From Tovey ER, Chapman MD, Platts-Mills TAE. *Nature* 1981; **289**: 592–3.

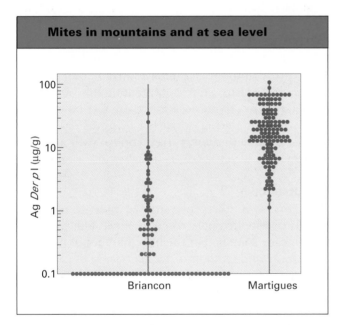

Fig. 3.4.5. Amounts of mite allergen (*Der p* I) on mattresses at high altitude (Briacon) and at sea level (Martigues). From Charpin D, Birnbaum J, Haddi E, *et al*. Altitude and allergy to house dust mites: a paradigm of the influence of environmental exposure on allergic sensitization. *Am Rev Respir Dis* 1991; **143**: 983–6.

Mite allergy at sea level and in mountains			
	Martigues (sea level)	**Briacon (3000 m)**	*p* value
House dust mites	16.7%	4.1%	<0.002
Cat dander	5.6%	3.3%	NS

Table 3.4.1. Percentage of skin reactions to house dust mites and to cat in school children from Martigues (at sea level) and Briacon (3000 m). From Charpin D, Birnbaum J, Haddi E, *et al*. Altitude and allergy to house dust mites: a paradigm of the influence of environmental exposure on allergic sensitization. *Am Rev Respir Dis* 1991; **143**: 983–6

thrive in *stuffed furniture*, *carpets*, and childrens' cloth dolls and *teddy bears*.

Differences between regions

House dust mites grow best in *warm areas with high humidity* (e.g. the tropics). The only areas that appear to be relatively spared of mite contamination are those with *very dry climates* (especially a cold climate) or those at *high altitudes* (>3000 m elevation) (Fig. 3.4.5; Table 3.4.1).

Differences between houses

Within the same geographical area, there are considerable differences between the size of mite populations in different houses. No mites occur in dwellings with a relative humidity below 45%, and

3.4.4), having the size of small pollen grains, are the cause of airway symptoms.

The highest concentration of mites are found in dust from the bed, especially from *feather pillows*, *eiderdowns* and *old mattresses*. But mites can also

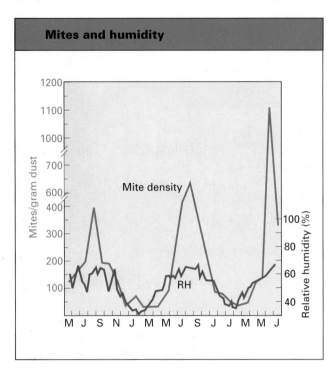

Fig. 3.4.6. Seasonal relationship between mite density in houses and indoor ambient relative humidity in a temperate zone in the Northern hemisphere. From Artien LG, Bernstein IL, Gallagher JS. Prevalence of house dust mites, *Dermatophagoides* spp, and associated environmental conditions in homes in Ohio. *J Allergy Clin Immunol* 1982; **69**: 527–32.

the size of the population will increase with increasing humidity. The *indoor humidity*, which varies with the degree of *ventilation* of the rooms, depends upon the *building construction*. The design of homes in the last 20 years, particularly the manufacture of *airtight, energy-efficient homes*, has led to significant increases in mite levels by reducing ventilation and increasing indoor humidity.

Seasonal changes

The seasonal changes in mite numbers are related to variations in the humidity. In temperate climates, the number of mites is *lowest in the winter* when artificial heating dries out the indoor air (Fig. 3.4.6). In the tropics, the mite population will *increase following the rainy season*.

Exposure as a risk factor

Data have shown a *dose–response relationship* between exposure to dust mite allergens for both sensitization and episodes of asthma. Exposure to ⩾2 µg of major allergen (*Der p* I) or to 100 mites per gram of dust is associated with an increased prevalence of *sensitization*, while a 10 µg (or 500 mites) exposure increases the risk of *symptomatic and acute asthma*.

Airborne allergen

As *mite faeces are large particles*, the quantity that becomes airborne is very low and is critically dependent on domestic disturbance. As soon as 30 minutes after disturbance (e.g. making the bed or vacuum cleaning) no or very little allergen is airborne. Major *exposure takes place at night* when we have our heads close to mite-infested material (i.e. pillow, blanket, mattress or sofa). This chronic exposure to mites contributes, imperceptively, to airway hyper-responsiveness and may trigger asthma in patients who have no awareness that house dust mites cause their asthma and rhinitis attacks. Conjunctivitis is not a problem as exposure occurs with closed eyes.

Storage mites

These mites are known pests of stored *foodstuff*. They are common in granaries, warehouses, food stores and farm stores. Storage mites are even more sensitive to desiccation than the house dust mites, their preferred condition being 25–30°C and >80% relative *humidity* (i.e. rooms with obvious dampness).

Occurrence

As sources of allergens, storage mites have been largely overlooked until recently. It was first shown in the Orkney islands that the huge number of mites, *in stored hay and grain*, is a frequent cause of allergy in farmers. Later, it was found that storage mites are more frequent than house dust mites *in tropical dwellings* and an important cause of asthma and rhinitis. This is partly due to the very high humidity, and partly because the same room is often used for sleeping, cooking and the storage of food.

Diagnosis

The recent recognition of storage mites as significant allergen sources has important diagnostic implications because they do not cross-react with the *Dermatophagoides* species. Extracts of the most important species of storage mites, *Glycophagus, Tyrophagus, Acarus*, are therefore necessary for an adequate allergy investigation in some parts of the world. When extracts of storage mites are not available, the diagnosis can be made by RAST.

Cockroaches

In *urban dwellings*, especially in *lower socioeconomic communities*, cockroaches are important indoor allergens and, in some inner city areas (e.g. Chicago, Washington, Atlanta and New York), a high proportion of asthma and rhinitis patients show a positive skin test to cockroach extract.

Major cockroach allergens, located in body parts, saliva and faeces, have now been identified and characterized. They are widely distributed in homes with the highest allergen levels being in kitchens and other food storage areas.

No studies on environmental control for cockroach allergens have, as yet, been reported. Unfortunately, there is reason to be pessimistic about the probable success of any such programme. Even though pesticides are widely available for the control of cockroaches, reinfestation is expected to be very common, particularly in the multi-unit dwellings that characterize inner-city housing. In our current state of knowledge, the following recommendations should be made for cockroach-sensitive patients: aggressive extermination from all units of a dwelling; careful attempts to reduce reinfestation; and good general housekeeping to help reduce sources of food for cockroaches.

A fruitful discussion
It is better to debate a question without settling it than to settle a question without debating it.

Joseph Joubert

3.5 Mammals and birds
Epidermals, saliva, urine and droppings

Key points

- There are cats or dogs in half of the homes in western countries.
- Allergy to cat and dog protein is a frequent cause of rhino-conjunctivitis and asthma.
- The major cat allergen (*Felix domesticus* I) is produced in salivary glands.
- Cats deposit allergen on their pelt by licking themselves.
- Cat allergen is continuously airborne as small particles.
- Cat-allergic patients often experience rapid onset of symptoms on entering a house with a cat.
- Cat allergens remain in a home for months after removal of the animal.
- In dogs, major allergens have been identified in saliva, epidermal scales and in urine.
- Urine from mice, rats, guinea-pigs and hamsters are potent allergen sources.
- As many as 20% of those who are occupationally exposed to these animals become sensitized.
- Allergy to horses is a decreasing problem.
- Allergy to cows is mainly a problem for farmers, veterinarians and cowboys.
- Allergy to bird droppings occurs in individuals having close contact with pigeons and budgerigars in poorly ventilated rooms.
- An IgE response results in asthma, while an IgG response to bird antigens is a cause of extrinsic allergic alveolitis.

Cats and dogs

Allergy to cat and dog proteins is a frequent cause of symptoms in patients with rhino-conjunctivitis and asthma. The frequency depends upon the size of the *pet population*, which is increasing in many countries. In North America and Northern Europe about half of all homes have at least one cat or dog.

The major cat allergen (*Felix domesticus* I) is produced predominantly in *salivary glands* and, to a lesser extent, in sebaceous glands of skin. Cats efficiently deposit allergen on the pelt by licking themselves. In dogs, major allergens have been identified in saliva, *epidermal scales* (epidermals or dander) and in urine. Hair, as such, is not allergenic.

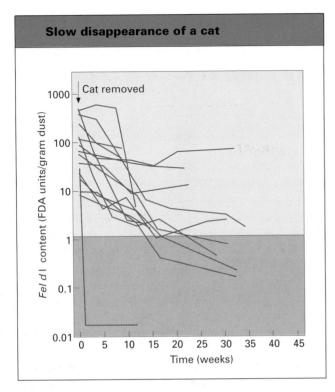

Slow disappearance of a cat

Fig. 3.5.1. Rate of decline of *Felix domesticus* I in household dust samples after cat removal. From Wood RA, Chapman MD, Adkinson NF, Eggleston PA. The effect of cat removal on allergen content in househod dust samples. *J Allergy Clin Immunol* 1989; **83**: 730–5.

Patients who are allergic to cats often report that they experience rapid onset of eye and airway symptoms when they enter a house with a cat. This phenomenon (which is almost never reported by mite-allergic patients) strongly suggests that cat allergen is continuously airborne as small particles, which fall slowly and can be kept airborne by minor air currents.

The cat allergen particles are sticky and become attached to walls, carpets and furniture, which provide a major reservoir of exposure for months after removal of the cat from the house. Thus, to assess the clinical importance of a pet, it may be necessary to observe the patient for some months after the pet has been removed and the house thoroughly cleaned (Fig. 3.5.1).

The latency period, the time it takes for a patient on entering a house with a cat to develop symptoms, lasts from a few minutes to some hours depending on the degree of exposure and sensitivity. Some low-grade allergic people will not experience symptoms from direct exposure but from an associated increase in non-specific reactivity due to long-term exposure to the allergen.

Rodents

Mice, rats, guinea-pigs and hamsters are widely used in *medical research* and have gained popularity as *pets*. They are potent allergen sources and constitute an increasing health problem.

Male rodents have permanent proteinuria and often spray their urine rather than just depositing it. In these animals, *urine* is the most potent allergen source. The dusty material in the cage is heavily contaminated and the physical activity of the animal releases large amounts of urinary proteins to the air. As many as 20% of those who are occupationally exposed to these animals become sensitized. Symptoms usually develop within the first year of exposure, and atopic subjects, especially those allergic to other mammals, have an increased risk of developing asthma (Table 3.5.1).

Screening of prospective employees by questionnaire and skin testing will reduce the need for compensation for occupational disability, but even subjects with a negative allergy history and skin test can become sensitized.

Horses

Allergy to horses is less of a problem than in earlier years. There are few horses in cities nowadays and there is less extensive use of horse hair in the manufacture of furniture, mattresses, padding and felts. People who ride as a hobby are exposed, and *indirect contact* through their clothes can precipitate symp-

Atopic status and development of allergy to laboratory animals		
	Atopic status (*n* = 51)	Non-atopic status (*n* = 89)
Asthma	18%	2%
Rhinitis and/or urticaria	12%	10%
No symptoms	70%	80%

Table 3.5.1. Relationship between symptoms provoked by laboratory animal exposures and atopic state before exposure. From Newman-Taylor AJ. Laboratory animal allergy. *Eur J Respir Dis* 1982; **63**(suppl 123): 60–4

toms in highly sensitive asthmatics. The cross-reactivity between *horse dander and serum* (tetanus vaccine) should be kept in mind.

Cows

Allergy to cows is mainly a problem for farmers, veterinarians and cowboys. The major allergens in *cow dander* are also found in beef, the concentration however, is very low, so, fortunately, cow dander-allergic subjects seldom get problems from eating. Processed hides are not allergenic but carpets made of animal hair contain considerable amounts of allergens, which are released slowly.

Birds

When extracts of feathers were earlier used for skin testing, it was noted that stored feathers, but not freshly plucked feathers, gave a positive reaction. It is now realized that the allergenicity of feather extracts is due mainly to contamination with mites.

Allergy to *bird droppings* occurs in individuals having close contact with birds in poorly ventilated rooms either for pleasure or financial gain. It is common among those keeping *pigeons* and *budgerigars* but uncommon in poultry breeders. An IgE antibody response results in *asthma*, while an IgG antibody response to bird antigens is a common cause of *extrinsic allergic alveolitis*.

The dog's Napoleon
Every man is a Napoleon for his dog. Therefore, dogs are so popular.

Aldous Huxley

3.6 Sensitizing agents in occupational asthma
High- and low-molecular weight sensitizers

Key points
- Occupational asthma is induced by a sensitizing agent inhaled at work.
- Non-sensitizing irritants can induce broncho-constriction in patients with pre-existing asthma.
- The prevalence of occupational asthma has increased over the last decades, representing 5% of adult-onset asthma.
- The introduction of highly reactive chemicals in the manufacture of synthetic materials (plastics) has increased the risk.
- In some industries, sensitization develops in as many as 20% of those exposed.
- High-molecular weight proteins act as allergens.
- Low-molecular weight chemicals can act as haptens or by a non-IgE dependent mechanism.
- Predisposing factors are heavy exposure, atopic status, bronchial hyper-responsiveness and smoking.
- In the case history, the relationship of symptoms to days at work, weekends and holidays is important.
- The history needs objective confirmation from serial records of peak expiratory flow (PEF) at work and at home.
- Skin testing or RAST are helpful in diagnosing allergy to proteins and to platinum salts.
- Inhalation challenge/exposure is needed for the diagnosis of sensitization to chemicals.
- This procedure is time-consuming and potentially hazardous.
- Challenge with chemicals usually induces both an early and a late response.
- Rats, mice and guinea-pigs are frequent causes of allergy in university research units and in pharmaceutical industry.
- Vapours from boiling of fish, crab and prawn results in sensitization of workers in fisheries.
- Enzymes, added to washing powders, may sensitize workers in the detergent industry.
- A massive load of organic dust in grain workers and pig breeders causes asthma and reduced lung function.
- Baker's asthma and rhinitis are due to allergy to wheat flour.

- Exposure to dust from green coffee, castor and soya bean can cause allergy and asthma.
- Byssinosis in workers in the cotton industry is due to inhalation of some concomitant of cotton dust.
- Isocyanates are widely used in the manufacture of plastics and other synthetic materials.
- About 5% of polyurethane foam makers, spray painters and plastics workers develop isocyanate-induced asthma.
- The pathogenesis is probably non-immunological but symptoms and pathology resemble those of atopic allergic asthma.
- Diagnosis is based upon history, identification of isocyanate in the working place and a bronchial challenge test.
- Acid anhydrides are used as hardening agents in the manufacture of epoxy resins (plastics, molding resins and surface coatings).
- Workers sensitive to fumes of acid anhydrides have IgE antibodies to anhydride human protein conjugates.
- Sawmill workers develop asthma due to a chemical, plicatic acid, in hardwoods, especially western red cedar.
- A diagnosis of red cedar asthma is based on a bronchial challenge test with plicatic acid.
- Plicatic acid induces bronchial hyper-responsiveness but mechanism of red cedar asthma is unsolved.
- Fumes of the pine resins, colophony, when used for soldering or as a glue, is a cause of asthma in workers in the electrical trades.
- Platinum salts are potent inducers of asthma among photographic workers and workers in metal refineries.

- Platinum salts can be used directly for skin testing.
- There are many irritants in work places (e.g. sulphur dioxide, nitrogen dioxide, ozone, ammonia and halogen gases).
- They induce episodes of asthma in those with bronchial hyper-responsiveness.
- Irritants provoke asthma within minutes and without a latent period.
- Inhalation challenge with a non-sensitizing irritant causes an immediate but not a late response.
- Long-term exposure to chemicals often results in persistent asthma.
- Early diagnosis and early removal from exposure is therefore important.

Definition

Occupational asthma is *induced by an agent inhaled at work*. It is often associated with rhinitis. From the point of view of compensation (in Britain) the definition of occupational asthma is 'asthma that develops after a variable period of symptomless exposure to a *sensitizing agent* encountered at work'. Patients with pre-existing asthma may develop bronchoconstriction at work after exposure to *irritants*. In clinical practice, it can be difficult to make a clear distinction between sensitizing agents and non-sensitizing irritants but there are some characteristic differences in the responses that they induce (Table 3.6.1).

Significance of occupational asthma

The prevalence of occupational asthma has *increased over the last decades*. Currently, it is thought that it represents about *5% of adult-onset asthma*, but the

Characteristics of sensitizing agents and irritants		
	Sensitizing agents	Non-sensitizing irritants
Symptoms occur only in subjects with hyper-responsive airways	No	Yes
Symptoms develop after a latent period	Yes	No
Early response to inhalation challenge	Yes	Yes
Late response to inhalation challenge	Yes	No
Induced increase of responsiveness	Yes	No

Table 3.6.1. Characteristics of the causes of asthma episodes in the working place

Risk of occupational sensitization	
Sensitizing agent	**Frequency**
Laboratory animals Enzymes	⩾20%
Platinum salts Prawn and crab processing	10–20%
Acid anhydrides Flour (baker's asthma)	5–10%
Isocyanate Western red cedar Gum	3–5%

Table 3.6.2. Frequency of sensitization to occupational sensitizers among exposed workers

percentage may be higher due to a generalized under-reporting of occupational diseases. In some industries, sensitization develops in as many as 20% of the exposed workers (Table 3.6.2). The agents reported to cause occupational asthma in the largest number of workers are isocyanates, laboratory animals, grain and wood dust.

The hazards encountered by farmers, bakers, and grain and cotton workers have been recognized for decades. Since World War II, the *manufacture of plastics* and other synthetic materials has introduced a series of *highly reactive chemicals* into factories, many of which have been associated with the development of asthma (Table 3.6.3).

Different types of agents and reactions

The causes of asthma in the working place can be classified on: 1, the molecular weight of the agents; and 2, the pathogenic response they elicit (Tables 3.6.4–5).

High-molecular weight proteins usually act as *allergens* inducing an IgE-mediated Type I reaction. In some occupations, the inhalation of large amounts of organic dust can cause asthma and reduced lung function by mechanisms that are not related to a specific allergen.

Low-molecular weight chemicals induce reactions which have many of the characteristics of an immunological reaction: 1, only a minority of the exposed workers become sensitized; 2, sensitization follows an initial symptom-free period; 3, bronchial histo-

pathology is similar to that of an allergic disease; and 4, an inhalation challenge test results in an early and a late response as well as increased non-specific responsiveness.

For some low-molecular weight chemicals, there is evidence of a formation of IgE antibody towards the complex of human protein and the sensitizing agent, which probably acts as a *hapten*. In other chemicals, specific IgE antibodies are not found, and these agents probably induce asthma through a non-IgE dependent mechanism.

Latent period

Sensitizing agents typically have a latent period between first exposure and debut of asthma. Some occupational allergens, such as laboratory mammals and platinum salts, are associated with short latent intervals, averaging from months to a few years. Isocyanates, have a latent interval averaging 2 years. At the longer end, those exposed to colophony have a mean latent interval of 4 years, and, in bakers, sensitization may occur for the first time more than 20 years after the first exposure.

Predisposing factors

Exposure to the sensitizing agent is obviously of importance and there seems to exist an *exposure-response relationship* with the most frequent sensitization in those most heavily exposed. Some molecules have a *high sensitizing potency*, and a considerable number of those exposed will develop an occupational disease (Table 3.6.2).

Patients with a *high atopic status* run an increased risk of developing IgE antibody and asthma to some of the occupational sensitizers. This association is best described for asthma caused by laboratory animals, flour and detergent enzymes. On the other hand, atopics seem to be at no greater risk than non-atopics of developing asthma on exposure to isocyanates and plicatic acid.

While atopic subjects run an increased risk of getting sensitized to occupational allergens and haptens, individuals with *bronchial hyper-responsiveness* have an increased risk of developing occupational asthma when they have become sensitized.

Tobacco smoking is associated with an increased risk of developing specific IgE and asthma caused by some agents inhaled at work (e.g. green coffee bean, acid anhydride and platinum salts). The mechanisms of this 'adjuvant effect' of tobacco smoking is unknown but it may be a consequence of injury to the

Agents that cause occupational asthma		
Class	**Agent**	**Occupation/Industry**
Animal proteins	Rodent urine Prawns and crabs Bovine proteins Egg white	Laboratory workers Prawn and crab workers Dairy workers Egg-processing workers
Mites and insects	Grain mites Fowl mites Locust	Granary workers, farmers and dock workers Poultry workers Research laboratory workers
Enzymes	*Bacillus subtilis* Papain Pancreatin	Detergent workers Food processors Pharmaceutical workers
Plant proteins	Grain dust Wheat and rye flour Cotton seed Psyllium Latex Gums	Granary workers, millers and dock workers Bakers and millers Cotton-seed oil producers, fertilizer workers and bakers Pharmaceutical workers and nurses Surgical glove manufacturers, nurses and doctors Printers, hairdressers and carpet workers
Isocyanates	Toluene diisocyanate Methylene diphenyl diisocyanate Hexamethylene diisocyanate	Polyurethane foam manufacturing Foundry workers Polyurethane foam Auto paint and plastics
Anhydrides	Phthalic anhydride Trimellitic anhydride	Plastics Epoxy resins, plastics, paints and coatings
Metallic salts	Platinum salts Nickel salts Chromium Stainless steel fumes	Platinum refining Metal plating Cement and tanning Welding operations
Wood dusts	Western red cedar	Carpenters and sawmill workers
Antibiotics	Penicillin	Pharmaceutical workers
Miscellaneous	Reactive dyes	Dye manufacture and use

Table 3.6.3. Some agents that frequently cause occupational asthma

airway mucosa, which is concurrent with the inhalation of novel antigens.

Pathology

The histopathology and pathophysiology of occupational asthma induced by allergens and haptens is *similar to that of atopic allergic asthma.*

Although IgE-mediated reactions do not seem to be responsible for sensitization to, for example, *isocyan-* *ate* and *western red cedar*, studies of bronchial biopsies, in patients with occupational asthma induced by these agents, have shown considerable similarities with atopic allergic asthma (Table 3.6.6).

At variance with patients with atopic allergic asthma, in whom the majority of T-cell clones are CD4$^+$ cells, the majority of T-cell clones derived from patients with isocyanate-induced asthma are CD8$^+$ cells.

Diagnosis

The diagnostic work has to be confined to a few centres as it is *difficult*, requiring detailed knowledge about working processes and the chemicals involved, and, ideally, measurement of potentially sensitizing agents in the air.

Case history

The diagnosis is usually, but not always, suggested by the history. Occupational asthma is most difficult to recognize in patients presenting with symptoms suggestive of chronic obstructive bronchitis. Cough

Classification of sensitizing agents
High-molecular weight proteins
IgE-mediated response (allergen)
Non-IgE-mediated response (rare)
Low-molecular weight chemicals
IgE-mediated response (hapten)
Non-IgE-mediated response

Table 3.6.4. Classification of the sensitizing agents that cause occupational asthma

and sputum production are often present, which may be due to the occupational disease alone or to the coincidental effects of *tobacco smoking*, which is often a confounding factor.

Some workers have classical *immediate reactions* within minutes of coming to work. *Late asthmatic reactions* are common, however. They typically start 4–8 hours after arrival at work but there is *great variability* and some do not start until the following night. The patterns of the daily reactions, composed of early and late responses, are superimposed on the normal *diurnal variation*. This makes it difficult to draw conclusions based on symptom variation within a 24-hour period.

Progression of symptoms with daily exposure is the most common pattern, and symptoms may present only at the end of each working week. Usually *symptoms improve during the weekend* but in chronic cases *improvement is only significant during holidays* and workers with severe occupational asthma may deteriorate to such a state that their *airway obstruction may appear fixed*. It neither varies greatly during days at work nor improves over short periods away from work. The start of recovery may be delayed for up to 1–2 weeks after leaving the work and may continue for months. Such patterns are particularly common in workers exposed to isocyanates and wood dust.

Table 3.6.5. Sensitizing agents and the reactions by which they induce occupational asthma

Occupational sensitizers and pathogenic reactions			
	IgE-mediated reaction		Non-IgE-mediated reaction
	Allergen	**Hapten**	
Laboratory animals Fish and crustaceans Enzymes Flour Bean dust Gums	+ + + + + +		
Acid anhydrides Platinum salt Penicillin		+ + +	
Grain dust Cotton dust Isocyanates Colophony Western red cedar			+ + + + +

Histopathology of isocyanate-induced asthma
Increased number of inflammatory cells
Increased number of eosinophils in all compartments
Eosinophils show signs of activation
Increased number of mast cells in the epithelium
Mast cells show signs of degranulation
Widened cellular spaces between basal epithelial cells
Thickened epithelial basement membrane
Normal number of lymphocytes
Lymphocytes show features of activation (increased expression of the IL-2 receptor)

Table 3.6.6. Bronchial biopsies from patients with occupational asthma induced by toluene diisocyanate have shown changes similar to those in atopic allergic asthma. Based on data from Bentley AM, Maestrelli P, Saetta M, *et al.* Activated T-lymphocytes and eosinophils in the bronchial mucosa in isocyanate-induced asthma. *J Allergy Clin Immunol* 1992; **89**: 821–8

Serial peak flow recordings

The history needs objective confirmation from serial records of peak expiratory flow (PEF) at work and at home. *Extensive measurements are necessary* (e.g. every 2 hours from waking to sleeping for 1 month) including weekends and, ideally, a 1–2-week holiday period. Self-recording *requires patient compliance and honesty.* A positive PEF record merely identifies the work as a source of the asthma and it may be of little help in finding the specific cause.

Skin testing and RAST

A precise diagnosis requires identification of the specific cause, but it is often difficult to be sure what a worker is exposed to. When the provoking agent is an *allergen*, a diagnosis can be based on *skin testing* or RAST. At present, skin testing or RAST with conjugates of hapten and body proteins are only of limited help in clinical practice.

Bronchial challenge and exposure testing

When it is necessary to support the case history of sensitization to *low-molecular weight sensitizers*, bronchial challenge testing is the best method of mak-

ing a precise aetiological diagnosis. However, inhalation testing is *time-consuming* and *potentially hazardous.* It should only be carried out by those with experience with occupational agents. The aim of the test is to expose the individual under single-blind conditions to the putative cause of his or her asthma in circumstances that resemble, as closely as possible, the conditions of his or her exposure at work.

It is necessary to measure lung function for 12 hours after the inhalation provocation. Workers with occupational asthma due to chemicals usually show a *dual response*, but an isolated late response, very rare in classic IgE-mediated disorders, can occur. The late response is associated with increased non-specific airway responsiveness, which, ideally, is measured before and 24 hours after challenge.

High-molecular weight agents

Proteins and other complex molecules of biological origin may be encountered in a wide variety of circumstances. These include agriculture, the storage and transport of crops, food production, the use of laboratory animals, the commercial exploitation of microbes as a source of food, antibiotics and enzymes. As a general rule, high-molecular weight molecules act as allergens.

Laboratory animals

Workers who are regularly exposed to *rats*, *mice* and *guinea-pigs* in the pharmaceutical industry, in university and research units, and in animal breeding facilities often develop allergic conjunctivitis, rhinitis and asthma (see Chapter 3.5).

Fish and crustaceans

Processing of several types of seafood can cause occupational asthma. During boiling of *fish*, *crab* and *prawn*, a vapour is released that results in sensitization of workers in fisheries.

Enzymes

Proteolytic enzymes from *Bacillus subtilis* are highly allergenic and when, in the 1960s, they were added to detergents to produce the so-called biological *washing powders*, a number of *workers in the detergent industry* developed IgE antibodies against these enzymes (alcalase and maxatase). Ocular and nasal symptoms often accompany and precede the onset of asthma. With better control of the environment in the work place, the incidence has now greatly diminished. The *consumers are not at risk* as the enzymes are added in a granulated or capsulated form that yields little dust.

Plant-derived enzymes, such as papain from papaya, are frequently used in food industries and can cause occupational asthma.

Grain dust and organic dust

Ramazzini, in 1713, made the observation that grain workers were almost all short of breath and rarely reach old age. Grain dust contains a mixture of many organic materials from seeds, fungi and insects, including the grain weevil and storage mites. In addition, the massive exposure of grain workers to bacterial and fungal endotoxins can cause fever and respiratory symptoms.

Pig breeders, who are exposed to large amounts of organic dust, frequently develop asthma and irreversibly reduced lung function (organic dust toxic syndrome). Apparently, the cause is more a massive load of inhaled organic matters than specific allergens, and the mechanism does not seem to be IgE dependent.

Flour

Rhinitis and asthma are common in millers and bakers, *baker's asthma*. The diseases are usually due to *allergy to wheat flour*, but there is considerable cross-reactivity between wheat, rye and barley proteins.

Bean dust

About 10% of workers exposed to the dust of the *green coffee bean* develop allergic symptoms. Fortunately, the allergenicity largely disappears in roasted coffee so passionate coffee drinkers are not at risk.

Asthma resulting from allergy to *castor bean* protein has been recognized for many years. It may develop in those working on the production of the oil, in people who live close to castor bean mills and in those using the dried residue of the beans as fertilizer.

Workers exposed to dust during transport and handling of unroasted *soya beans* can develop IgE-mediated asthma. A famous asthma epidemic in Barcelona was attributable to inhalation of dust generated by unloading of soya beans in the harbour.

Cotton dust

Workers employed in the initial processing stages (carding) of cotton, flax or soft hemp can develop asthma, *byssinosis*. It is a typical feature that the symptoms are initially confined to the first day of work after a weekend, Monday-morning asthma, and, with continued exposure, will persist for more and more days and become chronic.

Byssinosis is caused by some concomitant of the cotton rather than from the cellulose itself. Despite extensive studies, the cause of this important occupational disease remains to be fully elucidated. Suggested mechanisms are non-specific histamine release, endotoxin-like activity and allergy.

Low-molecular weight agents

The synthetic chemicals that can cause asthma when inhaled are relatively few in number but exposure to them occurs in a wide variety of industries. Isocyanates are the most important. They have a habit of turning up unannounced in all sorts of mixtures that supposedly do not contain them. The low-molecular weight sensitizers act as haptens and by yet unknown mechanisms.

Isocyanates

Since World War II, there has been an explosive increase in the use of isocyanates, predominantly *toluene diisocyanate (TDI)*, in a number of important industries. As isocyanates contain highly reactive –NCO groups, they react readily with hydrogen atoms in other compounds resulting in the formation of *polymerization products* (polyurethane). These products, as foams, surface coatings, adhesives, synthetic rubber and fibres, are used for upholstery, furniture, insulation material, packaging, paint and *plastics*.

High TDI concentrations, occurring when isocyanate-containing material is on fire, have a *direct irritant effect*. It can result in airway narrowing in all exposed subjects but, in particular, in those with hyper-responsive bronchi.

About 5% of workers, such as polyurethane foam makers, spray painters and plastic workers, who are exposed to low concentrations of isocyanate, will, following a latent period, develop occupational asthma. Once a subject is sensitized to isocyanate, very low levels may trigger an asthma attack.

The symptom response to inhalation of isocyanate is similar to that of allergen challenge, and the histopathological changes in the bronchi are similar to those of allergic asthma. Specific IgE antibody against isocyanate human protein complexes have been identified in only some 5–15% of the sensitive workers, and most investigators agree that *non-immunological mechanisms* are involved in the pathophysiology of isocyanate asthma; atopy is not a predisposing factor.

There is evidence that TDI can act as a partial beta agonist blocking the beta adrenoceptor, but this fails to explain the latent interval between exposure and the development of asthma, and the failure of TDI to provoke asthma in patients with bronchial hyper-responsiveness of other causes. At present, the mechanism of isocyanate-induced asthma is not known.

A diagnosis is based upon the case history, identification of isocyanate in the working environment and, as the most reliable diagnostic test, a dose–response *bronchial challenge*.

An *early diagnosis is important* because, once asthma has developed, many patients have *persistence of symptoms* even after they have been removed from exposure. The longer the duration of exposure of a sensitized worker, the lower the chance of cure.

Acid anhydrides

Acid anhydrides are widely used as hardening agents in the manufacture of *epoxy resins*, which have a wide range of applications for reinforced plastics, adhesives, molding resins, surface coatings, paints and encapsulation.

Workers who develop asthma and rhinitis on exposure to fumes of an acid anhydride have *IgE antibody* against anhydride human protein conjugates. IgE is directed against the anhydride *hapten* and against new antigenic determinants, formed by the conjugate.

Trimellitic anhydride, phthalic acid anhydride and other acid anhydrides show cross-reactivity, which vary from patient to patient.

All acid anhydrides have potent *irritant effects* on eyes and airways. Thus, at toxic level of exposure, it may be difficult to distinguish irritant from allergic symptoms.

Wood dust

Asthma due to *hardwoods*, especially *western red cedar*, develops in about 5% of exposed sawmill workers. The sensitizing agents are chemicals in the wood, especially *plicatic acid*.

A diagnosis of red cedar asthma cannot be based on skin testing. A bronchial challenge test with the responsible compound, plicatic acid, may be needed. It will commonly result in a *late bronchial response*.

The clinical feature of red cedar asthma is similar

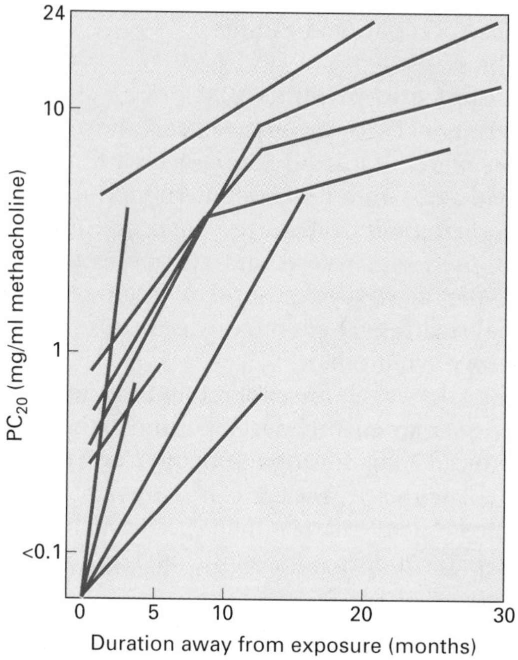

Fig. 3.6.1. Occupational exposure to western red cedar induces bronchial hyper-responsiveness in asthmatic workers. The figure illustrates the slow normalization rate of bronchial reactivity in nine workers after removal from exposure. Bronchial reactivity is measured as sensitivity to metacholine inhalation. A high PC_{20} indicates a low reactivity (normal). From Lam S, Wong R, Yeung M. Nonspecific bronchial reactivity in occupational asthma. *J Allergy Clin Immunol* 1979; **63**: 28–34.

to isocyanate-induced asthma. Exposed workers often develop *asthma during the night* and, because of this time lag, the relationship between exposure and symptoms can be overlooked. This is unfortunate because only half of the patients will recover completely when they leave the industry. The clinical presentation in the remainder resembles that of nonallergic or intrinsic asthma.

The exact pathogenic mechanism of red cedar asthma is not established but bronchial *hyper-responsiveness, induced by plicatic acid*, seems to play an important role (Fig. 3.6.1).

Colophony

Fumes of colophony, a natural pine resin, when *used for soldering* or as a glue, have been established as a cause of asthma in workers in the electric trades. Asthma resulting from colophony has many features of an allergic reaction but skin testing is negative and specific IgE is not demonstrated in serum.

Metallic substances

Platinum salts are more potent in inducing asthma than other metallic salts. Occupational disease from contact with complex salts of platinum has been described among *photographic workers* and workers in *metal refineries*. *Positive skin tests*, pointing to an allergic mechanism, are common, and platinum salts can be used directly as skin test reagents. Extremely small quantities of the complex salt are sufficient to cause a positive bronchial provocation test.

Asthma has been reported to occur in workers exposed to fumes of heavy metal salts of nickel, chromium and vanadium. Certain cases appear to be associated with specific IgE to metal human protein conjugates.

Non-sensitizing agents

Exposure to *irritants*, such as inert dust, sulphur dioxide, nitrogen dioxide, ozone, ammonia, halogen gases and hydrochloric acid, may lead to episodes of asthma in those with hyper-responsive airways. Typically, the non-specific stimuli provoke asthmatic reactions that generally occur *within minutes* of exposure and usually resolve within 1–2 hours of avoidance of exposure.

In contrast to the sensitizing agents, simple irritants provoke asthma *without a latent period*. In bronchial inhalation testing, the non-specific irritants provoke an immediate but *not a late response*.

Management and prognosis

It is of importance for an early diagnosis that the practising allergist and chest physician realize that a few per cent of their asthmatic patients have an occupational disease.

When workers are removed from exposure, bronchial hyper-responsiveness is reduced and asthma usually improves. However, as previously mentioned, cessation of exposure is not always associated with normalization of airway responsiveness and the disappearance of asthma. Following long-lasting exposure, in particular to small-molecular weight chemicals (e.g. isocyanates, anhydrides and plicatic acid), *asthma may persist* for several years, if not indefinitely, after avoidance of exposure to the initiating cause.

These observations emphasize the importance of *early diagnosis* and *early removal from exposure* in patients with occupational asthma. The removal from exposure should be complete for those sensitized to low-molecular weight agents.

Occupational rhinitis and asthma in researchers working with laboratory animals and in veterinarians may, as a second best, be prevented by minimizing their animal contact (wearing respiratory protection, most conveniently laminar flow equipment), and by drug treatment and immunotherapy.

An oversight of Hippocrates
To the questions recommended by Hippocrates, one more should be added: What occupation does he follow?
Bernardino Ramazzini
De Morbus Artificum, 1713

Further reading

Books

BERNSTEIN DI, BERNSTEIN M, CHAN-YEUNG M, MALO JL, eds. *Occupational Asthma* New York: Marcel Dekker, 1993: 1–714.

D'AMATO G, SPIEKSMA FTM, BONINI S, eds. *Allergenic Pollen and Pollinosis in Europe* Oxford: Blackwell Scientific Publications, 1991: 1–226.

GRAVESEN S, FRISVAD JC, SAMSON RA. *Microfungi* Copenhagen: Munksgaard, 1994: 1–168.

Articles

CHANG-YEUNG M, MCLEAN L, PAGGIARO PL. Follow up study of 232 patients with occupational asthma caused by Western Red Cedar (*Thuja plicata*). *J Allergy Clin Immunol* 1987; **79**: 7922–6.

CHANG-YEUNG M, MALO J-L. Aetiological agents in occupational asthma. *Eur Respir J* 1994; **7**: 346–71.

CHAPMAN MD. Manipulating allergen genes. *Clinc Exp Allergy* 1991; **21**: 155–6.

DEL PRETE GF, DE CARLI M, DÉLIOS MM, *et al.* Allergen exposure induces activation of allergen-specific Th2 cells in the airway mucosa of patients with allergic respiratory disorders. *Eur J Immunol* 1993; **23**: 1445–9.

DOWSE GK, TURNER KJ, STEWART GA, ALPERS MP, WOOLCOCK AJ. The association between *Dermatophagoides* mites and the increasing prevalence of asthma in village communities within the Papua New Guinea highlands. *J Allergy Clin Immunol* 1985; **75**: 75–83.

KORSGAARD J. Mite asthma and residency: a case control study of exposure of house dust mites in dwellings. *Am Rev Respir Dis* 1983; **128**: 231–5.

PLATTS-MILLS TAE, DE WECK A. Dust mite allergens and asthma: a worldwide problem. *J Allergy Clin Immunol* 1989; **83**: 416–27.

SAETTA M, DI STEFANO A, MAESTRELLI P, *et al.* Airway mucosal inflammation in occupational asthma induced by toluene diisocyanate. *Am Rev Respir Dis* 1992; **145**: 160–8.

SCHOU C. Defining allergens of mammalian origin. *Clin Exp Allergy* 1993; **23**: 7–14.

SPIEKSEMA FTM, KRAMPS JA, VAN DER LINDEN AC, *et al.* Evidence of grass-pollen allergenic activity in the smaller micronic atmospheric aerosol fraction. *Clin Exp Allergy* 1990; **20**: 273–80.

SPORIK R, HOLGATE ST, PLATTS-MILLS TAE, COGSWELL JJ. Exposure to house-dust mite allergen (*Der p* I) and the development of asthma in childhood. A prospective study. *N Engl J Med* 1990; **323**: 502–6.

VANDENPLAS O, MALO JL, SAETTA M, MAPP CE, FABBRI L. Occupational asthma and extrinsic alveolitis due to isocyanates: current status and perspectives. *Br J Ind Med* 1993; **50**: 213–28.

Part 4 Diagnosis of Allergy

4.1 Skin testing
The cornerstone in allergy diagnosis

Key points
- Skin testing is the primary tool of allergy diagnosis.
- The immediate wheal-and-flare reaction to an allergen is a measurement of mast cell fixed IgE antibody.
- The skin test results also depend upon mast cell releasability of mediators and the tissue sensitivity to them.
- The prick-puncture technique is preferred for clinical routine.
- If potent extracts are not available, the more sensitive intracutaneous test can be used when the prick test is negative.
- A positive and a negative control (histamine and diluent) should always be included.
- Standardized allergen extracts, having a consistent overall potency, are preferable.
- Antihistamine medication must be discontinued before testing.
- A prick test weal of 3 mm or larger is immunologically specific.
- A positive skin test occurs in 25–30% of unselected young adults.
- A positive test can be a sign of latent, subclinical or clinical allergy.

Principles
Direct skin testing is the oldest and still the most clinically useful test for measuring skin-sensitizing antibody, which, in humans, is identical to *IgE antibody*. When the allergen, introduced into the skin, interacts with mast cell bound IgE, it induces a *wheal-and-flare reaction* (oedema and erythema), which can easily be measured. Skin testing provides an estimate of the amount of IgE antibody, but the result also depends on the cells releasability of mediators, and of the tissue sensitivity to them.

Skin testing can be used as the principle tool for confirming suspected IgE-mediated disease in airways, skin and gut. IgE antibody, which may well be produced locally, is distributed to all parts of the body by plasma and tissue fluid; the *sensitization is generalized*.

Two methods can be used: prick testing and intra-

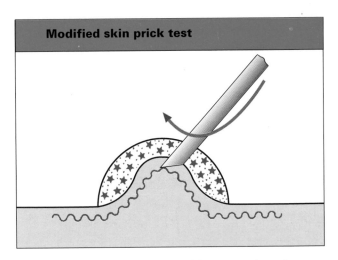

Fig. 4.1.1. The modified skin prick test consists of placing a drop of concentrated extract solution on the skin and pricking with a lifting motion through the drop.

cutaneous testing. A third method, scratch testing, has now largely been abandoned due to lack of precision.

Prick test
A drop of *glycerinated extract* (50% glycerol) is placed on the skin. The superficial layer is lifted with a needle, *modified prick test* (Fig. 4.1.1), or it is punctured by a 1 mm lancet, *prick-puncture test* (Fig. 4.1.2). Only about 5 µl is introduced into the skin, so the risk of anaphylactic reaction is extremely low. The test is quick and virtually painless. It has a better specificity than the intracutaneous test but the sensitivity is lower when concentrated and potent extracts are not available. The precision of the test can be improved when it is repeated, and preferably, the prick test is done *in duplicate*.

Intracutaneous (intradermal) test
About 0.02 ml of an *aqueous extract* from a 1 ml tuberculin syringe is injected superficially into the skin, giving a 3 mm bleb (Fig. 4.1.3). A low concentration, unlikely to produce a large reaction, is tested first, and subsequently, 10-fold dilutions are used to produce a 5–15 mm wheal reaction. The extracts used are 1000–10 000 times weaker than those used for prick testing. The test is highly sensitive but can induce irritant reactions. Intracutaneous testing is used more in the USA than in Europe.

Choice of test
The *prick-puncture test* is recommended for *initial screening* due to its simplicity, rapidity of perform-

Skin prick-puncture test

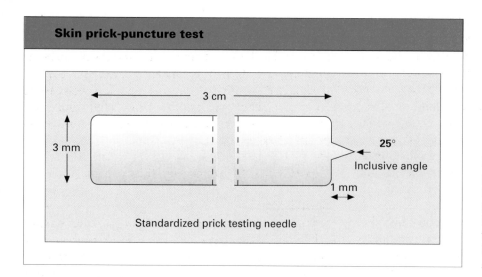

Fig. 4.1.2. Needle for prick-puncture test. This technique requires little operator skill and gives reproducible results. From Brown HM, Su S, Thantrey N. Prick testing for allergens standardized by using a precision needle. *Clin Allergy* 1981; **11**: 95–8.

Intracutaneous test

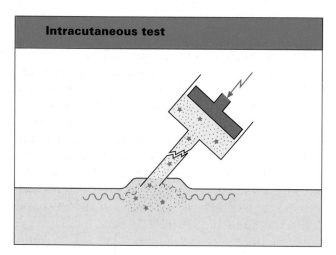

Fig. 4.1.3. Intracutaneous test consists of injecting a weak allergen extract superficially into the dermis.

ance, low cost and high specificity. It has several advantages over the intracutaneous test (Table 4.1.1.).

When a prick test is negative, some specialists proceed to the more sensitive intracutaneous test. If this is positive, the clinical significance of such a low-grade allergy is dubious. In general, the high sensitivity of the intracutaneous technique is only required when potent extracts are unavailable.

Negative and positive controls

Controls must be included whenever skin testing is performed. A *negative* control with the *diluent* is employed as patients, with dermographic skin, react to the trauma itself. A *positive* control with *histamine* (1 or 10 mg/ml for prick test and 0.01 mg/ml for intracutaneous test) is used to judge the reactivity of

the skin and to discover interfering medication. Repeated histamine testing, with calculation of the coefficient of variation, is also useful for judging the quality of the technique (coefficient of variation <20%).

Allergen extracts

Use standardized extracts

The concentration of an allergen extract is still occa-

Prick-puncture test versus intracutaneous test
In favour of the prick-puncture test
It is quicker, easier, cheaper and less painful
The risk of anaphylaxis is smaller
Testing can be finished on a single occasion
The specificity is higher
Occurrence of irritant reactions is lower
The extract is more stable
In favour of the intracutaneous test
The sensitivity is higher
The reproducibility is better

Table 4.1.1. Advantages of the prick-puncture test over the intracutaneous test

sionally given in weight/volume (w/v) or protein nitrogen units (PNU). Extracts with identical w/v or PNU labels can, in fact, vary considerably in allergen concentration, as the major allergens only constitute a small and variable percentage of the total protein. It is therefore advisable to use extracts that are standardized by *biological testing* (skin test titration) and *immunochemical methods* (RAST inhibition and crossed immunoelectrophoresis). They give the strength of the extract in *biological units* (BU/ml) or in *allergy units* (AU/ml).

Standardized, high-quality extracts that contain all of the important allergens and epitopes, present in the native material, have a *consistent overall potency*. Their use will allow comparisons between skin test results, obtained in the same patient tested at intervals or in different patients, which is of particular importance in *epidemiological studies*.

Loss of potency

Due to allergen adherence to glass surfaces, an aqueous extract loses activity rapidly *upon dilution* to low concentrations. This can be reduced by adding protein (human albumin) or detergent (Tween 20). However, a continuous loss of potency *during storage*, due to the preservative (phenol), is more serious with the *aqueous extracts*. Glycerol extracts, used for prick testing, are considerably more stable. All allergen extracts should be kept at refrigerator temperature (4°C) to delay loss of potency.

Factors influencing skin reactivity

Antihistamines depress skin reactivity considerably and treatment must be discontinued some days before testing (4 days are sufficient for most preparations but 4 weeks are needed for astemizole). Systemic steroids, given in anti-asthma dosages, have little effect on the immediate skin reaction but it is significantly reduced by topical steroid ointments.

The *test site* can also be of significance. Usually the back, or more conveniently, the forearm is used. On the forearm, avoid the skin near the cubital fossa and the wrist, and there must be at least 2 cm between the tests.

The whealing reaction decreases with *age*, but this can be accounted for by relating the allergen test to the histamine test.

Reading the skin reaction

The histamine reaction is maximal after 10 minutes and the allergen reaction after 15 minutes. A positive reaction is suggested by itching and erythema and confirmed by the typical wheal, which is both seen and felt. The largest diameter (D) and the diameter at right angles to this (d) are measured, and the reaction is expressed as D/2 + d/2. To obtain a permanent record, the wheal can be outlined by a felt-tipped pen and the markings transferred to squared paper by means of tape.

Significance of a positive test

Specificity

A prick test wheal of 3 mm or larger is *immunologically specific*, provided the extract is free from irritants (negative reaction in normal subjects). A negative prick test and a positive intracutaneous test point at a low-grade allergy provided an irritant reaction has been excluded.

Latent, subclinical and clinical allergy

A positive skin test in a symptom-free subject is regarded as evidence of *latent allergy* (no symptoms and no eosinophilia) or *subclinical allergy* (no symptoms and airway eosinophilia). A positive pollen test, for instance, in an asymptomatic subject indicates a 10-fold increase in the risk of developing hay fever. For a symptomatic patient, exposure to an allergen, causing a positive skin test, will usually be of *clinical significance*. However, a skin test can remain positive years after cessation of symptoms.

Food allergens

While the correlation between a positive skin test and allergen-induced symptoms is good for aeroallergens, it is poor for food allergens. Particular *caution* should, therefore, be used when interpreting skin tests for food. Only a fraction of patients with positive tests will react during a food challenge. This suggests that many patients having IgE antibodies to foods either do not react or have lost their clinical sensitivity. With food extracts, prick-puncture tests seem to be more reliable than intracutaneous tests for the latter can induce many *false positive reactions*.

When a commercial food extract gives a result, suspected of being *false negative, fresh materials* (milk, egg white, apples, etc.) can be used. For some foods (e.g. fruits) the prick-prick test is practical. The same lancet is used for pricking the food and then the skin.

Prevalence of positive skin tests

Prick testing with a limited number of common allergens (five to 10) can be used to determine the prevalence of atopy in a general population. A series of studies from different parts of the world have shown that the highest frequency of positive skin tests is in *young adults*. In this age group, about *25% have a positive test* but only about *10–15% develop symptoms*. The larger the skin reaction the higher the risk of allergic symptoms.

The magic of a diagnosis
Physicians think they do a lot for a patient when they give his disease a name.

Immanuel Kant

About doctors
They answered, as they took their fees:
'There is no cure for this disease'.

Hillaire Belloc

4.2 Measurement of specific IgE antibody
RAST and other tests

Key points
- RAST is a laboratory test for the determination of specific IgE antibody.
- The advantages of RAST include safety, a high degree of precision and standardization, and lack of dependence on skin reactivity and medication.
- The disadvantages include lack of immediately available results and high cost.
- RAST is mainly used as a supplement to skin testing when there is doubt regarding the clinical significance of the result.
- When a confirmatory test is needed, RAST is preferable to an allergen provocation test.

RAST (radioallergosorbent test) was the first laboratory test for the detection of *allergen-specific IgE antibody* in serum. The name RAST is still used as a term for all immunoassays for specific IgE antibody whether they use radioactive markers or not.

While *in vivo* tests measure IgE antibody, mast cell

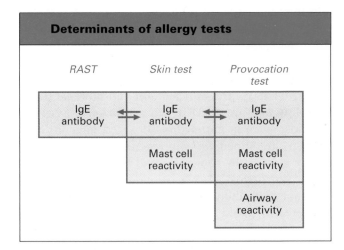

Fig. 4.2.1. Determinants of various allergy tests. All IgE antibody stems from the same circulating pool; only quantitative differences exist between IgE in serum, skin and airway. Theoretically, the major difference between these tests is that the bronchial test also depends upon non-specific tissue reactivity. In practice, the difference is confined to precision, sensitivity, specificity of the tests and variability of the parameter measured.

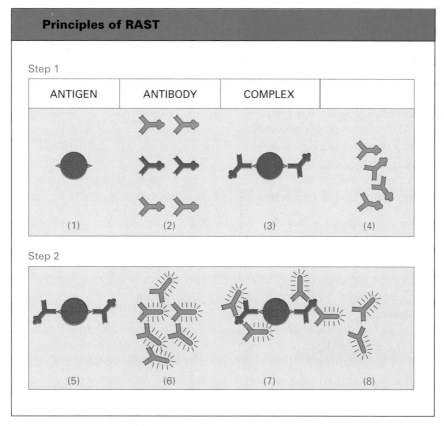

Principles of RAST

Step 1

ANTIGEN	ANTIBODY	COMPLEX	

(1)   (2)   (3)   (4)

Step 2

(5)   (6)   (7)   (8)

Fig. 4.2.2. RAST, used for the determination of IgE antibody, is a two-step immune reaction. *First step*: 1, the antigen is supplied by the manufacturer bound to a solid phase (immunosorbent); 2, the solid phase is incubated with the patient's serum; 3, IgE molecules with specificity for the antigen bind to the solid phase; and 4, unbound IgE is washed away. *Second step*: 5–6, labelled anti-IgE serum is added; 7, it combines with attached IgE; and 8, after unbound anti-IgE has been washed away, radioactivity (radioimmunoassay) or fluorescence (fluorescence immunoassay) of the solid phase is measured and used as a measure of the patient's serum level of specific IgE antibody.

releasability of mediators and tissue reaction to the mediators, *RAST measures circulating IgE antibody and nothing else* (Fig. 4.2.1).

Methods

Isotope method

The *allergen* is chemically *linked to a solid-phase support*, for instance a paper disc (Fig. 4.2.2). In this way, the allergen is easier to handle and more stable. The solid phase is *incubated with serum* from the patient. If IgE antibody is present, it will bind to the allergen. The solid phase is *washed* to remove the unbound protein. In the next stage, the disc is *incubated with anti-IgE antibody* labelled with a gamma-emitting *isotope*. All free anti-IgE is washed away and the radioactivity of the disc measured by a *scintillation counter*.

Fluorescence and enzyme methods

Radioimmunoassays are now increasingly being replaced by assays, which, for labelling of anti-IgE, use *fluorescence or enzyme instead of isotope*. The amount of fluorescent material bound to the solid phase is directly measured by *fluorometry*, while the enzyme is measured by *spectrophotometry* of a substrate, which changes colour upon enzymatic digestion. These methods are a *suitable alternative to radioimmunoassays* for laboratories that do not have isotope-counting facilities. Otherwise, they have similar advantages and disadvantages.

Correlation with other tests

There is an almost 100% correlation between *skin prick test* and RAST provided: 1, the same batch of allergen extract is used; 2, skin testing is carried out as end-point titration (determination of the lowest allergen concentration that gives a positive reaction); 3, the patient has a high degree of allergy; and 4, a reliable RAST method is used.

As the sensitive *intracutaneous test* will pick up all cases of low-grade allergy, the correlation between this test and RAST is relatively low. RAST relates closely to a positive *bronchial provocation test*.

While the classical RAST was a specific test with a relatively low sensitivity, a new and improved version (the Pharmacia CAP system) has both high specificity and increased sensitivity. In this system, the result can be quantified in kU/l according to a WHO reference system.

Advantages

1, The allergen used for testing is *easier to standardize* than allergen extracts used for skin testing, where batch to batch variation can be considerable. A RAST result shows little day-to-day and laboratory-to-laboratory variation. 2, The test does not depend on medication. 3, It can be carried out in patients with severe skin disease. 4, It is *completely safe*. 5, A serum sample can be frozen for exact comparison with later samples, and it is an *excellent tool for research*. 6, A variant of the test (RAST inhibition test) is valuable for the *standardization of allergen extracts*.

Disadvantages

1, The major disadvantage of RAST is the *cost*, which is only partly compensated for by increased diagnostic efficacy. 2, The result is *not immediately available*, which necessitates a second visit. 3, While RAST, when used in its classical form, is not as sensitive as skin testing, the sensitivity has improved with the modern version (the CAP system). 4, A very high level of total IgE (e.g. worm infestation and a few cases of atopic dermatitis) can cause a false positive result because small amounts of IgE molecules are trapped on the immunosorbent in a non-specific manner, but this problem seems to be eliminated in the new generation of RAST. 5, When immunotherapy is based on RAST and not on skin testing, extracts from different manufacturers may be used for diagnosis and for treatment.

Diagnosis of inhalant allergy

RAST as an alternative to skin testing

RAST is preferable to skin testing in the following cases: 1, the skin shows *dermographism*; 2, *antihistamines* cannot be discontinued; 3, there is a *widespread skin disease*; and 4, in patients who have had *very severe reaction* to the allergen in question (venom, penicillin and some occupational allergens).

RAST can be used as a primary tool by the general practitioner when there is *a single specific question* (e.g. allergy to a dog? or, allergy to pollen?). The specialist will use RAST primarily in cases of *rare allergens* (e.g. occupational allergens) as it is expensive to have an extract that is used for skin testing only a few times a year. Also, some allergens may not be available as extracts of adequate quality in a geographical region.

RAST as a supplement to skin testing

When a skin prick test is clearly positive and in accordance with the history, RAST or provocation testing may add no more information than would repetition of the skin test on the other arm. When there is doubt about the significance of a skin test, another type of test can be added, providing the result will be of consequence for the therapeutic decision. When *a confirmatory test* is needed, RAST is preferable to allergen provocation, because it is cheaper, safer and more precise.

Diagnosis of food allergy

RAST testing can provide useful supplementary information in the difficult evaluation of food allergy. In some cases, it gives a closer agreement with clinical findings than does skin testing, although both procedures usually produce more positive results than can be supported by the history and elimination/provocation diets. In particular, patients with atopic dermatitis often have a positive RAST to foods without clinical relevance.

The correlation between history and RAST is good for patients with severe food-induced symptoms and less good for those with mild and atypical symptoms. It also depends on which allergens are involved. Reliable results are obtained with fish, shrimps, nuts, peanuts and egg. Interpretation of a positive RAST to cereal grains and soyabean extract is difficult due to a high incidence of a positive test to these allergens in patients with a negative history.

Multi-allergen IgE antibody test

Recently a modification of the IgE antibody test, the multi-allergen antibody test, has been developed. The test is performed by using an immunosorbent that has several allergens coupled to it. The sensitivity of the multi-allergen method (Phadiatop) is comparable to single allergen methods (RAST). It is a cost-effective screening procedure, which is capable of identifying atopic allergic patients better than is the measurement of total IgE.

The leucocyte histamine-release test

This test can identify circulating allergen-specific IgE antibody in allergic patients by preincubating their sera with basophils from non-sensitized subjects and measuring the histamine release. The test is, at present, primarily used for research purposes. It has found limited clinical application because of the requirement of fresh blood cells and the limited number of allergens that can be tested using a single aliquot of blood.

It is hard to write a textbook
What is written without effort is read without pleasure.
Samuel Johnson

4.3 Allergen provocation test
— in bronchi, nose and eye

Key points
- Allergen provocation of bronchi, nose and eye is useful for the study of pathophysiology and pharmacodynamics.
- Allergen provocation, however, differs fundamentally from natural exposure (dosage and airway deposition).
- The bronchial response to allergen challenge depends upon specific allergy and non-specific responsiveness to released mediators.
- A bronchial challenge test is tedious and observation for 12 hours is necessary.
- It can be clinically useful for diagnosing allergy to those haptens that cannot be used for skin testing and RAST.
- Controlled inhalation exposure testing is of diagnostic value in occupational asthma.

Historical background
Previously, when badly characterized allergen extracts were used for intracutaneous testing, false positive reactions due to irritants were frequent. This resulted in a number of futile attempts at immunotherapy. Critical investigators found that the risk of misinterpretation of the skin results could be reduced when a positive test was confirmed by allergen provocation testing or allergen challenge of the diseased organ.

The situation has improved in recent decades as better characterized allergen extracts, without low-molecular irritants, have become available. In addition, RAST can now be used when confirmation of a positive skin test is needed.

Theoretical background

Information about a certain organ?
The argument put forward in favour of a provocation test is that this is the only way to obtain direct information about the significance of a specific allergen for a disease in a certain organ. Although there is some logic in this assumption, there are also arguments against it. It implies that fixation of IgE to mast cells differs in different tissues. IgE antibody, however,

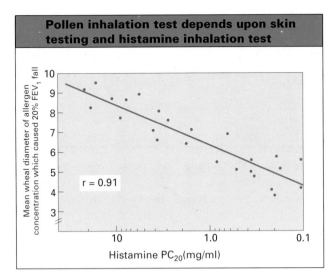

Fig. 4.3.1. This figure illustrates that the result of a pollen inhalation test can be predicted, to a high degree, by skin reactivity to allergen and bronchial responsiveness to histamine. From Cockcroft DW, Ruffin RE, Frith PA, *et al.* Determinants of allergen-induced asthma: dose of allergen, circulating IgE antibody concentration and bronchial responsiveness to inhaled histamine. *Am Rev Respir Dis* 1979; **120**: 1053–8.

circulates to all parts of the body, and there is no reliable evidence that specific sensitization can be localized to a single organ. The provocation test response of the bronchi to an inhaled allergen is more likely to reflect the patient's general sensitivity to that allergen than to prove the existence of the specific illness, asthma (Fig. 4.3.1).

Provocation versus exposure

A bronchial provocation test with *pollen grains* will not cause bronchoconstriction in pollen-allergic asthmatics, simply because the large pollen grains will not reach the bronchi. Provocation with *pollen extract*, on the other hand, can cause bronchoconstriction, even in hay fever patients who are never troubled by asthma in the pollen season.

These findings can be related to some fundamental differences between a *provocation test* in the laboratory and *natural exposure*. 1, In the provocation test, 1–2 μm droplets, inhaled through the mouth, will reach all parts of the airway; during natural exposure, the 20–30 μm large pollen grains are trapped in the nose. 2, Daily exposure in the pollen season consists of 15 000 'mini provocations'; a provocation test in the laboratory, on the other hand, will expose the airway to a total allergen dose corresponding to days or weeks of exposure during the season.

Determinants

The response to an allergen provocation test depends upon a number of factors: 1, the strength of *allergen extract*; 2, *deposition in the airway*, which is abnormal and variable in symptomatic asthmatics; 3, the number of *bronchial mast cells*, their content of mediators and their releasability; 4, the *non-specific responsiveness* of the bronchi to the released mediators; and 5, current *medication*.

It follows that the variability of the inhalation test is acceptable only in an almost symptom-free asthmatic who can do without medication. Usually, it is not the patient who causes diagnostic problems. A test can be *false positive* due to irritancy, hyperventilation and random bronchoconstriction. *False negative* tests are rare when potent extracts are used.

Correlation to other tests

The agreement between skin test, RAST and bronchial provocation test *depends upon the allergen* and *the degree of allergy*. The correlation is good when the allergen is potent, of high quality and the skin reaction is large. Small skin reactions, however, are usually not associated with positive RAST or provocation test.

Method

A number of *precautions* must be strictly followed to ensure the safety of the procedure, which should only be carried out in hospital under careful medical supervision. *Asymptomatic patients* are studied when the baseline FEV$_1$ is at least 80% of the predicted value. Testing of a symptomatic patient both increases the risk of severe asthma and of a false positive result.

An *aqueous extract* is made, preferably from a freeze-dried sample, using a diluent without preservative. Glycerinated extracts should not be used as they have a considerable tendency to elicit non-specific reactions. Starting with the diluent only, *increasing concentrations* of allergen are inhaled until a *20% fall in FEV$_1$* is attained. The concentration that gives a positive provocation is usually of the same order of magnitude as that causing a positive intracutaneous test. The top concentrations are avoided as they often contain sufficient irritants to elicit non-specific bronchial reactions. Patients must be kept under observation for at least 12 hours due to late responses.

Bronchodilators and *cromoglycate* are omitted

before testing. *Steroids can be continued*, although long-term inhaled use will increase the threshold.

Indication and limitation

A diagnosis of allergy to pollen and animals can be made with sufficient certainty by history, skin prick test and, eventually, RAST. *For mites and moulds*, there is seldom a convincing history to confirm a positive skin test. *If immunotherapy is considered*, it may be wise to increase the diagnostic certainty. For this purpose, RAST is preferable in most cases.

Allergen provocation can be used to *follow the effect of immunotherapy*, but a controlled setting, and repeated testing, is necessary to avoid false conclusions based on random variation. While it is questionable, in clinical routine, whether the therapeutic benefit justifies the effort of provocation testing, the procedure is *valuable for research*.

In recent years, this type of testing has been most useful in *identifying new allergens and haptens*, which cannot be detected by skin testing or RAST. This has an important place in *occupational medicine*.

Controlled exposure

Studies of occupational asthma have led to the development of a different type of bronchial provocation test, the controlled exposure. It consists of simple and safe techniques for simulating work exposure within the hospital environment. The patient is exposed to industrial gas, vapour or fumes in the same form and concentration as that encountered at work. Such tests may be the only way to confirm a specific sensitivity in *occupational asthma*.

Allergen provocation of the nose

Allergen can be given intranasally as an aqueous solution, a powder or by small filter paper disks soaked in allergen extract. The latter method is widely used for clinical work in Japan. Symptoms and signs can be recorded as number of sneezes, amount of secretion and change in nasal airway patency (nasal peak flow, rhinomanometry and acoustic rhinometry).

The nasal allergen challenge test is useful for the study of pathophysiology and the drug effect, but its role in clinical management of rhinitis is limited.

Allergen provocation of the eye

Dripping increasing concentrations of an allergen extract in one eye and the diluent in the other eye is an easy way of demonstrating conjunctival sensitivity. Itching and redness are recorded. Whether this test adds to the information obtained with careful skin testing, however, is dubious. Like the nasal provocation test, it serves more as a tool to investigate the pathophysiology and pharmacodynamics of an allergic disease (see Chapter 1.11).

Oeconomy and diagnosis
Before ordering a test decide what you will do if it is positive, or negative. If both answers are the same, don't do the test.

Arthur Bloch
Murphy's Law Book

4.4 Total serum IgE
An indicator of atopic status and allergy

Key points
- The serum level of total IgE depends on a genetic control of IgE production and on the synthesis of specific IgE antibodies.
- In atopic dermatitis, it is mainly a measure of the degree of atopy.
- In asthma/rhinitis, it reflects the severity and number of allergies and recent allergen exposure.
- As the serum IgE level is very low, sensitive immunoassays are required (radioimmunosorbent test (RIST), paper radioimmunosorbent test (PRIST) and the CAP system IgE).
- Normal values vary with age and selection of the reference population.
- Characteristically, there is a wide range and considerable overlap between non-atopic and atopic subjects.
- IgE measurements during infancy may predict the development of allergic symptoms.
- In adults, it is useful in equivocal asthma cases but of little help in rhinitis.
- Worm infestations are associated with very high levels of IgE.

Principles
IgE is produced by B lymphocytes and plasma cells distributed primarily in the lymphoid tissue adjacent to the respiratory and gastro-intestinal tracts. IgE, though synthesized near the location of allergen encounter, eventually becomes *homogeneously distributed* in body fluids and can be measured in the serum.

Babies of atopic parents have a higher total IgE level in cord blood (which is of fetal origin) than babies of non-atopic parents. However, the newborn has not yet been exposed to allergens, and specific IgE antibodies are not present in the serum. The newborn with an atopic predisposition is genetically coded as an IgE high-responder. The total IgE level in this case reflects the *atopic predisposition*.

Patients with atopic dermatitis often have elevated serum IgE, although IgE antibodies, of significance for their skin symptoms, cannot be identified. In these patients, the total IgE level is a measure of *atopic status*.

In hay fever, which is a monovalent allergy, it has been shown that as much as 25–50% of the total IgE is made up by IgE antibody to pollen. In this case, an increased total IgE level reflects the presence of specific IgE antibody and is an indicator of active *allergy*.

The serum level of total IgE is positively correlated to: 1, the state of atopy; 2, the number and degree of specific allergies; 3, the degree and duration of allergen exposure; and 4, the organs involved (skin + airway > skin > bronchi > nose). The serum IgE level correlates well with the severity of atopic dermatitis but poorly with the severity of airway symptoms.

Laboratory methods
IgE comprises less than 0.001% of the total circulating immunoglobulin in normal individuals. Since the serum concentration of IgE is extremely low, immunodiffusion methods, available for measurement of other immunoglobulins, are unsuitable.

Sensitive radioimmunoassays (RIA), and, later, fluorescence immunoassays (FEIA) and enzyme immunoassays (ELISA), have been developed to meet the need for a very sensitive method. The first test, utilized for measurement of IgE, was the *radioimmunosorbent test* (*RIST*). It was replaced by the more sensitive and precise *paper radioimmunosorbent test* (*PRIST*), which is a solid-phase immunoassay employing anti-IgE antibody coupled to an insoluble carrier (Fig. 4.4.1). The same main principle is now used in the *CAP system*, using either a radioimmunoassay or a fluorescence immunoassay.

Serum IgE values are generally expressed in international units (IU) per ml. One unit is equivalent to 2.4 ng of IgE (WHO reference standard).

Normal values

Newborns
Since maternal IgE does not cross the placenta, *umbilical cord levels* are normally very low (<0.5 IU/ml). In the first year of life, the relative rise in serum IgE is comparable to IgA but slower than IgG (Fig. 4.4.2).

Children and adults
Log-transformed serum IgE values from large populations are normally distributed (Fig. 4.4.3). The up-

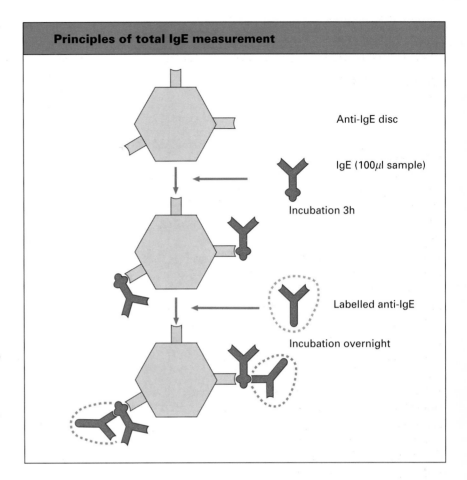

Fig. 4.4.1. Principles of the paper radioimmunosorbent test (PRIST). The solid phase is a cellulose paper disc to which anti-IgE antibodies are coupled. Patient serum is added and the IgE will be bound by the anti-IgE on the paper disc. After washing, radioactive-labelled anti-IgE is added and will bind to the patient's IgE, already bound to the solid phase.

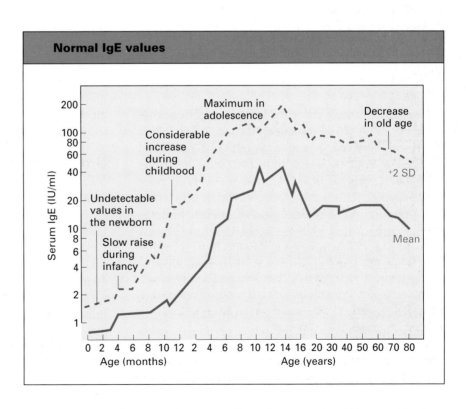

Fig. 4.4.2. Normal values for total serum IgE. —, geometric mean; – – – +2 SD.

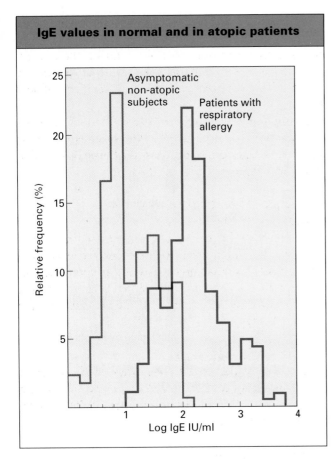

Fig. 4.4.3. The log distribution of the total IgE values in a normal reference group (blue line) and in adult atopic patients (red line). In this study, there was unusually good separation between normal and atopic subjects. From Zetterström O, Johansson SGO. IgE concentrations measured by PRIST in serum of healthy adults and patients with respiratory allergy. *Allergy* 1981; **36**: 537–47.

per *normal reference value* for IgE (geometric mean + 2 SD) is about 20 IU/ml under the age of 2 years, 100 IU/ml between 2 and 6 years, 150–200 IU/ml between 6 and 16 years, and 100 IU/ml in adults (Fig. 4.4.2). But *normal values vary widely* in published reports. This is largely due to differences in the study population. The definition of normal limits is further complicated by the observation that subjects without a personal history of allergy have a higher level when the family history is positive than when it is negative.

Prediction of allergy in infants?

A determination of total IgE has a predictive value with regard to the development of allergic disease during infancy. High IgE levels are present for

months before the appearance of clinical allergic disease. Such a screening, which can even be carried out on cord blood, has been recommended when both parents are atopic or if severe atopic disease is present in one parent/sibling. However, it was found that elevated cord blood IgE has a poor sensitivity and a low positive predictive value.

In any case, such practice would only be justified if it was followed by prophylactic measures. Many would argue that, in a newborn with a strong family history, any prophylactic measure felt to be effective should be instituted in view of the frequency with which allergic symptoms develop in this group. Thus, total IgE determination at birth or later during the neonatal period is not suitable for general allergy risk screening.

IgE levels in disease

Atopic dermatitis

Patients with mild atopic dermatitis (eczema) often have normal IgE levels. Patients with *marked eczema*, as a rule, have high IgE levels, especially when they also have *airway symptoms*. A high level is probably a reflection of a fundamental defect in the T lymphocyte function. It is usually associated with the formation of specific IgE antibodies of little importance for the skin disease.

Measurement of total IgE can be *of some help* in distinguishing between atopic dermatitis and other skin diseases. A value below 20 IU/ml in a symptomatic patient would indicate that atopic dermatitis is not present, and a value greater than 400 IU/ml is almost diagnostic when parasitic infestation is excluded. A slightly increased IgE value can be seen in other skin diseases.

Urticaria

IgE seldom plays a role in chronic urticaria, and measurement of IgE is *of no help*.

Gastro-intestinal symptoms

Patients with IgE-mediated allergy in the gastro-intestinal tract have immediate symptoms and are usually aware of their allergy. They avoid the allergen, and total IgE is therefore not elevated. Measurement of IgE can be *of some help* in small children with gastro-intestinal symptoms but not all of the chronic allergic symptoms from the gastro-intestinal tract are mediated by IgE.

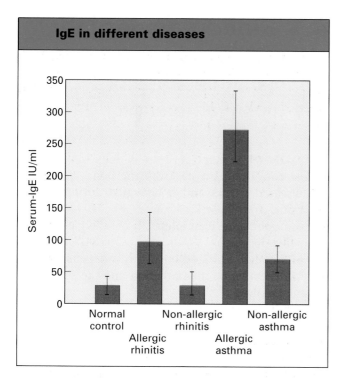

Fig. 4.4.4. Serum IgE levels in normal controls, and in patients with allergic and non-allergic disease. Courtesy of Dahl R, Department of Lung Medicine, Århus, Denmark.

Uncharacteristic airway symptoms

Allergy should be suspected when a child has recurrent 'airway infections' or 'wheezy bronchitis'. In such a case, measurement of IgE is often *a good guide* but a normal IgE level does not exclude allergy. The correlation between serum IgE and atopic disease is better *in children* than in adults; the test has little diagnostic value in an adult with vague airway symptoms.

Asthma

Serum IgE is significantly *elevated in 50–75%* of patients with allergic asthma (Fig. 4.4.4); it is found to be elevated more often in children than in adults. A high level is useful in prompting a further search for allergens in patient otherwise considered to have non-allergic disease. A level below 20 IU/ml is a strong indication that allergic asthma is not present, while a value over 100–150 IU/ml is highly suggestive of allergy. The severity of airway symptoms correlates well with the blood eosinophil count but poorly with the IgE level. This indicates that allergic inflammation is a more important determinant of the presentation of asthma than is the degree of atopy.

Rhinitis

In *seasonal allergic rhinitis*, the highest IgE level is reached after exposure to pollen during the season, but the level often remains within normal limits. An IgE assay is *not necessary* for management of hay fever.

Serum IgE is *elevated in about 25%* of patients with *perennial allergic rhinitis*. Measurement of IgE is valuable in children, but the test is of little or no value in adult patients with isolated rhinitis.

Allergic bronchopulmonary aspergillosis

These patients have elevated serum IgE that often reaches a very high level. Recurrences are associated with an increase that precedes clinical deterioration. Regular monitoring of total IgE is *important* as a measure of disease activity and the requirement for steroid therapy.

Worm infestations

Parasite infestation induces *very high levels* of serum IgE. This seriously *reduces the usefulness* of this test as an indicator of allergy in countries where worm diseases are frequent.

Other diseases

Because T cells regulate the production of IgE, T cell deficiencies may be associated with an increased IgE production. This can be the case with *Hodgkin's disease* and Wiskott–Aldrich syndrome. The very rare IgE-producing myelomas give extremely high IgE values.

Conclusions

The introduction of the IgE concept into allergy has had a profound influence on the development of the discipline. The introduction of *in vitro* procedures has increased the overall diagnostic precision. The results obtained by one allergist can now be understood and reproduced by others.

The IgE assay has its limitation, as many patients with atopic disease have IgE levels within the normal range. Patients with high serum IgE levels are easily recognized as atopics on the basis of clinical history and the results of skin testing. Measurement of total serum IgE is routine in many allergy clinics, but this practice can be questioned by the cost-conscious physician. It is a *valuable* examination when used with thought *in selected cases*.

4.5 Blood eosinophil count
—and soluble markers of allergic inflammation

Key points
- The eosinophil travels from the bone marrow to the diseased tissues and is activated during allergic reactions.
- Eosinophilia is characteristic of allergic and allergy-like diseases.
- The number of blood eosinophils depicts the severity of the allergic inflammation and the size of the organs involved.
- The allergic inflammation cannot be monitored by acute-phase proteins.
- Eosinophil and mast cell markers are potentially useful for monitoring allergic inflammation.
- Serum eosinophil cationic protein (ECP) is a measure of circulating activated eosinophils.
- Allergen challenge and exposure increase ECP levels.
- ECP correlates with the disease severity in asthma.
- A high ECP level can predict exercise-induced bronchoconstriction and a late bronchial response to allergen.
- The ECP level may be used as an indicator of steroid requirement, and ECP is reduced by oral and inhaled steroids.
- Serum ECP correlates with disease activity in atopic dermatitis.
- The serum level of tryptase, a mast cell marker, is elevated during anaphylactic reactions.

Blood eosinophil count

Kinetics
The eosinophil originates and matures in the *bone marrow*, then is released to the *blood stream* (see Chapter 1.10). After a mean circulation time of about 12 hours, it leaves the vessels and migrates, mainly to the skin, airway and gastro-intestinal tract, where it normally remains for a few days. The eosinophil is predominantly a *tissue cell* with a blood:tissue ratio of about 1:100.

Eosinophils in blood
Allergic reactions, with the release of cytokines and

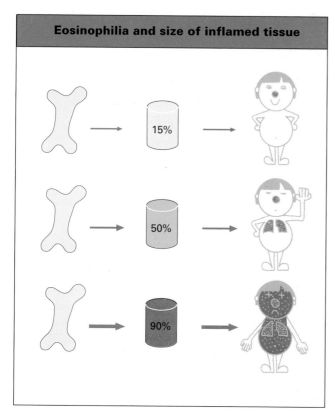

Fig. 4.5.1. The number of eosinophils transported from the bone marrow to the shock organ depends on its size. Therefore, blood eosinophilia is present in few rhinitis patients, in half the asthma patients and in the majority of patients with rhinitis, asthma and atopic dermatitis.

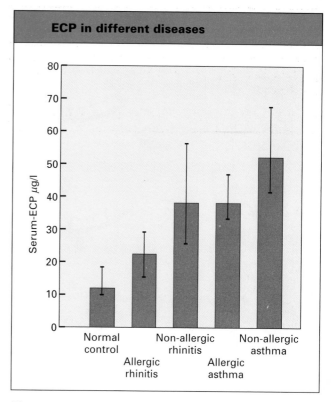

Fig. 4.5.2. Serum ECP can be used as a measure of the activated eosinophil population. This is higher in non-allergic disease than in allergic disease. From Dahl R, Venge P. Role of the eosinophil in bronchial asthma. *Eur J Respir Dis* 1982; **63**(suppl 122): 23–8.

eosinotactic factors in the tissue, stimulate the formation of eosinophils in the bone marrow and attract them from the blood. As the total number of extravascular eosinophils greatly outnumbers those in the blood, a determination of circulating eosinophils only gives a *transient picture* dependent on the actual ratio between *supply and demand*.

The degree of eosinophilia in blood gives information regarding the *severity* of the inflammation and the *size of the diseased organ*. When the latter is large (e.g. lungs or skin), the call-up of eosinophils from the bone marrow is considerable. Consequently, more asthmatic patients than rhinitis patients have blood eosinophilia (Fig. 4.5.1).

Normal values

In an adult population, without worm infestation, the upper limit for the normal is 350–400 eosinophils/mm³ in the morning and 400–450 in the afternoon. Norms for children are 50–100 cell/mm³ greater.

Allergic and allergy-like diseases

In asthma, eosinophilia is related to the disease as such and not to the presence of an IgE-mediated mechanism. The eosinophil count is generally higher in non-allergic than in allergic asthma (Fig. 4.5.2). There is a positive correlation between the *severity of asthma* and the number of blood eosinophils (especially of activated cells), so the eosinophil count is a useful guideline for the treatment of the disease, particularly in assessing the *requirement for steroids*.

Severe atopic dermatitis is often associated with eosinophilia, particularly in patients who also suffer from allergic airway disease.

Other diseases

Blood eosinophilia occurs in *worm infestation, Hodgkin's disease, periarteritis nodosa, Löffler's syndrome, hypereosinophilic syndrome*, a series of *skin diseases* and *drug allergy*. The elevation, in general, is slight in allergic disease (500–1500 cells/mm³), and moderate in non-allergic asthma and *bron-*

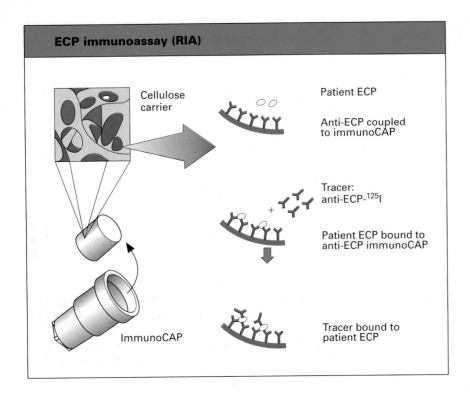

ECP immunoassay (RIA)

Cellulose carrier

Patient ECP

Anti-ECP coupled to immunoCAP

Tracer: anti-ECP-^{125}I

Patient ECP bound to anti-ECP immunoCAP

ImmunoCAP

Tracer bound to patient ECP

Fig. 4.5.3. In the Pharmacia CAP system, ECP RIA, the solid phase consists of a cellulose sponge placed in a plastic capsule. The radioactive tracer in the RIA can be replaced by a fluorescent agent (FEIA). A nearly identical system is used for determination of total IgE and of IgE antibody, as described earlier.

chopulmonary   aspergillosis   (1000–2000/mm³). Higher levels are suggestive of the other diseases mentioned.

Eosinopenic factors

Factors that reduce the number of eosinophils in the blood include acute *infection*, all types of *stress*, *fasting* more than 12–24 hours and *drugs*. The eosinopenic effect of *corticosteroids* is pronounced and well known; it may mask an eosinophilia. Oral steroids induce eosinopenia by systemic activity and by an anti-inflammatory effect in the bronchi with decreased eosinophil recruitment. Topical steroids predominantly induce a fall in the eosinophil count by the latter mode of action.

Soluble markers of allergic inflammation

The conventional way to assess and confirm an increased inflammatory activity in the body is to measure various acute-phase reactants (erythrocyte sedimentation rate, C-reactive protein, orosomucoid, etc.). However, the inflammation in atopic allergic disease does not give rise to increased synthesis of acute-phase proteins. In this type of inflammation, the eosinophil and the mast cell are the most notable cells. As they become activated, degranulate, and release mediators and proteins, measurement of these molecules in the circulation or other body fluids seems to be a rational way of making a diagnosis of allergic inflammatory reactions, in order to monitor disease activity and to adjust anti-inflammatory therapy.

Eosinophil markers – eosinophil cationic protein (ECP)

In allergic inflammation, eosinophils occur in increased numbers in blood, tissue and secretions, and they show signs of activation with release of their cytotoxic proteins, major basic protein (MBP), ECP, EPO and EPX. A commercially available immunoassay exists for the determination of ECP (Fig. 4.5.3). The amount of ECP measured in serum consists of *in vivo* released, free plasma ECP and *in vitro* released ECP from activated ('primed') eosinophils during coagulation.

ECP reflects asthma severity

In asthma, the ECP level in serum reflects the severity of the inflammation, and it correlates with the following disease activity parameters: 1, the lung function as evaluated by repeated PEF measurements; 2, the reactivity to inhaled histamine; 3, the tendency to develop exercise-induced bronchoconstriction (Fig. 4.5.4); and 4, the propensity for developing a late response to allergen challenge.

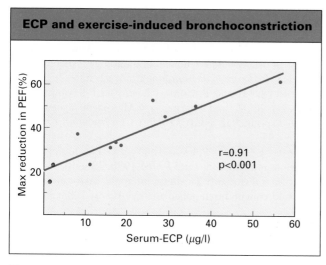

ECP and exercise-induced bronchoconstriction

r=0.91
p<0.001

Fig. 4.5.4. There is a positive linear correlation between the PEF reduction after exercise and the prechallenge serum ECP levels. From Venge P, Henriksen J, Dahl R. Eosinophils in exercise-induced asthma. *J Allergy Clin Immunol* 1991; **88**: 699–704.

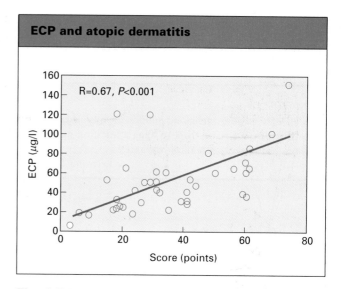

ECP and atopic dermatitis

R=0.67, P<0.001

Fig. 4.5.5. Correlation of serum ECP and the activity of atopic dermatitis expressed by clinical score points. From Czech W, Krutmann J, Schöpf E, Kapp A. Serum eosinophil cationic protein (ECP) is a sensitive measure for disease activity in atopic dermatitis. *Br J Dermatol* 1992; **83**: 1519–26.

Allergen exposure increases ECP

The ECP level is elevated during the late response to an allergen inhalation challenge. During the pollen season, there is an increase in serum and nasal lavage ECP. When mite-allergic asthmatic children stay at high altitudes in order to escape mite exposure, the ECP level decreases.

ECP and treatment

Inhaled steroids prevent both the late response to allergen and the associated increase in serum ECP. In clinical asthma, ECP decreases with the symptoms during treatment with inhaled steroid in a dose-dependent manner.

These findings indicate that the most important role for ECP measurement may be to serve as *an indicator of adequate steroid treatment* in order to avoid either over- or under-treatment.

Immunotherapy can also inhibit the ECP increase during the pollen season, which may be an important mode of action of the type of treatment.

ECP and atopic dermatitis

Studies on patients with atopic dermatitis have shown deposition of ECP in eczematous skin and elevated serum levels, which correlate with disease activity (Fig. 4.5.5). These studies suggest a pathogenetic role for cytotoxic eosinophil proteins in the skin lesions of atopic dermatitis, and indicate that

ECP measurements may be of clinical value in the evaluation of the disease activity and the need for anti-inflammatory treatment.

Problems

Although the use of ECP as a marker of allergic inflammation is a very tempting approach, it is too early to judge the clinical usefulness of this test, and there are some unanswered questions. 1, It is not definitely proven that ECP can give clinically more valuable information than repeated counting of eosinophils. 2, It is uncertain whether the examination of tissue fluid (sputum, BAL, nasal lavage fluid and skin blister fluid) can be more informative than the study of serum. 3, The blood sample must be handled in a strictly standardized way as the serum ECP level changes during coagulation.

Mast cell markers – tryptase

Histamine is an unreliable measure of mast cell/basophil degranulation. Tryptase, on the other hand, is a good indicator of mast cell degranulation. In can be identified in lavage fluid during the early response to allergen challenge in the airways, but, so far, studies during natural allergen exposure have failed to show increased values.

Raised serum values are found during anaphylactic reactions. With the exception of differentiating between an anaphylactic reaction and other systemic reactions, the measurement of tryptase has not yet shown clinical usefulness.

Also valid for allergy

In all affairs, love, religion, politics or business, it's a healthy idea, now and then, to hang a question mark on things you have long taken for granted.

Bertrand Russell

Further reading

ANONYMOUS, From the Board of Directors. American Academy of Allergy and Clinical Immunology. Allergen skin testing. *J Allergy Clin Immunol* 1933; **92**: 636–7.

BOUSQUET J, CHANEZ P, CHANAL I, MICHEL F-B. Comparison between RAST and Pharmacia CAP system: a new automated specific IgE assay. *J Allergy Clin Immunol* 1990; **85**: 1039–45.

BOUSQUET J, CHANEZ P, LACOSTE JY, *et al*. Eosinophil inflammation in asthma. *N Engl J Med* 1990; **323**: 1033–9.

DREBORG S, FOUCARD T. Allergy to apple, carrot and potato in children with birch pollen allergy. *Allergy* 1983; **38**: 167–171.

DREBORG S, FREW A. Position paper: allergen standardization and skin tests. *Allergy* 1993; **48**(suppl 14): 49–82.

EWAN PW, COOTE D. Evaluation of a capsulated hydrophillic carrier polymer (the ImmunoCAP) for measurement of specific IgE antibodies. *Allergy* 1990; **45**: 22–9.

HANSEN LG, HØST A, HALKEN S, *et al*. Cord blood IgE. III. Prediction of IgE high-response and allergy. A follow-up at the age of 18 months. *Allergy* 1992; **47**: 404–10.

KAPP A. The role of eosinophils in the pathogenesis of atopic dermatitis – eosinophil granule proteins as markers of disease activity. *Allergy* 1993; **48**: 1–5.

KJELLMAN NIM. IgE in neonates is not suitable for general allergy screening. *Pediatr Allergy Immunol* 1994; **5**: 1–4.

MAPP CE, PLEBANI M, FAGGIAN D, *et al*. Eosinophil cationic protein (ECP), histamine and tryptase in peripheral blood before and during inhalation challenge with toluene diisocyanate (TDI) in sensitized subjects. *Clin Exp Allergy* 1994; **24**: 730–6.

NACLERIO RM, NORMAN PS, FISH JE. *In vivo* methods for the study of allergy. In: Middleton E, Reed CE, Adkinson NF, Yunginger JW, Busse WW, eds. *Allergy. Principles and Practice* 4th ed. St Louis: Mosby, 1993; 595–627.

VENGE P. Soluble markers of allergic inflammation. *Allergy* 1994; **49**: 1–8.

Part 5 Gastro-intestinal Reactions and Food Sensitivity

5.1 The gastro-intestinal tract and immunology

Tolerance, IgA protection and IgE allergy

Key points

- Most protein antigens in the food are broken down by digestive enzymes.
- Anatomical and immunological barriers reduce absorption of protein antigens.
- Protein in mother's milk is absorbed in infants, but, at the age of 3 months, intestinal closure for antigens occurs.
- Gut-associated lymph tissue (GALT) consists of Peyer's patches, intra-epithelial lymphocytes, and lymphocytes in lamina propria.
- Peyer's patches are a major site of antigen entry into the GALT.
- Intra-epithelial lymphocytes are mainly CD8+ T cells, and antigen stimulation may induce immunological tolerance.
- Lamina propria T cells are mainly CD4+ cells and antigen stimulation induces IgG and IgE responses and inflammation.
- Antigen-stimulated T cells circulate and return to mucous-membrane-associated lymphoid tissue, preferentially to the tissue in which they encountered antigen (homing).
- APCs are follicular dendritic cells, interdigitating cells and macrophages.
- A secretory IgA response is protective, possibly reducing antigen penetration.
- A moderate IgG response, for example to cow's milk, is normal.
- An exaggerated IgG response, by a Type III-like reaction, may play a role in adverse reactions to food.
- An IgE response and a Type I reaction are important in allergic reactions to food.
- Activated T cells are present in the lamina propria in cow's milk allergy, but their pathogenetic role is uncertain.

Food allergy: a controversial subject

The concept that certain foods can produce abnormal reactions in susceptible individuals has a long history, the aphorism 'one man's meat is another man's poison' being attributed to Lucretius (100 BC). Nev-
ertheless, the idea of adverse reactions to food evokes considerable controversy. Some laymen and physicians relate every conceivable symptom (behavioural problems, hyperactivity in children, fatigue–tension syndrome in adults, irritable bowel syndrome, migraine, enuresis and otitis media) to 'food allergy', while some academicians think it a subject beyond the fringe of clinical credibility.

There is a wide discrepancy between the public perception of food-induced reactions and the medical profession's view of the problem. About 5% of an adult population claim that they react adversely to specific foods, but it is only a minority of these cases that can be confirmed by objective testing.

Antigen digestion and absorption

Protein antigens in food are initially acted on by stomach acid, and pepsin, pancreatic enzymes and intestinal peptidases. Many large molecules are broken down into small peptides and amino acids. Mucosal epithelial cell enzymes further degrade the absorbed peptides into amino acids.

The amount of antigenic material absorbed is limited by *anatomical barriers* (mucus layer and epithelium) and by *immunological barriers* (secretory IgA). Digestion and barrier mechanisms may reduce the antigen access to the immune system.

In immature mucous membranes, the epithelial cells can, by endocytosis, take up macromolecules without decomposing them, and protein molecules are, in unchanged form, transported to the portal circulation. This property is important in the absorption of maternal immunoglobulins, but it diminishes at about the age of 3 months, when intestinal closure for antigens is said to occur. However, small amounts of intact protein can be absorbed in adults.

The intestinal immune system

An immunologist may picture the gastro-intestinal tract as a tube of epithelium that separates highly immunogenic antigens in the lumen from immunoreactive cells in the surrounding lamina propia. Indeed, the gastro-intestinal mucosa contains most of the lymphoid tissue in the body and the gut lumen is filled with dietary and bacterial antigens. Normally the intestinal immune system steers a delicate course between undesirable extremes of immune incompetence and hypersensitivity; it is remarkable how the mucosal immune system is capable of producing an effective immune response without destroying the fragile mucosal barrier.

While the airway of an atopic individual is sensitized by nanograms of inhaled allergens (see Chapter 3.1), the gastro-intestinal tract is daily loaded with grams of allergenic material.

Lymphocytes

There exists a common mucous-membrane-associated lymphoid tissue (MALT) of which the gut-associated lymphoid tissue (GALT) is the quantitatively most important part. Basically, GALT has three components: 1, Peyer's patches; 2, intra-epithelial lymphocytes; and 3, lymphocytes in the lamina propria.

Peyer's patches

These organized lymphocyte aggregates are believed to be a major site of antigen entry into the mucosal immune system. Peyer's patches, in a number of 20–30, occur in the more distal gut regions (ileum), which is below the principal digestive sites in the proximal gut.

A Peyer's patch consists of a germinal centre (particularly with B cells), a parafollicular area (with T cells) and a dome area (Fig. 5.1.1). The patches are covered by a specialized epithelium (follicle-associated epithelium) containing M cells (microfold cells). These thin epithelial cells pinocytose macromolecules and allow them to traverse the epithelial barrier and closely contact the macrophages and T cells. M cells, which lack MHC class II molecules, cannot present antigen but merely provide close physical contact.

Intra-epithelial lymphocytes

Such cells are frequent in the gut where they occupy 10% of the total epithelial cell mass. They are all T cells and the majority (around 80%) have the supressor-cytotoxic phenotype (CD8+). Studies have indicated suppressor and memory functions for these cells and they do not appear to be cytotoxic.

Intra-epithelial T cells have now been identified as a specific lymphocyte population, recognition being based on their expression of a specific membrane receptor (human mucosal lymphocyte receptor or HML-1). These cells are frequently seen in close association with antigen-presenting macrophages, which lie in the lamina propria adjacent to the basement membrane of the epithelium (Fig. 5.1.1).

Antigen presentation for the intra-epithelial CD8+ suppressor T lymphocytes will result in a down-regulation of the immune response and possibly in the development of immunological tolerance (see later).

Lamina propria lymphocytes

The lamina propria contains both B and T cells; the majority of the T cells are of the helper phenotype (CD4+). Thus, while the function of T cells in the epithelium is suppressive, the predominant function of lamina propria T cells is immunological help, implying a potentiality for an IgG or IgE response and subsequent risk of mucosal inflammation.

Lymphocyte traffic and circulation

Once activated by antigen in the gut, B and T cells migrate to the mesenteric lymph nodes and, subsequently, enter the systemic circulation via the thoracic duct (Fig. 5.1.1). The lymphocytes then extravasate from blood to tissue, exhibiting a remarkable selective migratory return to the tissues in which they originally encountered antigen. This process, called *homing*, is due to expression of a lymphocyte homing receptor (CD44), which binds selectively to ligands on endothelial cells in the mucous membrane of the gut.

Many similarities exist between the mucosal lymphoid tissue of the gut and that of organs, such as the airways, salivary glands and breast. Lymphocytes from any of these sites will populate all mucosa-associated lymphoid tissue, with a preference for the organ of origin, and MALT can be considered as a functional unit within the immune system.

Antigen-presenting cells

There are numerous APCs in the gut; their presence may be due to the high level of dietary antigen at this site. There are different types of APCs: 1, follicular dendritic cells, which facilitate B-cell responses and occur within the germinal centres of Peyer's patches; 2, interdigitating cells, which facilitate T-cell responses and occur diffusely throughout the lamina propria, within parafollicular regions and beneath the dome epithelium of Peyer's patches; and 3, macrophages.

The intestinal immune response

Antigen presentation by these cells may mediate: 1, an IgA response; 2, an IgG response; 3, an IgE response; 4, a T-cell response; and 5, tolerance (Fig. 5.1.2).

IgA response – normal protection

B lymphocytes, presented for antigen in the Peyer's patches, generate a predominantly IgA immune response, once back in the gut. The number of IgA-

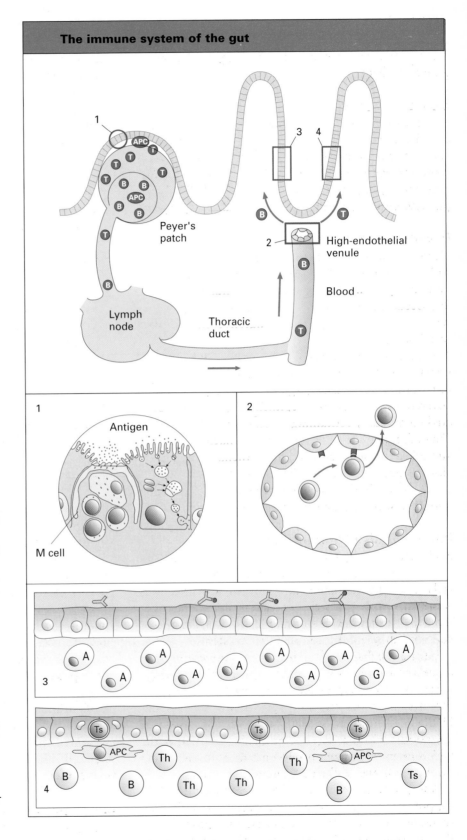

The immune system of the gut

Fig. 5.1.1. 1, Antigen is taken up by M cells in the epithelium and is presented for the immune system in a Peyer's patch. Proteins, ingested by other epithelial cells, are broken down to peptides by lysosomal enzymes. Activated lymphocytes travel via the lymphatics to regional lymph nodes and in the thoracic duct to the blood. 2, They 'home' selectively in mucosal blood vessels due to 'homing receptors' with affinity for ligands in high-endothelial venules. 3, The homing lymphocytes develop into IgA-producing plasma cells, and secretory IgA binds antigens in the surface mucus layer. 4, Intra-epithelial lymphocytes, which are of the CD8+ T suppressor type, are in close contact with APCs. The lamina propria lymphocytes are both B and T cells, with a predominance of CD4+ T helper cells.

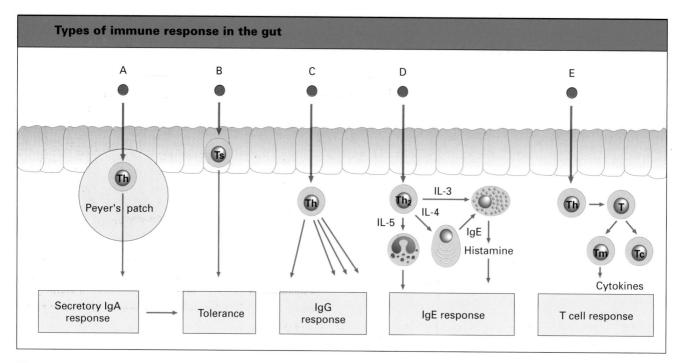

Fig. 5.1.2. (A) Antigen recognition in a Peyer's patch results in a protective secretory IgA response. (B) Antigen presentation for the intra-epithelial CD8+ T suppressor cells results in the development of specific tolerance to the antigen. (C–E) Excessive antigen exposure, and/or a defective epithelial barrier, facilitates antigen presentation for T helper cells in the lamina propria. (C) A normal IgG response or an excessive and pathogenetic IgG response. (D) Stimulation of Th₂ cells in lamina propria results in IgE formation. The inflammatory events are deduced from changes in the skin and airways. (E) A pathogenic T cell response, which, by cytotoxic effector cells and cytokines, contributes to tissue damage in inflammatory intestinal diseases.

producing plasma cells in the lamina propria (85%) far exceeds the numbers synthesizing IgM (10%), IgG (4%), IgD (<1%) and IgE (<<1%).

Secretory IgA, as the major immunoglobulin isotype at mucosal surfaces, serves to protect the mucosa from colonization and invasion by infectious agents. Its role is clearly protective and, as it cannot fix complement or bind to mast cells, it plays little or no role in harmful hypersensitivity responses.

Secretory IgA antibody can *combine with antigen on the epithelial surface* and, in this way, it probably plays a role in *reducing allergen penetration* (Fig. 5.1.1).

The IgA immune system is poorly developed at birth; the number of IgA-producing cells and the concentration of secretory IgA increase slowly during childhood.

IgG response – Type III hypersensitivity

Normal response. Normally, small amounts of dietary proteins can appear antigenically intact in the circulation so the ingestion of food antigens (e.g. cow's milk protein) will result in an IgG immune response. Indeed, all healthy people develop and maintain high levels of IgG antibodies to specific food antigens, and circulating immune complexes, between IgG and dietary antigens, are regularly found after meals. Such immune complexes are rapidly cleared by the reticulo-endothelial system and are, in the majority of cases, of no pathological significance.

Exaggerated response. When antigen or antibody is in excess, there can, at least in theory, be a deposition of immune complexes in blood vessels, skin, kidney and joints (serum sickness or Arthus'-type reaction).

Some observations suggest that IgG-mediated, Type III-like reactions can play a primary role in some cases of adverse reactions to foods, and a secondary role in inflammatory bowel diseases, due to the increased epithelial permeability. The pathogenic role of IgG, however, is difficult to evaluate as IgG antibodies to food occur as a normal phenomenon.

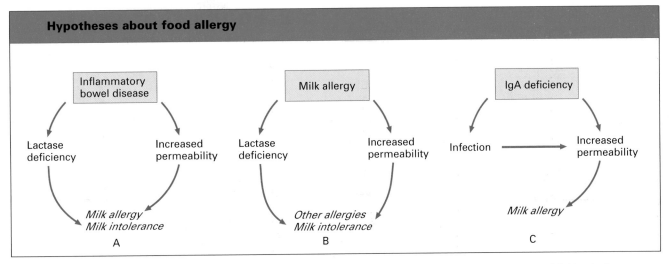

Hypotheses about food allergy

Fig. 5.1.3. Hypotheses for the pathogenesis of food allergy and its inter-relationships with other enteropathies. (A) An inflammatory bowel disease increases the epithelial permeability and with that the risk of food allergy, for example to milk. Mucosal damage and lactase deficiency result in lactose and milk intolerance. (B) Food allergy as an example of an inflammatory disease, which starts a vicious circle. (C) IgA deficiency increases the risk of food allergy.

IgE response – Type I hypersensitivity

Little is known for certain about the pathogenesis of IgE-mediated, allergic gastro-intestinal diseases. However, mast cells, which are of the MC_T or mucosal mast cell type, are certainly involved (Fig. 5.1.2). In favour of this statement is the observation of increased levels of plasma histamine following a positive oral food challenge.

The release of histamine and other inflammatory mediators may have a profound effect on gut function. There occurs an outpouring of mucus, and an increase in epithelial permeability and intestinal movement, leading to diarrhoea.

T-cell response

With large numbers of MHC class II⁺ APCs in the lamina propria adjacent to CD4⁺ T helper cells, antigen crossing from the gut lumen may be able to initiate a primary T-cell response, consisting of development of effector cells and cytokine production.

Experimental studies suggest that T cell activation can induce histological lesions, and there is little doubt that T cells can be involved in intestinal pathology. However, the direct evidence for T-cell immunity as a cause of the lesion in food-sensitive enteropathies is scant. Activated T cells (CD25⁺) are present in the lamina propria in cow's milk protein allergy, coeliac disease and Crohn's disease.

Oral tolerance

The induction of immunological tolerance by an orally introduced antigen is a well-established phenomenon in experimental animals. Various effector mechanisms have been described and one of them is the antigen induction of CD8⁺ T cells with suppressor function in the intestinal epithelium. Although there is no unequivocal evidence for the role of intra-epithelial lymphocytes in the development or maintenance of oral tolerance, their phenotype and proximity to both MHC class II⁺ APCs in the epithelium and the underlying mucosal immune system make them likely candidates.

Development of allergy

Why some individuals develop food allergy is unknown but it usually occurs within *the first months of life*, and exposure to potent allergens in this 'vulnerable period' seems to be of importance. Antigen absorption and stimulation of lymphocytes in the lamina propria is probably facilitated by: 1, *increased permeability* of the mucous membrane; and 2, *immaturity of the immune system*, with a physiological *IgA deficiency* (Fig. 5.1.2). Closure of the mucous membrane and maturation of the immune system during the first months of life may also explain the high remission rate of food allergy during childhood.

It is known that excessive uptake of dietary antigens, for example during an *inflammatory bowel disease*, increases the formation of IgG antibody, and IgE-mediated food allergy increases gut permeability. However, there is no definite proof that increased uptake of antigen plays a role in the development of food allergy, although it is a likely hypothesis (Fig. 5.1.3).

A miracle!
For the immunologist it is a miracle how man can survive the process of eating.

JF Soothill
Childrens' Hospital, London

5.2 Foods that cause adverse reactions
Milk and eggs most important

Key points
- Adverse reactions to food consist of food allergy and food intolerance (no immunological aetiology).
- Sensitizing allergens are usually those that are ingested frequently, and are heat and acid stable.
- Cow's milk, causing gastro-intestinal, skin and airway symptoms, is a prime offender in infancy, while milk allergy is rare in adults.
- Allergy to hen's eggs (egg white) is important, especially in children.
- Fish contains very potent allergens (50% react to all and 50% tolerate some species).
- Eating fish can, within minutes, cause angioedema, urticaria, gastro-intestinal symptoms, asthma and anaphylactic reactions.
- Wheat, rye and barley are occasionally involved in allergic reactions in which gastro-intestinal symptoms predominate.
- The peanut is a potent allergen capable of eliciting life-threatening anaphylactic reactions.
- Soyabean products, used in a growing number of foods, can cause allergic reactions.
- Shellfish are noted for their tendency to cause violent allergic reactions of the urticaria/angioedema type.
- Cashew nut can cause severe anaphylactic reactions.
- Hazel nut causes itching in the mouth and throat in birch-pollen-allergic patients.
- Fresh fruit and vegetables often cause 'oral allergy syndrome' in pollen-allergic patients.
- Beverages often precipitate symptoms in the gastro-intestinal tract, skin and airways by a variety of mechanisms.
- Sulphite, added to salad bar lettuce, can cause life-threatening asthma and anaphylaxis.
- Foods can contain biologically active agents (e.g. histamine in dark-flesh fish).

Terminology
It is common knowledge that some people become ill, repeatedly and predictably, when they eat certain foods. Laymen will usually call this 'food allergy'. As adverse reactions to food can be based both on an immunological and on a non-immunological mech-

anism, the physician should try to distinguish between *food allergy* (immunological aetiology proven or likely) and *food intolerance* (immunological aetiology unproven or unlikely).

Food antigens

In principle, virtually any food can cause adverse reactions but, in practice, the number of quantitatively important foods is limited.

Sensitizing antigens or allergens are usually *those which are ingested frequently* so the local diet influences the prevalence of specific food hypersensitivity. Allergy to peanuts and to soyabeans is, for example, more frequent in the USA than in Europe.

Foods are complex mixtures of a series of allergenic molecules; they are less well described than inhalant allergens. Food allergens are *water-soluble proteins*, with molecular weights in the range of 10–40kDa, and most allergens are *heat and acid stable*. Some fruits and vegetables, however, only cause symptoms in the mouth and throat, because they loose their allergenicity on acid and enzymatic digestion.

Cow's milk protein

Cow's milk is a prime offender in *infancy*, causing *gastro-intestinal, skin and airway symptoms*. It remains a major cause of allergy into early childhood, while allergy to milk is rare in adulthood.

There are at least 20 proteins in cow's milk but only five are of special allergenic significance. These include β-lactoglobulin, α-lactalbumin, casein, bovine serum albumin and immunoglobulins. Reaction to a single allergen is exceptional; two or more proteins are usually involved. Of great importance is β-lactoglobulin, which is *resistant to heating* so cooking milk will seldom reduce its allergenicity.

Patients allergic to cow's milk are not usually allergic to beef protein (although there is albumin in a rare steak) or to inhalation of cow dander but they will react to *goat's milk*.

IgE antibody can be demonstrated in most patients with clinical sensitivity to cow's milk protein. It is postulated that precipitating *IgG antibody* plays a role in some cases, but it is difficult to prove as development of IgG antibodies is a normal response.

Hen's eggs

Together with cow's milk, eggs are of outstanding importance both in nutrition and in allergy, especially in children. The major allergens, *ovomucoid and ovalbumin*, are contained in the egg white, while egg yolk only contains some minor allergens. Like β-lactoglobulin in milk, ovomucoid is *resistant to heat*, acid and proteolytic enzymes, while ovalbumin is relatively heat labile. Most allergic persons will therefore react to both raw and cooked eggs. Patients allergic to egg usually tolerate chicken meat but not *vaccines grown on egg*.

Fish

Fish contains *very potent allergens* and a challenge test can be dangerous. The major allergen in cod muscle (allergen M or *Gad c* I) was the first allergen to be isolated as a pure fraction. Fish contains both common allergens and species-specific allergens. About 50% of fish-allergic patients react to all species, while 50% tolerate some species of fish. Fish allergens are *resistant to heat* and the patients react both to raw and cooked fish.

The diagnosis of fish allergy is easy as all cases are *IgE mediated*. Eating fish can, within minutes, cause angioedema, urticaria, gastro-intestinal symptoms, asthma and anaphylactic reactions. Inhaled emanations from fish, such as steam from cooking, causes asthma in very sensitive patients. Even kissing a person who has had a fish meal can cause problems.

Cereals

Cereal grains (wheat, rye, barley, oat, corn and rice) account for 70% of the world's food protein. They are occasionally involved in allergic reactions in which gastro-intestinal symptoms predominate.

Wheat, rye and *barley* all belong to the same family and they exhibit pronounced cross-reactivity.

Wheat flour protein consists of about 20 allergens so individual variability is considerable. Digestion with proteolytic enzymes in the gastro-intestinal tract markedly reduces the allergenicity of wheat protein. Wheat flour proteins can cause three types of disease: 1, gluten enteropathy (coeliac disease); 2, inhalant allergy (baker's asthma); and 3, food allergy. A patient with inhalant allergy may not react to ingestion of the allergen and vice versa.

Corn (maize) allergy is rare but problematic to manage as corn products are used in a wide variety of foods (processed meats, peanut butter, jam and jelly, cheese, ice-cream, biscuits, cakes and sweets).

Rice belongs to another tribe and sensitization is rare. Rice forms the staple diet of one-half of the world's population but very little has been published on allergy to rice.

Legumes

Legumes are seed plants, which include peanuts, soyabeans, peas, lentils and beans.

Peanuts

The peanut, which is not a nut, has long been noted as a *potent allergen* capable of eliciting life-threatening *anaphylactic reactions*. Unfortunately, the peanut maintains its allergenicity after roasting. While the allergen is obvious in roasted peanuts and in peanut butter, it can be hidden from the patient as a nutritional supplement added to a series of foods.

Soyabean

The soyabean is an increasingly important source of protein. Soya products are being used *in a growing number of foods* (e.g. burgers and pre-cooked meals), and it can be difficult for the patient to identify the allergen and avoid exposure. Soya is a potent allergen, which can cause anaphylaxis in exquisitely sensitive individuals.

Shellfish

Shellfish include two families; crustaceans (shrimps, prawns, crabs, lobsters and crayfish) and molluscs (clams, scallops, oysters and mussels). Most important are the *crustaceans*. Allergens in this family are usually shared by all or most of the members. Crustaceans are noted for their tendency to cause violent allergic reactions of the *urticaria/angioedema* type and occasional anaphylactic reactions. The reaction is *IgE mediated* and the diagnosis is easy, usually made by the patient.

Nuts

Nuts will often give rise to *IgE-mediated allergy*. Reactions to cashew nut are *occasionally anaphylactic*, and deaths have been described. Allergy to hazel nut (and walnut) is very common in subjects with *birch pollen allergy*. The main symptom is *itching in the mouth and throat*.

Fruits and vegetables

The symptoms of allergy to fruits and vegetables are usually confined to the *mouth and throat*, probably due to enzymatic digestion in the gastrointestinal tract. Many of these allergens are *heat-*

Allergen cross-reactivity	
Pollen	**Fruit/vegetable/nut**
Birch	Hazel nut Apple Peach Cherry Walnut Pear Almond Plum Kiwi Potato peel Brazil nut Cashew nut Tomato Carrot
Grass	Bean Lentil Green pea
Mugwort	Celery Parsley Chives Banana Melon Parsnip Vermouth*
Ragweed	Watermelon Honey dew melon Cantaloupe Banana Zucchina squash Cucumber

Table 5.2.1. Common sensitivities to fruit and vegetables in pollen-allergic subjects due to common epitopes. *Contains the pollen allergen

labile and loose their activity when cooked, frozen or tinned.

This *'fruit-and-vegetable syndrome'* or *'oral allergy syndrome'* is frequent in pollen-allergic patients due to common epitopes (Table 5.2.1). Patients with *birch pollen allergy* are often sensitive to fresh *apple, peach, pear, carrot* and others, in various combinations; scraping *new potatoes* can cause sneezing or wheezing. *Ragweed-allergic subjects* will often report itching in the throat from eating *banana and melon*, and *mugwort allergy* is associated with reactions to celery.

Citrus fruits are common causes of skin rashes, especially around the mouth, in infants and children with atopic dermatitis.

Beverages

Alcoholic drinks often precipitate symptoms in patients with disease of the gastro-intestinal tract, skin and airways. They contain a series of *biologically active molecules*, dyes, preservatives (SO_2) and, occasionally, allergens. In the general population, *alcoholism* is a far more common cause of gastro-intestinal symptoms and diarrhoea than food allergy or intolerance.

Diarrhoea in children and youngsters, drinking large amounts of fruit juice, may be due to an osmotic effect of the fructose ('toddler's diarrhoea'). Soft drinks often contain a high concentration of artificial dyes, allowing 'lemonades' to be used for challenge tests.

Food additives

Tartrazine and other dyes

Tartrazine (yellow dye no. 5) has been accused of causing urticaria, angioedema and deterioration of atopic dermatitis, urticaria and asthma. However, it has been very difficult to confirm this by controlled challenge tests.

Sulphites

The Romans burned sulphur to produce SO_2, which was then bubbled through wine to prevent further fermentation and inhibit microbial contamination. Today, sulphites, which liberate SO_2, are widely used in foods as preservatives and as an antioxidant to inhibit browning in food. There are high contents of sulphites in *salad bar lettuce*, *wine*, *dried fruits*, citrus juice and dried potatoes.

Exposure to large amounts of sulphites is most likely to occur *in restaurants*, where many foods, especially salads, are sprayed or otherwise treated with sulphites to maintain a fresh appearance. Sulphited lettuce, for example, appears to be particularly provocative because there is nothing in lettuce to react with a sulphiting agent and transform it into a more innocuous substance.

While most asthmatics with hyper-responsive airways can react with bronchoconstriction to large doses of sulphites, a small subgroup reacts with *life-threatening asthma or anaphylaxis* to low doses. Such exquisitely sensitive patients typically have a history of one or more severe reactions in restaurants ('salad bar syndrome').

Benzoates and parabens

These two preservatives are both added to various foods. Their use has occasionally been associated with urticaria and asthma but intolerance to these preservatives is probably rare. Parabens are also widely used as antimicrobial agents in pharmaceutical and cosmetic creams, and there is an extensive literature on paraben-induced allergic contact eczema (Type IV allergy).

Monosodium glutamate

Seaweed has long been used throughout Asia in food preparation to enhance flavour. The active component is monosodium glutamate, which is now widely used as a flavour enhancer in a variety of manufactured and restaurant food. Its use is no longer limited to Asian cooking.

Adverse reactions to large amounts of monosodium glutamate, for example in Wonton soup, was first described as the 'Chinese restaurant syndrome'. Symptoms consisted of headache, a burning sensation along the neck and back, chest tightness, nausea and sweating. It was later shown that some asthmatic patients react with bronchoconstriction to monosodium glutamate, *'Chinese restaurant asthma'*. It is probably due to a neuroexitatory effect that monosodium glutamate causes symptoms and asthma. The onset of symptoms is often delayed for some hours after the meal.

Biologically active agents

Foods often contain biologically active molecules. Large amounts of free *histamine* occur in tuna fish, mackerel, other fish with dark flesh and old cheese. Certain foods have a *histamine-releasing activity* (strawberries, tomatoes and oranges). *Lectins*, found in a series of vegetables, fruits and cereals, can cause histamine release by non-specific binding to mast cell fixed IgE. Other *vasoactive amines* (tyramine and phenylethylamine), which are found in chocolate, red wine and old cheese, can cause headache and urticaria. Also *toxins* and *micro-organisms* must be considered causes of food-induced symptoms.

Gluten intolerance

Gluten-induced enteropathy (coeliac disease and sprue) usually presents in the first year of life, but milder cases are often first diagnosed in adults. The patients have a persistent *intolerance to the gluten protein, gliadin*. The disease is *associated with an IgG response* to this protein. Recent evidence strongly indicates that *T cell activation* plays a role in the pathogenesis and in tissue damage. Interestingly, there is an over-representation of a certain HLA type (A1, B8 and DRw17), often associated with autoimmune disease. The diagnosis is based on the *malabsorption symptoms*, an *intestinal biopsy* (atrophy of intestinal villi) and clinical improvement on a *gluten-free diet* (no wheat and no rye).

Lactase deficiency

In a *hereditary form*, this is a rare cause of lactose intolerance and enteropathy. An *acquired deficiency* is more common; it is secondary to mucosal damage, found in patients with inflammatory changes in the intestine (milk allergy, gluten intolerance, ulcerative colitis and kwashiorkor). Lactase deficiency, lactose intolerance and associated milk-induced gastro-enteropathy will disappear following successful treatment of the underlying disease.

Prolonged milk avoidance in adults is a common cause of lactose intolerance (atrophy of the lactase-producing system). The majority of adult African and Asian people produce very little lactase and cannot tolerate the quantities of cow's milk that are commonly consumed in Europe and North America.

Poison or allergy?

What's one man's poison, signor, is another's meat and drink.

Lucretius, 100 BC
Love's Cure

5.3 Food-induced symptoms and diseases
– in gastro-intestinal tract, skin and airways

Key points
- Symptoms caused by food allergy typically involve more than one organ system.
- Food allergy is more important in children than in adults.
- Cow's milk is an important cause of gastro-intestinal symptoms in infants (vomiting, colic and diarrhoea).
- Milk sensitivity occurs in 2% (challenge test) to 6% (case history) of all infants.
- Allergy to cow's milk develops in infancy and usually disappears in childhood.
- Other food allergies develop later and may continue indefinitely.
- Anaphylaxis may be caused by milk, egg, peanuts, soyabean, nut, shellfish, fish and sulphites.
- It can have a delayed onset (1–2 hours) and only develop when food consumption is followed by exercise.
- Unfortunately, the first symptoms, pruritus in the mouth and throat, are often neglected by the patient.
- About 30% of atopic dermatitis children and 10% of asthmatic children appear to have some adverse reactions to food.
- In atopic dermatitis, foods may induce itching and urticaria but they are not the cause of eczema and skin dryness.
- Food allergy is a frequent cause of acute urticaria/angioedema but a very rare cause of chronic disease.
- Occasional ingestion of an allergenic food can cause an acute attack of asthma, which can be fatal.
- Daily ingestion of food as a cause of chronic airway symptoms occurs occasionally in infants but rarely in adults.
- Rhinitis almost never occurs as the only manifestation of food allergy or intolerance.

Organs involved
Food-induced symptoms are not limited to the gut, and *food allergy* is not synonymous with *gastro-intestinal allergy*. The *gastro-intestinal tract* is affected in most cases; the *skin* is frequently involved and the *airways* is occasionally involved. Involvement of

more than one organ system is typical of food sensitivity. Symptoms attributed to food allergy/intolerance are legion but in many instances the cause–effect relationship has been poorly documented. This chapter will be confined to symptoms, and diseases, which have been associated with food, in studies using controlled challenge tests.

Frequency

A positive case history of cow's milk-induced symptoms occurs in 6–8% of all infants, but studies using controlled challenges have shown milk sensitivity in only 2%. About 10% of *asthmatic children* and 30% of *atopic dermatitis children* appear to have some adverse reactions to food. The frequency *decreases considerably with age*, and food reactions are rare in adults. While a considerable number of people have occasional episodes of food-induced symptoms, it is seldom that adverse reactions to food account for symptoms occurring daily.

Natural history

Allergy to cow's milk *develops in infancy*, while allergy to fruit usually makes its first appearance in adolescence. Sensitivity to some foods *often disappears with age*, especially cow's milk (90% at 3 years of age), soyabean (90% at 5 years) and eggs (50% at 5 years), whereas sensitivity to others, such as fish, shellfish, peanuts and nuts, usually persists.

Anaphylaxis

Causes

Almost any food may cause anaphylactic reactions but those most commonly responsible are *milk, egg, peanuts and soyabean* in children, and *peanuts, nut, shellfish and fish* in adults. In the USA, peanuts are one of the most common food allergies and probably the most common cause of death by food-induced anaphylaxis. As a very potent allergen, peanuts can produce allergic reactions in milligram quantities.

The only food additive for which there is substantial evidence of causing fatal anaphylaxis is *sulphites.*

A small subset of cases of food-induced anaphylaxis occurs only when exercise follows food consumption, usually within 2 hours, *exercise-and-food anaphylaxis.*

Clinical features

An anaphylactic reaction can occur without any forewarning, but the food has often caused minor symptoms on an earlier occasion. Reactions can occur when a patient ingests a known allergen as a 'hidden additive' to a dish.

Symptoms can have an explosive *onset within minutes* or can be *delayed for up to 1–2 hours* after ingestion of the offending food. The *first symptoms* are usually *pruritus in the mouth and throat*. Unfortunately, patients may *neglect these symptoms*, which soon may be followed by *symptoms from the gut* (nausea, emesis, abdominal pain and diarrhoea), *the skin* (generalized pruritus, urticaria and angioedema), or *the airways* (sneezing, hoarseness and bronchospasm). *Circulatory collapse* and death may occur rapidly. The risk of death due to a food reaction is considerably increased *in asthma patients*.

Gastro-intestinal symptoms

Cow's milk, is by far the most important cause of gastro-intestinal symptoms. When breast-fed infants are weaned on to cow's milk adverse reactions will occur in about 2%. The most striking symptom is *vomiting*, followed by *abdominal cramps*, *diarrhoea* and screaming ('colic'). Recurrent vomiting and chronic diarrhoea can result in *failure to thrive*. In severe cases, *malabsorption* develops due to destruction of intestinal villi. Extreme sensitivity can occur with anaphylactic shock following a few drops of cow's milk. The importance of gastro-intestinal symptoms decreases considerably with age, and food allergy/intolerance is a rare cause of gastro-intestinal symptoms in adults.

The oral allergy syndrome

Oral symptoms are both *the most frequent* and *the first event* in an IgE-mediated reaction to food. *Itching* in the mouth occurs within minutes and is followed by *swelling* of the lips, mouth, throat and, perhaps, by a *circumoral rash* in infants. These symptoms are often produced by ingestion of fresh food, especially *nuts, fruits and vegetables* (which cross-react with pollens).

Atopic dermatitis

Many patients with atopic dermatitis have *positive skin tests* to food allergens. It is generally accepted that IgE-mediated food allergy can play a role in atopic dermatitis, but there is considerable *controversy* between dermatologists and allergists as to the percentage of patients affected and the significance of foods for the expression of symptoms and disease.

It may be a compromise to say that the *symptoms can be made worse* by the ingestion of certain foods in about 30% of children with atopic dermatitis. However, although ingestion of foods can induce *pruritus, skin rash and urticaria*, it is *not the cause of chronic eczema* and dry skin. Consequently, an elimination diet will not cure the patients and will rarely make them symptom-free.

Urticaria and angioedema

While most cases of *acute urticaria* can be ascribed to food allergy, this is rarely the case in *chronic urticaria* (probably only a small percentage). These patients usually believe that ingestion of food is the cause of their symptoms, and it is the physician's job to inform them that this is probably not the case.

A reaction to *NSAIDs* is a well-known cause of acute urticaria, such patients may, in rare cases, also react to dyes and preservatives in food.

Foods with a high content of *vasoactive peptides, histamine and histamine-liberators* (fish with dark flesh, strawberries and old cheese) can provoke symptoms in patients with chronic urticaria.

Asthma and rhinitis

When ingestion of an allergenic food causes asthma, it can either be: 1, *by absorption* of allergen, which reaches the airways with the circulation; 2, by an effect of mediators released in the gut; or 3, *by inhalations* of volatile food molecules.

Occasional ingestion of an allergenic food can cause an *acute attack of asthma*, which may be part of an anaphylactic reaction.

Daily ingestion of the food may result in *chronic airway symptoms*. This happens mainly *in infants and children* who suffer from asthma and atopic dermatitis. Food as a cause of chronic asthma decreases rapidly with age and seems to be very *rare in adults*.

Rhinitis almost never occurs as the only manifestation of food allergy or intolerance.

In conclusion, the role of food allergy in causing daily airway symptoms should not be overestimated, but a few food-sensitive asthma patients run a risk of dying from food allergy.

Non-pharmacological management
It is our duty to remember at all times that medicine is not only a science, but also the art of letting our own individuality interact with the individuality of the patient.
Albert Schweitzer

5.4 Diagnosis of food allergy and intolerance
Trial diet and double-blind food challenge

Key points
- First of all, exclude other diagnoses, for example gluten intolerance and lactose intolerance.
- Testing for food sensitivity is very time-consuming and demanding.
- When no particular food is incriminated, the diagnostic work will be difficult and a negative result the rule.
- Testing is relevant in infants with gastro-intestinal symptoms, in children with atopic dermatitis and chronic asthma, and in a few adults with severe disease.
- The usefulness of skin testing and RAST varies with symptoms and allergens.
- The diagnostic work consists of a run-in period, a diet period and food challenge.
- A food challenge test is required when symptoms improve on the trial diet.
- Testing is started with an open food challenge, and this is sufficient in infants.
- In older children and adults, a positive challenge should be followed by a double-blind challenge in order to avoid bias.
- Double-blind, placebo-controlled food challenge (DBPCFC) is the gold standard in diagnosing food allergy and intolerance.
- Whenever possible, the result of challenge is based on recording of objective signs.
- Early symptoms are reliable, while isolated late symptoms are not.
- DBPCFCs have taught us that:
  most case histories are inaccurate;
  the number of important foods is restricted to milk, egg, peanuts, nuts, soyabean, wheat, fish and shellfish;
  food-induced symptoms are confined to the gastro-intestinal tract, skin and airways.

Differential diagnosis
The symptoms of gastro-intestinal allergy can, in infants and children, be mimicked by a variety of other clinical entities. Vomiting can be secondary to *gastro-intestinal reflux* and *pyloric stenosis*. Functional bowel disorders, infections and organic diseases must be ruled out as the cause of diarrhoea.

Of particular importance is the distinction between wheat protein allergy and gluten intolerance, and between milk protein allergy and lactose intolerance.

The distinction between *gluten intolerance* and allergy to wheat protein can be difficult. The diagnosis of gluten intolerance is favoured by severe malabsorption and marked atrophy of the intestinal villi. The diagnosis of wheat protein allergy is supported by symptoms in other organs and by the demonstration of IgE antibody.

Breast milk is tolerated by allergic infants but not by those with *lactose intolerance*. An abnormal lactose tolerance test can be secondary to milk allergy, but it will be normalized when the child has been on a cow's milk-free diet for some weeks.

Indications for testing
It is important to consider carefully the selection of patients for testing. On the one hand, proper testing for adverse reactions to food is *time-consuming and demanding* for both the patient and the physician. On the other hand, an uncertain diagnosis may lead to *unnecessary therapeutic diets*.

When there is a *suggestive case history* of immediate reactivity to a single food, the chance of obtaining a positive result is good. When no particular food is incriminated and *no history* of a reaction to meals is obtainable, the diagnostic work will be difficult and a negative result the rule.

The *history* can be so *evident* that further testing is unnecessary, for example when an otherwise symptom-free person has repeatedly had angioedema after eating shrimps. However, experience has shown that apparently obvious case histories are not necessarily correct when checked by controlled challenges.

Patients who are often tested are: 1, *infants with significant gastro-intestinal symptoms* and suspicion of cow's milk sensitivity when weaned off mother's milk; 2, *children with atopic dermatitis and chronic asthma*; and 3, *selected adults* with the same diseases in a *severe form* (Table 5.4.1).

Pollen-allergic patients with sensitivities to cross-reacting *fruits and vegetables* need information about possible sensitivities, and further examination is not indicated.

Some adults with *atypical symptoms and a firm belief* in food allergy come to the physician in order to have their own opinion confirmed. An attempt to obtain an objective result in these circumstances is

Testing for food sensitivity—pros and cons
In favour of testing
Disease in infants and children
Severe chronic symptoms from gut, skin or airways
Symptoms from more than one organ system
An (apparently) obvious case history
A history of a life-threatening reaction where there is uncertainty about the offending food
Patients who loose ground when on an exclusion diet
Against testing
Disease in middle-aged and old patients
Mild, trivial symptoms
Atypical symptoms
Symptoms from a single organ
An (very) obvious case history
A convincing history of life-threatening reaction to a food that can be easily avoided
Food sensitivities related to pollen allergy

Table 5.4.1. Arguments in favour of and against testing for food sensitivity

doomed to failure, and the physician is well advised to avoid challenging these patients.

Case history
A thorough history is important for deciding whether further examination is indicated, for identifying the suspected food and for selecting a suitable trial diet and challenge substance (Table 5.4.2).

Physical examination
In infants, particular attention should be paid to *weight* and *height* (repeated measurements), well-being or irritability, wasting of the buttocks and other signs of malnutrition.

Demonstration of IgE antibody
The *usefulness of allergy testing is limited* for the following reasons: 1, foods, as allergen sources, are poorly standardized and contain a multitude of allergens, insufficiently mapped; 2, the allergen content varies with the state of the food: fresh/stored, raw/cooked; 3, some ingested allergens are deactivated in the stomach and gut; 4, demonstration of IgE antibody can be without clinical relevance; and 5, IgG antibody is possibly responsible for allergy in a few cases.

In principle, a *skin prick test* and *RAST* give identical results. RAST can be better standardized, but it can be influenced by very high levels of total IgE (false positive result).

For fish allergen, the correlation between a positive skin prick test/RAST and clinical sensitivity is almost 100%. The usefulness of tests for IgE antibody to other types of food varies. Wheat protein, for example, gives results that correlate well with the symptoms in baker's asthma but poorly with those of atopic dermatitis.

Some allergens in commercial extracts may be inactive, so it is recommended that they be supplemented by fresh foods. It is easy to make a prick test through, for example, a drop of milk, egg white or juice from an apple, or by simply pricking the food and the skin with the same lancet (the prick-prick test).

Diagnostic principles
It is necessary for a diagnosis of food sensitivity that: 1, symptoms have occurred after ingestion of the food; 2, they disappear when the food is not ingested; and 3, they recur upon controlled challenge.

The case history
Identify suspected food
Precise description of symptoms
Severity of symptoms
Time between ingestion and symptoms
Quantity of suspected food causing symptoms
Number of episodes
Reproducibility of reaction
Review of current diet

Table 5.4.2. The case history in food sensitivity

Different types of elimination diets
Breast milk (contains lactose)
Amino acid formula (Elemental 028)
Milk protein hydrolysate (Nutramigen, Profylac)
Soyabean formula (Mull-soy)
Dye-free diet
Gluten-free diet

Table 5.4.3. Different types of elimination diets

Therefore, the diagnostic work consists of three steps: 1, a full diet; 2, an elimination diet; and 3, food challenge.

Diagnostic trial diet

The diagnostic work is started with daily symptom recording during a 2-week *run-in period* on a normal and varied diet.

If the patient has significant symptoms in this period, it is followed by a 2-week *trial diet period* without the suspected food. The choice of the trial diet is based on patient age and symptoms, the suspected food item and the result of skin prick testing (Table 5.4.3).

If the *symptoms improve significantly* (ideally disappear) during the diet period, a challenge test with the suspected food is the next step. This requires that the symptoms are stable and that the disease activity is as low as possible. Otherwise, it is better to postpone the challenge.

Food challenge

Open challenge

An open challenge will be *sufficient in infants* who are unbiased. *In other patients*, an open challenge can be *a first step* in the investigation. If the challenge is negative, testing can be stopped. Otherwise, it is necessary to continue with blinded challenges.

Blinded challenge

In older children and adults, *double-blind, placebo-controlled food challenges* (DBPCFCs) are recommended for the following reason. Chronic urticaria, atopic dermatitis and asthma have a multifactorial pathogenesis, and an unpredictable course with rapid

deterioration and improvement. The biased patient, firmly attached to his or her belief, and an uncritical physician run a considerable risk of relating a spontaneous change of symptoms to the elimination or reintroduction of a suspected food. In recent years, it has been convincingly shown that more than 50% of all diagnoses will be incorrect unless they are based on DBPCFC (Table 5.4.4; Fig. 5.4.1), which is now considered *the gold standard* in diagnosing food allergy and intolerance.

DBPCFC is *very time-consuming* and *involves a certain risk*. Challenge should only be carried out by trained personnel and at a location with full facilities for cardio-respiratory resuscitation. If, in the rare case, it is justified to challenge with a food suspected of having caused an anaphylactic reaction, it must be done with utmost caution.

Evaluation of the challenge is based on subjective symptoms and, whenever possible, *objective signs*. *Early symptoms*, occurring within 2 hours, are usually IgE mediated. Late symptoms (2–24 hours) may be due to other immunological reactions, or the mode of action remains obscure. While a late reaction can follow an early reaction, it is *questionable whether an isolated late reaction does exist* (with the exception of gastro-intestinal symptoms in infants). In most cases, it may be a *coincidental worsening* of the symptoms. In a chronic disease with fluctuating

Food challenge testing
Symptoms have to improve significantly during a 2-week trial diet
Patient is symptom-free or in steady state
Obtain dry food; wet food can be freeze dried. Alternatively hide fresh food in Elemental 028 and blackcurrant juice
Have your pharmacy fill the suspected food into opaque (glucose) capsules
Administer initially 20–2000 mg, depending on the suspected degree of sensitivity; in infants, have the suspected food hidden in the diet by a nurse
If no reaction occurs within 2 hours, increase the dose twofold daily until 8000 mg is attained
A full meal with the suspected food included

Table 5.4.4. Method of double-blind food challenge

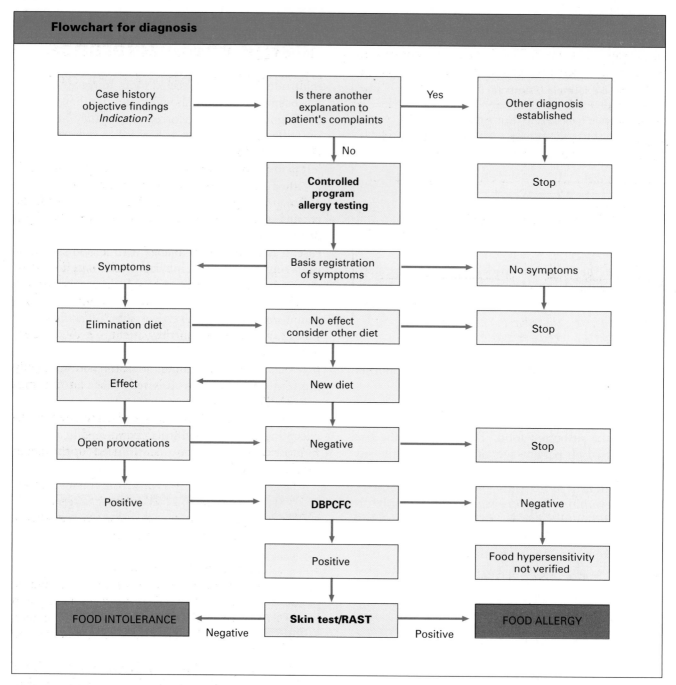

Fig. 5.4.1. Flowchart for a controlled programme for diagnosing food allergy and intolerance. From Bindslev-Jensen C. Food allergy and intolerance. In: Mygind N, Naclerio RM, eds. *Allergic and Non-allergic Rhinitis. Clinical Aspects* Copenhagen: Munksgaard, 1993: 46–50.

symptom activity, food challenge tests can be extremely *difficult to interpret*, and sometimes a conclusive result cannot be obtained.

Even a gold standard has its weaknesses. A single, negative DBPCFC cannot completely rule out the possibility that repeated ingestion of food or ingestion together with, for example, physical exercise may be the cause of symptoms. In addition, the use of capsules excludes the study of oral symptoms.

Experience with DBPCFC has given valuable information about adverse reactions to food: it has confirmed some and refuted other clinical observations.

1, Most case histories are inaccurate. 2, It is unusual for more than two to three foods to cause symptoms in the single patient. 3, The number of foods causing reactions is largely restricted to a short list: milk, egg, peanuts, nuts, soyabean, wheat, fish and shellfish, which account for more that 90%. 4, Reproducible food-induced symptoms are confined to the gastrointestinal tract, skin and airways. 5, Isolated late reactions have been difficult to document.

A good wish
May you live all the days of your life.

Jonathan Swift

A dilemma for everybody
Life can only be understood backwards; but it must be lived forwards.

Søren Kierkegaard

5.5 Management of food allergy and intolerance
Elimination of the offending food

Key points
- The diagnosis should be as certain as possible, as it is difficult to adhere to an elimination diet.
- When a diagnosis has been firmly established, the patient is informed about the elimination diet by a dietician.
- It is easier to avoid 'hidden' allergens when meals are prepared at home, using fresh material, than when prepacked meals are bought in a supermarket or when meals are prepared in restaurants.
- The strictness of the diet should be balanced against the sensitivity of the patient and the severity of the symptoms.
- Served a meal of uncertain composition, highly sensitive patients can be advised to use an oral mucosa challenge test.
- Milk hydrolysate formulae are given to cow's milk-allergic infants, weaned from breast-feeding.
- It is important to reconsider the need for the diet at regular intervals.
- Patients, who have experienced life-threatening attacks, need adrenaline for self-administration.
- H_1 antihistamines have some effect on oral allergy symptoms, skin itching and urticaria.

Principles and counselling
It is a general principle that *the diagnosis should be as certain as possible*, as it is difficult, annoying and can be expensive to adhere to a strict elimination diet. In addition, it can impair nutrition in infants and children.

When a diagnosis has been firmly established, the patient is informed about the *elimination diet*, how to avoid the offending food and how to replace it. This counselling is best given by *a professional dietician*, who knows the pitfalls associated with the increasingly complex composition of mass-produced, prepacked food. As a general rule, it is easier to avoid 'hidden' allergens and additives when *meals are prepared at home*, using fresh material, than when *prepacked meals* are bought in a supermarket. Most problematic are *restaurant meals*. Unfortunately, an enquiry in the kitchen as to the ingredients of the meal and the use of food additives is not always reliable.

It is another general principle that the *strictness of the diet* should be *balanced against the sensitivity* of the patient and the severity of the symptoms. Some patients need not be very strict about the diet as they can tolerate small amounts of the food. In their case, there is a dose–response relationship at work, and a reduction of habitual intake may suffice. Other patients, who are highly sensitive and have had serious reactions, must adhere painstakingly to the diet. They can be advised to use an *oral mucosa challenge test* if they are served a meal of uncertain composition. If chewing a small amount of the food and keeping it in the mouth for a few minutes results in oral pruritus, the dish must not be eaten. The chewed food should not be swallowed and the mouth carefully rinsed.

Therapeutic diet

In cow's milk-allergic infants, weaned from breast-feeding, the safest replacement is hypo-allergenic *milk hydrolysate formulae*, but they are expensive. For that reason, soya preparations are sometimes used as first-line substitutes, but this implies a risk of sensitization.

In adults, a single food can be replaced without increasing cost but a diet may limit social life and reduce the quality of life.

Food additives (e.g. dyes and preservatives) can never be completely avoided but a diet can reduce their amount significantly. It is recommended that the patient *prepares his or her own food* from fresh raw materials and avoids prepacked factory food. It is necessary to develop the habit of reading food labels in the supermarket.

It is important to reconsider the need for the diet at regular intervals. Patients often adhere to a diet, prescribed many years ago, that is no longer required. Challenge tests should be repeated at suitable intervals to avoid this occurring. This is of particular importance in the first years of life because of the *transient nature of adverse food reactions in children*. In infants and young children, it is important to eliminate as few foods, for as short a period of time as possible, due to the risk of malnutrition.

Drug therapy

Anaphylaxis is treated with *adrenaline* (see Chapter 12.2), and patients, who have experienced life-threatening attacks, need adrenaline for self-administration.

H₁ antihistamines have some effect on oral allergy symptoms, skin itching and urticaria, but the patient must not use it for the prevention of anaphylaxis while violating the prescribed diet.

Oral sodium cromoglycate has been tried in patients with severe reactions to food allergens. The effect is not convincing, the treatment is expensive, and it is not without adverse effects.

Immunotherapy has no proven effect on the symptoms of food allergy.

> A strict diet, for example?
> There are some remedies worse than the disease.
> Publilius Syrus

Further reading

Books

Husby S, Halken S, Høst A. Food allergy. In: Klurfeld DM, ed. *Human Nutrition – a Comprehensive Treatise. Nutrition and Immunology* volume 8. New York: Plenum Press, 1993: 25–49.

Metcalfe DD, Sampson HA, Simon RA, eds. *Food Allergy. Adverse Reactions to Foods and Food Additives.* Oxford: Blackwell Scientific Publications, 1991: 1–418.

Articles

Anderson JA. The clinical spectrum of food allergy in adults. *Clin Exp Allergy* 1991; **21**(suppl 1): 304–15.

Brunner M, Walzer M. Absorption of undigested proteins in human beings: the absorption of unaltered fish protein in adults. *Arch Intern Med* 1928; **42**: 173–9.

Fuglsang G, Madsen C, Saval P, Østerballe O. Prevalence of intolerance to food additives among Danish school children. *Pediatr Allergy Immunol* 1993; **4**: 123–9.

Harvey J, Jones DB. Human mucosal T-lymphocyte and macrophage subpopulations in normal and inflamed intestine. *Clin Exp Allergy* 1991; **21**: 549–60.

Metcalfe DD, Sampson HA. Workshop on experimental methodology for clinical studies of adverse reactions to food and food additives. *J Allergy Clin Immunol* 1990; **86**: 421–442.

Nørgaard A, Skov PS, Bindslev-Jensen C. Egg and milk allergy in adults: comparison between fresh foods and commercial allergen extracts in skin prick test and histamine release from basophils. *Clin Exp Allergy* 1992; **22**: 940–7.

Samson HA, Mendelson L, Rosen JP. Fatal and near-fatal anaphylactic reactions to food in children and adolescents. *N Engl J Med* 1992; **327**: 380–4.

Part 6 Skin Diseases

6.1 The skin: structure and function

Epidermis, dermis and subcutaneous layer

Key points

- Skin diseases are very frequent and they often have an immunological or allergic background.
- The skin consists of epidermis and dermis resting on a layer of subcutaneous fat.
- Epidermis, with its stratum corneum, is of great importance as a physical barrier.
- The epidermis has a thickness varying from 0.05 mm on the eyelid to 1.5 mm on the palm of the hands.
- Eczema is often localized to regions with thin skin.
- The epidermal lipid barrier protects against transepidermal water loss and dryness of the skin.
- This function is impaired in atopic dermatitis.
- The lower cellular layer of epidermis contains keratinocytes, Langerhans' dendritic cells and melanocytes.
- Keratinocytes produce keratins, which are very resistant to physical and chemical impacts.
- When damaged, they can produce cytokines and form a setting for leucocyte infiltration and inflammation.
- Langerhans' dendritic cells are very potent antigen-presenting cells; they also carry Fc receptors for IgE.
- Dermis contains an extensive, complex vasculature used for thermoregulation.
- Dermis is a dense connective tissue, consisting of collagen, blood vessels, interdigitating dendritic cells and some mast cells.
- Sensory nerve fibres terminate in the upper papillary layer of the dermis.

Skin symptoms occur in everybody at some point during their lifetime, and skin diseases are very frequent. The general practitioner will, among 10% of his or her patients, be confronted with a dermatological problem, and skin diseases often have an immunological or allergic background.

This chapter will outline some aspects of the structure and function of the skin that can be related to atopic dermatitis, urticaria, angioedema and contact eczema.

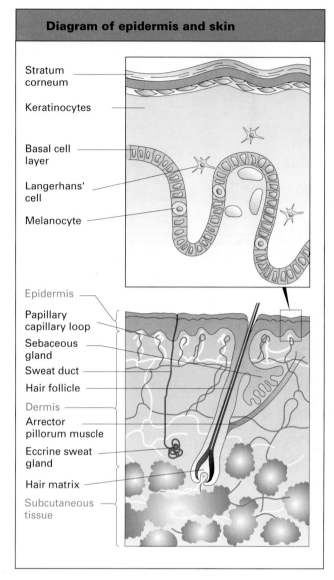

Diagram of epidermis and skin

Stratum corneum

Keratinocytes

Basal cell layer

Langerhans' cell

Melanocyte

Epidermis

Papillary capillary loop

Sebaceous gland

Sweat duct

Hair follicle

Dermis

Arrector pillorum muscle

Eccrine sweat gland

Hair matrix

Subcutaneous tissue

Fig. 6.1.1. The anatomy of the epidermis and of the skin in full thickness.

The skin (cutis) (Figs 6.1.1–2) is considered in terms of two principal layers: *epidermis* and *dermis*. Beneath is the *subcutaneous layer*, mainly consisting of fat and vessels.

Epidermis

Two layers

The epidermis has an average thickness equal to that of paper, varying from 0.05 mm on the eyelid to 1.5 mm on the palms of the hands. It is a stratified epithelium composed of two major layers (Fig. 6.1.1): 1, the *stratum corneum* consisting of dead keratin-filled keratinocytes embedded in lipids like a 'brick-

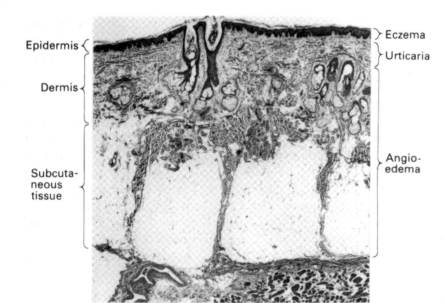

Fig. 6.1.2. Section of the skin (× 25) showing epidermis, dermis and subcutaneous fat. Note the different localization of the diseases.

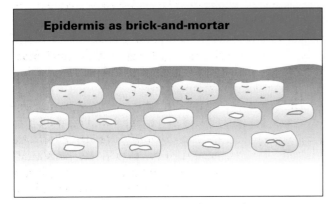

Fig. 6.1.3. Epidermis can be looked upon as a brick-and-mortar layer. Dying keratinocytes secrete 'laminar bodies', which contain skin lipids, and they embed themselves in a 'mortar' of water-impermeable lipids. The dead keratinocytes ('bricks') are filled with keratins.

and-mortar' wall (Fig. 6.1.3); and 2, the lower cellular layer consisting of living keratinocytes, Langerhans' dendritic cells and melanocytes.

Keratinocytes produce keratins, which are insoluble proteins very resistant to physical and chemical impacts. *Melanocytes* produce melanin, which is delivered to keratinocytes and determines our pigmentation. *Langerhans' dendritic cells* form the first defence of our immune system against the environment. There are no blood vessels in the epidermis.

Desquamation

It normally takes 1 month for a keratinocyte to travel from the basal layer to the surface, where approximately one cell layer is shed daily ('food for mites').

When epidermal thickness is constant, desquamation is in steady-state with cell proliferation in the basal layer. The mitotic rate may be dramatically increased by inflammation, such as eczema, and *scaling* follows.

Protective function

The epidermis has a mechanical protective function. It forms a barrier preventing the entrance of micro-organisms, toxic substances and drugs. These functions are largely due to the thin flexible layer of keratinized cells forming the stratum corneum. The protective function depends upon the *thickness of stratum corneum*. It is thickest on the plantar and palmar areas and thinnest on the eyelids and cheeks. The skin is also thin on the forehead, flexor surfaces and abdominal wall. Allergic contact dermatitis is often localized to regions with thin skin, because the distance between surface antigens and the immune system is short. The protective function is impaired by epidermal diseases, such as eczema.

Lipid barrier

The lipid barrier in stratum corneum determines our transepidermal water loss and the *water content of the skin*. The epithelial lipid barrier is resistant to daily wear-and-tear, but it can be damaged by intense and prolonged contact with *detergents and irritants*. *Atopic persons*, with previous or present eczema, have an *impaired epidermal lipid barrier* and structural changes of their skin surface.

The impairment of the barrier function will lead to an increased water loss, and to dryness and '*chap-*

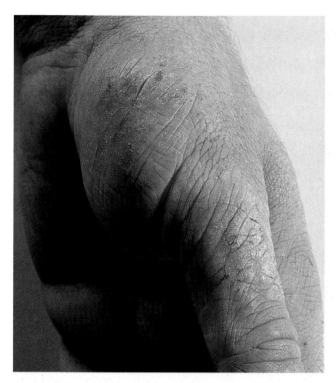

Fig. 6.1.4. Chapping as a sign of impaired barrier function with increased water loss and skin dryness. The skin is vulnerable, and irritant eczema easily develops.

ping' of the skin (Fig. 6.1.4). This is the first step towards irritant eczema, as the skin becomes less resistant to further irritation and more penetrable for antigens. It will take at least 2–3 days to repair a damaged lipid barrier.

Chapping can be prevented by regular use of an emollient, which inhibits increased water loss and, thus, leads to an increased amount of water in the epidermis.

Keratinocytes

Keratinocytes form about 90% of the cells in the epidermis. Through their adhesion (desmosomes) they create the physical structure of the epidermis. When damaged, they can *release cytokines* (TNF, IL-1, IL-6 and IL-8). They can also express adhesion molecules when exposed to IFNγ from activated T lymphocytes. Thus, damaged keratinocytes can form a setting for leucocyte infiltration and inflammation.

Melanocytes

Cells that synthesize melanin comprise about 10% of the cells in the basal layer of the epidermis. The percentage is the same in all races, but melanocytes of dark people make more melanin. They extend their area by long cytoplasmatic processes. Their function can be damaged by epidermal disease and trauma (scratching) leading to hypopigmentation.

Langerhans' cells

Epidermis contains 1–3% of dendritic cells, which are very potent *antigen-presenting cells* (APCs) through their expression of MHC class II molecules and their cytokine production. They also carry Fc receptors for IgE, which can be demonstrated in persons with increased plasma IgE levels. They are more potent as APCs than monocytes and macrophages. They travel to regional lymph nodes and are important in our immune surveillance system.

Dermis

Dermis ('leather') is a dense connective tissue, mainly consisting of *collagen*. The upper papillary layer of the dermis interdigitates with the epidermis and contains vascular loops. There is an excess of *blood vessels*, because *thermoregulation* is a cardinal function of dermal vasculature, which also plays an important role in inflammation.

The master cell of the dermis, the *fibroblast*, produces collagen (90% of dry weight) and elastic fibres (2% of dry weight). *Interdigitating dendritic cells* are the APCs of the dermis. *Mast cells* (7–10 cells/mm²) lie along the blood vessels and are important players in urticaria. There are also scattered leucocytes, lymphocytes and plasma cells.

Subcutaneous tissue

The subcutaneous fat layer varies in thickness and shapes our bodies, to an extent, attracting sculptures and artists. Besides its aesthetic role, the subcutaneous fat functions as a heat insulator and a reserve depot of calories. It contains vessels that may participate in angioedema and vasculitis.

Nerves

Sensory fibres

The skin is a major sense organ, where sensory nerves terminate in the upper papillary layer of the dermis. This explains why urticaria, which is localized to this area, itches, while angioedema, in the lower dermis and subcutis, does not (Fig. 6.1.2).

Itching, defined as the desire to scratch, is the sensation of greatest importance to patients with skin disease. Although sensations of itch and pain are transmitted by the same unmyelinated fibres, the nerve impulse frequency in itching is appreciably lower than in pain. By scratching, the pruritic patient substitutes pain for itch, replacing the slow, maddening impulses with faster, more tolerable ones.

Autonomic fibres

The skin is richly supplied with efferent, autonomic nerves. Sympathetic, adrenergic nerves contract the smooth muscle in blood vessels and hair erector muscles. Cholinergic fibres innervate the eccrine sweat glands and are instrumental in producing sweat. The sebaceous glands are mostly free of autonomic innervation and depend on endocrine stimuli for function.

Don't worry, be happy
He who fears to suffer, suffers from fear

French proverb

6.2 Atopic dermatitis I: aetiology and pathogenesis
Dry skin with B- and T-cell abnormalities

Key points

- Atopic dermatitis is a chronic, relapsing eczema in children.
- The skin shows two cardinal abnormalities: excessive dryness and a markedly reduced threshold for itching.
- In the acute phase, the lesions are exudative, whereas the chronic phase is characterized by a dry lichenified eczema.
- Although many patients develop IgE antibody, an allergic reaction is not a major cause of symptoms.
- Atopic dermatitis is apparently not a truly allergic disease and its cause is unknown.
- Skin dryness is possibly due to an abnormal lipid synthesis in epidermis.
- The mechanical barrier in the skin is defective and the transepidermal water loss is increased.
- There are immunological abnormalities both within the B- and T-lymphocyte system.
- Many patients have increased total serum IgE consisting of allergen-specific IgE and 'no-sense IgE'.
- CD4$^+$ T cells accumulate in eczematous skin and show sign of activation.
- There is an imbalance between Th2 cells and Th1 cells, favouring IgE synthesis.
- Skin mast cells are increased in number.
- Skin eosinophils are increased in number and they release ECP.
- The skin shows non-immunological abnormalities, probably related to dysfunction of the autonomic nervous system.
- This is visualized by an abnormal reaction to acetylcholine and by white dermographism.

Characteristics of the disease

Atopic dermatitis is largely *a disease of children*. It is a *chronic, relapsing eczema* characterized by extreme *itching* leading to persistent *scratching*. In the acute phase, the lesions are often exudative, implicating secondary infection, whereas the chronic phase is characterized by dry, lichenified eczema.

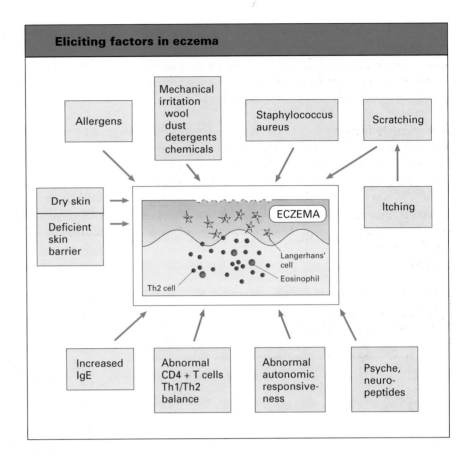

Fig. 6.2.1. Factors that elicit symptoms and aggravate the atopic eczema.

Many patients develop IgE antibody to common environmental allergens, but, in contrast to the other two atopic diseases, an antigen–antibody reaction is not considered a major cause of symptoms in atopic dermatitis, which apparently is *not a truly allergic disease*. The role played by IgE antibody is unclear and the cause of the disease is unknown. Several factors can, however, influence the intensity of the atopic eczema (Fig. 6.2.1).

Abnormal skin structure and fatty acid metabolism

The texture of the skin of patients with atopic dermatitis differs from that of normal persons, visualized by scanning electron microscopy (Fig. 6.2.2). In the abnormal skin, *the mechanical barrier and the epidermal lipid barrier are defective*, and *the transepidermal water loss is increased*.

Some data seem to relate these abnormalities to intake and metabolism of fatty acids. 1, Animals fed a diet deficient in essential fatty acids suffer from increased transepidermal water loss and symptoms similar to those of atopic dermatitis. 2, Patients with atopic dermatitis have reduced enzymatic metabolism

of linolenic acid. 3, The content of various lipids in atopic skin and plasma differs from that of normal controls.

Immunological abnormalities

The most significant biological changes in atopic dermatitis are found in the immune system, both within the B- and T-lymphocyte system (Table 6.2.1).

It is characteristic of the immunological parameters that they range from normal to dramatically changed. The degree of abnormality, as a rule, parallels the clinical severity of the disease.

B lymphocytes

Their number in peripheral blood is within the normal range. *Total serum IgE* is increased in one-third of patients with eczema only, and in two-thirds of patients with eczema and allergic rhinitis/asthma. Many of these patients do not have specific IgE antibodies, meaning that most of their IgE is 'no-sense IgE'. A defective regulatory system for IgE production is the likely explanation for the production of 'no-sense IgE'. Obviously, some of the patients also synthesize *specific IgE towards allergens*.

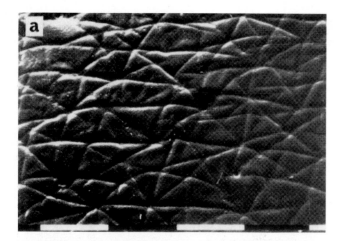

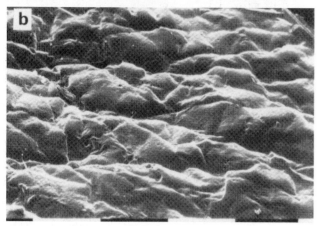

Fig. 6.2.2. Scanning electron micrographs of (a) normal and (b) dry atopic skin. From Linde YW, Bengtsson A, Lodén M. Dry skin in atopic dermatitis. *Acta Derm Venereol (Stockh)* 1989; **69**: 315–19.

T lymphocytes

Patients with atopic dermatitis have a normal or slightly decreased number of T lymphocytes in the blood, but the number of *activated T cells is increased*. This is shown by an increased level of soluble IL-2 receptors in plasma (Table 6.2.1), as activated T cells express receptors for IL-2.

A skin biopsy from atopic eczema will show an *accumulation of CD4+ T cells* both in dermis and, to a lesser extent, in epidermis (Fig. 6.2.3). When skin biopsies are stimulated by antigen *in vitro*, the T cells proliferate and T-cell clones can be established. The majority of these clones have a Th2 profile. Thus, it is likely that the increased IgE in atopic dermatitis is a consequence of an imbalance between CD4+ T cell subpopulations in the skin, where atopic patients have more *Th2 cells* than Th1 cells (Fig. 6.2.4).

Other cell types

IgE can be shown on the surface of *Langerhans' cells* in patients with elevated plasma IgE. However, this phenomenon is not specific for atopic dermatitis.

The number of *mast cells* is almost doubled in eczematous skin. *Basophils* from the patients have increased release of histamine after stimulation with anti-IgE antibody *in vitro*. The pathogenic significance is unknown.

The number of *eosinophils* is increased in the blood and skin, where they may form up to 10% of the infiltrating cells. They secrete *ECP* and other me-

Table 6.2.1. Some of the immunological changes observed in atopic dermatitis

Immunological changes in atopic dermatitis			
	Change	**Tissue**	**Frequency**
Cells			
B lymphocytes	Normal	Blod	
T lymphocytes	Decreased	Blood	1/10
CD4+ T cells	Increased	Skin	All
Eosinophils	Increased	Blood	1/2
Mast cells	Increased	Skin	All
Immunoglobulins			
IgE	Increased	Serum	1/3–2/3
Mediators			
Soluble IL-2 receptors	Increased	Serum	2/3
IL-4 : IFNγ ratio	Increased	Skin lymphocytes	?
Histamine release	Increased	Blood basophils	2/3

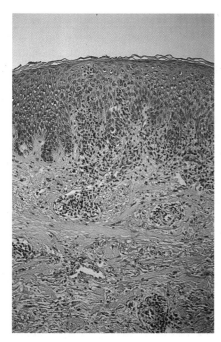

Fig. 6.2.3. Skin biopsy from atopic dermatitis showing cell accumulation (T lymphocytes and eosinophils) in epidermis and dermis.

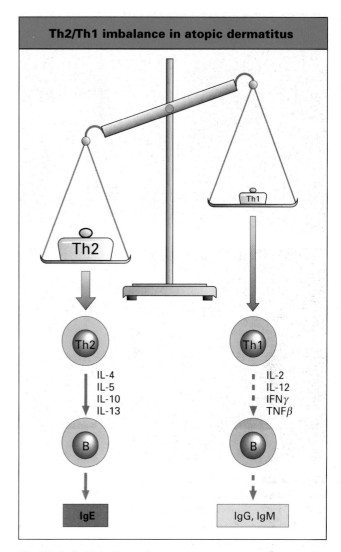

Fig. 6.2.4. This figure illustrates the balance supposed to be relevant for IgE production in atopic patients. There seems to be an increased number of Th2 cells associated with atopy.

diators, which are increased in serum. The changes reflect the disease activity.

The cellular changes in atopic dermatitis are fully compatible with what is observed in allergic contact dermatitis.

Autonomic abnormalities

Patients with atopic dermatitis have non-immunological abnormalities of involved and uninvolved skin, probably related to dysfunction of the autonomic nervous system. When the parasympathetic neurotransmitter, acethylcholine (or its analogue methacholine), is injected into the skin, it produces vasodilatation and an erythematous flare in normal persons, but blanching in eczema patients. This so-called paradoxical vascular response is also demonstrated by scratching the skin with a fingernail. In the patients, the erythematous line, normally produced, is quickly replaced by a white line, *white dermographism* (Fig. 6.2.5).

Szentivanyi has proposed a *beta adrenergic blockage theory* in which there exists a diminished cell responsiveness to beta adrenergic stimulation as a basic abnormality in atopic patients. However, there are strong arguments against this hypothesis, for example the normal levels of adenylate cyclase and of phosphodiesterase in lesional skin (see Chapter 9.4).

Itching

While H$_1$ antihistamines can eliminate itching in urticaria, these drugs have little or no effect in atopic eczema. Consequently, *histamine is not the mediator of itching in eczema*. It is *probably a cytokine* released from T cells and perhaps other cell types as well. The marked efficacy of steroids in inhibiting cytokine release from T cells and itch in eczema gives support to this statement.

Scratching and eczema

The skin of patients with atopic dermatitis shows two cardinal abnormalities: excessive dryness and a markedly reduced threshold for itching. It was earlier be-

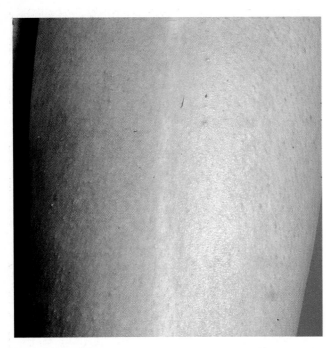

Fig. 6.2.5. White dermographism as a sign of autonomic dysfunction.

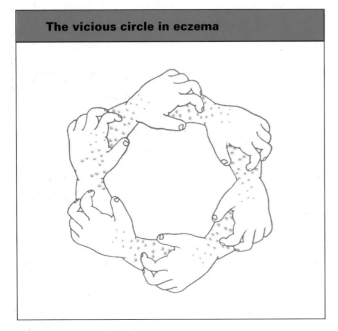

Fig. 6.2.6. The vicious circle in eczema. Itching results in scratching, which causes more eczema and itching. By courtesy of Kjell Aas.

closely related to itching and scratching. All stimuli that increase itching and scratching will worsen the disease and a vicious spiral is started (Fig. 6.2.6).

> **Dr Mayo's prayer**
> Lord, deliver me from the man who never makes a mistake, and also from the man who makes the same mistake twice.
>
> William J Mayo

lieved that scratching was the only cause of the eczematous lesion: 'It is not the eruption that is itchy, but the itchiness that is eruptive.' Although it is now known that unscratched skin is abnormal, it is still true that the pathogenesis of the eczematous lesion is

6.3 Atopic dermatitis II: clinical presentation
Itching – the primary feature

Key points
- The incidence of atopic dermatitis has increased from 3% to 15% during the last 3 decades, and the cause is unknown.
- Atopic dermatitis develops within the first 3 years of life in 90% of patients.
- Symptoms disappear during childhood in 80% but relapse in 10–20% at the end of the teenage years.
- About 25–50% of all children with atopic dermatitis develop irritant hand eczema as adults.
- Itching, leading to scratching and excoriations, is the cardinal symptom, and it is not histamine mediated.
- In the acute phase, papules, vesicles and exudation predominate.
- In the chronic phase, the dry skin becomes lichenified, fissurated and excoriated.
- In the infantile stage, the cheeks and scalp are first affected.
- In the childhood stage, the flexural sides of elbows and knees are typically involved.
- In the adult stage, head-and-neck dermatitis is often added.
- The diagnosis is based on history, physical examination and, in atypical cases, it can be supported by laboratory tests.
- Allergy testing is positive in 50–75%, and a similar percentage develop allergic rhinitis or asthma.
- While food allergy can induce an urticarial rash, it is not the cause of chronic eczema.
- Itching and eczema can be induced and aggravated by skin irritation, wool, dust, heat, sweating, stress and infection.
- During an acute exacerbation, oozing is a sign of bacterial infection with *Staphylococcus aureus*.
- Viral skin infections are also frequent complications to atopic dermatitis, especially eczema herpeticum.

Increased prevalence rate
The incidence of atopic dermatitis has *increased considerably* during the last 3 decades from about 3% in 1960 to about 15% in 1992 (Fig. 6.3.1). The increase has been observed in several countries (Scandinavia,

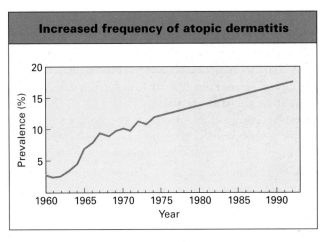

Fig. 6.3.1. Incidence of atopic dermatitis in Denmark.

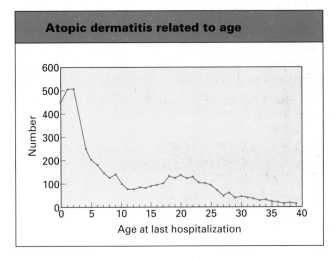

Fig. 6.3.2. Age at last hospitalization for atopic dermatitis in Denmark during 1977–92 (*n* = 5049).

the UK and Japan). There is no proof that the increase is related to environmental factors, such as air pollution or tobacco smoking.

Genetics
The increased prevalence rate is surprising because the disease is *strongly influenced by genetic factors*. In a large, Danish twin study, dizygotic twins had concomitant expression of atopic eczema in 21% of cases, whereas homozygotic twins had a concordance rate of 86%. The disease occurs equally in both sexes and can be inherited from both mother and father. No gene locus has so far been found for the disease.

Course
Atopic dermatitis occurs *predominantly in childhood* and disappears usually during growth ('immunological maturation'?) (Fig. 6.3.2). In 90% of the patients,

it develops within the first 3 years of life, and the more severe the disease the earlier the first appearance of symptoms. *Symptoms usually disappear*, and 80% of the patients become symptom-free during childhood. However, a relapse is seen in 10–20% at the end of the teenage years.

Even though the eczema has disappeared, the atopic person will continue to have dry skin, and 25–50% of the patients will develop *irritant hand eczema*.

Itching

Itch is a *cardinal symptom* of atopic dermatitis. It can *lead to severe excoriations*, as the need for scratching the skin is irresistible. The patient feels that the itch is only relieved once the epidermis has been 'opened'.

Itch is not a constant symptom. It arises most commonly when the patient becomes tired in the afternoon and at night. Its intensity is reflected in the disturbance of sleep leading to a significant strain on parents, who will have to take care of the child almost every night. The child becomes irritable and unhappy.

Eliciting factors

There are several factors that can induce exacerbations of eczema (see Fig. 6.2.1). *Intolerance to foods* is often manifested as eczema around the mouth in children eating oranges and tomatoes. *Food allergy* is less common than expected. It may induce an urticarial rash but it is not the cause of chronic eczema.

Skin irritation from certain textiles, especially *wool*, is a common and well-known eliciting factor. Physical factors, such as *heat* and *dust*, especially dust from concrete and from houses under repair, will irritate the skin. *Sweating* will aggravate itching, and as a result, the patient may stop sport activities. Both *hot, humid weather* and *cold, dry weather* are badly tolerated by the patient, but avoidance is difficult. In young adults, *stress* is a common eliciting factor.

Staphylococcus aureus is the most important contaminating bacteria in atopic skin. Its stickiness to the dry skin is 20 times higher compared to non-atopic skin. Staphylococci are the most common bacteria causing *impetigo*, and they are the main cause of *acute oozing exacerbations* of atopic eczema. Certain phagotypes produce exotoxins that exhibit either a *superantigen effect*, that is, they can directly stimulate certain subtypes of T cells, or they can

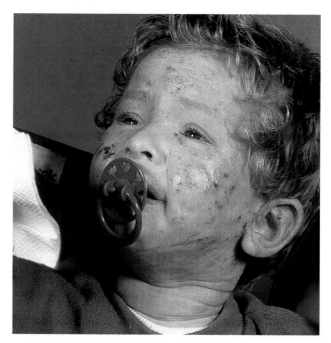

Fig. 6.3.3. Infant with excoriated eczema in the face.

release enzymes (serine proteases), which can induce a cytokine response in mononuclear cells (IL-1 and IL-8).

Infantile stage

Atopic dermatitis, in contrast to seborrhoeic dermatitis, rarely begins earlier than 2 months of age. Typically, the *scalp and cheeks* are first affected by a pruritic erythema with papules, vesicles, exudation and, always, excoriations (Fig. 6.3.3). During exacerbations, the lesions spread to the neck, trunk, arms and legs.

Childhood stage

This stage is a continuum from the early stage. It tends to be more localized, characteristically involving the *flexural sides of elbows and knees* (Fig. 6.3.4). Involvement of the wrists, ankles, neck and head, with painful fissures around the ear lobes, also occurs. During exacerbation, spreading may occur to all regions except the palms and soles. The extensive scratching often leads to pronounced *lichenification* (Fig. 6.3.5).

Atopic winter feet is a special form of atopic dermatitis, where the skin becomes extremely dry, scaling and exhibits painful fissuring.

Adult stage

The distribution of eczema is largely as in childhood.

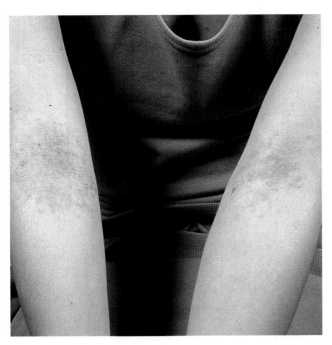

Fig. 6.3.4. Child with dry eczema, typically localized to the flexural sides of elbows and knees.

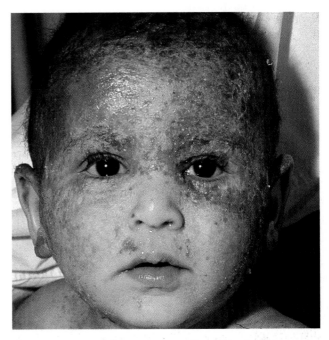

Fig. 6.3.6. Oozing eczema complicated by infection with *Staphylococcus aureus* and impetigo.

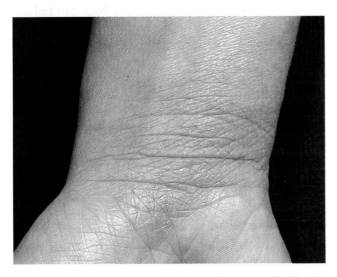

Fig. 6.3.5. Skin of patients with atopic dermatitis shows lichenification, which features an increase in visibility of normal skin markings, hyperlinearity and thickening of the skin.

A special form is *head-and-neck dermatitis*, where eczema is most pronounced in air-exposed regions. Type I allergy to *Pityrosporum orbiculare*, which is a common skin fungus, has been considered as an aetiological factor, but the effect of anti-fungal therapy is disappointing.

Dryness of the skin continues to be a problem and there is often large areas of lichenification with

fissures. *Irritant hand eczema* develops in a large proportion of the patients.

Contact urticaria to food products, especially oranges and tomatoes, often occurs around the mouth.

Complications

Bacterial skin infections are by far the most frequent complication, which must be suspected whenever the eczema starts to ooze (Fig. 6.3.6). Bacterial culture from atopic eczema will reveal the presence of *Staphylococcus aureus* in 95% of cases, even though there may be no clinical sign of infection. Thus, the presence of these bacteria on the skin is intimately connected to the disease, atopic dermatitis.

Viral skin infections are also frequent complications. The most severe is *eczema herpeticum*, where a sudden, abrupt vesicular eruption occurs in the face (Fig. 6.3.7). It is important to start treatment with specific anti-viral compounds even on suspicion of this complication. Some patients with severe atopic dermatitis will also suffer from pox virus infections, normally seen in children (molluscum contagiosum), or warts, both ordinary warts and condylomata.

Associated diseases

Atopic dermatitis is a harbinger of *allergic rhinitis or asthma* in 50–75% of the patients. *Atopic kerato-*

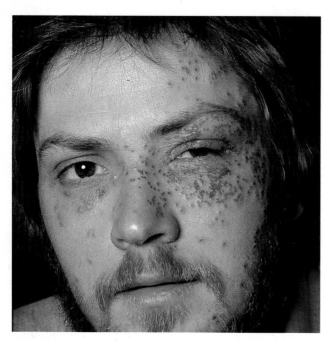

Fig. 6.3.7. This patient with atopic dermatitis developed eczema herpeticum after contact with a friend who had a 'cold sore'.

conjunctivitis can be a troublesome complication in severe cases (see Chapter 7.3). *Subcapsular cataracts* have been reported in about 5%, usually young adults. It can also be induced by systemic steroid usage.

Diagnoses

The history and the physical examination will be sufficient in most patients. Laboratory tests may be helpful in selected cases.

Physical examination

The skin is *dry and pale*. The distribution of the eczematous lesions is characteristic, and the excoriations and lichenification may be extensive. Eczema, which shows *oozing*, is heavily infected with *Staphylococcus aureus*. *Enlarged lymph nodes*, localized to the area of eczema (and infection), are frequent and should not cause unnecessary worry.

Height and weight measurements are important, as children may show growth retardation resulting from severe disease and/or dietary restrictions.

Laboratory tests

Serum IgE and blood eosinophils can give some indications about the severity of the disease. Skin culture for microbiological examination is of little value, because *Staphylococcus aureus* are almost always present. If children are on a strict diet, anaemia should be ruled out.

Allergy examination

Allergy testing reveals positive reactions in 25–50% of the patients with eczema only, and in about 75% of patients with eczema and airway symptoms. Positive reactions to *foods* occur, especially in infants and young children, but it must be borne in mind that these antibodies may be of little direct significance for the eczema. Testing is mainly indicated to identify allergies of importance for airway disease.

It is possible that *aero-allergens* may play a role in eliciting *allergic contact eczema* (a Type IV reaction). *House dust mite* antigen has been most studied, and various investigators have found a positive patch test in 5–50% of patients with atopic dermatitis. The exact clinical role of this Type IV reaction is not known because intervention studies are lacking.

Contact urticaria (a Type I reaction) can also be the result of direct contact with an allergen, for example when mite allergen is rubbed into excoriated skin at night.

Atopic dermatitis patients may develop allergic contact eczema to *nickel*, perfume, lanoline and even topical steroid, which may complicate the clinical picture and the treatment.

Differential diagnosis

Seborrhoeic dermatitis in infancy can resemble atopic dermatitis. The correct diagnosis of seborrhoeic dermatitis can usually, but not always, be made from the following characteristics: 1, age of onset before 2 months of age; 2, pruritus is minimal; 3, the lesion consists of thick, greasy scales; 4, the scalp is the primary region; 5, the nappy region is involved; and 6, laboratory tests are normal.

Metabolic disorders and *immunodeficiencies* can present with eczema, and may initially be mistaken for atopic eczema.

To learn or to be taught?
Personally, I am always ready to learn, although I do not always like being taught.

Winston Churchill

6.4 Atopic dermatitis III: dietary management
For prevention? For treatment?

Key points
- There is good evidence that breast-feeding can postpone the development of atopic dermatitis.
- It is uncertain whether it can be prevented.
- Exclusive breast-feeding is recommended for 4–6 months in infants of atopic parents.
- For the treatment of atopic dermatitis, it is generally agreed that elimination diets, at the most, play a minor role.
- An eczema patient on a diet does not become symptom-free, as does a hay fever patient avoiding pollen.
- However, some children do improve on a diet.
- A diagnostic elimination diet is made based on case history and skin testing/RAST.
- Many positive skin reactions/RASTs to food are without clinical relevance.
- Noticeable improvement during the diet period is followed by challenge tests.
- Clinical food sensitivity often diminishes or disappears with age.
- An elimination diet need not necessarily be lifelong.

A controversial subject
Whether certain foods should be eliminated from the diet of infants and children with atopic dermatitis remains a hotly debated subject. Many *allergists* are convinced that the disease in a number of patients is exacerbated by foods. Many *dermatologists* are equally convinced that dietary manipulation is futile. It is possible that allergists and dermatologists see different subpopulations of patients. However, it is generally agreed that elimination diets, at the most, *play a minor role*. An eczema patient on a diet does not become symptom-free, as does a hay fever patient avoiding pollen. While food allergy and intolerance can cause urticarial rashes in some patients, it is not the cause of the dry, itchy skin or the chronic eczema.

Prevention
There is now good evidence from controlled studies that breast-feeding can postpone the development of atopic dermatitis, but it remains uncertain as to whether it can be prevented. Thus, the present evidence favours a recommendation of *exclusive breast-feeding* for 4–6 months in babies of parents with severe atopic disease. Delayed introduction of solid foods, known to be highly sensitizing, is advisable.

Treatment
When a patient/parent observes that a food repeatedly evokes skin symptoms, the diagnosis of either allergy or intolerance is easy. It is then up to the patient to balance the strictness of the diet against the severity of the disease. Without such history, diagnosis of an offending food is uncertain and time-consuming. Skin testing and RAST may give some guidelines but many positive reactions are without clinical relevance. It is bad advice to base a diet on skin testing or RAST and to tell the patient/parent that this must be adhered to indefinitely. When further examination is indicated, and the patient/doctor motivated, the next step is a *diagnostic elimination diet*. This is best given at home, as the hospital environment itself often improves the condition.

Noticeable improvement during a diet period is followed by *challenge tests*, which are preferably conducted in a double-blind, placebo-controlled fashion, as described in Chapter 5.4. This time-consuming diagnostic work is confined to selected patients with severe symptoms.

Clinical sensitivity often diminishes or disappears with age (usual for milk, often for egg and seldom for fish), and an elimination diet need not necessarily be lifelong. Food items may be more symptom eliciting during severe exacerbations than during periods of light or no eczema.

A single passage
I shall pass through this world but once; any good things therefore that I can do, or any kindness that I can show to any human being, or dumb animal, let me do it now. Let me not defer it or neglect it for I shall not pass this way again.

John Galsworthy

6.5 Atopic dermatitis IV: medical management
Control of dryness, itching and infection

Key points
- The therapeutic principles are avoidance of irritants and control of skin dryness, itching and infection.
- Daily use of a skin moisturizer is necessary.
- An emollient containing urea increases the water-binding capacity of epidermis but it stings.
- Itching is diminished by cold, and the patient should use low temperatures as a remedy.
- H$_1$ antihistamines have effect on urticarial symptoms but not on eczema.
- A bedtime dose of a sedative antihistamine is helpful in children who scratch during sleep.
- Topical corticosteroids are the most successful agents available for the treatment of atopic dermatitis.
- Steroid efficacy and adverse effects depend upon epidermal thickness.
- An acute exacerbation is treated for 1–2 weeks with a potent group III or II steroid preparation.
- This treatment is followed by the low-potency group I preparation, hydrocortisone.
- Hydrocortisone is also used for mild eczema, in children and in areas with thin skin (e.g. face, neck and groin).
- Correct usage not only makes life more tolerable for the child, but can also reduce scratch-induced damage to the skin.
- In severe atopic dermatitis, some skin atrophy from steroids is the price to pay for control of itching.
- Tars are the next most useful anti-inflammatory drugs but they smell and discolour.
- Various types of light therapy can improve atopic dermatitis.
- Skin infection with *Staphylococcus aureus* is treated with water and mild soap, antimicrobial bath and systemic antibiotics.

Therapeutic principles
Avoidance of irritants and provoking factors is a primary treatment principle, but, as a general rule, this will not suffice to control the disease. General skin care and medical treatment is necessary to make the disease bearable and permit the patient to maintain a normal life pattern. Treatment is directed against *skin dryness, itching, inflammation* and *infection.*

Skin dryness
It is important that the patient, in good and in bad periods, on a routine, daily basis uses a *skin moisturizer,* always after bathing and dish-washing. A lotion is useful for generalized application and a cream for localized application. Ointments are reserved for very dry, thickened and fissurized skin.

Emollients containing low-molecular agents (urea or salts) can, by osmolar forces, increase the water-binding capacity of epidermis and prevent loss of moisture. However, such products can cause stinging and induce skin irritation, especially on skin with excoriations and fissures.

In principle, an emollient under occlusion is most efficient in inhibiting transepidermal water loss, but atopic skin under occlusion will loose its thermoregulatory capacity and become too warm, which will aggravate the itch.

Water on the skin will shortly improve skin hydration and bath therapy using *bath with oil* can be recommended. Baths are preferable to showers, and the water temperature should be temperate and not hot. A long, hot shower may worsen the condition.

The disease can be aggravated by *bathing in fresh water*, which dehydrates the skin, while swimming in sea water and beach life during the summer often have markedly beneficial effects.

Therapy of skin dryness in an atopic patient is a delicate balance between *application of water* and *improved holding capacity of water* in the skin without irritating it or disturbing its thermoregulation.

Itching
Cold is very effective in diminishing itch, which is worsened by heat. The patient should therefore be advised to use low temperatures as a remedy: use light clothing, low room temperature, especially in the bedroom, cold bed linens, a walk in the cold evening air, cold showers, etc.

H$_1$ antihistamines are very commonly used. They are beneficial in eczema patients who also have urticarial symptoms, but antihistamines do not improve the itch elicited from T cell activation or other forms of cytokine-mediated skin inflammation. How-

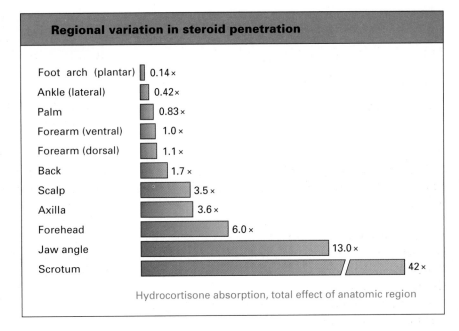

Fig. 6.5.1. Regional variation in the percutaneous penetration of a corticosteroid. From Maibach Hl. *In vivo* percutaneous penetration of corticosteroids in man and unresolved problems of their efficacy. *Dermatologica* 1976; **152**(suppl 1): 11–25.

ever, a *bedtime dose* of a *sedative antihistamine* is helpful, especially in small children who scratch during sleep. They can wear soft cotton mittens at night to reduce scratching. The fingernails are trimmed.

Topical corticosteroids

Since their introduction in 1952, topical steroids have revolutionized dermatological therapeutics. As they suppress inflammation and itching, they are *the most successful agents* currently available for the treatment of atopic dermatitis.

Topical steroids are divided into *four categories* based on their vasoconstrictor effect in normal human skin, and their biological potency in skin diseases. This system helps the doctor in choosing preparations of adequate efficacy.

Drug penetration

Stratum corneum acts as a reservoir for topically applied steroids, which, after a single application, are released over a period of many hours to the dermis, where the most pronounced inflammation is present.

Both the efficacy of treatment and the risk of skin atrophy depends upon steroid penetration and, with that, *epidermal thickness*. The palms and eyelids must therefore be treated differently. Penetration also increases with skin hydration, and absorption of steroids is highest in the *moist areas* (Fig. 6.5.1).

Adverse effects

Penetration through the epidermis to dermis means absorption into the circulation, but systemic side effects are confined to extreme cases, when general therapeutic rules have not been followed.

The major problem is local adverse effects, which will follow regular long-term use of topical steroids (Table 6.5.1). These adverse effects, such as *atrophy* of both the epidermis and dermis, can be severe and disfiguring. The risk depends on the potency of the steroid molecule, the thickness of the skin and the length of the treatment.

Therapeutic principles

It is considerably more difficult in the skin than in the airways to balance between inadequate disease

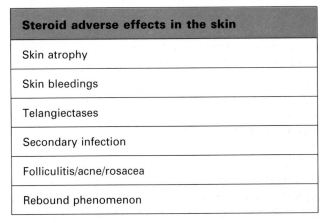

Table 6.5.1. Corticosteroid adverse effects in the skin

Use of topical steroids in atopic dermatitis
Face and genital area
Group I only (hydrocortisone)
All other areas
Group III (severe eczema) or group II (moderate eczema) – twice daily for 1–2 weeks
Reduce to lower potency group – once to twice daily for 1–2 weeks
Group I (hydrocortisone) on remaining eczema spots – once daily for 1–2 weeks as required

Table 6.5.2. A guideline for the use of topical steroids for exacerbations of atopic dermatitis

Patient instruction in the use of topical steroids
Protect your fingers with plastic gloves
Only apply the cream/ointment to active areas
Apply it in a thin layer
Use the cream once or twice daily, preferably after a bath
Always treat over as short a period as possible
Always use the least potent steroid that can control the disease
Be very cautious with the use of steroids other than hydrocortisone on the face and neck
Never use a steroid cream simply as a moisturizer

Table 6.5.3. Patient instruction for topical use of corticosteroids

control and adverse effects, due to the different side effect profiles that steroids have in these organs.

Important for optimal treatment is knowledge about the hierarchy of steroid preparations (group I–IV) and of the highly varying skin thickness and sensitivity to steroids in different regions (Fig. 6.5.1).

It is an important principle to *start treatment with a relatively potent steroid* molecule and, as soon as disease control has been achieved, to change to a less potent preparation. In this way, eczema and itching are effectively controlled, the total amount of potent steroid is relatively low, and the disease will not flare-up once treatment is stopped.

Use of the very potent group IV preparations are confined to severe exacerbations, supervised by a dermatologist. Group IV should not be used in the face or in children (outside a specialist ward), as permanent disfiguring changes can result.

Group III and group II preparations are given for 1–2 weeks during acute exacerbations. In order to prevent a flare-up and recurrences, treatment with potent preparation should not be stopped abruptly but be followed by a weaker preparation (Table 6.5.2).

The low-potency hydrocortisone in group I, used following more potent preparations, is preferred for mild eczema, in children and in sensitive areas with thin skin (e.g. face, neck and groin).

Practical use

Topical steroids are used *once or twice daily*. The evening application is most important as it gives relief for itching during the night.

Thorough *patient instruction* in the use of a steroid preparation is important (Table 6.5.3). It is also of importance that the doctor prescribes adequate amounts of medication and notes the frequency of prescriptions. One gram of cream will cover an area of approximately 10 by 10 cm; 30–60 g are needed for the entire body.

Misuse

Steroid creams are often misused, that is, underused, overused or used in a wrong way. The doctor must realize that *compliance is poor* in many cases. Most parents are reluctant to use steroids in their children, and *underuse* is the rule. By inappropriate use, they also get the impression that 'steroids don't help after all, because the eczema immediately comes back'. The doctor must explain and convince the parents that correct usage not only makes life more tolerable for the child, but can also reduce scratch-induced damage to the skin.

Overuse of potent preparations resulting in permanent disfigurement occurs most frequently in countries where such preparations are available over-the-counter. In severe cases of atopic dermatitis, some adverse effects from steroids must be accepted as a price for controlling intolerable itching, which will otherwise lead to more or less permanent damages, such as severe lichenification.

Tars

Tars are the next most useful drugs to steroids due to their *anti-inflammatory and anti-proliferative activities*. Their odour and colour are objectionable to some patients, but it must be emphasized that their effect is not associated with a risk of long-term side effects. Due to irritancy, tar preparations are *not used during acute exacerbations*, and treated skin should not be exposed to direct sunlight, because of the risk of burns. *Tar baths* in combination with topical steroids may induce long-term remissions in patients with severe atopic dermatitis.

Light therapy

Sunlight will often improve atopic dermatitis, although patients with active eczema have an increased sensitivity to large amounts of sun (and heating of the sun). *PUVA therapy*, which includes ultraviolet A light and the oral administration of psoralens, is an efficacious therapy in adults with severe eczema. *UVB light therapy* is more difficult to handle because it irritates the eczema. *UVA therapy* (solarium) can also be beneficial.

Systemic anti-inflammatory treatment

In general, systemic therapy should not be used in children, but restricted to selected adults. *Systemic steroids* should not be used to treat atopic dermatitis except when the eczema turns into *erythroderma*. *Cyclosporin* has a documented effect, but eczema relapses immediately after cessation. The drug has serious adverse effects, including kidney damage, and it is very expensive. *Azathioprine* seems to have some effect, but well-conducted trials are lacking. *IFNγ* has proven its clinical effect in a double-blind, placebo-controlled study, but it was not able to reduce serum IgE.

Skin infection

Staphylococcus aureus is present in nearly all skin areas with atopic eczema. When eczema becomes oozing, it is a sign of infection, which should be treated. The best way to keep a low number of staphylococci on the skin is *water and soap*, even

Topical antibacterial therapy
Regular, daily use of water and mild soap
Bath therapy in water with chlorhexidine 0.005%
Bath therapy in water with *potassium permanganate* (only in hospital)

Table 6.5.4. Topical antibacterial therapy of atopic dermatitis

though soap carries a skin defatting and irritating effect. It has been shown that eczema activity is reduced through regular use of mild soap on a daily basis. In more severe cases, antimicrobial bath therapy should be recommended (Table 6.5.4). *Systemic antibiotics* are to be recommendeed in eczema with severe oozing. *Erythromycin or dicloxacillin* is preferred because the staphylococci are often resistant to penicillin.

Final comments

Atopic dermatitis is a true *conundrum of allergy* in the broad sense of the word. It demonstrates reactions of immunological specificity, that is, an allergen reacting with the relevant epitope on a T lymphocyte or an IgE antibody. At the same time, it carries aspects in which simple physical, mechanical, chemical, microbial and psychological factors are important for the elicitation of symptoms. It represents *inflammation* in which the inducing factor may be one among many. It may represent the *clinical expression of immunological, developmental immaturity*, in which a genetic background, probably related to ectodermal tissues, carries the basic factor(s) for all observed immune deviations.

Savings
The best thing to save for your old age is yourself.
LS McCandless

Just one more year
No one is so old as to think he cannot live one more year.
Cicero

6.6 Urticaria I: aetiology and pathogenesis
Mast cell release of histamine

Key points
- Urticaria is a disseminated eruption of migrating itching wheals.
- A wheal is a flat, pale-red elevation caused by oedema in the upper part of the dermis.
- The wheal-and-flare reaction, visualized by allergy skin testing or a mosquito bite, is the lesion of urticaria.
- Histamine is the principal mediator of urticaria.
- Histamine release in the skin will lead to itching and increased vascular permeability.
- The mast cell is the key cell in urticaria.
- A vast array of factors can trigger mast cells to release their mediators and induce urticaria.
- An abnormal responsiveness to physical stimuli is characteristic for urticaria (dermographism).
- A variety of chemical compounds can directly elicit mast cell degranulation (e.g. drugs, toxins, foods and food additives).
- Viral infections may be accompanied by urticarial symptoms, but the pathomechanisms are not known.
- Parasitic infections are commonly accompanied by urticaria via Type I reactions.
- Type I reactions to food (e.g. shrimps, crab, shellfish, nuts, fruit and egg) is a common cause of acute urticaria.
- Type I reactions to aero-allergens can also result in contact urticaria.
- Type II reactions can cause an urticarial rash during mismatched blood transfusions.
- Type III reactions, manifested by urticaria, fever and arthritis, are induced by the injection of serum or drugs.
- Complement activation is an important part in immune-mediated urticaria in autoimmune and malignant diseases.

Definition
Urticaria (nettle rash or hives) is a disseminated eruption of migrating, itching wheals.

Wheals
A wheal is a flat, pale-red elevation caused by oedema in the *upper part of the dermis*. The size varies from 0.2 to 10 cm or more. It is evanescent, develops within minutes and disappears within 24 hours. Physiologically it mimics *Lewis triple response* to histamine, as described in 1927 by Sir Thomas Lewis: 1, initial erythema of the injection site is due to vasodilatation; 2, this is followed by a swelling (wheal) due to increased vascular permeability, exudation and oedema; and 3, erythema (flare) is formed in a larger area due to axon reflex vasodilatation. The *wheal-and-flare reaction* is the lesion of urticaria, and is visualized by allergy skin testing or a mosquito bite.

Histamine
Histamine is the *principal mediator* of urticaria. It is on a molar basis released in large quantities compared with leukotrienes and prostaglandins. It is preformed in the mast cell granules from where a number of stimuli will lead to its release. Histamine release in the skin causes itching and increased vascular permeability.

Mast cells
The mast cell is the *key cell* in urticaria. Mast cell subsets and content of mediators are described in Chapter 1.9. The number of cells in urticaria is usually within normal limits, although some investigations have shown a slightly increased number. In urticaria pigmentosa, huge focal accumulations of mast cells are found in the skin.

Why urticaria suddenly occurs and then, in most cases, spontaneously disappears is not known. It implies that the skin mast cells are somehow changed. It could be due to the fact that malfunctioning mast cells are distributed from the bone marrow for a certain period of time. So far, no experimental evidence exists for this hypothesis.

A vast array of factors can trigger mast cells to release their mediators and induce urticaria.

Causes of histamine release

Physical stimuli
An abnormal responsiveness to physical stimuli is characteristic for urticaria. Most frequent is traumatically induced urticaria (dermographism). In some patients, urticaria is selectively induced only by one of the physical stimuli: pressure, cold, sun and heat. While the trigger factors differ, histamine release seems to be the common step in the pathogenesis (Fig. 6.6.1).

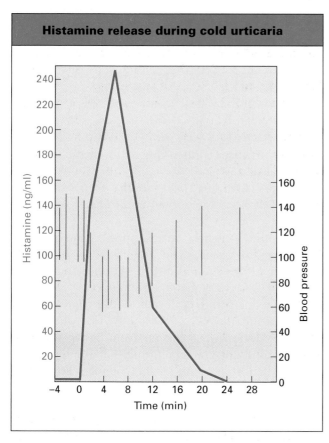

Histamine release during cold urticaria

Fig. 6.6.1. Histamine release and blood pressure recordings obtained after challenge of a cold urticaria patient by placing one hand in ice water for 4 minutes. Time zero is when the hand is removed from ice bath. From Kaplan AP. Mediators of urticaria and angioedema. *J Allergy Clin Immunol* 1977; **60**: 324–32.

Chemical stimuli

A variety of chemical compounds can directly elicit mast cell degranulation. They range from *drugs*, such as acetylsalicylic acid and NSAIDs, morphine, codeine, polymyxin, tubocurarine, radiocontrast media, and antibiotics, including penicillin, to *toxins* from plants (nettles), goblets, jellyfish ('Portuguese Man-of-War') or insects.

Food additives, like flavouring agents, antioxidants, dyes or preservatives, can elicit urticaria via a direct effect on mast cells. *Foods* may cause urticaria by their content of histamine (fish with dark meat), by a direct effect on mast cells and by an immune specific mechanism.

Infections

Many *viral infections* are accompanied by urticarial symptoms. The pathomechanisms are not known,

but may involve cytokine-mediated changes of mast cell membrane permeability. There is an overlap to immune-mediated mediator release because the development of antigen–antibody complexes can induce a Type III-mediated urticaria as seen in cryoglobulinaemia.

Parasitic infections are commonly accompanied by urticarial reactions at the local site of skin penetration ('cercarial itch') and, later, via toxins or Type I-mediated reactions.

Type I reactions

IgE-mediated allergy to food (e.g. shrimps, crab, shellfish, nuts, fruit and egg) is a common cause of *acute urticaria* and of urticarial flare-up in patients with atopic dermatitis. Minute skin trauma and direct contact with an aero-allergen (e.g. lying on a grass lawn, playing with a dog or sleeping in a mite-populated bed) can induce *contact urticaria*.

A Type I reaction is a rare cause of chronic urticaria. Recently, autoantibodies to the IgE receptor (FcεR1) was identified, in a few patients, as the cause of severe chronic urticaria.

Type II reactions

Circulating IgG antibody (from recipient) reacts with cell-fixed erythrocyte antigen (from donor), complement is activated and a cytolytic Type II immune reaction develops; urticaria is caused by anaphylatoxin (C3 and C5). This mechanism has been clearly delineated in the case of urticarial and anaphylactic reactions to blood, plasma or immunoglobulins.

Type III reactions

Serum sickness, originally defined as an adverse reaction to the injection of animal serum, may also follow the administration of various drugs. It occurs 7–14 days after the first medication and is manifested by urticaria, fever and arthritis.

Complement activation

Activation of the complement cascade is an important part in immune-mediated urticaria, including anaphylaxis and *autoimmune diseases*, such as systemic lupus erythematosus or rheumatoid arthritis. In these diseases, urticaria may be an accompanying or herald symptom. Quite often this type of urticaria is somewhat different, because whealing has a more prolonged and less fluctuating course. Thus, a single wheal may be present for 24–72 hours. Histological examination will often reveal a leucocytoclastic vasculitis. Urticaria in malignant disorders is probably elicited via similar mechanisms.

Consolation to us all

Whenever I have found out that I have blundered, or that my work has been imperfect, and when I have been contemptuously criticized, it has been my greatest comfort to say hundreds of times to myself that I have worked as hard and as well as I could, and no man can do more than this.

Charles Darwin

6.7 Urticaria II: classification
The largest group is idiopathic

Key points
- Acute urticaria is often due to an allergic reaction to a food or a drug.
- Chronic urticaria (>1 month) is divided into various disease categories according to eliciting factors.
- Idiopathic urticaria forms approximately three-quarters of all chronic urticaria cases.
- Traumatically induced urticaria or dermographism occurs in 5% of the general population.
- Cholinergic urticaria develops after heat exposure and sweating.
- The eruption is different from other types of urticaria and appears as multiple, small papules.
- Cold urticaria occurs within minutes after challenge with cold air or water.
- In a few cases, cold urticaria is secondary to cryoglobulinaemia.
- Solar urticaria is a rare disorder in which brief exposure to light causes the development of urticaria.
- Pressure urticaria is characterized by deep, painful lesions occurring after application of pressure.
- Allergic urticaria constitutes a large percentage of the acute but not of the chronic forms.
- Urticaria pigmentosa is a rare disease with accumulations of mast cells (mastocytosis).
- Angioedema is the deeper equivalent of urticaria.
- It presents as a large swelling with diffuse borders, and the skin over the swelling appears normal.
- While urticaria itches, angioedema is felt as tenderness.

Acute or chronic
Acute urticaria is arbitrarily defined as urticaria of less than 1 month's duration. Many patients experience only one major attack of a few days duration elicited by ingestion of food or intake of drugs, including pain killers or penicillin. Many drugs may, in particular, elicit a urticarial rash in connection with a febrile illness for which the drug is administered.

Chronic urticaria is defined as urticaria of *more than 1 month's duration*. Clinically, it does not differ from acute urticaria. Chronic urticaria is divided into

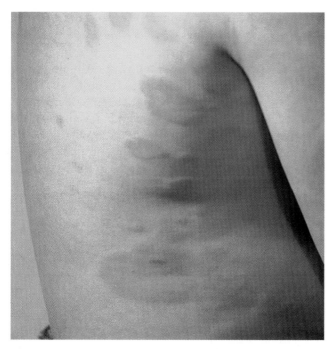

Fig. 6.7.1. Clinical presentation of urticaria.

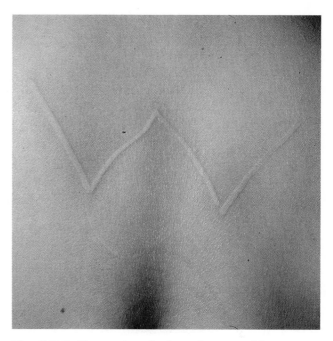

Fig. 6.7.2. Traumatic urticaria or dermographism ('writing on the skin').

various disease categories according to the clinical picture and possible eliciting factors.

Idiopathic urticaria

This group forms 75% of all cases with chronic urticaria. Urticaria can involve any area of the trunk, extremities or face (Fig. 6.7.1). The typical lesions appear abruptly, change in shape within hours and *persist less than 24 hours.* They move to other areas and may relapse in the same skin area after a few days. The wheals may be continuously present or relapse with intervals of days or weeks. Apart from itching, some patients feel a burning, painful sensation in the skin. It is a significant sign that patients with urticaria *do not excoriate their skin.* If scratch marks are seen, the diagnosis should be reconsidered.

Physical urticaria

A significant number of urticaria patients react abnormally to physical stimuli. Most frequent is traumatically induced urticaria or *dermographism.* Linear whealing develops when the skin is firmly stroked with a blunt-pointed instrument or a fingernail (Fig. 6.7.2). The pathogenesis resembles that of Lewis' triple response. It is the commonest form of physical urticaria, occurring in about 5% of the general population. Sometimes, it manifests itself as *swelling under tight-fitting clothing.*

Cholinergic urticaria

This disease is also known as *generalized heat urticaria* and develops after *heat exposure and sweating* (hot bath, vigorous exercise, pyrexia and anxiety). *The eruption is different* from other types of urticaria and appears as multiple, small, 1–3-mm sized papules surrounded by areas of erythema. The stimuli have the common feature of being mediated by cholinergic nerves. Injection of acetylcholine produces a similar eruption in these persons. Their mast cells appear to have an increased sensitivity to this neurotransmitter.

Cold urticaria

Attacks will occur within minutes after challenge, which includes a marked drop in air temperature, bathing or swimming, cold foods and liquids. The lesions are often maximal after rewarming. In a few cases, cold urticaria is mediated by IgE antibody. It may also be secondary to *cryoglobulinaemia* in association with myelomatosis, systemic lupus erythematosus, cold agglutinin syndrome or syphilis.

Solar urticaria

This is a rare disorder in which brief exposure to light causes the development of urticaria in the exposed skin area. Some forms are antibody mediated, and other types are metabolic disorders in which protoporphyrin acts as a photosensitizer.

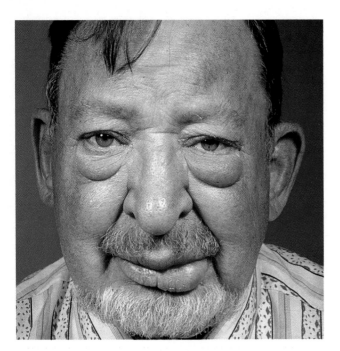

Fig. 6.7.3. A patient with facial angioedema.

Pressure urticaria
Pressure urticaria is a rare variant of physical urticaria. It is characterized by *deep painful lesions* occurring immediately or hours after application of pressure. The symptoms can be pronounced in palms and feet.

Allergic urticaria
Allergic reactions account for a large percentage of *acute urticaria*, but, contrary to common belief, they rarely explain the daily symptoms in the chronic forms.

Urticaria pigmentosa
Urticaria pigmentosa is a rare disease that is most often confined to the skin, where accumulations of mast cells are seen in reddish-brown macules, which, on scratching, shows dermographism. The disease may occur during early childhood, but then tends to disappear spontaneously. It can also occur in adults where the symptoms then persist lifelong. Intestinal symptoms occur quite frequently.

Angioedema
Angioedema (Fig. 6.7.3) is the *deeper equivalent of urticaria*; it is concomitant in pathophysiology with urticaria, and they often occur together. It is, like urticaria, caused by increased vascular permeability and oedema formation. While the lesion in urticaria is localized to the upper part of the dermis, angioedema is confined to the *lower part of the dermis* and the *subcutaneous tissue*.

It presents as a large swelling with diffuse borders; the skin over the swelling appears normal. While urticaria itches, angioedema is felt as tenderness. It can occur in all parts of the skin and may also involve the larynx, mouth and pharynx. Pressure urticaria can resemble angioedema. A rare, unique type is hereditary angioedema (see Chapter 6.9).

On education
Of all treasures knowledge is the most precious, for it can neither be stolen, given away, or consumed.

Hitopadesa

6.8 Urticaria III: diagnosis and treatment

H₁ antihistamines are effective

Key points

• Urticaria is common, affecting 10–20% of the population at some time in their lives.
• The majority of cases present as isolated acute urticaria to foods and drugs.
• Chronic urticaria is most common in middle-aged women, and spontaneous improvement is the rule.
• The typical lesion appears within minutes and persists less than 24 hours.
• Wheals enlarge by peripheral extension to become confluent, with resulting bizarre geographic configurations.
• Although the lesions itch, patients with urticaria do not excoriate their skin.
• Allergy testing may give information of value in acute urticaria but very seldom in chronic urticaria.
• In selected cases of chronic urticaria, a diagnostic elimination diet can be justified.
• Laboratory examinations include erythrocyte sedimentation rate, blood eosinophils, liver and kidney tests, antinuclear antibodies, urine analysis, chest X-ray and stool examination.
• A skin biopsy, to exclude vasculitis, is indicated in atypical chronic urticaria when the single lesion persists for more than 24 hours.
• Simple challenge tests are available for the diagnosis of physical urticarias.
• Treatment consists of avoidance when possible.
• Non-sedating H₁ antihistamines are very effective in 80–90% of the patients.
• As a general rule, oral steroids should not be used.

Urticaria is common, affecting 10–20% of the population at some time in their lives. The majority of cases present as isolated *acute urticaria* to foods and drugs. The cause is obvious and most of these patients are not seen by a physician.

Chronic urticaria is most common in middle-aged women (Fig. 6.8.1). Spontaneous improvement is the rule even in cases of quite long duration (Fig. 6.8.2).

Disease history

In the search for a causative factor, the disease history is most important and should be detailed. Specific

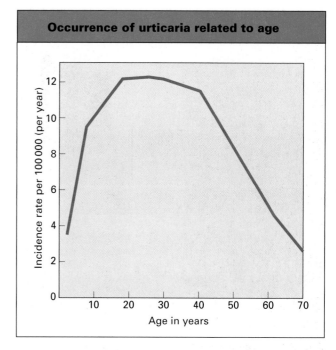

Fig. 6.8.1. Occurrence of urticaria related to age. From Champion R, Roberts S, Carpenter R, Roger J. Urticaria and angio-oedema. A review of 544 patients. *Br J Dermatol* 1969; **81**: 588–97.

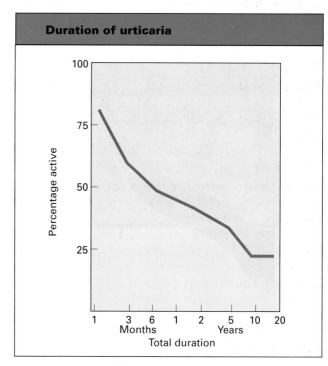

Fig. 6.8.2. Duration of urticaria (mean with 95% confidence limits). From Champion R, Roberts S, Carpenter R, Roger J. Urticaria and angio-oedema. A review of 544 patients. *Br J Dermatol* 1969; **81**: 588–97.

Causes and types of chronic urticaria		
Cause	**Total number**	**Percentage**
Idiopathic urticaria	1657	72
Physical urticaria	370	16
Cholinergic urticaria	88	3.8
IgE-mediated allergic urticaria	79	3.4
Urticarial vasculitis	48	2.1
Other disorders	30	1.0
Infections	24	1.0
Hereditary angioedema	12	0.5

Table 6.8.1. Causes of chronic urticaria in 2310 patients investigated at a dermatological department in the UK. Idiopathic urticaria is the most common form, even though extensive investigational procedures were performed. From Champion RH. Urticaria: then and now. *Br J Dermatol* 1988; **119**: 427–36

enquiry is directed to ingestion of *acetylsalicylic acid* (also for coronary disease) and to foods. Also, enquire about febrile illness, travel to tropical areas, vaccinations, medical therapy, and how long the wheals remain in one site of the skin.

Malignant diseases, especially lymphomas, can be associated with itching and urticarial eruptions.

Physical examination

A full medical examination is indicated where symptoms and signs of underlying diseases are considered. Urticaria is an easy clinical diagnosis where the shape of the individual lesions may give significant help to the diagnosis, such as in cholinergic urticaria, pressure urticaria, angioedema and urticaria pigmentosa.

Wheals vary in size, and enlarge by peripheral extension to become confluent, with resulting bizarre geographic configurations. The colour is bright red in acute, and more dusky red in chronic, urticaria. It *disappears on pressure* from a glass slide. This is a useful test for making the distinction between erythema and bleeding.

Allergy examination

Almost every patient with urticaria believes that he or she has an allergic disease and the patient's demand for an allergy examination is therefore considerable.

In *acute urticaria* skin tests or RAST may give information of value, although the results correlate poorly with food-induced disease.

Table 6.8.1 documents that only a few per cent of patients with *chronic urticaria* will have their disease because of specific allergy. Therefore, time-consuming and expensive work on allergy examination is only justified in exceptional cases.

Diet

In selected cases of chronic urticaria, a diagnostic elimination diet can be justified in order to know whether food allergy or intolerance is of significance. Provided the diet leads to significant clinical improvement, which can be documented by a diary record of symptoms of wheals and itch, oral provocations with food additives, flavours, colouring agents and acetylsalicylic acid should be performed (see Chapter 5.4). Unfortunately, a positive result leading to a helpful therapeutic elimination diet is very rare.

Laboratory examinations

Dependent upon the history and the medical examination, laboratory examinations could include sedimentation rate, a complete blood count, including circulating eosinophils, liver and kidney tests, antinuclear antibodies, complement assays, cryoglobulin determination, urine analysis and chest X-ray. The stools should be examined for parasites and ova, if the history suggests worm infestation or the blood eosinophil count is raised.

Skin biopsy

There are *few perivascular cells* in acute urticaria,

some in chronic urticaria and *many in vasculitis*. The cellular infiltrate is of a mixed type, including lymphocytes. In leucocytoclastic vasculitis, where wheals last for up to 72 hours, neutrophils are prominent. Skin biopsies are, in general, not of diagnostic help in urticaria, with the exception of atypical, chronic cases where the single lesion persists for more than 24 hours. The diagnosis of urticaria pigmentosa (mastocytosis) can be confirmed by biopsy.

Skin challenge tests

Dermographism is demonstrated with a blunt instrument or a fingernail. It is fairly common in chronic urticaria and is always present in urticaria pigmentosa. The *ice-cube test* can confirm the diagnosis of cold urticaria. It simply consists of placing an ice-cube on the skin for 10 minutes. A *light test*, using a monochromatic light source and varying wave lengths, is an accurate test for solar urticaria. Protoporphyrin and coproporphyrin are measured in such cases. An *exercise test*, which provokes sweating, is a readily available method of producing cholinergic urticaria.

Treatment

Avoidance of causative factors is the first therapeutic principle, and it is feasible regarding drugs and most food items.

Suppression of symptoms is the second principle, and H_1 *antihistamines* are the drug of choice. The new *non-sedating H_1 antihistamines* listed in Table 6.8.2 are all highly effective, and they have fairly similar effect/side effect profiles (see Chapter 8.6).

Yet, in 10 to 20% of the cases of chronic urticaria, H_1 blockers may not be efficacious indicating that mediators other than histamine can be important in the pathogenesis of the disease.

Pressure urticaria is usually resistant to antihistamine therapy, but cetirizine, in double or triple dosage, which may then introduce sedation, has a significant effect in some patients.

Injections of adrenaline have an effect in cases of universal eruption and should be used when it is associated with anaphylaxis.

Oral corticosteroids, in rather high doses, may also have some effect. As a general rule, *steroids should not be used* for urticaria, which is a self-limiting, non-life-threatening disease. However, when chronic urticaria severely interferes with the quality of life, prednisolone 20–30 mg daily may be justified for a

H₁ antihistamines	
Generic name	**Recommended dosage**
Acrivastine	8 mg t.i.d.
Astemizole	10 mg o.d.
Cetirizine 10 mg o.d.	
Loratadine	10 mg o.d.
Terfenadine	120 mg o.d.

Table 6.8.2. Non-sedating antihistamines with proven efficacy for chronic urticaria

short period of time. In some patients with pressure urticaria, systemic steroids may be the only efficacious therapy.

Wrong and right
Lord, where we are wrong, make us willing to change, and where we are right, make us easy to live with.

Peter Marshall

6.9 Hereditary angioedema
Lack of functional C1 inactivator

Key points
- Hereditary angioedema is a genetic disorder in which the function of C1 inactivator is markedly reduced.
- Many stimuli can activate complement and C1 activator is the 'break' of this activation.
- When the 'break' is deficient, complement activation can occur after minimal stimulation.
- Generation of kinins by complement activation is most important for the formation of angioedema.
- The disease usually starts in childhood.
- Angioedema can involve all parts of the skin, the upper airway and the gastro-intestinal tract.
- The attack can occur spontaneously or as the result of a minor trauma.
- Due to laryngeal involvement, the mortality was previously high.
- Dental extraction and tonsillectomy/adenoidectomy can provoke life-threatening oropharyngeal oedema.
- Involvement of the intestinal mucosa causes alarming abdominal colic.
- A history of recurrent swellings, starting during childhood, and a positive family history suggest the diagnosis.
- It can be confirmed by measurement of C1 inactivator (total and functional levels).
- The acute attack is treated with adrenaline and intubation when needed.
- Successful prevention of the attacks can be attained with anti-fibrinolytic agents or androgenic derivatives.
- In every case, dental work and tonsillectomy/adenoidectomy need pretreatment.

Definition
Angioedema is 'giant urticaria', occurring as large swellings in the *deeper parts of the dermis* and subcutaneous tissue or in mucous membranes. *Hereditary angioedema* is a genetically dominant disorder in which the function of a plasma protein, the inhibitor of the first component of complement, is markedly reduced.

Mechanism
Many stimuli, such as antigen-antibody reactions and trauma, can activate the first factor of complement, C1 to $C\bar{1}$, also called C1 esterase. *C1 esterase inhibitor* (C1 inhibitor or *C1 inactivator*) is the 'break' of this activation (Fig. 6.9.1). When the 'break' is deficient, complement activation can occur after minimal stimulation. $C\bar{3}$ and $C\bar{5}$ (anaphylatoxin) are generated, but, in contrast to urticaria, histamine is of little significance for the formation of oedema. Most important is the generation of *kinins* from activated C2 (Fig. 6.9.1). Other mechanisms may also play a role, as C1 inactivator acts as an inhibitor in the *blood-clotting* and *fibrinolytic system*.

Clinical presentation
The disease *runs in families* and often, but not always, it *starts in childhood*. It is characterized by recurrent, circumscribed swellings, which can involve all parts of the skin, the upper airway and the gastro-intestinal tract — isolated or together.

The attack can occur *spontaneously* or as a result of a minor *trauma*. *Dental extraction* and *tonsillectomy/adenoidectomy* are of particular importance, as they often provoke oropharyngeal oedema, which, untreated, can lead to lethal airway obstruction.

Subcutaneous oedema varies in size from a few centimetres to involvement of an entire limb. It develops over the course of a few hours and persists for some days. The lesion is not itchy but can be tender. Usually, the attack is *not associated with urticaria*.

Laryngeal involvement is life-threatening and, previously, the mortality was high. A sensation of fullness in the throat, dysphagia and voice change are warning signals.

Involvement of the intestinal mucosa causes nausea, vomiting and severe *abdominal colic*, alarming for the surgeon. The abdomen is tender but seldom rigid, owing to the lack of peritoneal involvement.

Diagnosis
A history of recurrent swellings, starting during childhood, and a positive family history (negative in 20%) suggest the diagnosis. Compared with idiopathic angioedema, a characteristic feature of the disease is involvement of the gastro-intestinal tract.

The serum level of C4 is usually diminished during symptomatic and asymptomatic periods. This is a readily available screening test. C2 is only diminished during an attack. The most *specific test* is an assay for

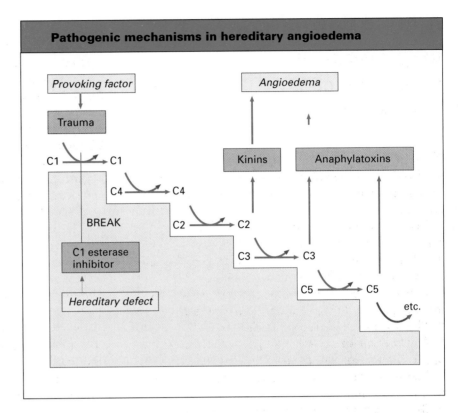

Fig. 6.9.1. Illustration of complement activation as a pathogenic mechanism in hereditary angioedema. When the 'break' is deficient the process is readily activated. Note, this staircase model is so simplified that it is not, strictly speaking, correct. Complement activation is an extremely complicated business.

C1 inactivator. A significantly reduced (>50%) or absent level confirms the diagnosis. Approximately 15% of the patients have a normal level, but the protein is non-functioning. Thus, a *functional test* for C1 inactivator is necessary when the total level is normal.

When angioedema of the above clinical and biochemical type first appears in an adult, it may be secondary to a *lymphoma* with an unusual complement utilization profile. The *acquired form* shows a depressed level of C1, which can be used to distinguish it from the hereditary form.

Treatment and prevention

Intermittent administration of subcutaneous *adrenaline* may reduce the formation of oedema but not reverse the swellings. Antihistamines are of no, and high-dose corticosteroids of little, benefit. It is important to call upon the otologist and anaesthetist when the throat and larynx is involved and to persuade the surgeon not to operate when the gastrointestinal tract is involved. *Intubation* is preferable to tracheotomy as the disease abates in 2–3 days. But these procedures are often unnecessary today, because attacks can be prevented and reduced by specific treatment.

Successful *prevention* of the attacks was first reported with *anti-fibrinolytic agents* (epsilon-aminocaproic acid and tranexamic acid). These agents can also be efficient in a few cases of severe idiopathic angioedema.

Androgenic derivatives not only prevent attacks of swelling but also induce synthesis of C1 inactivator, which returns to normal or almost normal levels together with C4. Danazol and stanozolol, having relatively little virilizing effect, are preferable and appear to have no unwanted side effects in men and in postmenopausal women.

Attacks in many patients are sufficiently mild or infrequent not to require long-term treatment. In every case, *dental work* and *tonsillectomy/ adenoidectomy* need pretreatment with antifibrinolytic or androgenic agents, perhaps fresh plasma, and post-surgical observation.

Health and wealth
Many men spend the first half of their lives expending health to gain wealth and the second half of their lives expending wealth to gain health.

Ernest W Dunbar

A good advice
It is our responsibilities, not ourselves, that we should take seriously.

Peter Ustinov

6.10 Allergic contact eczema
— and irritant eczema

Key points
- Contact eczema is caused by irritants (two-thirds) or by cell-mediated allergy (one-third).
- Histologically, it is characterized by accumulation of activated CD4+ T cells and microvesicle formation in epidermis.
- Irritants probably induce inflammation by up-regulation of cytokines in the skin.
- Contact eczema is quite common, and it has probably increased in prevalence, being a concomitant of atopic dermatitis.
- Contact eczema is most frequent among women between 20 and 40 years of age.
- In the acute phase, severely itching microvesicles develop in the epidermis.
- In the chronic phase, scaling and dryness of the skin are dominant.
- Contact eczema occurs in the face, neck, lower legs and, in particular, the hands.
- It develops predominantly in areas of 'thin epidermis' (between the fingers, on the dorsal side of the fingers and hands).
- The course of the disease is often chronic with acute relapses.
- The diagnosis is based on clinical history and examination.
- Skin patch testing is needed in order to discover possible allergies.
- Nickel is the most common cause of allergy, and ear-piercing is a risk factor.
- Occupational contact eczema develops in persons with a high impact of irritants on their skin.
- An endogenous form of eczema is characterized by vesicles in the palms, including the palmar side of the fingers.
- Therapy includes avoidance of allergens and irritants, and topical steroids.

Definition
Contact eczema is defined as eczema caused by contact with the environment. Most often, contact eczema is caused by irritants, which elicit the skin inflammation. However, in one-third of patients, a cutaneous cell-mediated allergy is found. The ability

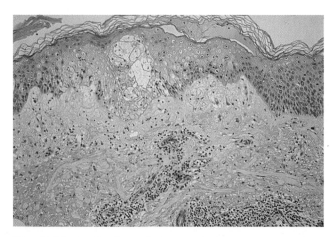

Fig. 6.10.1. Histological picture of contact eczema. Note the accumulation of lymphocytes (activated CD4+ T cells), some of which show migration into the epidermis, where a microvesicle is formed.

to develop contact eczema is somehow related to predisposition; in particular, patients with atopic dermatitis are at risk.

Contact eczema and immunity
Contact eczema is, histologically, an accumulation of activated CD4+ T lymphocytes in the superficial parts of the stratum papillare of dermis. Some lymphocytes migrate into the epidermis, where microvesicles are formed (Fig. 6.10.1). The Langerhans' cells of epidermis and the interdigitating cells in the stratum papillare are very potent antigen-presenting cells for T lymphocytes. Thus, the microvesicle formation in epidermis probably occurs around the Langerhans' cells.

Contact eczema resembles, both clinically and histologically, a true cell-mediated immune reaction, including expression of cytokines, chemokines and adhesion molecules. A Type IV allergic reaction can be demonstrated in approximately one-third of patients using epicutaneous patch testing (Fig 6.10.2).

Inflammation induced by irritants
How can irritants induce inflammation? At present, this is not known. It is likely that irritants in predisposed individuals will up-regulate both cytokines and chemokines, leading to an accumulation of T lymphocytes in the skin. This propensity is correlated with atopy. The following cytokine cascade has been found following the impact of certain irritants to human skin: IL-1, IL-8 and TNF, followed by the occurrence of T-lymphocyte-derived cytokines, such as IL-2, IL-4 and IFNγ.

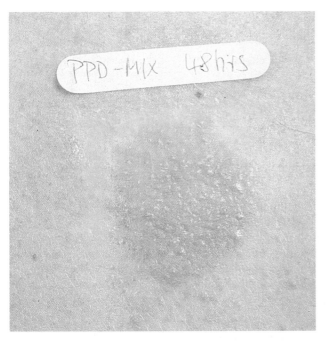

Fig. 6.10.2. Epicutaneous patch test showing vesicles, redness and infiltration as a sign of acute, vesicular contact eczema. This reaction is a sign of cell-mediated immunity in the patient towards the antigen in question.

Hand eczema in patients with previous atopic disease	
Atopic dermatitis hospitalized patients (*n* = 549)	41%
Atopic dermatitis out-patients (*n* = 406)	25%
Respiratory atopy (*n* = 222)	5%
Normal controls (*n* = 199)	4%

Table 6.10.2. Hand eczema among patients with previous atopic disorders. From Rystedt I. Hand eczema in patients with history of atopic manifestations in childhood. *Acta Derm Venereol (Stockh)* 1985; **65**: 305–12

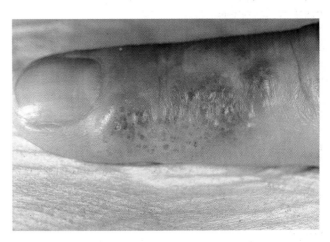

Fig. 6.10.3. Finger with acute eczema. Note that scaling is not prominent. The reaction resembles the acute eczema seen in a positive patch test.

Epidemiology

Contact eczema is quite common. Table 6.10.1 shows the prevalence of hand eczema in two large epidemiological studies performed in Sweden 2 decades apart. The suggested rise in prevalence is probably real and secondary to the increase of atopic dermatitis. As many as 25–50% of children with atopic dermatitis will develop irritant hand eczema during adult life (Table 6.10.2).

Prevalence of hand eczema			
Age (years)	Number investigated	Year	Prevalence (%)
>10	110 000	1964	2.8*
20–65	20 000	1983	5.6†

Table 6.10.1. Epidemiology of hand eczema in two major Swedish studies. *From Agrup G. Hand eczema and other dermatoses in South Sweden. *Acta Derm Venereol (Stockh)* 1969; **49**(suppl 61). †From Meding B, Swanbeck G. Prevalence of hand eczema in an industrialized city. *Br J Dermatol* 1087; **116**: 627–34

Clinic

The word 'eczema' or '*ekzein*' is greek and means 'to boil over'. The patient feels that her or his skin is 'boiling' from itching.

Contact eczema is most frequent among women (two-thirds), and occurs typically between 20 and 40 years of age. In the initial acute phase, severely *itching microvesicles* develop in the epidermis (Fig. 6.10.3). They are, in the chronic phase, followed by *scaling and dryness* of the skin (Fig. 6.10.4).

Contact eczema occurs in skin that is in contact with the outer world (face, neck, hands and lower legs), but contact eczema is almost synonymous

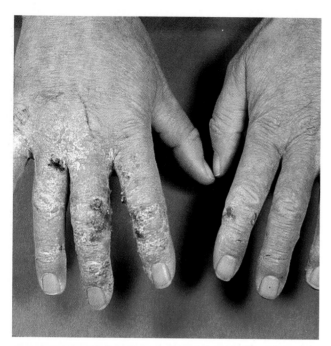

Fig. 6.10.4. Chronic eczema, where scaling is prominent but where vesicles are only seen in smaller areas at the border of the lesions. Use a magnifier to see the vesicles. Note that the eczema is localized to skin with thin epidermis, that is, a short distance between the environment and the immune system.

with hand eczema. Symptoms typically *develop in areas of 'thin epidermis'*, that is where the distance between the environment and the immune system is minimal. This means that contact eczema develops *between the fingers*, on the *dorsal side of the fingers*, and hands, and at the volar side of the wrist.

The duration of the disease is often chronic. Initial

The top-10 list of epicutaneous allergies		
Allergen	**Women (%)**	**Men (%)**
1 Nickel	11.1	2.2
2 Tiomersal	3.1	3.6
3 Perfume	1.0	1.1
4 Cobalt	1.4	0.7
5 Formaldehyde resin	1.0	1.1
6 Balsam of Peru	1.4	0.7
7 Colophony	1.0	0.4
8 Isotiazoliones	1.0	0.4
9 Chromium	0.3	0.7
10 Thiuramix	0.3	0.7

Table 6.10.3. The top-10 list of epicutaneous allergies in a general population. From Nielsen NH, Menné T. Allergic contact sensitization in an adult Danish population. *Ugeskr Læger* 1994; **156**: 3471–4

acute outbreaks of eczema is followed by prolonged periods with scaling, itching and 'sensitive skin', with acute relapses intermingled (Fig. 6.10.5).

Diagnosis

The diagnosis is based on clinical history and examination. Patients with eczema in the face, neck, on the hands or lower legs of more than 3 months duration should be patch tested in order to discover possible allergies.

Contact allergy

Table 6.10.3 shows the top-10 list of allergens among the general population in Denmark. Patients with

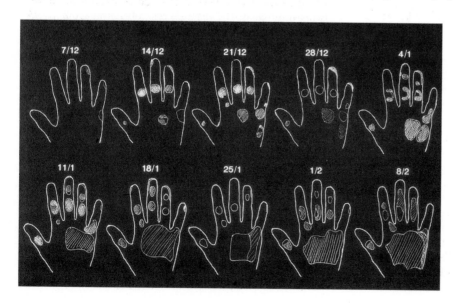

Fig. 6.10.5. Drawing of how an irritant contact eczema develops and spreads during a 2-month period in a violin player. Note that the disease occurred in the winter time, when contact eczema is most pronounced.

Ear-piercing and risk of nickel allergy	
	Positive nickel skin patch test (%)
Ears pierced (*n* = 692)	13
Ears not pierced (*n* = 268)	1

Table 6.10.4. A total of 960 unselected Swedish school girls aged 8–15 years were patch tested irrespective of previous or present skin disease. From Larsson-Styme B, Widström L. *Contact Dermatitis* 1985; **13**: 289–98.

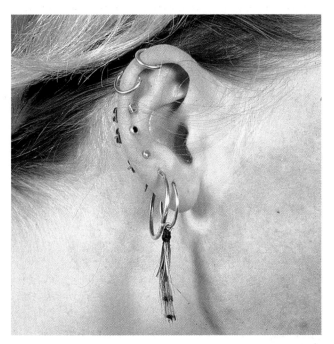

Fig. 6.10.6. Ear-piercing considerably increases the risk of nickel allergy and contact eczema.

eczema will have significantly higher incidences of contact allergy. Nickel is the most common cause of allergy, especially in women. This is related to the fact that ear-piercing is a common phenomenon in society (Table 6.10.4). Approximately half of the girls with nickel allergy will later develop eczema (Fig. 6.10.6).

Occupation and contact eczema

Occupational contact eczema is quite common. It develops in persons with a high impact of irritants on their skin. It is advisable to tell children with severe

Occupation and risk of hand eczema	
Occupation/industry	Prevalence of hand eczema (%)
Cooks and sandwich makers	10.9
Hairdressers	9.0
Packing industry	6.2
Furniture industry	6.0
Mechanics	5.3
Bakers	4.7
Meat industry	3.2
Fishing industry	2.7
Laboratory technicians	2.6
Cleaning assistants	2.4

Table 6.10.5. Prevalence of hand eczema in different occupations. By courtesy of Lars Halkier-Sørensen

atopic dermatitis that they should avoid jobs listed in Table 6.10.5.

Differential diagnosis: pompholyx

Eczema of the hands is not necessarily contact eczema. It is important to realize that eczema in the palms, including the palmar side of the fingers, is an *endogenous form of eczema*, which is associated with smoking (75%), predisposition for atopy (50%) and nickel allergy (20%). The mechanisms behind these associations are unknown. The disorder is called *vesicular eczema of the hands*, *pompholyx* (Greek for 'bubble') or *dyshidrotic eczema* (misnomer) and forms approximately 5% of hand eczema. This endogenous disease develops between 30 and 50 years of age. It is characterized by cyclic episodes of sudden eruption of severely itching vesicles as seen *in the palmar skin* – often without known external skin irritation. Within a week, it is followed by scaling, dryness, development of fissures and erosions. The itch is diminished, but the pain from damaged skin will increase (Fig. 6.10.7). A new relapse will occur within 2–8 weeks.

Any skin impingement, such as washing the hands, washing the hair, cooking and house cleaning, will irritate the skin and aggravate the symptoms. However, even if the patient goes on sick leave, new relapses will occur.

Quite commonly, contact allergies will arise towards rubber and/or chromium because the patient protects the hands using rubber or leather (chromium) gloves.

Patch testing is therefore relevant in order to help

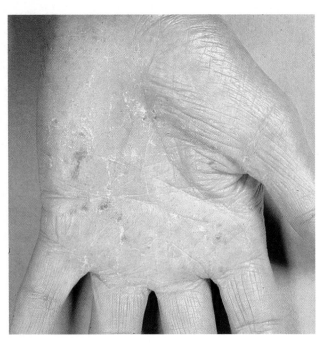

Fig. 6.10.7. The endogenous form of eczema, which is more or less a symmetrical affection of palmar (and sometimes also plantar) skin. The eczema is in a more or less chronic stage. However, areas with vesicles can be seen.

the patient to avoid eliciting allergens. The disease can quickly become a mixture of pompholyx of endogenous origin, contact allergy and irritant eczema. The course of the disease may be severe and year long. Very often, eczema also occurs in the plantar skin.

Therapy

Treatment strategies include *avoidance of allergens and irritants*, which may be difficult. *Topical glucocorticosteroids* are very efficacious due to their anti-inflammatory activities. Potent steroids should be used once or twice daily until the vesicular eruption is subdued, which may take 1–3 weeks. Then intermittent therapy with mild steroids should be applied. Emollients will help prevent skin dryness.

The endogenous form of eczema is difficult to treat. In severe cases, systemic therapy may be necessary using PUVA (psoralens and UVA light) or methotrexate, whereas systemic steroids should be avoided.

In research work
We learn more from things that disagree with our hypothesis than from those which don't.

Karl Popper

Further reading

BERTH-JONES, J, GRAHAM-BROWN RAC. Placebo-controlled trial of essential fatty acid supplementation in atopic dermatitis. *Lancet* 1993; **341**: 1557–60.

DORNER W, BAYLOCK KW, HANIFIN JM, HOLDER WR, JENSEN GT. Guidelines of the care for atopic dermatitis. *J Am Acad Dermatol* 1992; **26**: 485–91.

DREBORG S, ed. Postgraduate course: atopic dermatitis. *Pediatr Allergy Immunol* 1991; **1**(suppl 2): 1–48.

HANIFIN JM, RAJKA G. Diagnostic features of atopic dermatitis. *Acta Derm Venereol (Stockh)* 1980; **92**(suppl 44).

ORFAN NA, KOLSKI GB. Angioedema and C1 inhibitor deficiency. *Ann Allergy* 1992; **69**: 167–72.

SAMPSON HA. Atopic dermatitis. *Ann Allergy* 1992; **69**: 469–479.

THESTRUP-PEDERSEN K, GRØNHØJ C, RØNNEVIG J. The immunology of contact dermatitis. A review with special reference to the pathophysiology of eczema. *Contact Dermatitis* 1989; **20**: 81–8.

WAHLGREN C-F. Pathophysiology of itching in urticaria and atopic dermatitis. *Allergy* 1992; **47**: 65–75.

Part 7 Eye Diseases

7.1 The eye and immunology

Immunodeficiency of the eyeball

Key points
- It is essential for normal vision that the optical axis passes through transparent media only.
- Therefore, the cornea, anterior chamber, lens and vitreous body all lack lymphatics, blood vessels and inflammatory cells.
- It follows that the eyeball is immunologically deficient.
- The anterior chamber, lens and vitreous body are inaccessible to micro-organisms and safe due to their location.
- The cornea, exposed to the environment, is protected by a structural defence, the blinking mechanism, tears, and the immune system in the conjunctiva.
- The conjunctiva is fully immunologically equipped with lymphocytes and neutrophils, but eosinophils are normally absent.

- The distribution of mast cells indicates where Type I allergic diseases are most frequent in the eye.
- Their number is high in the conjunctiva and lids, but very low in the lacrimal glands and eyeball.
- Allergic conjunctivitis is a prevalent Type I allergic disease.
- Vernal kerato-conjunctivitis is a rare atopic disease with a Type I allergic component.

Local immunodeficiency
It is essential for normal vision that the optical axis passes through *transparent media* only (Fig. 7.1.1). One can therefore understand why the cornea, anterior chamber, lens and vitreous body all lack lymphatics, blood vessels and inflammatory cells. It follows that *the eyeball is immunologically deficient*, and the tissues of the eye cannot normally raise an inflammatory response.

Immunological isolation
The *lens* is in immunological isolation; it is full of antigens, capable of inciting an immune response in the body, but inflammation does not occur in the intact lens, as neither antibody nor lymphocytes have access to the tissue.

In the *cornea*, the tight junctions between the

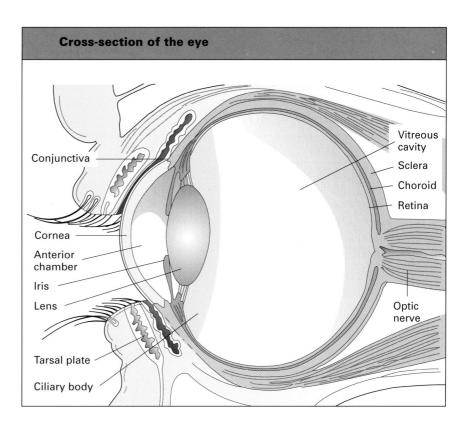

Fig. 7.1.1. Section of the orbit to demonstrate the target organs involved in immunological eye diseases. Type I allergic reactions are confined to the conjunctiva, but the cornea can be secondarily afflicted.

Cross-section of the eye

Conjunctiva
Vitreous cavity
Sclera
Choroid
Retina
Cornea
Anterior chamber
Iris
Lens
Optic nerve
Tarsal plate
Ciliary body

Distribution of mast cells in the eye

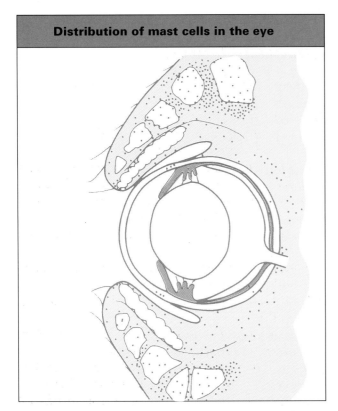

Fig. 7.1.2. Diagrammatic representation of mast cells in ocular tissues of the rat. Note the density of cells in the lids and conjunctiva, which contain about 95% of the mast cells in the eye. The total number of mast cells in the human eye is estimated at 50 million. From Allansmith MR. *The Eye and Immunology* Saint Louis: The CV Mosby Company, 1982: 1–209.

epithelial cells keep out many macromolecules, so it takes several days for antigens and antibodies to penetrate the tissue. Although antigen–antibody reactions can take place in the cornea, they will *not result in inflammation*, as mast cells are absent, neutrophils cannot be recruited and no lymphocytes patrol the tissue. Many patients have obtained secondary benefit from this physiology, as it results in a 90% success rate for corneal transplantation.

Alternative defence systems

Anterior chamber, lens and vitreous body

Only sterile environments will allow an immunologically deficient tissue to remain unpunished, unless alternative defence systems exist, and they fortunately exist in the eye. The inside of the eyeball is, generally, *inaccessible to micro-organisms*. The an-

terior chamber, lens and vitreous body are safe due to their location.

The cornea

The cornea, on the other hand, is in contact with the environment and its content of potential invaders. It is provided with a dual defence mechanism: 1, an efficient *structural defence* of tight junctions between the squamous epithelial cells; and 2 the *blinking mechanism* together with the flushing action of the tears.

'Immunological war'

Immune protection of the cornea is provided by the surrounding conjunctiva, and the tears offer an additional supply of antibodies. According to Mathea Allansmith, Department of Ophthalmology, Harvard University: 'These elements fight excellently and protect the cornea in most limited skirmishes. Occasionally, an all-out immunologic war occurs, and the privileged "cornea castle" is invaded by inflammatory soldiers dragging their transportation lines of blood vessels and lymphatics with them. Sometimes these immunologic wars are so severe that the war is won, but the cornea left so scarred as to blind the patient'.

Conjunctiva

As the *conjunctiva defends the cornea* so vigorously, it follows that it must be fully immunologically equipped. This implies a risk both of inflammation and of allergy.

Lymphocytes and *neutrophils* are normally found in the conjunctiva. As in all other exposed mucosal membranes, they are attracted to the epithelial surface to defend the tissues against invaders. *Eosinophils*, on the other hand, are generally absent in the normal conjunctiva. The number of *mast cells* is high in the conjunctiva and lids, but very low in the lacrimal glands and approaching zero in the eyeball. The distribution of this cell type (Fig. 7.1.2) indicates where Type I allergic diseases are most frequent in the eye.

Type I allergic reactions

The Type I allergic reaction in the ocular tissues is bothersome because the eye is functionally so critical and its disorders obvious. *Allergic conjunctivitis* is the eye disease, which, with the greatest certainty, can be called a Type I reaction. *Vernal kerato-conjunctivitis* is an atopic disease with a significant

Type I allergic component. Only these two diseases are regularly seen by the allergist and will be described, but many eye diseases have an immunological background.

A short life can be long
Life isn't the days that have passed but the days you remember.

Pavlenko

7.2 Allergic conjunctivitis
Pollen and animal protein

Key points
- Allergic conjunctivitis is a common disease, associated in most cases with allergic rhinitis.
- Eye symptoms are generally more frequent and troublesome in seasonal than in perennial disease.
- Histamine is responsible for the principal symptom, itching, which leads to eye rubbing.
- Redness and irritation are caused by histamine and by rubbing.
- Tearing can be reflex-initiated from the conjunctival and the nasal mucosa.
- Oral H_1 antihistamines can relieve the itching within 30 minutes.
- Topical H_1 antihistamines give immediate relief, which lasts 12 hours with levocabastine.
- A vasoconstrictor is often added to the antihistamine eye drops in order to counteract redness.
- The patient should use the drops instead of, and not after, rubbing the eyes.
- Prophylactic treatment with cromoglycate every 3–4 hours can reduce the symptoms.
- Patients may obtain immediate relief from a simple eye bath with saline.
- Short-term systemic steroids can be used when eye and nose symptoms are severe.
- Immunotherapy may be considered in severe cases.

Allergic conjunctivitis is usually part of allergic rhino-conjunctivitis. In any affected individual, either the ocular or the nasal symptoms may predominate. Conjunctivitis is generally a more prominent component of seasonal than of perennial disease, and more significant in allergy to animal protein than in mite allergy. This is because we are exposed to mites with our eyes closed, and because the heavy mite faeces particles are airborne for much shorter periods of time than the small particles of, for example, cat protein.

As *seasonal allergic conjunctivitis* and *perennial allergic conjunctivitis* are non-sight-threatening diseases, they are usually treated by general practitioners and allergists and are rarely seen by ophthalmologists.

Pathogenesis

The allergen dissolves quickly in the tear film and makes contact with IgE antibody affixed to *mast cells* in the *conjunctiva*. The released *histamine* and other biochemical mediators are directly responsible for the symptoms and signs of allergic conjunctivitis. Histamine dropped into the eye produces *itching* and *redness*, indistinguishable from hay fever symptoms. This indicates that histamine is the most important mediator substance, and H_1 antihistamine has the most marked effect in allergic conjunctivitis. *Tearing* can be *reflex-stimulated* from both the conjunctival and the nasal mucosa. Irritation of the nose causes transient conjunctival vasodilatation, but not itching.

Symptoms and signs

Eye *itching* is one of the most troublesome symptoms of hay fever and interferes profoundly with daily life (personal experience). The pruritus is mainly localized to the medial ocular angle, where the pollen grains are concentrated by blinking. *Rubbing* gives immediate relief and satisfaction but, alas, it is short-lasting; the itching returns with renewed vigour and a vicious spiral is started. As a result, conjunctival blood vessels are dilated and the eye becomes *red* and irritated.

It is important to make a distinction between the intense itching, characteristic of allergic conjunctivitis, and irritation and smarting of the eye, which result from non-specific 'smog conjunctivitis'.

The ocular *discharge* in hay fever is watery, occasionally with a mucoid component. The *cornea is not involved*, in contrast with vernal kerato-conjunctivitis, so there is no intense photophobia. Slight, transient photophobia may occur in allergic conjunctivitis after vigorous eye rubbing.

Treatment

As pollen exposure cannot be avoided during the season, treatment is necessary. H_1 *antihistamines* relieve the itching; the tablets are effective after 30 minutes and usually last for 24 hours. Topical application gives immediate relief, which, for levocabastine, can last 12 hours. Antihistamine *eye drops* are often combined with a *vasoconstrictor*, to counteract redness. It is important to tell the patient to use the drops instead of, and not after, rubbing the eyes. Otherwise the drops will cause considerable smarting due to the preservative added.

Prophylactic treatment with *cromoglycate* can be administered every 3–4 hours. This will reduce the symptoms somewhat, with the cost being the only known contra-indication. Some patients obtain immediate relief from the eye drops; this is probably due to a washing-out of allergens. A simple *eye bath with saline* will produce the same effect.

As the cornea is not involved, *corticosteroids* are to be *avoided*, unless all other treatment has failed. A 2-week course of corticosteroids can then be justified. As most of these patients have severe nasal symptoms too, systemic rather than local administration is advisable. It is a sound principle that *only ophthalmologists prescribe steroid eye drops* due to their potential for causing serious adverse effects.

Immunotherapy can reduce, but seldom eliminate, the symptoms of pollen conjunctivitis. It is used together with pharmacotherapy in severe cases.

The conditions of research work
The great tragedy of science – the slaying of a beautiful hypothesis by an ugly fact.

Thomas Huxley

7.3 Vernal kerato-conjunctivitis

– and atopic kerato-conjunctivitis

Key points

- Vernal kerato-conjunctivitis is an atopic disease characterized by intense itching and giant papilla.
- The disease is chronic with exacerbations during spring and summer.
- Although skin testing is usually positive, allergen exposure only accounts for a few of the symptoms.
- The disease is rare; it is more frequent in warm than in temperate regions.
- The patients are usually boys below the age of 10 years.
- The disease, as a rule, resolves within 5–10 years.
- There is intense and persistent itching, thick ropy discharge, marked photophobia and, in severe cases, impaired vision.
- Examination of the eye reveals giant papillae of the upper conjunctiva and keratitis during exacerbations.
- Topical steroids are necessary but are reserved for acute exacerbations with corneal involvement.
- Supportive treatment consists of cromoglycate, H_1 antihistamines, antibiotics, surgery, ice compresses and good lid hygiene.
- The differential diagnosis is giant papillary conjunctivitis, in contact-lens wearers, and atopic kerato-conjunctivitis.
- Atopic kerato-conjunctivitis is a chronic disease of young adults with atopic dermatitis involving the eyelids.

Vernal kerato-conjunctivitis is a *chronic* inflammation of the conjunctiva characterized by *giant papilla* of the upper tarsal conjunctiva. There are intermittent *exacerbations*, which are often *seasonal*, during which keratitis may develop.

As symptoms are severe and the disease may be sight-threatening, an *ophthalmologist* should always be involved.

Atopic disease

The following characterize vernal kerato-conjunctivitis as an atopic disease: 1, the majority of patients (about 75%) have a *family history*; 2, they have *other atopic diseases*; 3, they have raised serum *IgE* level, 4, they have multiple *positive skin tests*; and 5, the pathology is consistent with an atopic disease: conjunctiva contains many degranulated mast cells, *eosinophilia* can be demonstrated in ocular discharge, and the histamine level in a conjunctival washing is elevated.

Allergic disease?

Vernal kerato-conjunctivitis cannot, strictly speaking, be classified as an allergic disease, as allergy only appears to account for occasional exacerbations and not for the daily chronic symptoms. The disease corresponds to atopic dermatitis in this respect, the spontaneous course being similar, *commencing early in life* and, as a rule, *resolving within 5–10 years*.

Symptoms

The disease is *rare*, and more frequent in warm than in temperate regions. The symptoms usually start in the warm season ('vernal' means spring), and tend to become chronic, with seasonal exacerbations. The patients are usually boys below the age of 10 years.

The most prominent symptom is *intense itching*, which is persistent and distressing: 'I want to scratch my eyes out'. Although *eye rubbing* should be discouraged, it is an inevitable consequence, and adds to the *redness* and burning irritation in the eyes. A sensation of a foreign body is common. The *mucoid discharge*, especially in periods of exacerbations, is thick and ropy.

Keratitis, with intense *photophobia* and reduced visual acuity, is frequent. The cause of the keratitis is unclear, as the cornea has no mechanisms with which to express allergy.

Signs

When a patient presents with active disease, the conjunctiva is hyperaemic, oedematous, and its surface appears milky. The diagnosis can be confirmed by everting the upper tarsal plate. This will show *papillary hypertrophy* with a typical 'cobblestone' appearance (Fig. 7.3.1). The inflammatory cells in the papillae are mainly lymphocytes (CD4$^+$ T cells), mast cells and eosinophils.

During exacerbations, the ophthalmologist can detect a keratitis, which takes the form of *punctate epithelial keratitis* on the upper part of the cornea. In severe cases, these epithelial lesions may become confluent, and an *ulcer* develops. It is difficult to heal as it becomes covered by a hard *plaque* of mucus and

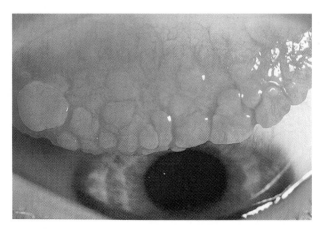

Fig. 7.3.1. Upper tarsal conjunctiva in vernal kerato-conjunctivitis. The upper lid has been everted to reveal typical papillary hypertrophy. From Buckley RJ. Conjunctivitis – diagnosis and treatment. In: Holgate ST, Church MK, eds. *Allergy* London: Gower Medical Publishing, 1993: 20.1–8.

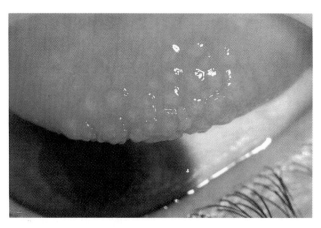

Fig. 7.3.2. Upper tarsal conjunctiva in giant papillary conjunctivitis in a contact-lens wearer. The appearance is similar to that of vernal kerato-conjunctivitis, but there is no corneal involvement. From Buckley RJ. Conjunctivitis – diagnosis and treatment. In: Holgate ST, Church MK, eds. *Allergy* London: Gower Medical Publishing, 1993: 20.1–8.

fibrin. If the ulcer persists, vascularization with *scarring* and some loss of vision will occur.

Differential diagnosis

A distinction must be made between vernal keratoconjunctivitis and other diseases with papillary hypertrophy. *Trachoma* must be considered in some countries and lens-associated *giant papillary conjunctivitis* (Fig. 7.3.2) in others; the latter occurs in *contact-lens wearers* and is probably an immunological reaction to deposits on the lens.

Treatment

Patients and doctors should be prepared for a *long battle*. As nearly all patients recover spontaneously within 5–10 years, management primarily aims at bringing the patient through these difficult years without permanent visual impairment from disease or from treatment. Cases where the disease starts after puberty have a less optimistic prognosis.

Topical corticosteroids are necessary for acute exacerbations of keratitis. All other treatment, psychological support included, must be vigorous. In general, immunotherapy to airborne allergens is of little help.

Management of itching

As in atopic dermatitis, H_1 *antihistamines* have generally been disappointing, but they may give some relief from the itching. *Crushed-ice* compresses for the ocular region are a good substitute for eye rubbing.

Cromoglycate

Cromoglycate drops are not a wonder treatment for this disease (Table 7.3.1), but, as this atoxic drug can reduce the need for steroids, continuous treatment (4–6 times/day) is *advisable*, especially during the pollen season.

Corticosteroids

Steroids, applied topically, are exceedingly valuable agents when the dosage is adjusted according to the severity of the disease. Their use is generally *confined to exacerbations* affecting the cornea; at these times,

Cromoglycate in vernal kerato-conjunctivitis			
Response	**Mild disease**	**Moderate disease**	**Severe disease**
Full control	19	0	0
Partial control	19	35	11
Useful response	1	6	8
No response	0	1	0

Table 7.3.1. Response to cromoglycate drops in 100 patients with vernal kerato-conjunctivitis. Open assessment over a 4-year treatment period. From Buckley RJ. Long-term experience with sodium cromoglycate in the management of vernal kerato-conjunctivitis. In: Pepys J, Edwards AM, eds. *The Mast Cell* Kent: Pitman Medicals, 1973: 518–23

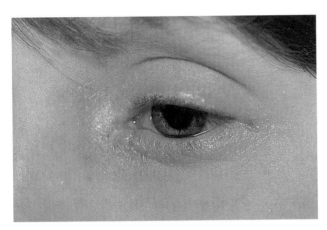

Fig. 7.3.3. The thickened lid margins and eczematous skin in atopic kerato-conjunctivitis. From Buckley RJ. Conjunctivitis – diagnosis and treatment. In: Holgate ST, Church MK, eds. *Allergy* London: Gower Medical Publishing, 1993: 20.1–8.

the patient may require steroid drops every 1–2 hours during the day and ointment applied at night. Ointments may be helpful when tear production is profuse, as steroid drops can be diluted to the point of ineffectiveness. As there is a *risk of serious adverse effects* (glaucoma, cataract and herpetic keratitis), the quantity of steroid medication should be kept as low as possible, and its use always supervised by an *ophthalmologist*.

Other measures

Surgical removal of a mucus plaque on the cornea, known as *superficial keratectomy*, is occasionally required. *Antibiotic therapy* will be indicated for bacterial complications. Both inflammation and exudation require good *lid hygiene*. A mild soap, such as a baby shampoo, diluted from full strength, is an effective lid cleaner.

Atopic kerato-conjunctivitis

This is a chronic and very distressing disease of young adults with atopic dermatitis, who develop facial eczema involving the eyelids (Fig. 7.3.3). The cornea may be subject to epithelial defects, scarring and vascularization. Atopic kerato-conjunctivitis can be thought of as an adult equivalent to vernal kerato-conjunctivitis, and treatment is similar. The thickened lid margins are often infected with *Staphylococcus aureus*, and antibiotics are frequently needed.

Further reading

Books

ALLANSMITH MR. *The Eye and Immunology.* Saint Louis: The CV Mosby Company, 1982: 1–209.

Articles

ABELSON MB, GEORGE MA, GAROFALO C. Differential diagnosis of ocular allergic disorders. *Ann Allergy* 1993; **70**: 95–109.

BIELORY L, FROHMAN LP. Allergic and immunologic disorders of the eye. *J Allergy Clin Immunol* 1992; **89**: 1–15.

BONINI S, BONINI S, BUCCI MG, et al. Allergen dose response and late symptoms in a human model of ocular allergy. *J Allergy Clin Immunol* 1990; **86**: 869–76.

BONINI S, TOMASSINI M, BONINI S, CAPRON M, BALSANO F. The eosinophil has a pivotal role in allergic inflammation in the eye. *Int Arch Allergy Immunol* 1992; **99**: 354–8.

BUCKLEY RJ. Vernal keratoconjunctivitis. *Int Ophthalmol Clin* 1989; **29**: 303–8.

BUCKLEY RJ. Diagnosis and treatment of atopic eye diseases. *Clin Exp Allergy* 1992; **22**: 887–8.

BUTRUS SI, OCHSNER KI, ABELSON MB, SWARTZ LB. The level of tryptase in human tears. An indicator of activation of conjunctival mast cells. *Ophthalmology* 1990; **97**: 1678–84.

CIPRANDI G, BUSCAGLIA S, PESCE G, et al. Deflazacort protects against late-phase but not early-phase reactions induced by the allergen-specific conjunctival provocation. *Allergy* 1993; **48**: 421–30.

CIPRANDI G, BUSCAGLIA S, PESCE G, CANONICA GW. Allergic subjects express intercellular adhesion molecule-1 (ICAM-1 or CD54) on epithelial cells of conjunctiva after allergen challenge. *J Allergy Clin Immunol* 1993; **91**: 783–92.

FOSTER CS, RICE BA, DUTT JE. Immunopathology of atopic conjunctivitis. *Ophthalmology* 1991; **98**: 1190–6.

FRIEDLAENDER MH. Current concepts in ocular allergy. *Ann Allergy* 1991; **67**: 5–10.

MAGGI E, BISWAS P, DEL PRETE G, et al. Accumulation of Th-2 like helper T cells in the conjunctiva of patients with vernal kerataconjunctivitis. *J Immunol* 1991; **146**: 1169–1174.

MORGAN SJ, WILLIAMS JH, WALLS AF, et al. Mast cell numbers and staining characteristics in the normal and allergic human conjunctiva. *J Allergy Clin Immunol* 1991; **87**: 111–116.

PROUD D, SWEET J, STEIN P, et al. Inflammatory mediator release on conjunctival provocation of allergic subjects with allergen. *J Allergy Clin Immunol* 1991; **85**: 896–905.

TUFT SJ, KEMENY MD, DART JKG, BUCKLEY RJ. Clinical features of atopic keratoconjunctivitis. *Ophthalmology* 1991; **98**: 150–8.

Part 8 Rhinitis

8.1 Structure and function of the nose

Heating, humidification and filtration

Key points

• The internal nose consists of narrow, slit-like passages, giving close contact between the inhaled air and the nasal mucosa.
• The mucous membrane supplies water (many glands) and heat (high blood flow) to the inhaled air.
• Nervous regulation of venous sinusoids permits the nose to adjust itself to changing demands.
• The shape of the nasal cavity facilitates deposition of particles, particularly those of large size, and water-soluble gases.
• The mouth is an adequate substitute for the nasal air conditioner under normal basal conditions.
• Breathing through the nose is preferable, when subjects with hyper-responsive airways are exposed to environmental challenges.

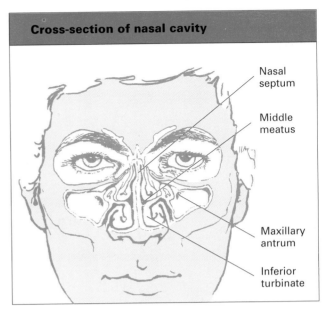

Fig. 8.1.2. Cross-section through the nasal cavities, showing turbinates and the slit-like passages. From Proctor DF. The upper respiratory tract. In: Fishman AP, ed. *Pulmonary Diseases and Disorders* New York: McGraw-Hill, 1980: 209–23.

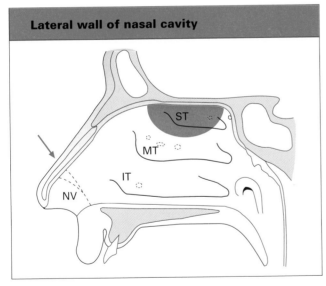

Fig. 8.1.1. Lateral wall of the nasal cavity. The nasal vestibule (NV) and the olfactory region (blue area), which in humans occupies 10 cm², as compared with 170 cm² in the German shepherd dog. The openings from the naso-lacrimal duct and paranasal sinuses are under the inferior (IT), middle (MT), and superior turbinates (ST). The arrow points to the internal ostium.

Structure

The internal nose consists of, on each side, the nostril (vestibule) and the *nasal cavity*. The vestibule and cavity are separated by the *internal ostium* (nasal valve). This, the narrowest part of the whole airway (0.3 cm² on each side), is positioned at the lower border of the lateral nasal cartilage (which can be reached by a finger).

The nasal cavities are deeper than suggested by the visible nose, the length being 10–12 cm from the tip of nose to the pharyngeal wall (Fig. 8.1.1). Due to the prominence of the three nasal turbinates, each of the two cavities is a *narrow slit* only 2–4 mm wide (Fig. 8.1.2). This complex arrangement indicates that the nose is more than a simple conductive airway, and this is confirmed by the fact that it accounts for 50% of the total resistance to airflow in the airways.

Functions

The anatomy of the nose is important for its functions (Fig. 8.1.3): 1, *airway*; 2, *heating, humidification* and *filtration* of inhaled air, which protect the delicate structures of the lower airways; 3, the *sense of smell*, which is vital for many animal species; for humans it is important for the pleasure of eating and drinking; and 4, *conservation of exhaled*

Functions of the nose

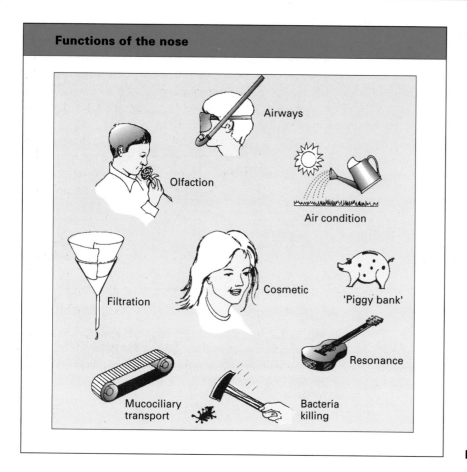

Fig. 8.1.3. Functions of the nose.

water and heat in the relatively cold anterior part of the nose; due to this 'piggy bank' function, the body saves 100 ml water/day.

Airway

The nose, and not the mouth, is the first part of the natural airway, a fact often forgotten by pulmonary physiologists. Airflow in the nose is rapid, about 3 m/s. At the internal ostium, it is 15 m/s, and during a sniff it can easily reach the speed of a hurricane (>30 m/s).

During exercise, a switch from nasal to oro-nasal breathing occurs when the ventilation is about 35 l/min. Oral breathing occurs earlier in rhinitis patients with partly blocked noses.

Regulation of nasal patency

The width of the nasal passages, important for airflow and conditioning, is actively regulated by sympathetic nerves acting on the venous sinusoids. The *sympathetic tone* in the nose normally changes from one nostril to the other in a 2–4 hour cycle. This *nasal cycle* is only noted by subjects with an anatomical

The nasal cycle

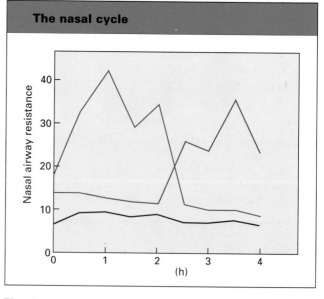

Fig. 8.1.4. The nasal cycle of changing congestion and decongestion in the two nasal cavities. Right cavity (blue); left cavity (red); both cavities (black).

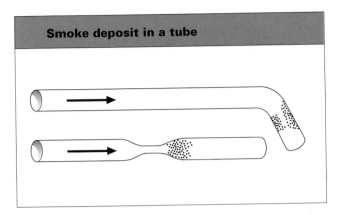

Fig. 8.1.5. Deposits are left by smoke passing through a tube behind a bend and a constriction due to impingement and turbulence. From Proetz AW. *Applied Physiology of the Nose*. Saint Louis: Annals Publishing Company, 1953.

abnormality (deflected septum) or swollen mucous membrane (rhinitis) (Fig. 8.1.4).

Filtration

The following are of importance for the filtration function: 1, particles impinge against the mucosa due to *bending of the airstream* in the nose; and 2, turbulence behind the *narrow entrance* to the cavity promotes particle deposition (Figs 8.1.1 & 8.1.5).

Particles

The efficacy of the nasal filter *depends upon the size* of the inhaled particles. Very few particles larger than 10 μm will penetrate the nose and the upper airways (pollen grains are 20–30 μm), while most particles smaller than 2 μm (mould spores) bypass the nose (Fig. 8.1.6).

Deposited particles are cleared from the nose within 30 minutes by *mucociliary transport*. Before nasal mucus is swallowed, a large part has passed over the adenoids (Fig. 8.1.7), where inhaled antigens are brought in close contact with, and can stimulate, the immune system.

Gases

The nose also acts as a 'gas mask' by retaining 99% of inhaled *water-soluble gases*. It is important that the common pollutants, ozone (outdoors from cars), sulphur dioxide (outdoors and indoors from fossil fuels) and formaldehyde (indoors from building materials and fabrics), only reach the lower airways in small amounts as they are strong irritants.

Air conditioning

The nose has good design features for an air conditioner: 1, the *slit-like shape* provides close contact between inhaled air and mucous membrane; 2, heat exchange is facilitated by *large arterial blood flow* (50% of the total blood flow runs in arterio-venous anastomoses); 3, the nasal mucosa has a *high secretory capacity* (100 000 glands on each side); and 4, the width of the cavity can quickly be adapted to demands by change in the degree of contraction in the *large venous sinusoids* ('pseudo-erectile tissue') (Fig. 8.1.8).

– in the nose

Air at room temperature, inhaled through the nose, is warmed to 30°C (86°F) by the time it reaches the pharynx, and it is almost saturated with water. When cold air (0°C, 32°F) is inhaled, its pharyngeal

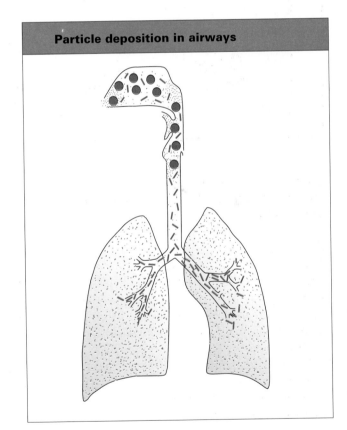

Fig. 8.1.6. Airway deposition of inhaled particles depends on the aerodynamic diameter. The 25 μm large pollen particles (large round dots) are deposited in the upper airway, causing allergic rhinitis. Inhalation of the smaller *Cladosporium* spores (about 5 μm (short bars)) provokes asthma due to deposition in the bronchi. The small *Micropolyspora faeni* (2 μm (small points)) are a cause of allergic alveolitis.

Mucociliary transport in the nose

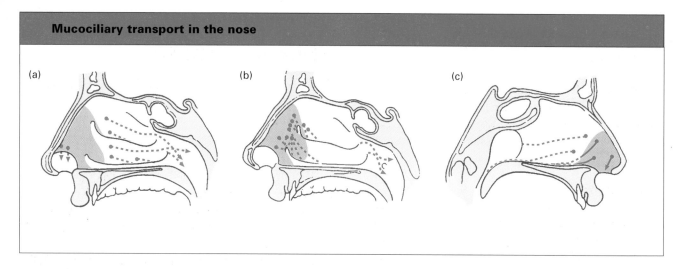

Fig. 8.1.7. (*Above.*) Pattern of mucociliary transport in the nose. (a) The course of mucus flow on the lateral wall in the ciliated area and in the very front of the nasal cavity. (b) The course of flow on the lateral wall in the non-ciliated area (grey area). (c) The course of mucus flow on the septum. From Hilding AC. Phagocytosis, mucous flow and ciliary action. *Arch Environ Health* 1963; **6**: 61–71.

Nasal mucous membrane

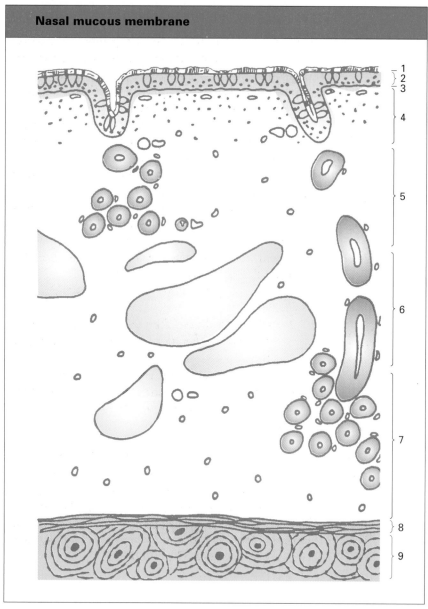

Fig. 8.1.8. Diagram of the mucous membrane on the inferior turbinate: 1, secretion layer; 2, ciliated pseudostratified columnar epithelium; 3, basement membrane; 4, cell-rich subepithelial layer; arterio-venous anastomoses and glandular ducts are indicated; 5, superficial glandular layer; 6, middle layer, containing large venous sinusoids; 7, profound glandular layer; 4–7, lamina propria ('submucosa'); 8, periosteum; and 9, bone.

temperature is about 25°C (77°F). Thus, 'a single sniff can change Scandinavian winter to Mediterranean summer'.

– in the mouth

The mouth can condition inspired air at room temperature as effectively as the nose does cold air, but effectiveness decreases with the degree of mouth opening.

– and asthma

Inability to breathe through the nose is unpleasant and potentially harmful during exposure to environmental challenges, especially in subjects with asthma and *hyper-responsive airways*. During exercise, oral breathing and hyperventilation can cause bronchoconstriction due to bronchial heat loss, this is partially prevented if nasal breathing can be maintained.

Impaired function

Impaired function of the nasal air conditioner can have various causes: 1, reduced nasal breathing (nasal blockage); 2, reduced wall contact with inhaled air (e.g. when polyps block the upper part of the cavity and surgical turbinectomy has created an airway in the lower part of the nose, transforming the normal slit-like passage into a tube); and 3, drying of the mucous membrane and atrophy of the glands (atrophic rhinitis).

Anatomy of the nose
If Cleopatra's nose had been shorter, the whole face of the earth would have changed.

Blaise Pascal, 1623–62
Penses II

The dirty organ
The nose is in fact one of the most dirty organs in the body and should be washed daily with anti-septic solutions.

Editorial
Br Med J, 1895

8.2 Pathogenesis of allergic rhinitis
Surface mast cells, histamine and reflexes

Key points
- Allergic reactions in the nose are frequent, as inhaled allergens are trapped in the nasal filter.
- Allergic inflammation is characterized by accumulation of Th2 cells, mast cells of the MC_T type and eosinophils.
- The allergen interacts with mast cell attached IgE, and the number of epithelial mast cells is increased in allergic rhinitis.
- Released histamine causes symptoms by a direct effect on vascular histamine receptors (oedema formation).
- It also stimulates sensory nerves and induces reflex-mediated sneezing and hypersecretion.
- Histamine accounts for the immediate allergic symptoms in the nose, but not for the late inflammatory reaction or the increase in reactivity.
- Stimulation of adrenergic fibres in sympathetic nerves contracts blood vessels.
- Stimulation of cholinergic fibres in the parasympathetic nerves causes hypersecretion.
- Reflexes running in the trigeminal nerve and in efferent parasympathetic fibres are important for nasal physiology and pathophysiology.
- The role of peptidergic nerves is not clear at present.
- Both allergic and non-allergic rhinitis is characterized by increased reflex activity and a hyper-reactive mucous membrane.
- This seems to be the only abnormality in a subgroup of patients (no eosinophilia), while another subgroup has both increased reactivity and inflammation (eosinophilia).

Allergen deposition in the nose
The nose is the site of more allergic symptoms and illnesses than any other organ. They result from its effective *filtering action* for allergens in the inhaled air. Particles (e.g. pollen grains trapped in the nose) induce the release of mediator molecules very fast and symptoms can be provoked within minutes.

Allergic inflammation

A characteristic feature of allergic inflammation is the local accumulation of inflammatory cells, including CD4+ T lymphocytes of the Th2 type, mast cells of the MC_T type and eosinophils. The interaction between these cells, described in detail in Part 1, is summarized in Fig. 8.2.1.

Surface mast cells

There are now a series of observations showing that histamine and other mediators are released predominantly from cells *near the epithelial surface*. The surface mediator cells mainly consist of mast cells (MC_T) and some basophil leucocytes; their number is *increased in allergic rhinitis*.

Histamine

Histamine is definitely the most important mediator of allergy in the nose, in contrast to the bronchi. Histamine 1, *directly* stimulates cellular histamine receptors, which cause vasodilatation, oedema formation and exudation of plasma to the airway lumen,

and 2, acts *indirectly*, via reflexes, to account for sneezing and watery hypersecretion (Fig. 8.2.2).

Because the surface mediator cells release histamine close to sensory nerve endings, they hold a key position in the *double amplification system*, consisting of mast cell degranulation and reflex activation.

The importance of reflexes in the first part of the airway can, teleologically, be understood; if sneezing and hypersecretion are considered protective mechanisms, they warn against and expel harmful inhaled agents. *Stimulation of a small mucosal area* results in an instantaneous and vigorous *response from the entire nasal lining*. It is the misfortune of hay fever patients that this sensitive alarm system is triggered by harmless pollen grains.

The clinical effect of H_1 antihistamines clearly demonstrates the role played by histamine. It accounts for the great majority of sneezing and associated watery hypersecretion, while it seems to play a minor role in nasal blockage and no role in hyper-responsiveness.

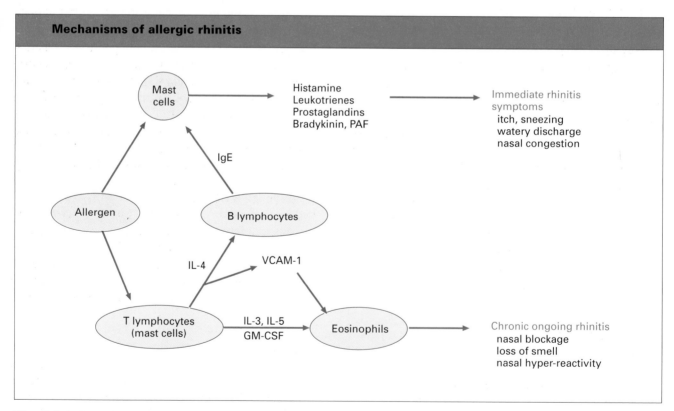

Mechanisms of allergic rhinitis

Fig. 8.2.1. Hypothesis on the immunological background of the inflammation in allergic rhinitis. IL-4, produced by Th2 cells and by mast cells, promotes B-cell isotype switching in favour of IgE. In addition, IL-4, by promoting increased expression of VCAM-1 on vascular endothelium, may also, together with IL-3, IL-5 and GM-CSF, selectively recruit eosinophils. By courtesy of Stephen Durham, National Lung and Heart Institute, London.

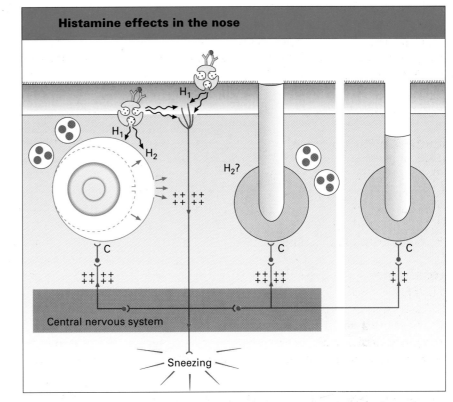

Fig. 8.2.2. Histamine acts directly on vascular histamine receptors causing vasodilatation (H_1 and H_2 receptors), plasma exudation and oedema formation (H_1 receptors). Glands possess histamine H_2 receptors, but their significance in the airways is unknown. Histamine stimulates sensory nerves (H_1 receptors) and initiates a parasympathetic reflex via cholinoceptors (C), which results in hypersecretion and transient vasodilatation, also on the contralateral side. From Mygind N. Mediators of nasal allergy. *J Allergy Clin Immunol* 1982; **70**: 149–59.

Other cells and mediators

Mast cells in the nose, as in other organs, release histamine, *arachidonic acid metabolites* and a series of other putative mediator substances. They probably act in concert with histamine and with a number of other mediators and cytokines released from other cell types and from plasma during the late inflammatory response to allergen (Table 8.2.1). The relative importance of these putative mediators is not known in detail because specific antagonists are not available.

Non-allergic mechanisms

In rhinitis, allergic as well as non-allergic, the effector cells in the blood vessels and the glands are under the control of the autonomic nervous system.

Sympathetic nerves

There are an abundance of *adrenergic fibres* around the *blood vessels*, while the sympathetic innervation of the glands is sparse and insignificant (Fig. 8.2.3). Stimulation of the adrenergic fibres releases noradrenaline, which acts both on *alpha adrenoceptors* (marked vasoconstriction) and on beta$_2$ adrenoceptors (slight vasodilatation). Adrenergic stimulation therefore results in *vasoconstriction*.

Alpha adrenoceptor *agonists* (sympathomimetics) are used as nasal decongestants. Alpha adrenoceptor *antagonists*, drugs that inhibit the release of noradrenaline, some *antihypertensives* and *psychosedatives* increase nasal airway resistance. These drugs can cause a '*dry nasal blockage*'. Beta$_2$ adrenoceptor agonists (bronchodilators), as weak vasodilators, do not increase nasal airway resistance when used orally.

Parasympathetic nerves

Cholinergic fibres are found close to blood vessels, but they are particularly numerous around the *glands* (Fig. 8.2.4). Stimulation of these fibres releases acetylcholine; this neurotransmitter stimulates secretion and causes transient vasodilatation by stimulation of *cholinoceptors*. The hypersecretion, but not the nasal blockage, is inhibited by atropine.

Peptidergic nerves

There is increasing evidence that non-adrenergic, non-cholinergic nervous mechanisms play a role in nasal physiology and pathophysiology. Recent studies of the nose have shown that a growing number of neuropeptides coexist with the classical neurotransmitters, noradrenaline and acetylcholine, in the same neurones (Fig. 8.2.5). The exact role of these

Allergic rhinitis symptoms and proposed mediators

Symptom	Pathological feature	Proposed mediator
Pruritus	Sensory nerve stimulation	Histamine (H_1)
Sneezing	Sensory nerve stimulation, somatic reflex and expiratory muscle contraction	Histamine (H_1)
Rhinorrhoea	Sensory nerve stimulation and cholinergic glandular reflex	Histamine (H_1)
	Direct effect on glands	Histamine (H_2) Leukotrienes – and other secretagogues
	Direct effect on goblet cells	Surface irritants
Nasal obstruction	Vasodilatation	Histamine (H_1) Histamine (H_2) Leukotrienes Prostaglandins? VIP?
	Extravasation and oedema formation	Histamine (H_1) Leukotrienes? Prostaglandins? PAF? Substance P?
Hyperirritability and hyper-responsiveness	Increased sensitivity of nerve endings	Not histamine
	Increased responsiveness of vasculature and glands	Eosinophil products?

Table 8.2.1. (*Above.*) Proposed mediators and pathological features behind the symptoms of allergic rhinitis. PAF, platelet activating factor; VIP, vasoactive intestinal polypeptide

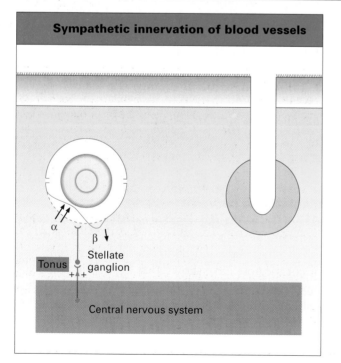

Sympathetic innervation of blood vessels

α

β

Tonus

Stellate ganglion

Central nervous system

Fig. 8.2.3. There is a continuous impulse traffic (tonus) in efferent sympathetic fibres to the blood vessels, keeping them partially constricted by stimulation of alpha adrenoceptors and beta adrenoceptors, which have opposite actions. (The postganglionic fibres emerge from the stellate ganglion in the neck and reach the nose along the arteries.) From Mygind N. Mediators of nasal allergy. *J Allergy Clin Immunol* 1982; **70**: 149–59.

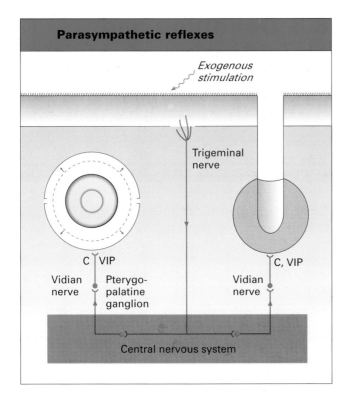

Fig. 8.2.4. The afferent sensory nerves to the nose run in the trigeminal nerve. The efferent parasympathetic fibres are derived from the facial nerve; the synapse between preganglionic and postganglionic fibres is located to the pterygopalatine ganglion. Most of the preganglionic fibres travel via the nerve of the pterygoid canal (the vidian nerve). Parasympathetic stimulation of glands and blood vessels is mediated via cholinoceptors (C) and receptors for vasoactive intestinal peptide (VIP). Inhaled ambient air, due to its unphysiological condition, slightly stimulates the sensory nerves in the nose. The resulting parasympathetic reflex activity may cause mild hypersecretion and insignificant vasodilatation, not noted by normal subjects. From Mygind N. Mediators of nasal allergy. *J Allergy Clin Immunol* 1982; **70**: 149–59.

neuropeptides, however, is not clear at present and is difficult to study because specific antagonists are not available.

Reflexes

The afferent sensory fibres, running in the *trigeminal nerve*, are part of a reflex arc, with efferent parasympathetic fibres in the *vidian nerve* (Fig. 8.2.4).

The sensory nerves in the nose are more exposed to stimulation from polluted and *ambient inhaled air* than are the bronchial nerves. It seems likely that there is constant reflex activity, which stimulates glandular activity, modulates vascular tone and nasal

patency. These reflex changes can quickly adapt the air-conditioning function of the nose to the steadily changing demands of the environment. They may also readily trigger nasal symptoms, and a certain degree of symptoms can be considered as an expression of *normal nasal physiology*.

Hyper-responsiveness

An allergen challenge test will increase the nasal responsiveness. This phenomenon, called *nasal priming*, has a clinical equivalent. Rhinitis patients react with nasal symptoms on exposure to a series of everyday stimuli, while even normal subjects react on exposure to large amounts of dust, high levels of inhaled irritants and very cold air. The *non-specific*

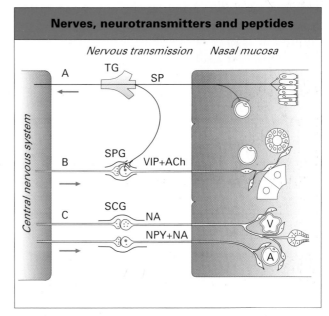

Fig. 8.2.5. Schematic illustration of the principle peptidergic innervation of the nasal mucosa in relation to 'classical' autonomic pathways. (A) Sensory nerve fibres from the trigeminal ganglion containing substance P (SP) with nerve endings under and within the epithelium as well as around the blood vessels. (B) Cholinergic fibres synapse in the sphenopalatine ganglion (SPG), and release acetylcholine (ACh) and vasoactive intestinal peptide (VIP) around glands and blood vessels. (C) Sympathetic adrenergic fibres synapse in the superior cervical ganglion (SCG). They innervate arteries, release noradrenaline (NA) and neuropeptide Y (NPY), while the venous sinusoids (V) principally have an adrenergic innervation. From Uddman R, Änggård A, Widdicombe JG. Nerves and neurotransmitters in the nose. In: Mygind N, Pipkorn U, eds. *Allergic and Vasomotor Rhinitis. Pathophysiological Aspects* Copenhagen: Munksgaard, 1987: 50–62.

hyper-responsiveness is characteristic of both allergic and non-allergic rhinitis. In the research laboratory, it can be measured by *histamine and methacholine challenges*. These tests can distinguish between groups of rhinitis patients and normal controls, but there is considerable overlap between the groups. At present, such tests are not used for the diagnosis of rhinitis.

In theory, three different diseases

Three types of non-infectious rhinitis can theoretically be delineated. 1, *Allergic rhinitis*, which is now well characterized with regards to aetiology and pathogenesis. 2, A non-allergic but '*allergy-like*' disease with eosinophil inflammation and hyper-responsiveness but of unknown aetiology. 3, A non-allergic, non-inflammatory disease with increased responsiveness to exogenous stimuli as the only abnormality. Some of these patients also have exaggerated responses to cooling of their fingers and toes. The disorder may be considered a *variant of normal nasal physiology* or, in popular terms, 'maladjustment of the nasal air conditioner'.

Paradoxical noses

The nose is man's most paradoxical organ. It has it's root above, its back in front, its wings below, and one likes best of all, to poke it into places were it doesn't belong.

Diffenbach, 1831

8.3 Definition and classification of rhinitis
Infectious, allergic and non-allergic

Key points
- All subjects occasionally have nasal symptoms, and quantitative measures are necessary to distinguish between a normal and a diseased state.
- Rhinitis can be defined as a combination of sneezing, discharge and blockage, lasting ≥1 hour on most days.
- First, exclude other diseases and structural abnormalities.
- Second, make a distinction between purulent and non-purulent disease.
- Third, separate allergic from non-allergic patients.
- Fourth, if possible, characterize non-allergic rhinitis as eosinophilic or non-eosinophilic.

Normal or disease?
The definition of bronchial asthma has plagued chest physicians and allergists for years, so it is not surprising that the definition and classification of rhinitis, involving aetiological criteria (infectious or allergic), has caused even more confusion. In addition, it is difficult to make a clear-cut distinction between a normal and a diseased state, as all subjects occasionally have nasal symptoms. Consequently, *quantitative measures* are necessary to distinguish between a normal or diseased state. Somewhat arbitrarily, rhinitis can be defined as a combination of *sneezing, discharge and blockage* (not blockage alone), lasting *≥1 hour* on most days. Thus, mild nasal symptoms lasting <1 hour/day are considered to be normal.

Simple classification of rhinitis
Seasonal allergic rhinitis (hay fever)
Perennial allergic rhinitis
Perennial non-allergic rhinitis

Table 8.3.1. Simple classification of non-infectious rhinitis for clinical routine diagnosis

Table 8.3.2. Characteristics of perennial non-allergic rhinitis sub-groups

Perennial non-allergic rhinitis		
	Eosinophilic subgroup	Non-eosinophilic subgroup
Nasal eosinophilia	+	−
Nasal polyps	+/−	−
Hyperplastic sinusitis	+/−	−
Asthma	+/−	−
NSAID intolerance	+/−	−

Infectious (purulent) or non-infectious (non-purulent)?

Infectious rhinitis can be confused with non-infectious rhinitis. As a matter of clinical routine, a diagnosis of viral or bacterial disease is not based on identification of the specific micro-organism but on the macroscopic character of the nasal discharge (± purulency), preferably supported by microscopy (± neutrophilia).

Seasonal or perennial?

Seasonal allergic rhinitis is a generally accepted term for pollinosis or hay fever. However, pollen allergy is perennial in the tropics, and in temperate zones a seasonal increase of symptoms can be caused by allergy to mites.

Allergic or non-allergic?

The diagnosis of *inhalant allergy* can usually be agreed when the history and skin test results are combined. This is not the case with *food allergy*, which is a controversial subject and a very rare cause of isolated rhinitis.

The term perennial *non-allergic rhinitis* is used for a chronic, non-infectious disease of unknown aetiology (Table 8.3.1). *Idiopathic rhinitis* is an alternative term, preferable to *vasomotor rhinitis*, which incorrectly implies a specific pathogenesis.

Eosinophilic or non-eosinophilic?

Perennial non-allergic rhinitis is a heterogeneous syndrome consisting of at least two subgroups. One is characterized by nasal secretion eosinophilia, frequent occurrence of polyps, non-allergic asthma and a good response to pharmacotherapy. These

Differential diagnoses
Mechanical factors
Septal deviation
Abnormal ostiomeatal complex
Nasal polyps
Foreign body
Tumours of nose and sinuses
Tumours of the nasopharynx
Congenital choanal atresia
Meningocele/encephalocele
Adenoidal hypertrophy
Infections
Viral infection (common cold)
Bacterial infection
Sinusitis
Leprosy
Immunodeficiency
Primary ciliary dyskinesia
Miscellaneous
Rhinitis medicamentosa
Cocaine abuse
Pregnancy
Antihypertensive drugs
Wegener's granulomatosis
Cystic fibrosis
Leak of cerebrospinal fluid

Table 8.3.3. Other causes of nasal symptoms

characteristics are lacking in the other subgroup (Table 8.3.2). However, a distinction between eosinophilic and non-eosinophilic rhinitis can only be made by the few clinicians who use nasal cytology as a routine examination.

Differential diagnosis

Congenital choanal atresia can be a cause of unilateral obstruction, with discharge, in an infant (Table 8.3.3), but a *foreign body* is much more common at that age. *Enlarged adenoids* are a frequent cause of mouth breathing.

Septal deviation is another well-known cause of nasal obstruction; it is often bilateral (S-shaped deviation). A nasal blockage, developing in an adult, cannot be ascribed exclusively to septal deviation unless the patient has had a trauma with fracture (rowdies, sportsmen and boxers). However, the swollen mucous membrane of rhinitis can make a septal deviation clinically significant, giving the patient a combined problem. A septal deviation with a spur, resulting in contact between septal and lateral mucous membranes ('*kissing mucous membranes*'), causes irritation, and induces reflexes and rhinitis

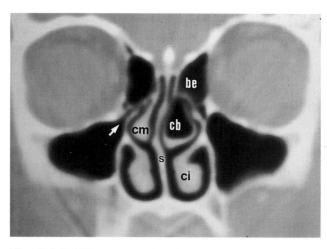

Fig. 8.3.2. CT-scan imaging of an air-filled middle turbinate, concha bullosa, which may be a cause of nasal symptoms, especially a sensation of congestion. From Stammberger H. Rhinoscopy. In: Mygind N, Naclerio RM, eds. *Allergic and Non-allergic Rhinitis. Clinical Aspects* Copenhagen: Munksgaard, 1993: 51–7.

symptoms (Fig. 8.3.1). Other anatomical abnormalities, such as an air-filled middle turbinate, *concha bullosa* (Fig. 8.3.2), can also cause nasal symptoms, especially blockage.

Malignant tumours in the nose, paranasal sinuses or nasopharynx and *Wegener's granulomatosis*, usually start with uncharacteristic symptoms. A first diagnosis of perennial rhinitis is not uncommon in these cases.

> **The problem of classification**
> It is very seldom that diseases are found pure and unmixed, as they are commonly described by authors; and there is almost an endless variety of constitutions.
>
> Matthew Baille

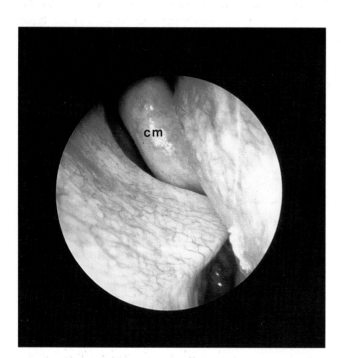

Fig. 8.3.1. A septal spur can, by contact, irritate the mucous membrane and induce reflex-mediated symptoms, especially sneezing and rhinorrhoea. From Stammberger H. Rhinoscopy. In: Mygind N, Naclerio RM, eds. *Allergic and Non-allergic Rhinitis. Clinical Aspects* Copenhagen: Munksgaard, 1993: 51–7.

8.4 The case history in rhinitis

Diagnosis and assessment of severity

Key points
- Give a detailed description of nasal symptoms, qualitatively and quantitatively.
- Are there allergic diseases in first-degree relatives?
- Does the patient have symptoms from skin or bronchi?
- Is the patient exposed to allergens at home or at work?
- Are there animals in the home?
- How is the bedroom arranged?

Family history
The patient is asked about the presence of allergic rhinitis, bronchial asthma and atopic dermatitis in *first-degree relatives* (all humans have a sneezing uncle or a wheezing aunt).

Social and environmental factors
Occupation and *working environment* must be known in case the patient is exposed to occupational allergens, irritants, extreme temperatures or large amounts of dust. In some occupations, even moderate rhinitis symptoms can seriously compromise work capacity (e.g. opera singers, pilots, priests, teachers or telephone operators). The home environment is discussed with particular reference to the *bedroom* and *exposure to animals*.

Asthma and dermatitis
For accurate characterization of a rhinitis patient, it is important to describe all symptoms from the airways and the skin, both past and present. Persistent *dry cough* and *exercise-induced wheeziness* indicate involvement of the bronchial mucosa and may be a forerunner of asthma.

Description of nasal symptoms
The patient is questioned specifically about the following symptoms. 1, *Itching in the nose*, distinct from irritation in the nostril (vestibulitis). 2, *Sneezing*. 3, *Nasal discharge*, either running from the nostril, easily blown out or cleared with difficulty by sniffing and swallowing as 'post-nasal drip'. It is important to know whether the discharge is opaque and milky/coloured (purulent) or clear and watery/mucoid (non-purulent). 4, *Nasal blockage*, which can be bilateral, unilateral or alternating from side to side. 5, *Mouth breathing*, especially at night, and its consequences, which are sore throat, snoring, disturbed sleep (for the entire family), daytime fatigue and, perhaps, sleep apnoea. 6, *Nasal voice*, and its significance at work. 7, *Reduced sense of smell* and 'taste'. 8, *Eye symptoms* – itching as distinct from smarting and irritation. 9, *Sinusitis symptoms*, consisting of nasal blockage, nasal irritation secondary to sinus pathology, nasal congestion, which is a feeling of stuffiness of the head due to pathology of the ostiomeatal complex, and closure of the ostia to the paranasal sinuses with changed pressure in the sinuses.

The physician must relate the symptoms to the *psyche* of the patient, as some individuals have an unusual awareness of nasal symptoms and seem to complain disproportionately.

Severity of symptoms
Symptoms can show *seasonal variations*, and be *perennial*, *chronic* or *intermittent*. Most patients have mild to moderate symptoms, but, in severe cases, the disease can interfere with the patient's daily activities, school or work performance.

Quantitative criteria are necessary to distinguish a minor disorder from a significant disease requiring further examination and therapy. The average *number of sneezes*, *number of nose blowings* and *daily duration of symptoms* are useful measures of severity. Most reliable is a detailed recording of symptoms on a diary card over a 2-week period.

Trigger factors
Enquiry is made, if the patient suspects any *causative factors*, as to whether the symptoms vary with *location* or change during week-ends or holidays.

It is rare for the case history to point convincingly to specific causes other than *pollens* and *animals*. Questioning about reactions to *acetylsalicylic acid*, especially in patients with polyps, is obligatory.

Most patients with perennial rhinitis will report that exposure to cold air, dust, fumes, paint, polluted air, printing ink, washing powder, hot spicy food and alcoholic beverages can precipitate or aggravate the symptoms. In most cases, they act as *non-specific irritants*.

Directions for sneezing
before the King and Queen
You must *not* sneeze. If you have a vehement cold, you must take no notice of it; if your nose-membranes feel a great irritation, you must hold your breath; if a sneeze still insists upon making its way, you must oppose it by keeping your teeth grinding together; if the violence of the repulse breaks some blood vessels, you must break the blood vessels—but *not* sneeze.

Francis Burney, 1785

8.5 Examination of the nose

A matter of course in chronic rhinitis

Key points
• The face will often show characteristic signs in children with perennial allergic rhinitis.
• Rhinoscopy is important for the diagnosis of septal deviation, nasal polyps and for routine assessment of the patient.
• In severe cases, endoscopy and CT-scan imaging are necessary for the exact diagnosis of anatomical abnormalities and sinus disease.
• Nasal patency is estimated by rhinoscopy and, for research, by rhinomanometry or acoustic rhinometry.
• Microscopy of nasal smears can be helpful for classification of the disease, and to determine whether an exacerbation is caused by infection (neutrophils) or by allergy (eosinophils).

Face and outer nose
Many children with long-standing allergic rhinitis can be recognized by their facial characteristics and mannerisms (Fig. 8.5.1). There is often a discoloration ('dark circles' or 'shiners') and oedema ('bags') under the eyes (Fig. 8.5.2). If nasal obstruction is severe, the typical open-mouthed 'adenoidal' face is seen ('allergic gaper'). This can predispose the child to a high-arched palate, overbite and malocclusion (Fig. 8.5.2). Frequent upward rubbing of the nose to alleviate itching, '*the allergic salute*', results in the development of a transverse '*nasal crease*' across the lower third of the nose (Fig. 8.5.3).

Rhinoscopy
Inspection of the nasal mucosa should be a matter of course, at each visit, in patients with chronic nasal symptoms.

Note is taken of the position of the septum, the appearance of the *mucous membrane*, and the presence and character of *secretions*, *polyps* and other abnormalities. 'Palpation' with a cotton-tipped applicator can give additional information about the nature of the mucousal changes (a motile polyp or a firm, swollen middle turbinate).

In chronic perennial rhinitis, allergic and non-aller-

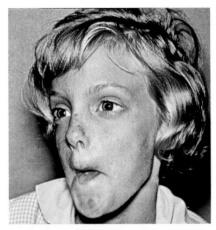

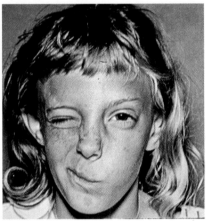

Fig. 8.5.1. Mannerisms for relief of nasal itching. From Marks MB. *Stigmata of Respiratory Tract Allergens* Kalamazoo: The Upjohn Company, 1972.

gic, the mucous membrane is typically *pale-bluish, boggy and wet* (Fig. 8.5.4), while it is usually reddened in acute infections, although this distinction is not absolute.

The presence of a septal perforation should raise the possibility of previous surgery, cocaine abuse, Wegener's granulomatosis, aggressive nose picking or, in the rare case, it may be an adverse effect of intranasal steroid therapy.

Routine use of a *vasoconstrictor spray* is necessary to improve the view, disclose small polyps, and to make a distinction between vascular engorgement and other causes of obstruction.

Modern rhinologists find that use of a speculum and a mirror provides limited information; they prefer a flexible or a rigid *endoscope*. It is a simple examination, which is obligatory in patients with unilateral symptoms, haemorrhagic secretions or pain. Together with *CT-scan imaging*, endoscopy

provides an excellent tool for the precise diagnosis of anatomical abnormalities, nasal polyps and sinusitis (Fig. 8.5.5).

Nasal patency

In routine clinical examination, nasal patency is estimated during *rhinoscopy*. While normal rhinoscopy strongly suggests normal patency, many patients with rhinoscopically abnormal noses have normal nasal airway resistance. About 50% of the general population have some rhinoscopic abnormality, usually a slightly deflected septum.

Recording of flow–pressure curves are, in research work, used for objective and quantitative measurement of nasal airway resistance, *rhinomanometry*. *Acoustic rhinometry*, a new and promising method, may be clinically useful as it is quick, simple and

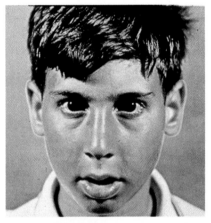

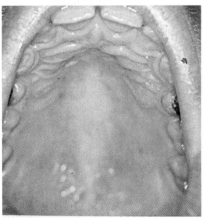

Fig. 8.5.2. 'Allergic shiners' and 'oedema bags' in a boy with perennial allergic rhinitis since infancy (upper part). Chronic mouth breathing has resulted in an 'adenoidal face' and a high arched palate (lower part). From Marks MB. *Stigmata of Respiratory Tract Allergens* Kalamazoo: The Upjohn Company, 1972.

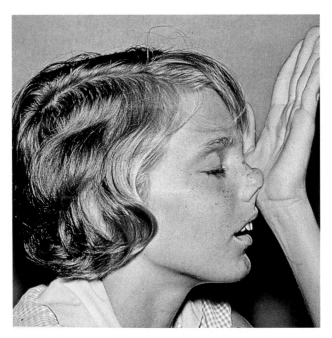

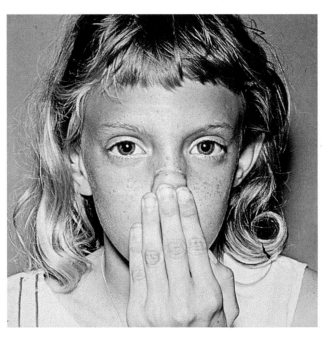

Fig. 8.5.3. The 'allergic salute' (*left*) and resulting 'nasal crease' (*right*). From Marks MB. *Stigmata of Respiratory*

Tract Allergens Kalamazoo: The Upjohn Company, 1972.

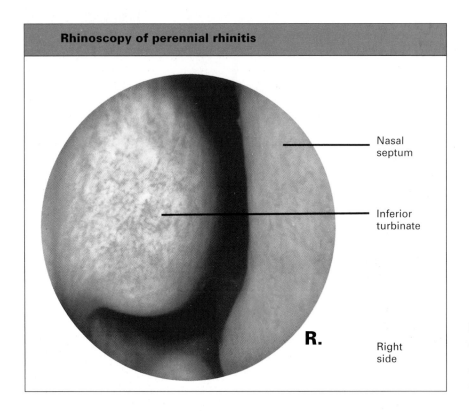

Rhinoscopy of perennial rhinitis

Nasal septum

Inferior turbinate

R.

Right side

Fig. 8.5.4. In perennial rhinitis, allergic as well as non-allergic, the mucous membrane of the inferior turbinate is typically swollen, wet and of a pale-bluish colour.

requires minimal patient collaboration. Control of airway patency is dynamic; no method of measurement can offer more than a snapshot of the rapid and considerable changes that occur.

Repeated measurements of *nasal peak flow* (expiratory or, preferably, inspiratory) can also give information of value and is used in clinical trials.

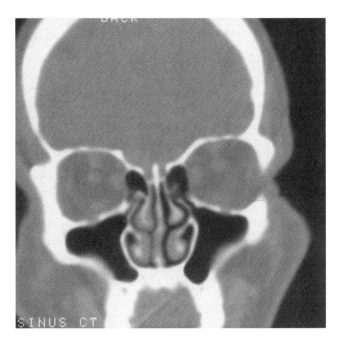

Fig. 8.5.5. A CT-scan of the nose and paranasal sinuses gives an excellent presentation of soft and hard tissues. Note how the mucous membrane in the nose takes shape after the surrounding structures, creating a slit-like air passage. There is good visualization of the position of the opening of maxillary sinuses into the superior part of the nose under the middle turbinate (middle meatus).

Nasal cytology

Collection of specimen

A *wiped smear* can be obtained by a tightly wound cotton swab. It is introduced two to three times into each side, and the mucosa is scraped with a firm, rolling movement. As the cells are often unevenly distributed, it is important to get *as much secretion as possible*. The swab must reach *into the posterior part* of the nose, as a smear, taken from the anterior part, will only contain squamous cells in watery discharge.

Better specimens and more reproducible results can be obtained with a *disposable plastic curette* (Rhinoprobe) or a *cytology brush*. For research purposes, cells in nasal lavage fluid can be quantified reliably in a counting chamber and identified in a cytospin preparation.

Staining and microscopy

For diagnostic purposes, staining for eosinophils and metachromatic cells is sufficient. When a *rapid method* is used (Table 8.5.1), the specimen is ready for microscopy within minutes. For research purposes, nasal samples are suitable for staining with a

Staining of nasal smear for eosinophils
May–Grünwald and Giemsa stains
Cover the slide with May–Grünwald stain
Add six drops of Giemsa stain after 30–45 seconds
Rinse in water from the tap after 30–45 seconds
Quick decoloration with alcohol–if necessary
Rinse in water
Hansel stain
Cover the slide with Hansel stain (two alcoholic stains: 1:500 eosin and 1:200 methylene blue)
Add distilled water after 30–45 seconds
Quick decoloration in alcohol
Rinse in water
Wright stain
Dip several times in equal parts of ether and alcohol
Cover the slide with Wright–Giemsa stain
Add a similar amount of distilled water after 30–45 seconds
Rinse in water after 30–45 seconds

Table 8.5.1. Quick staining methods for eosinophils in nasal smears

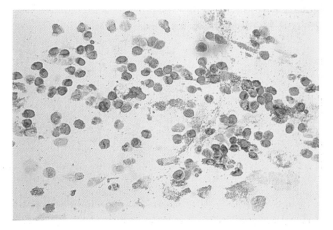

Fig. 8.5.6. Eosinophilia in a nasal smear as seen in allergic rhinitis and non-allergic eosinophilic rhinitis.

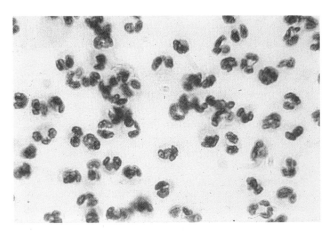

Fig. 8.5.7. Neutrophilia in a nasal smear as seen in viral and bacterial infection. A certain degree of neutrophilia is normal, probably due to air pollution.

series of monoclonal antibodies to demonstrate subsets of cells.

More than 10% of eosinophils is suggestive of allergic rhinitis or the non-allergic eosinophilic rhinitis, but the judgement of a trained microscopist is often more valuable than an exact percentage. As the *cells often appear in clumps*, the entire smear must be studied before it can be considered negative (Figs 8.5.6–7). The cytological examination of a nasal smear is useful only if you are trained, do it frequently, take care to obtain sufficient material and *do the microscopy yourself*. At present, only a few specialists use nasal cytology in routine diagnosis.

A spiritual nose
Instinct is the nose of the spirit.

Emile de Girardin

8.6 Antihistamines
H₁ receptor antagonists

Key points
- Histamine exerts its actions in tissue by binding to histamine H_1, H_2, and H_3 receptors; H_1 is most important in allergy.
- The classical or first generation of sedating H_1 antihistamines have largely been replaced by the second generation of non-sedating/slightly sedating compounds.
- H_1 antihistamines are rapidly absorbed and are metabolized by the hepatic cytochrome P system.
- Many second generation H_1 antihistamines also possess anti-allergic activity, but the clinical significance of this is uncertain.
- Overdosing with terfenadine and astemizole can cause serious ventricular arrhythmias, which can also result from drug interaction.
- H_1 antihistamines have a good effect on itching, sneezing and watery discharge, but a poor effect on nasal blockage.

Histamine, synthesized in 1907, was so named because of its occurrence in animal and human tissues ('*histos*' is Greek for tissue) and its amine structure. While histamine has a series of well-defined effects contributing to the pathophysiology of allergic diseases, its normal physiological role has not been precisely defined.

Histamine H₁ and H₂ receptors – and H₃

Histamine exerts its actions in the tissues by binding to and stimulating histamine receptors in the cell membrane. They have been defined pharmacologically as H_1, H_2 and H_3 receptors. It is possible that more than one subtype of the H_1 receptor exists. Recently, the genes encoding for the H_1 and H_2 receptors have been cloned, and their molecular structure is now being characterized.

Histamine has, via *H_1 and H_2 receptors*, a series of well-defined effects on several cell types and tissues, summarized in Table 8.6.1.

More recently, an *H_3 receptor* was described, mainly localized to central nervous system (CNS) tissue. It has also been identified in perivascular nerve terminals, where it may regulate sympathetic tone. Neither H_1 nor H_2 receptor antagonists exert any

Effects of H_1 and H_2 receptor stimulation
H_1 receptor
Stimulation of sensory nerves
Contraction of bronchial smooth muscles
Contraction of intestinal smooth muscles
Increased permeabililty of post-capillary venules, extravasation and oedema formation
H_1 and H_2 receptors
Dilatation of blood vessels
H_2 receptor
Stimulation of gastric glands
Stimulation of airway glands (relative importance uncertain)
Effect on basophils, eosinophils and lymphocytes (significance for allergic reactions not known)

Table 8.6.1. Histamine has, via H_1 and H_2 receptors, effects on several cells and tissues

marked effects on histamine-induced nasal blockage, suggestive perhaps of a role for the H_3 receptor in controlling vascular congestion in the nose.

First and second generation H_1 antagonists

The classical or *first generation* H_1 antihistamines were introduced in 1942. A long series of compounds have been synthesized and marketed, but they have all had, to a varying degree, a *sedating* effect. *Chlorpheniramine* and *clemastine* are examples of drugs that cause relatively little sedation and have the highest therapeutic index in this group. When they are administered, as *a single dose at bedtime*, sedation is minimized and can be tolerated by some patients.

The marked sedative effect of *hydroxyzine* and *cyproheptadine* is used in patients with atopic *dermatitis* for the treatment of itching and scratching at night.

In the early 1980s, a *second generation* of non-sedating or marginally sedating antihistamines was introduced (Fig. 8.6.1). The dose–response curves for

wanted and unwanted effects are better separated for the second than for the first generation of drugs (Fig. 8.6.2).

Some characteristics of the more widely used drugs are summarized in Table 8.6.2. There seems to be only minor differences between the efficacy of these drugs in the recommended doses. The adverse effect profile of the drugs differ somewhat and will be discussed later.

The introduction of the second generation H_1 receptor antagonists has been an important progression in the management of rhino-conjunctivitis and urticaria. Antihistamines, often available over the counter, are the most frequently used remedy for these afflictions.

More recently, H_1 antagonists for topical use in eye and nose have been introduced.

Pharmacology of H_1 antagonists

Pharmacokinetics

The drugs are *rapidly absorbed* from the gastro-intestinal tract, and peak plasma concentrations are achieved in 1–2 hours.

Most of the drugs are metabolized in the hepatic *cytochrome P-450* system. As many metabolites are active H_1 antagonists, the plasma half-life of the parent drug is poorly predictive of the duration of action. Usually, inhibition of the wheal-and-flare reaction considerably outlasts that calculated by measuring plasma half-life values.

Plasma half-life is prolonged in patients with hepatic dysfunction and in patients concomitantly receiving drugs that are metabolized by the same cytochrome P-450 enzyme (see later).

Cetirizine is not metabolized and is excreted unchanged in the urine. Its elimination half-life is prolonged in elderly patients and in patients with impaired renal function.

While the first generation agents readily cross the *blood–brain barrier*, second generation drugs do this with difficulty as they are less lipophilic.

Pharmacodynamics

Competitive H_1 receptor blockage

All of the available antagonists are competitive inhibitors of histamine interaction with the H_1 receptor, with the exception of *astemizole*, which binds irreversibly and indefinitely to the receptor.

Onset of the antihistamine effect begins within 1

H₁ receptor antagonists

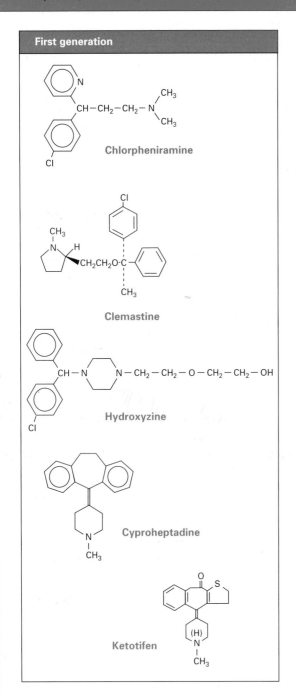

First generation

Chlorpheniramine

Clemastine

Hydroxyzine

Cyproheptadine

Ketotifen

Second generation

Terfenadine

Astemizole

Cetirizine

Loratadine

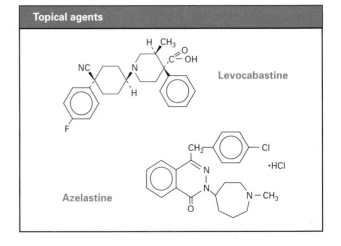

Topical agents

Levocabastine

Azelastine

Fig. 8.6.1. Structural formula of some H₁ antagonists.

First and second generation H₁ histamine antagonists – dose–response curves

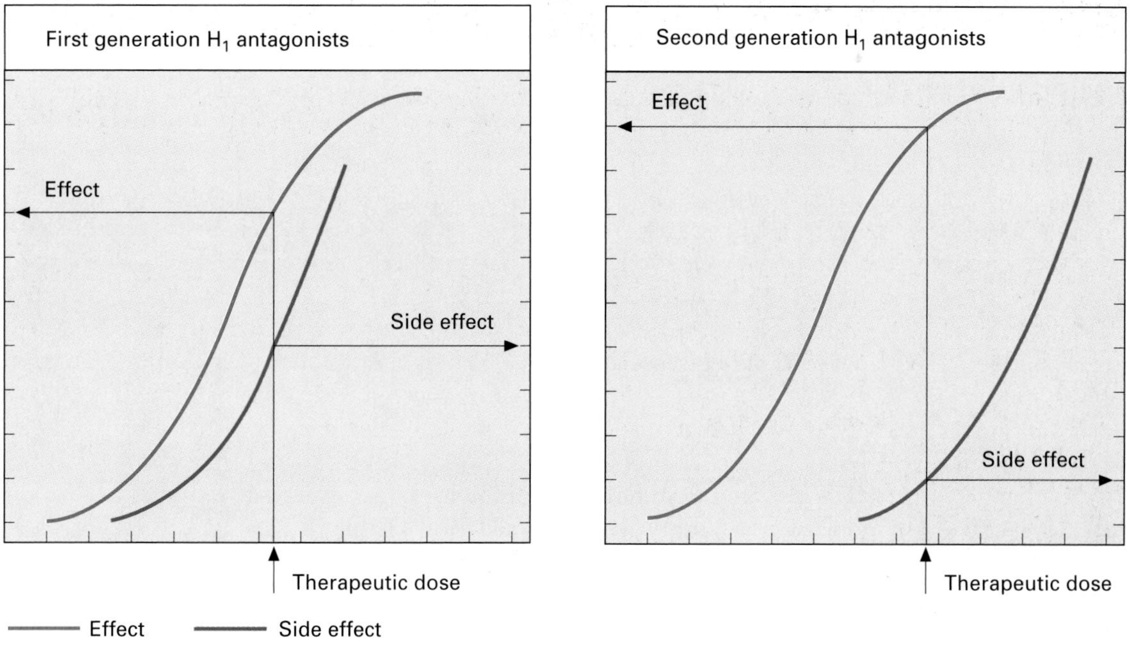

First generation H₁ antagonists

Effect

Side effect

Therapeutic dose

—— Effect —— Side effect

Second generation H₁ antagonists

Effect

Side effect

Therapeutic dose

Fig. 8.6.2. Schematic representation of the position of dose–response curves for wanted effect (symptom reduction) and unwanted side effects (sedation most important) for first and second generation H₁ antagonists. The figures are constructed and are not based on experimental data.

Second generation H₁ receptor antagonists				
	Astemizole (10 mg once daily)	**Cetirizine (10 mg once daily)**	**Loratadine (10 mg once daily)**	**Terfenadine (120 mg once daily)**
Clinical effect	+++	+++	++(+)	++(+)
Suitable for p.r.n. use	No	Yes	Yes	Yes
Additional effect	Anti-allergic effect?	Inhibition of eosinophil migration?	Anti-allergic effect?	Anti-allergic effect?
Metabolism/ excretion	Hepatic	Renal	Hepatic	Hepatic
Plasma half-life	9.5 days	11 hours	8.3 hours	4.5 hours
Sedation	–	(–)*	(–)*	–
Risk of weight gain	+	–	–	–
Risk of cardiac arrhythmias	+	(–)	(–)	+

Table 8.6.2. Characteristics of four widely used, non-sedating H₁ antagonists in the dosage recommended by the manufacturer. A precise drug comparison is not possible because full dose–effect and dose–side effect curves are not available. *Sedating in a dose-dependent manner, beginning at 10–20 mg for cetirizine and at 20–40 mg for loratadine. The few patients who become sedated from 10 mg cetirizine may benefit from halving the dose (and the price)

hour of oral administration of the compound. However, astemizole is an exception: there is a lag of some hours before maximum H_1 blockage occurs and, therefore, it is not suitable for usage on an as-needed basis.

The drug effect continues for many hours, and it is usually sufficient to give the second generation preparations in *a single daily dose*, even in children who have a short plasma half-life. An exception is *acrivastine* which needs to be given three times daily. As this results in poor patient compliance, the use of this drug is confined to patients with mild disease and occasional symptoms.

As an H_1 antihistamine acts as a pharmacological and not as a physiological antagonist, it cannot reverse tissue changes already induced by histamine. Therefore, H_1 receptor antagonists is preferably given *before an allergic reaction* in order to achieve maximum efficacy at the time of need.

In the nose, binding of the antagonist to H_1 receptors on sensory nerve endings is the most likely explanation of the pronounced effect on itching, sneezing and watery rhinorrhoea, although such receptors have not directly been identified. While histamine can increase vascular permeability and vasodilate by stimulating vascular H_1 and H_2 receptors, the poor effect of H_1 antagonists on nasal blockage in rhinitis suggests either that histamine makes little contribution to this symptom or that other histamine receptor subtypes are of importance.

Anti-allergic effect

Laboratory studies have indicated that some H_1 antihistamine preparations, sedating (ketotifen, azelastine, oxatomide) as well as non-sedating (terfenadine, loratadine, astemizole), inhibit immunogenic mediator release from mast cells, and perhaps other cells; this inhibition is referred to as the 'anti-allergic effect'. Some H_1 antagonists appear to be antagonists to other putative mediators as well (leukotrienes, PAF and serotonin). Cetirizine inhibits the influx of eosinophils in the skin but not in the nose.

Although these results are interesting, it is difficult to say what they mean for the practical management of allergic disorders. Clinical trials have, in general, failed to demonstrate superiority of H_1 antihistamines, which are claimed to have additional 'anti-allergic' effects. Until such data are produced, we prefer to consider an antihistamine as an antihistamine.

Adverse effects

Sedation

In a considerable number of patients, the *first generation* H_1 antagonists will cause sedation, impairment of cognitive and psychomotor functions, diminished alertness and slow reaction time. Although these CNS effects tend to diminish with continuous use, they have severely limited the use of the first generation antihistamines. Patients taking these drugs must be warned not to drive a car or to operate machinery.

When the *second generation* H_1 receptor antagonists are given in the manufacturers recommended dose, the incidence of sedation and impairment of CNS functions is similar to that seen with placebo. However, a few sensitive persons may experience sedation (Table 8.6.2).

It is clinically important that the second generation of H_1 antagonists, unlike their predecessors, can be associated with alcohol, benzodiazepines or other CNS depressant drugs.

The relative lack of sedative effects of the second generation drugs may be due to their relatively poor penetration into the CNS. It has also been postulated for some drugs that they have a preference for peripheral rather than central histamine H_1 receptors.

Unfortunately, too many patients are still, by routine or economy, treated with first generation drugs and suffer from their adverse effects. A businessman will loose his initiative, an artist his creativity and a driver his safety.

Other adverse effects

Many of the first generation drugs possess other pharmacological activities, especially an *anti-cholinergic effect*. The second generation preparations have a more specific affinity for the H_1 receptor, and they lack anti-cholinergic activity, with mequitazine as an exception.

Drug allergy is very rare when H_1 antagonists are given orally. It is more common when an antihistamine is applied to the skin and, for that reason, antihistamine ointments and creams are not recommended by dermatologists. To date, there have been no reports of local sensitization occurring following their topical use as eye drops or nasal spray.

Increased appetite and *weight gain* can be a problem with cyproheptadine, ketotifen and astemizole. It is difficult to understand how astemizole, which does not cause sedation, can reach the centre for appetite regulation in the brain.

Cardiac arrhythmias

Deliberate overdosing with *terfenadine and astemizole* has resulted in serious cardiovascular events, including *QT prolongation, torsades de pointes* and other *ventricular arrhythmias*, cardiac arrest and death. Probably, the drugs exert an action on the heart similar to that of quinidine.

Similar adverse effects have been described in a few patients taking ordinary doses of terfenadine together with *ketoconazole*. This anti-fungal drug markedly inhibits the metabolism of terfenadine, as both molecules are metabolized by the same *cytochrome P-450* enzyme (3A4) (Figs 8.6.3–4). This enzyme system is also responsible for the biotransformation of *erythromycin*, other macrolide antibiotics, itraconazole and, probably, astemizole.

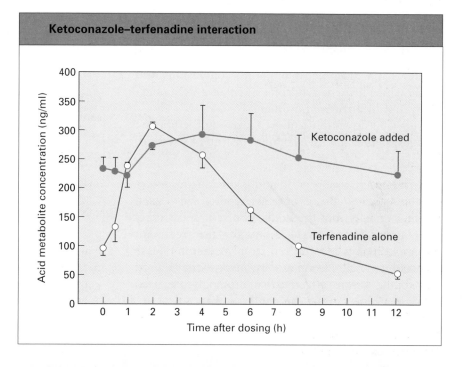

Fig. 8.6.3. Concomitant administration of ketoconazole markedly increases the plasma level of terfenadine, which can reach arrhythmogenic levels. Each point represents a mean of six subjects (±SEM). From Honig PK, Wortham DC, Zamani K, *et al.* Terfenadine–ketoconazole interaction. *JAMA* 1993; **269**: 1513–18.

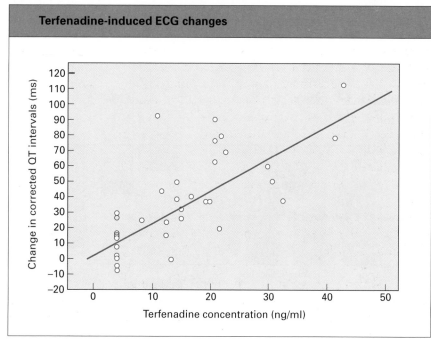

Fig. 8.6.4. Linear correlation between plasma concentration of terfenadine and electrocardiogram (ECG) change in QT interval ($p = 0.0001$). From Honig PK, Wortham DC, Zamani K, *et al.* Terfenadine–ketoconazole interaction. *JAMA* 1993; **269**: 1513–18.

In order to avoid high plasma levels of terfenadine and astemizole and to eliminate the risk of life-threatening cardiac arrhythmias, the guidelines in Table 8.6.3 must be adhered to.

The terfenadine–ketoconazole example, first disclosed after years of extensive use of the drug, gives support to the sound principle of always using topical treatment whenever possible.

Intoxication

In acute poisoning with first generation H_1 antagonists, their central excitatory effects constitute the greatest danger. The symptoms include excitement, hallucination, flushing, dry mouth, convulsions and death, which give the syndrome a remarkable similarity to that of atropine poisoning.

It is well known that children, even on therapeutic dosages, can react with excitation instead of sedation.

Topical preparations

Eye drops have a very good and instantaneous effect on itching. They also counteract redness when used prophylactically, but the addition of a vasoconstrictor (Antistin-Privin) is necessary for the treatment of an eye that is already red from mediator release and rubbing. The H_1 antagonist, *levocabastine*, used twice daily, is more effective than cromoglycate, used four times daily, in the eye and nose (Fig. 8.6.5).

Eye drops containing preservative (benzalkonium chloride) will cause some stinging and irritation; this is acceptable to most patients provided that they have not rubbed their eyes before medication. Tell the patient to use the drops in the eye *instead of rubbing.*

Levocabastine and *azelastine nasal sprays* offer quick relief of itching and sneezing, and, when used

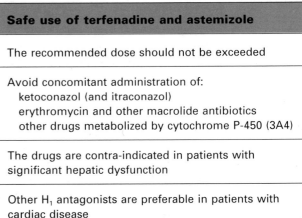

Safe use of terfenadine and astemizole
The recommended dose should not be exceeded
Avoid concomitant administration of: ketoconazol (and itraconazol) erythromycin and other macrolide antibiotics other drugs metabolized by cytochrome P-450 (3A4)
The drugs are contra-indicated in patients with significant hepatic dysfunction
Other H_1 antagonists are preferable in patients with cardiac disease
Discuss the potential risks with the patient

Table 8.6.3. Measures to eliminate the risk of serious cardiac arrhythmias in the use of terfenadine and astemizole

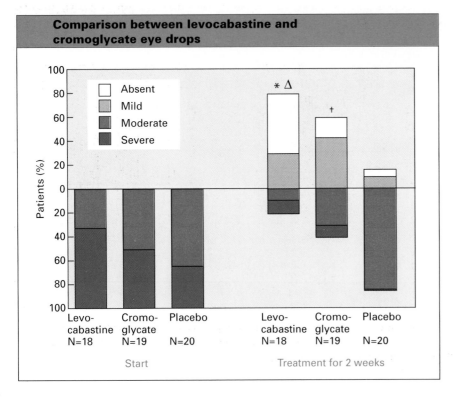

Fig. 8.6.5. Severest nasal symptom (for a given patient at a given point) at the start of the study and after 2 weeks of treatment. $p < 0.05$ for levocabastine versus cromoglycate, $p < 0.001$ for levocabastine versus placebo, and $p = 0.07$ for cromoglycate versus placebo. From Schata M, Jorde W, Richarz-Barthauer U. Levocabastine nasal spray better than sodium cromoglycate and placebo in the topical treatment of seasonal allergic rhinitis. *J Allergy Clin Immunol* 1991; **87**: 873–8.

twice daily, they can prevent the development of these symptoms. Their place in the management of allergic rhinitis has not yet been delineated. Probably, they are most useful in mild hay fever and before exposure to a known allergen.

Clinical effect in allergic rhinitis

Allergen challenge
Pretreatment with an H_1 antagonist before allergen challenge has: 1, a marked effect on itching and sneezing; 2, a moderate effect on rhinorrhoea; 3, little or no effect on blockage during the early-phase response (Fig. 8.6.6); 4, no significant effect on the late-phase response; and 5, no effect on the increased mucosal responsiveness.

Seasonal allergic rhino-conjunctivitis
H_1 antagonists have an established and valued place in the symptomatic treatment of pollen allergy. As the time for exposure to pollen is usually known, it is possible to take the drug before an anticipated allergic reaction, thereby achieving maximum efficacy. The antihistamines have a *good effect on itching in the eye and nose*, and on *sneezing and watery discharge*, but a *poor effect on nasal blockage*. They are therefore often combined with a vasoconstrictor.

Perennial rhinitis
Generally, H_1 antihistamines are less effective in chronic, *perennial allergic rhinitis*, characterized by nasal blockage, than in hay fever. Patients with *perennial non-allergic rhinitis*, associated with sneezing, watery discharge and local eosinophilia, may respond to antihistamines, but these drugs are of little or no help in patients with pronounced nasal blockage and nasal polyps.

Clinical effect in other allergic diseases

Asthma
H_1 antihistamine pretreatment reduces the early response to allergen challenge (50%) and slightly reduces the response to exercise (20%). Antihistamines are *not prescribed for the treatment of asthma*, but, when used for pollen rhino-conjunctivitis, they may provide *relief for mild asthma symptoms*.

Urticaria
H_1 receptor antagonists are *first-line medications* in the treatment of urticaria (see Chapter 6.8).

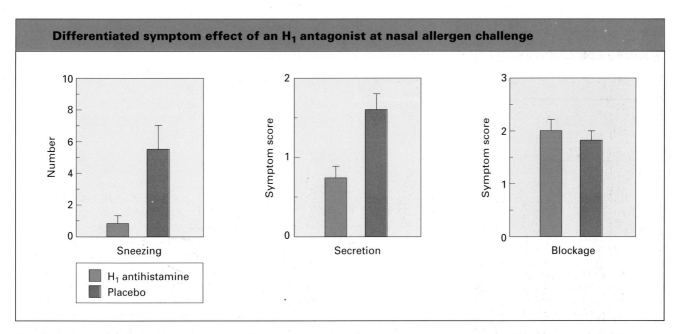

Fig. 8.6.6. Nasal symptoms at a nasal challenge with allergen following local pretreatment with the H_1-blocker levocabastine. Adapted from Holmberg K, Bake B, Blychert L–O, Pipkorn U. Effects of topical H_1 and H_2 receptor antagonists on symptoms and local vascular reactions induced by nasal allergen challenge. *Allergy* 1989; **44**: 281–7.

Atopic dermatitis

While *sedating antihistamines* have a well-established role in relieving itching and scratching at night, the results with the second generation drugs have been disappointing (see Chapter 6.5).

Anaphylactic shock

H$_1$ antagonists have only a *subordinate and adjuvant role* to adrenaline in the treatment of systemic anaphylaxis. The *combined use of H$_1$ and H$_2$ preparations* is more effective than an H$_1$ antagonist alone in *preventing* a systemic allergic reaction, for example to a drug or radiocontrast media.

Other conditions

Insect bites and ivy poisoning respond well, especially when medication can be taken prophylactically. Many *drug reactions* attributable to allergic phenomena, particularly those characterized by itch and urticaria, respond to therapy with H$_1$ antagonists. While these drugs give some relief for *the oral allergy syndrome*, gastro-intestinal allergies are seldom benefited.

Art and science

All too often art and science are being looked upon as two distinctly different, almost opposite domains of the human mind. I have never quite understood why. Both are aimed at improving the quality of life. Both are demanding a deep understanding of human endeavour. Both are following the path of discovery that has no end.

Paul Janssen
Janssen Pharmaceutical

8.7 Intranasal corticosteroids
Basic anti-inflammatory therapy

Key points

- The modern steroid sprays are highly effective in the nose in doses not associated with systemic side effects.
- They control nasal symptoms in most hay fever patients, but concomitant use of non-steroidal eye drops is necessary.
- Most patients with perennial rhinitis and nasal polyps also benefit from intranasal steroids, predominantly those patients with nasal eosinophilia.
- There exists no contra-indication to a 2–3-month course of treatment for hay fever.
- Regular use in children with perennial rhinitis should be restricted to severe cases, not controlled by other means.
- Blood-stained crusts and epistaxis can occur, but widespread use for 2 decades has not disclosed any serious damage to the mucous membrane.

Glucocorticosteroids (steroids) are currently the *most potent medication* available for the treatment of allergic and non-allergic rhinitis. The effect of intransal steroids is based on local activity; the administration of the equivalent amount of drug orally produces no benefit. The introduction of intranasal steroids is one of the best examples of how the therapeutic index of a medication can be dramatically improved when it is administered topically (Fig. 8.7.1).

Initially reserved as a second-line agent, the role of intranasal steroid is now changing. In a recent 'International Consensus Report on the Diagnosis and Management of Rhinitis', intranasal steroids were considered first-line therapy in moderate to severe cases of hay fever, perennial allergic rhinitis in adults, and perennial non-allergic rhinitis.

Mechanisms of action

Steroids have a broad range of anti-inflammatory effects, which have been studied in detail in the human nose. Intranasal steroid therapy has the following effects: 1, reduced synthesis of *Th2-type cytokines* and, probably secondary to this action, reduction in the numbers of: 2, antigen-presenting *Langerhans'*

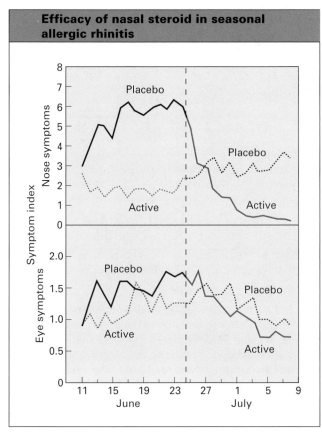

Fig. 8.7.1. The effect of beclomethasone dipropionate nasal aerosol is marked on nasal hay fever symptoms but absent on eye symptoms. This shows that the mode of action is local and not systemic. From Mygind N. Local effect of intranasal beclomethasone dipropionate aerosol in hay fever. *Br Med J* 1973; **4**: 363–6.

cells, 3, *epithelial mast cells* (of the MC_T type), 4, mucosal *eosinophils*, and 5, *circulating progenitor cells* (Figs 8.7.2–5).

Drugs and drug administration

A steroid applied to the nasal mucosa will be absorbed into the circulation, but steroid molecules, which are first-pass deactivated in the liver, have a local effect in the nose at a dosage not associated with a significant risk of systemic side effects. *Beclomethasone dipropionate* (Fig. 8.7.1), introduced in 1974, was the first of the modern potent steroids used topically in the nose. *Flunisolide, budesonide, triamcinolone acetonide*, and *fluticasone propionate* followed later. There does not seem to be any major difference between these molecules with regard to efficacy and side effect profile. Thus, the steroid hierarchy, known in dermatology, does not seem to exist in the nose.

Local therapy can be given as a *freon-propelled aerosol* of a micronized powder from a pressurized canister or as an aqueous suspension/solution from a *metered-dose pump spray*. The pump spray gives the best intranasal drug distribution (Figs 8.7.6–7). Recently, budesonide became available as a *pure-powder formulation* delivered from a multi-dose device.

A *once daily* medication is sufficient in most cases and has good patient compliance. Twice daily medication can be tried in severe cases and during exacerbations.

Clinical effect

Seasonal allergic rhinitis

Symptom relief can be achieved within 12 hours and be maximal after 2–4 days. A steroid spray controls nasal symptoms in the majority of patients, but, as for

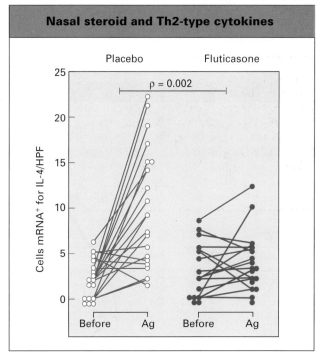

Fig. 8.7.2. Effect of fluticasone propionate on the number of cells in the nasal mucosa expressing mRNA for IL-4. Data are shown from baseline (before) and at 24 hours after allergen challenge (Ag) following 6-week treatment with fluticasone propionate (closed circles) or placebo (open circles). From Masuyama K, Jacobson MR, Rak S, *et al*. Topical glucocorticoid (fluticasone propionate) inhibits cells expressing cytokine mRNA for interleukin-4 in the nasal mucosa in allergen-induced rhinitis. *Immunol* 1994; **82**: 192–9.

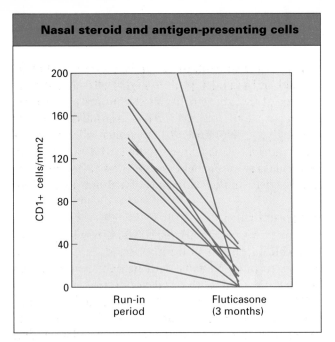

Fig. 8.7.3. The number of Langerhans' cells (CD1+ cells) in the nasal epithelium of patients with perennial allergic rhinitis before and during fluticasone propionate therapy. From Fokkens WJ, Godthelp T, Holm AF, *et al*. Effect of 3 months' nasal steroid therapy on nasal T cells and Langerhans cells in patients suffering from allergic rhinitis. *Allergy* 1995; **50**(suppl 23): 21–4.

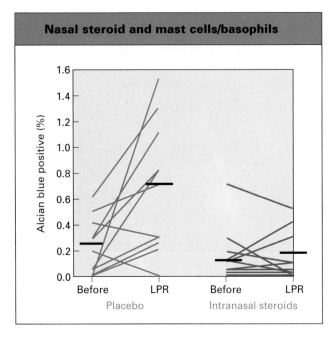

Fig. 8.7.4. Influx of mast cells and basophils (alcian blue positive cells) after nasal allergen challenge in allergic subjects. The late phase LPR is 3–11 hours after antigen challenge. Placebo versus intranasal steroid treatment late-phase, $p < 0.001$. From Bascom R, Wachs M, Naclerio RM, *et al*. Basophil influx occurs after nasal antigen challenge: effect of topical corticosteroid pretreatment. *J Allergy Clin Immunol* 1988; **81**: 580–9.

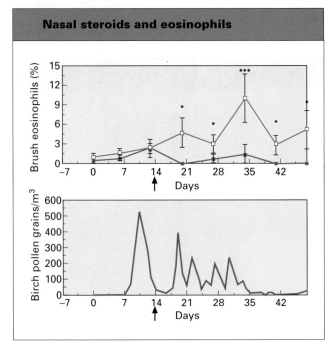

Fig. 8.7.5. Proportion of eosinophils harvested from the nasal mucosa prior to and during the pollen season. Open squares, mean ± SEM for placebo group. Filled squares, values obtained during budesonide treatment. The arrow indicates start of treatment. *$p < 0.05$, ***$p < 0.001$, for comparisons active versus placebo. From Klementsson H, Svensson C, Andersson M, *et al*. Eosinophils, secretory responsiveness and glucocorticoid-induced effects on the nasal mucosa during a weak pollen season. *Clin Exp Allergy* 1991; **21**: 705–10.

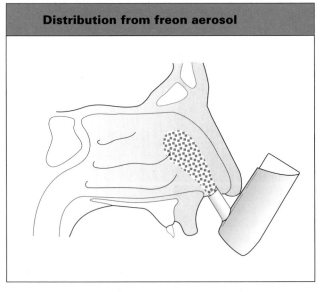

Fig. 8.7.6. A freon-propelled aerosol is frequently used for intranasal medication. It is easy to use, but the drug distribution is second to that of a pump spray.

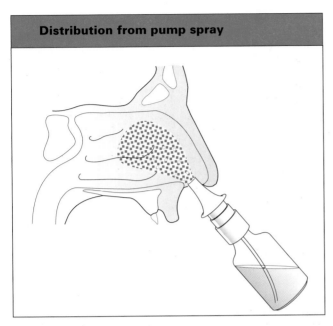

Fig. 8.7.7. A metered-dose pump spray gives a good drug distribution in the nose.

any type of treatment, there can be a symptom breakthrough at the pollen peak in highly allergic patients.

Topical treatment of nasal symptoms necessitates a *prescription for eye drops* (antihistamine or cromoglycate, *not steroids*). In pollen allergy, intranasal steroids may also reduce the increase in bronchial responsiveness during the season and have a mild effect on the symptoms of asthma (Fig. 8.7.8).

Perennial rhinitis

Patients with perennial *allergic* rhinitis will get considerable improvement from a steroid spray; the same applies to most patients with perennial *non-allergic* rhinitis and those with nasal *polyposis*.

The major reason for the lack of efficacy of a nasal steroid spray in some patients (Table 8.7.1) is its inability to gain access to the site of inflammation when nasal blockage is pronounced. In these cases, a short course of systemic steroid will increase the number of *responders*. However, a subgroup of pa-

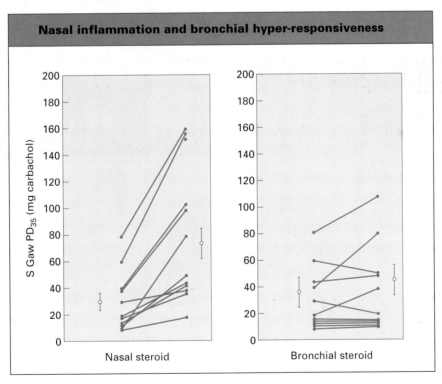

Fig. 8.7.8. Patients with allergic rhinitis without asthma but with bronchial hyper-responsiveness were in a double-blind design treated with beclomethasone dipropionate 400 µg in the nose (left) or as bronchial inhalation (right). While the provoking dose of carbachol (similar to methacholine), necessary to cause a 35% fall in lung function, increased significantly ($p < 0.001$) following nasal medication, bronchial administration had no significant effect. Thus, when inflammation is localized to the nose, airway responsiveness seems only to be reduced when anti-inflammatory therapy is directed to the inflamed nasal mucosa. From Aubier M, Clerici C, Neukirch F, Herman D. Different effects of nasal and bronchial glucocorticoid administration on bronchial hyperresponsiveness in patients with allergic rhinitis. *Am Rev Respir Dis* 1992; **146**: 122–6.

Treatment failures	
Cause	**Measure**
The disease is not steroid responsive	Try other therapies
The spray is used to give immediate relief	Better patient information
The spray is used in a blocked nose	Occasional use of vasoconstrictor, or short-term systemic steroid
Fear of local adverse reactions	Rhinoscopy every 3–6 months
Treatment with pressurized aerosol stopped due to haemorrhagic crusting	Change to pump spray or powder, reduce dosage
Treatment stopped due to immediate sneezing	Continue; this symptom will often improve with time

Table 8.7.1. Causes of a negative treatment result with a steroid spray

tients with perennial non-allergic rhinitis are *non-responders* to any type of steroid treatment. *Nasal eosinophilia* usually predicts a good result while neutrophilia predicts treatment failure.

In perennial rhinitis and nasal polyposis, a 2–4-week treatment may be necessary to obtain full symptom relief. In these chronic conditions, an improvement can last for weeks to months after discontinuation of the treatment. Apparently, some vicious circle is broken.

When symptoms are under full control, the dose can be adjusted according to the clinical response. The goal should be to use the lowest dose that provides full efficacy. Treatment may be discontinued, for example for 1 month every 12 months in adults and every 6 months in children, in order to ensure that therapy is still required.

Patient instruction

Always explain to the patient that this spray does not give immediate relief and that it must be used on a *regular basis*. In hay fever, it is preferable to start as soon as the patient experiences the first symptoms.

Adequate *mucosal distribution* of the drug in the nose is of importance for its efficacy and patients must be instructed not to use the spray in a blocked nose or nostril.

Adverse effects

As many patients have a negative bias to steroids, the

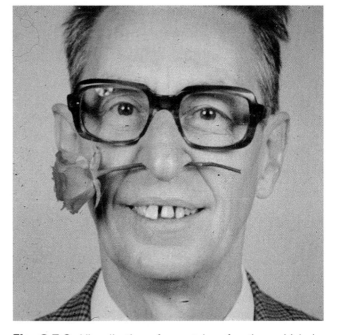

Fig. 8.7.9. Visualization of a septal perforation, which, in the rare case, may be a side effect of intranasal steroid therapy. Photo taken by Dr Bob Wentges, Niejmegen, Holland.

real risk of adverse effects should be discussed at the time the prescription is given.

Irritation and sneezing immediately after spraying are frequent but rarely a problem. They usually diminish with time because they are more a conse-

Intranasal steroid versus antihistamine

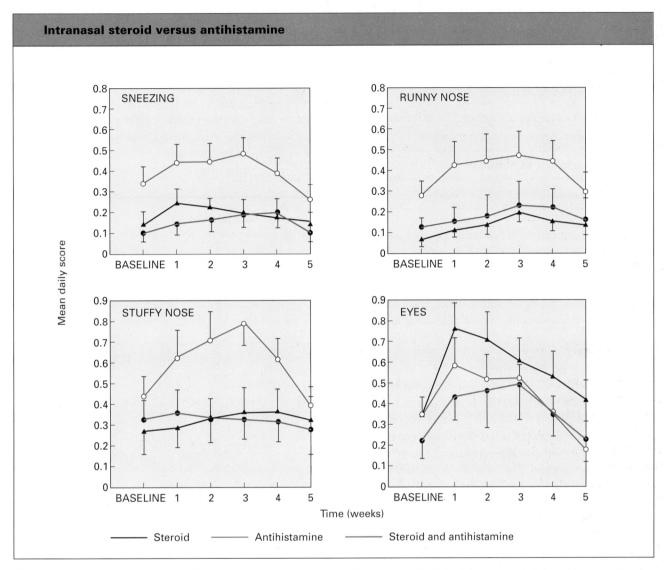

Fig. 8.7.10. Mean daily nose and eye symptom scores (±SEM) before and throughout the ragweed-pollen season: beclomethasone dipropionate nasal spray alone; astemizole alone; beclomethasone dipropionate plus astemizole (filled circle). From Juniper EF, Kline PA, Hargreave FE, Dolovich J, Comparison of beclomethasone dipropionate aqueous nasal spray, astemizole, and the combination in the prophylactic treatment of ragweed pollen-induced rhinoconjunctivitis. *J Allergy Clin Immunol* 1989; **83**: 627–33.

quence of mucosal hyper-responsiveness than a true adverse effect.

A modern steroid spray for the nose, used in correct dosage, will *not cause systemic side effects* although the drug is absorbed. However, when a patient receives steroids by various routes, all contributions will be additive. A dose of steroid sprayed into the nose will have more systemic activity than when inhaled. More of the drug reaches the absorbing, airway mucosa in the nose (20–50%) than when delivered to the lower airways (10–20%).

Dryness in the anterior part of the nose, *blood-stained crusts* and even *epistaxis* can occur but are not progressive and are seldom troublesome. Dose reduction, use of an ointment in the nostril and change to an aqueous solution or a powder formulation can be helpful in these cases. As modern steroid sprays have been widely used for 20 years without any report of the development of atrophic rhinitis, this risk seems to be negligible. A few cases of a *septal perforation* associated with use of intranasal steroids have been reported (Fig. 8.7.9). Candida

Perennial use of nasal steroids in children
Allergen avoidance carried out
Cromoglycate and antihistamine tried and found inadequate
Daily symptoms of significance for the child
The daily dose as low as possible
Medication given once daily in the morning
Regular checks

Table 8.7.2. Use of nasal steroids for perennial allergic rhinitis in children

overgrowth does not occur in the nose, and viral and bacterial infections do not change their frequency or severity.

Pros and cons

The *marked efficacy* of intranasal steroids for treating allergic rhinitis is indisputable. It exceeds that of H_1 antihistamines (Fig. 8.7.10) and cromoglycate.

The major limitation of nasal steroid therapy lies in the *lack of effect on eye symptoms* and the relatively *slow onset of action*. The use of nasal steroids is therefore confined to regular medication in patients who have daily nasal symptoms.

It is understandable that there is a public bias against steroids as such, but 20 years of experience has shown that intranasal steroid treatment is at least as safe as other types of medication for rhinitis.

Safety in children

While there is no reason to question the safety of intranasal steroids in adults, their use in children and during pregnancy is still a question of debate.

When a child is treated with an 'adult dose', given as 200 µg twice daily, very sensitive methods (kneemometry) can detect a reduction of short-term growth. This is not the case when treatment is confined to a single dose given in the morning. While intranasal steroids can be used freely in hay fever with a short season, their perennial use in children should not be first-line treatment (Table 8.7.2).

Safety during pregnancy

In principle, no medication can be considered as 100% safe during pregnancy, especially during the

first trimester. The following rules are advisable: 1, increase restrictiveness in the prescription of any drug; 2, prefer topical to systemic administration; and 3, prefer an old and widely used drug to a recently marketed drug.

When treatment is definitely needed, a saline douche and cromoglycate may be tried initially. If they are unsuccessful, topical nasal steroids, given in the recommended dosage, have not been associated with any teratogenic or other adverse effects.

True also for allergy books?
History books which contain no lies are extremely dull.
Anatole France

8.8 Systemic corticosteroids and rhinitis

Only for short-term use

Key points

- In severe cases, short-term use (2 weeks) of systemic steroids is a valuable supplement to other therapies.
- A short course can break vicious circles and give prolonged relief.
- Treatment can be given orally or as a depot-injection.
- In hay fever, oral medication is, in principle, preferable as it can be adjusted to the pollen count.
- In perennial rhinitis and nasal polyposis, it is an advantage of depot-injections that they put the control of treatment in the hands of the doctor.
- The treatment is safe provided that there is at least a 3-month interval between courses.
- Systemic steroids should not be given for rhinitis in children or pregnant women.

Principles of therapy

As the risk of adverse effects from systemic corticosteroids depends largely on the duration of treatment, it is a principle that *only short-term therapy* (2 weeks) is used in rhinitis. When the rules, given in Table 8.8.1, are followed, the use of systemic steroids can be both safe and useful in rhinitis.

Preparations

Steroids can be given *orally* (prednisolone, 5–25 mg/

Systemic steroids for rhinitis
Only short-term therapy (2 weeks)
Not used more frequently than every 3rd month
Not used instead of other treatments, but in addition to a basic medication, which has proved to be insufficient
Not given to children, pregnant women or patients with known contra-indications

Table 8.8.1. Principles for safe use of systemic steroids for rhinitis

day) or as a *depot-injection* (e.g. methylprednisolone, 40–80 mg/injection). Oral treatment is confined to 2 weeks, which approximately corresponds to the activity of a single injection.

Depot-injections are often used, and occasionally misused, in the treatment of allergic rhinitis. General practitioners, using this form of therapy, argue that clinical experience has shown that one to two injections are free of serious adverse effects. However, it must be remembered that an injection of 80 mg methylprednisolone corresponds to 100 mg prednisolone, and that continuous release during the day will suppress the hypothalamic–pituitary–adrenal (HPA) axis more than a single oral dose given in the morning. Almost all *specialists recommend oral medication*. Table 8.8.2 summarizes arguments and counter arguments.

Seasonal allergic rhinitis

When other treatments are inadequate in hay fever, the patient can be supplied with *prednisolone tablets* (5–10 mg in the morning during troublesome periods). Oral steroid medication has the advantage over depot-injections in that treatment can follow the pollen count. In this way, unnecessary medication during rainy periods can be avoided.

Some general practitioners treat hay fever, with a short season, successfully with a single injection. Although this may not be optimal pharmacotherapy, it is difficult to justify any major criticism of such a procedure.

Perennial rhinitis and nasal polyposis

Systemic steroids, in contrast to topical treatment, reach all parts of the nose and the paranasal sinuses. Short courses in patients with severe perennial rhinitis or nasal polyposis can be helpful. This treatment can be used to open up a blocked nose before topical therapy and when there is a temporary failure of spray treatment, for example after a common cold. Systemic steroids have a marked effect on nasal blockage (Fig. 8.8.1).

Contra-indications

Contra-indications to systemic steroids are glaucoma, herpes keratitis, diabetes mellitus, psychic instability, advanced osteoporosis, severe hypertension, tuberculosis or other chronic infection. As mentioned, systemic steroids are not used for rhinitis in children or during pregnancy.

Oral steroid or depot-injection?
In favour of oral medication
Cheap
The dosage can be adjusted to the changing need for treatment, for example during a pollen season with a highly varying pollen count
Medication once daily causes minimal suppression of the HPA axis
In favour of depot-injection
A number of placebo-controlled trials have proven the dosage used to be effective (there are no such studies for oral treatment and the dosages used vary considerably)
An injection places the treatment in the hands of the physician, and patient compliance is no problem
The use of an injection in a patient with a chronic disease ensures that he or she cannot convert what was intended to be intermittent therapy to continuous treatment
In a busy out-patient clinic, it may be easier to communicate the strict rules for the use of steroids to all personnel and patients, when an injection is to be given than when tablets are to be prescribed
A relatively small total dose is given and some steroid side effects may relate to the total dose more than to the frequency of medication
Suppression of the HPA axis for a few weeks does not imply any clinical risk of Addisonian crises
The only controlled comparison between oral and injected steroid in rhinitis showed a therapeutic index in favour of the depot-injection

Tabel 8.8.2. Arguments in favour of oral medication and of depot-injection of steroids for the treatment of rhinitis

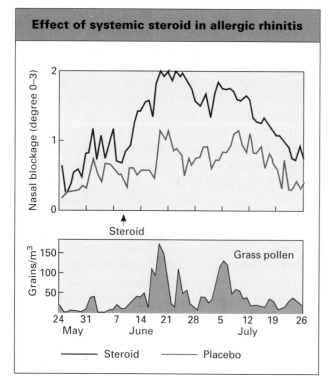

Fig. 8.8.1. A depot-steroid injection (80 mg methylprednisolone) has a marked and long-lasting effect on nasal blockage in hay fever and perennial rhinitis. From Borum P, Grønborg H, Mygind N. Seasonal allergic rhinitis and depot injection of a corticosteroid. *Allergy* 1987; **42**: 26–32.

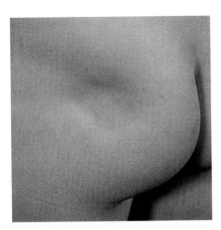

Fig. 8.8.2. Skin depression over subcutaneous necrosis, which developed following a depot-injection of corticosteroid. From Wahn U, Seger R, Wahn V. Pädiatrische Allergologie und Immunologie in Klinik und Praxis. Stuttgart: Gustav Fischer, 1994: **1**: 1–573.

Side effects

The side effects from a 2-week treatment are few and mild. Depot-injections can, in rare cases, cause a depression over the injection site (Fig. 8.8.2). Some authors recommend depot-injections into swollen nasal turbinates and polyps, but this must be discouraged as blindness has been reported.

Science = common sense!
Science is, I believe, nothing but trained and organized common-sense.

Thomas Huxley

A presidential advice
It is common sense to take a method and try it. If it fails, admit it frankly and try another.

Franklin D Roosevelt

8.9 Cromoglycate in allergic rhinitis
Non-steroid anti-inflammatory treatment

Key points
- Cromoglycate and nedocromil were originally considered to be mast cell stabilizing agents.
- These drugs have a moderate anti-inflammatory effect in allergic mucous membranes.
- In the eye and nose (and bronchi), they can be used prophylactically before allergen exposure.
- The drugs give a variable degree of symptom amelioration in allergic rhino-conjunctivitis.
- Their short duration of action necessitates frequent medication, which impairs patient compliance.
- The main indication for daily use is perennial allergic rhinitis in children.

Mode of action
Cromoglycate (sodium cromoglycate, cromolyn in USA) is used prophylactically in the nose, eye and bronchi. Animal studies have indicated that this molecule inhibits allergen-induced release of mediators from mast cells. This led to the concept that cromoglycate acted through mast cell stabilization and to its classification as an *'anti-allergic'* compound. Subsequent development led to the synthesis of *nedocromil sodium*, which is more potent than cromoglycate. Although these compounds have a clinical effect in allergic rhinitis, it is uncertain whether their beneficial effect relates primarily to an action on nasal mast cells or to an action on other cellular components. Their effect has also been attributed to an effect on sensory neural stimulation.

Seasonal allergic rhinitis
Placebo-controlled studies have demonstrated the superiority of cromoglycate to placebo in hay fever (Fig. 8.9.1), but not all trials have identified clear benefit. Cromoglycate seems to be a more useful drug *in the eye* than *in the nose*, as the more active steroids have serious adverse effects when used in the eye, but not when applied to the nose. It is advisable to start treatment as soon as pollens occur in the air and before significant symptoms have developed.

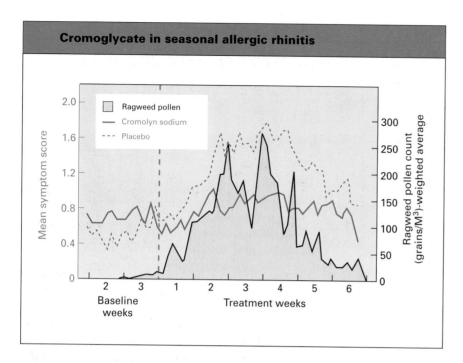

Fig. 8.9.1. Daily symptom scores for rhinorrhoea in ragweed-allergic patients treated with 4% cromoglycate (cromolyn) nasal solution or placebo. From Handelman NI, Friday GA, Schwartz HJ *et al*. Cromolyn sodium nasal solution in the prophylactic treatment of pollen-induced seasonal allergic rhinitis. *J Allergy Clin Immunol* 1977; **59**: 237–42.

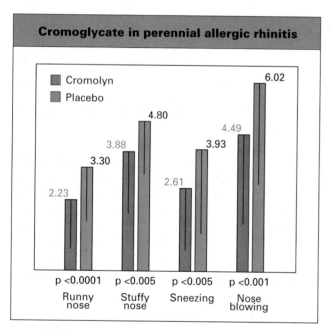

Fig. 8.9.2. Daily symptom scores (mean −SD) in 34 adult patients with perennial allergic rhinitis, receiving either 4% cromoglycate or placebo, six times daily. From Cohan RH, Bloom FL, Rhoades RB, Wittig HJ, Haugh LD. Treatment of perennial allergic rhinitis with cromolyn sodium. *J Allergy Clin Immunol* 1976; **58**: 121–8.

Perennial allergic rhinitis

The overall symptom reduction is about 25–30% with the least benefit on nasal blockage (Fig. 8.9.2). There is a variability in the response, and, based on clinical experience, it has been proposed that most clinical benefit is seen in patients who fulfil the following criteria: 1, an obvious *allergic* aetiology; 2, local eosinophilia; 3, predominance of *sneezing*; 4, short duration of the disease; and 5, *young age*.

The drug is more valuable in *children* than in adults as children usually have uncomplicated allergy. Most paediatricians reserve the more potent steroid sprays for children with severe symptoms, not controlled by cromoglycate.

The drug is well suited for occasional use before exposure to allergens (animals). In symptomatic patients, no immediate symptom relief will be evident. The *prophylactic* nature of the treatment must be explained to the patient.

Drug administration

Cromoglycate is available for nasal insufflation as a powder preparation (10 mg/capsule) and as a 2–4% metered-dose pump spray (2.6–5.2 mg/dose). Due to its relatively short duration of action, the drug is administered every 4 hours; this can lead to poor patient compliance. Nedocromil is now available in some countries as a 1% nasal spray.

Adverse effects

Cromoglycate is completely atoxic; the price is the only contra-indication. Nedocromil has a bitter taste.

Combined therapy

Clinical experience has indicated that the benefit from cromoglycate can be added to that of immunotherapy and antihistamines, but it seems unlikely that combined usage of cromoglycate and a topical steroid will be more effective than the steroid alone.

Cheap therapy without adverse effects
The physician's best remedy is Tincture of Time.
Bela Schick

8.10 Alpha adrenoceptor agonists
Nasal decongestants

Key points
- Alpha adrenoceptor agonists contract blood vessels and act as nasal decongestants.
- Topical application is more effective than oral administration.
- Ephedrine from a drop-bottle gives a good distribution in the nose, of particular importance for sinusitis.
- The more potent and long-acting xylometazoline/oxymetazoline given from spray bottles are easy to use, and to abuse.
- Regular use must be limited to 7–10 days due to the risk of rhinitis medicamentosa.
- Combined oral preparations of an alpha agonist and an antihistamine are widely used for allergic rhinitis.
- These two types of drugs have effects that supplement each other, and their side effects on the CNS tend to be mutually neutralizing.
- Oral decongestants must be used with care in children and in adults with heart disease, hypertension or prostatism.

The use of vasoconstrictors is rooted in antiquity. Ephedrine is the active constituent of Ma huang, a Chinese herbal medicine, which has been used for more than 5000 years. It was introduced into modern medicine in 1927 and was soon followed by other sympathomimetic agents, given orally or intranasally, to reduce nasal obstruction. The total use of nasal decongestants is huge and the misuse is considerable.

Background
The blood vessels of the nasal mucosa have a *rich sympathetic innervation*, which determines vascular congestion and nasal patency. During normal conditions, sympathetic activity maintains the venous sinusoids contracted at about 50% of the maximal contractile state. On exercise, sympathetic activity is increased, resulting in vasoconstriction and an increase in nasal patency. A similar effect is obtained by administration of the sympathomimetic drugs.

Topical vasoconstrictors

Mode of application

Application of a large volume of a weak solution from a *drop-bottle/pipette* gives a good distribution over the nasal mucosa, particularly important in the treatment of sinusitis. Instruction in the correct usage is necessary as improperly instructed patients will bend the head backwards and pour the solution along the nasal floor into the nasopharynx (Fig. 8.10.1).

It is easy to use (and abuse) a *plastic bottle nebulizer*, and the dosage delivered varies considerably depending upon the force used to compress the bottle. Its use is *prohibited in children*; some parents will turn it upside down and empty the bottle into the child's nose and severe intoxication may result.

A *metered-dose pump spray*, which is now widely used, is preferable to a plastic bottle nebulizer as it delivers an exact dosage.

Effect

Patients like the quick onset of action and the pronounced effect. However, although the nasal airway is opened, it does not mean that normal physiological conditions, characterized by slit-like passages, are re-established. Often, a wide tunnel is opened in the lower part of the nose while the upper part is still blocked.

Choice of drug

The vasoconstrictor effect of *ephedrine* is moderate, short lasting and tachyphylaxis develops rapidly. *Xylometazoline* and *oxymetazoline* control nasal congestion better than ephedrine, and their prolonged action (6–8 hours) is of importance for treatment of nocturnal blockage.

Indications for use

Patients, not guided by a physician, tend to use a vasoconstrictor spray for all types of rhinitis, which is unjustified.

In *perennial rhinitis*, it must be used with caution as there is a considerable risk of abuse and the development of rhinitis medicamentosa. A vasoconstrictor spray can be used: 1, when the patient starts a basic treatment with topical steroid in order to ensure optimal drug distribution in the nose; 2, when the patient has upper airway infection and sinusitis; and 3, on special occasions when nasal blockage can have detrimental consequences (e.g. important business meetings, air travel and dates).

Nasal congestion is most pronounced in the supine position, and nasal blockage with mouth breathing results in snoring and *disturbed sleep*. If a patient regularly uses a vasoconstrictor spray before going to bed, he or she should be told only to use it on one side and to change sides every day.

Side effects

Long-term treatment with an intranasal alpha adrenoceptor agonist causes more symptoms than it relieves. It results in the development of *rhinitis medicamentosa* (the 'nose-drop-nose'), which is characterized by rebound congestion, increased nasal

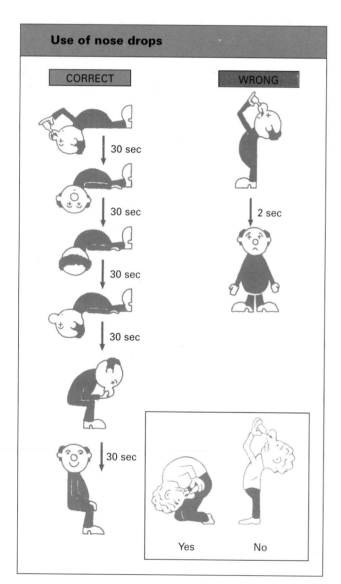

Use of nose drops

CORRECT   WRONG

30 sec

30 sec   2 sec

30 sec

30 sec

30 sec

Yes   No

Fig. 8.10.1. Illustration of correct and incorrect use of a vasoconstrictor delivered from a pipette or a drop-bottle. Inset courtesy of Ian MacKay, London.

irritability, hyper-reactivity and a feeling of burning and dryness in the nose.

Possible *pathogenic factors* are as follows. 1, The high concentration of agonist at the receptor site, which results in down-regulation of vascular adrenoceptors. This may lead to reduced responsiveness to endogenous catecholamines, which participate in normal physiological regulation of the vascular tone. 2, An alpha adrenoceptor agonist does not normalize nasal blood flow, as it contracts both veins and arteries, resulting not only in increased patency but also in local hypoxaemia. 3, Prolonged spraying of the preservative, benzalkonium chloride, may increase mucosal irritability and reactivity.

Regular use of intranasal vasoconstrictors is limited to *7–10 days*, and they must be prescribed with caution in patients with chronic disease. Carefully given information is the best way to prevent rhinitis medicamentosa. The latter is often treated with a short course of *steroids*, although there is no current documentation of the benefit of this treatment.

Oral vasoconstrictors

Effect

Oral medication with alpha adrenoceptor agonists has *less effect on nasal patency* than topical treatment, but it can be used regularly *without risk of rhinitis medicamentosa*. In addition, it reaches all parts of the nasal and sinus mucosa.

Side effects

It is not elegant pharmacotherapy to constrict every blood vessel in the body in order to treat a stuffy nose, and the dosage needed is at the borderline of that which causes other *systemic side effects*. Dosing must be precise and oral vasoconstrictors should be used with caution in children (psychotic episodes) and elderly gentlemen (prostatism). There are many *contra-indications* (coronary disease, hypertension, thyrotoxicosis, glaucoma, diabetes mellitus, and use of monoamine oxidase inhibitors). Systemic side effects, such as restlessness, insomnia, tremor, tachycardia and palpitations, are frequent.

Choice of drug

Pseudoephedrine and *phenylpropanolamine* (norephedrine) are preferable to ephedrine as they have fewer CNS effects.

Combined preparations

It is logical to combine *H₁ antihistamines and alpha adrenoceptor agonists* for two reasons: 1, the antihistamines have a good effect on sneezing and rhinorrhoea and the alpha agonist has a good effect on blockage; and 2, the CNS stimulatory effect of the alpha agonist may counteract sedation from the antihistamine.

While combined preparations may be useful in allergic rhinitis, there is *considerable overuse* of these 'common cold tablets' in diseases in which they have no, or only marginal, effect (colds, influenza, sinusitis and otitis media).

Fatal for rodents

A drug is a substance that, when injected into a rat, produces a scientific paper.

8.11 Cholinoceptor antagonists
Anti-rhinorrhoea therapy

Key points
* Watery discharge is mediated via cholinergic receptors in nasal glands.
* Isolated watery rhinorrhoea rarely responds to antihistamines or steroids.
* The quantity can be reduced by topical application of the anti-cholinergic drug, ipratropium bromide.
* Ipratropium is effective in perennial rhinitis-, cold air- and hot spicy food-induced rhinorrhoea and in the common cold.
* The dosage must be adjusted to the severity of symptoms in order to optimize efficacy and minimize adverse effects (i.e. dryness in the nose).

Watery rhinorrhoea can be excessive and it is then a very annoying symptom. When it is not associated with sneezing, there is rarely a good response to antihistamine or steroid therapy. As there is good evidence that watery rhinorrhoea is mediated via cholinergic receptors in nasal glands, use of a cholinoceptor antagonist is a logical choice.

Drug administration
Ipratropium bromide (ipratropium) is preferable to atropine, as quarternary amines are poorly absorbed after topical application to mucosal surfaces and are slow to cross the blood–brain barrier. Ipratropium is, at present, delivered from a pressurized aerosol, soon to be replaced by an aqueous pump spray.

The usual recommendation is to give a fixed dose of ipratropium four times daily. However, symptoms vary considerably from patient to patient and during

Use of ipratropium spray
Determine the severity of the disease (tissues/day during 1 week)
Match the dosage to symptom severity
Give one large dosage early in the morning
Administer smaller doses p.r.n. during the day

Table 8.11.1. Optimal use of ipratropium nasal spray

Patient selection
Adults
Clear nasal discharge >1 hour each day
No major problem with nasal blockage
No known allergic basis for the rhinitis
No satisfactory response to antihistamine or steroid spray

Table 8.11.2. Selection of patients for ipratropium therapy

Limitations of ipratropium
No effect on itching, sneezing and blockage
Only effects fluid formed in glands (not tears, sinus secretion, goblet cell secretion, condensed water or exudation)
Effects only watery rhinorrhoea; no effect on purulent secretions
Reduces physiological secretory activity with local side effects (nasal dryness)

Table 8.11.3. Limitations of the usefulness of ipratropium nasal spray

the day. Usually, rhinorrhoea is most pronounced in the morning, while glandular secretion is low during the night. It may therefore be preferable to *individualize the treatment*, by giving one large dose in the morning, and later only when needed, especially before exposure to known provoking factors (Table 8.11.1). Ipratropium is effective within 30 minutes and the effect is long-lasting (8–12 hours).

Clinical efficacy
In patients with *perennial non-allergic rhinitis* with *watery rhinorrhoea as a dominant symptom*, the regular use of an ipratropium spray can reduce nasal discharge by 40%, but careful selection of patients is necessary (Table 8.11.2). Although ipratropium is effective in allergic rhinitis, it is preferable to use antihistamines or steroids, which, in contrast to ipratropium, also counteract itching and sneezing (Table 8.11.3).

The spray can inhibit rhinorrhoea induced by *cold air* ('skier's nose') and by *hot spicy food* ('gustatory rhinitis'). It also reduces watery discharge during the first days of a *common cold*.

Side effects

Apparently ipratropium reduces both reflex mediated and basic secretory activity in the nose. Significant reduction of severe attacks of rhinorrhoea can therefore cause a *sensation of nasal dryness* at other times. When marked morning symptoms are treated with a high dosage, the long-lasting activity of the drug in the nose can result in dryness in the evening and at night, if secretory activity is low. In which case, a *saline spray* is helpful.

There is only today, tomorrow does not exist

As to the method of work, I have a single bit of advice which I give with the earnest conviction of its paramount influence in any success which may have attended by efforts in life—*take no thought for the tomorrow*. Live neither in the past nor in the future, but let each day's work absorb your entire energies, and satisfy your widest ambition.

William Osler

8.12 Seasonal allergic rhinitis
Hay fever

Key points

- Seasonal allergic rhinitis or hay fever is caused by pollen allergy.
- There are three groups: tree, grass and weed pollen, with seasons in spring, summer and autumn, respectively.
- Hay fever is a common disease, affecting 10% of the total population.
- It often starts in childhood, is most frequent in adolescence, improves in middle age and is seldom a problem in elderly people.
- Symptoms are itching of the eyes, nose and throat, repeated sneezing, watery discharge and nasal congestion.
- Asthma can occur at the peak of the season.
- The symptoms are related to the pollen count.
- The diagnosis of hay fever is easy and skin testing is necessary only in selected cases.
- Treatment must be active in order that the patient can live a normal life.
- Occasional symptoms are treated with antihistamines, which can also be used for continuous therapy when eye symptoms are prominent.
- A nasal steroid spray is more effective on nasal symptoms, especially blockage.
- Topical treatment of nasal symptoms requires the use of eye drops (antihistamine or cromoglycate).
- Short-term systemic steroids can be added at the peak of the season in severe cases.
- Immunotherapy should be considered in those patients who do not respond adequately to drug treatment.

Seasonal allergic rhinitis, or more correctly rhino-conjunctivitis, is caused by pollen allergy. It can be complicated by seasonal allergic asthma. The old term '*hay fever*' relates to the observation, made more than one hundred years ago, that nasal symptoms develop on exposure to flowering grass fields, 'fever' implying a disease rather than pyrexia. Pollen allergy is also called *pollinosis*.

Pollens

Pollen grains, as relatively large particles, impinge

against the eye, are trapped in the nasal filter and do not reach the lower airway in any significant number. However, pollen asthma can be induced by allergen-containing dust. The most important sources of pollen allergens are *trees*, *grasses* and *weeds*, which, in the northern hemisphere, have seasons in *spring*, *summer* and early *autumn*, respectively (see Chapter 3.2).

The length of the pollen season varies considerably from place to place. When the patient is allergic to tree, grass and weed pollen, the season is long and the disease resembles perennial rhinitis.

Prevalence

Pollinosis is, world wide, the most common expression of IgE-mediated allergy (worm infestations excluded). Although seasonal allergic rhinitis, from a clinical point of view, is a well-defined disease, it is less so in epidemiological terms. This is because the clinician will only see the tip of the iceberg, the troubled patient, in his office. Many allergic persons have no or few symptoms, and this may explain why the frequency figures in the literature vary considerably. A reasonable average figure for *cumulative prevalence* (have and have had) of symptomatic hay fever is *10–15%*. However, only about 2% of a general population will use a hay fever remedy during the pollen season. These data support the clinical impression that many patients are under-treated or not treated at all for what they believe is a 'prolonged summer cold'.

Natural history

The majority of cases present during childhood and adolescence. The disease tends to worsen for the first two to three seasons, remain stationary for 2–3 decades, *improve in middle age* and seldom be a problem in the elderly. The pollen count can vary considerably from season to season. It is therefore difficult to judge, in a few seasons, the spontaneous course of the disease and the result of therapy.

Hay fever patients have a two- to three-fold increased risk of developing *perennial asthma*. It has been claimed, but not proven, that this risk can be reduced by immunotherapy with pollen extract.

Symptoms

Rhino-conjunctivitis

The pollen-exposed patient is constantly aware of the nose due to *itching* and *watery rhinorrhoea*. This is

disturbing at work and annoying during social activities. The itching results in serial *sneezing* (five to 25 sneezes), and the rhinorrhoea necessitates constant use of a handkerchief (the nose can produce 10 ml per hour). *Congestion* gives the patient a nasal voice and makes him feel 'stuffy' in the head. *Itching of the soft palate* indicates that the mucociliary system has transported pollen allergen to the nasopharynx. Some patients get referred *itching in the ears* due to the common innervation of the pharyngeal mucosa and the ear.

While irritation of the nasal mucosa can cause running eyes, *itching of the eyes* is due to a local allergic reaction and is characteristic of allergic conjunctivitis. It leads to eye rubbing, and a vicious circle is started, ending with red and smarting eyes.

Asthma

Some patients, especially those with severe rhino-conjunctivitis, develop bronchial symptoms at the peak of the pollen season. Mild symptoms are frequent but acute severe asthma can occur. Patients with *seasonal allergic asthma* often have bronchial hyper-responsiveness all year round and an increased risk of developing perennial asthma.

Pollen count and symptoms

The severity of eye and nose symptoms varies with the daily pollen count (given on the radio and in newspapers), while the correlation is less obvious for asthma. The pollen count is usually *high in sunny, dry weather* and low in cold, rainy periods.

The pollen count varies considerably from place to place, although pollen grains can fly several miles with the wind. It is *high on farmland* and in valleys, and low by the sea and on mountains. It is *higher in the country* than in the city; symptoms can be severe in a *summer cottage*, while they are negligible in a flat on the 10th floor. A *bicycle ride* or a car drive with open windows is an effective way of sampling pollen in the eyes and nose. Symptoms are invariably provoked by *cutting the lawn* and also the hedge, which harbours pollen dust on the leaves.

Diagnosis

Diagnosing hay fever is easy. A patient will often suspect pollen allergy, especially when the daily pollen count has drawn his or her attention to the possibility. In mild cases with a short season, the case history will suffice for diagnosis and treatment.

When needed, *skin prick testing* is usually sufficient

Table 8.12.1 Treatment of seasonal allergic rhinitis according to Lund *et al.* Lund VJ. International consensus report on the diagnosis and management of rhinitis. *Allergy* 1994; **49**(suppl 19): 1–34

Treatment of seasonal allergic rhinitis
Mild disease or with occasional symptoms
Oral non-sedating H₁ antihistamine (when symptomatic) or Antihistamine or cromoglycate topically to eyes or nose or both
Moderate to severe disease with prominent nasal symptoms
Topical nasal steroids plus Antihistamine or cromoglycate topically to eyes
Moderate to severe disease with prominent eye symptoms
Oral non-sedating H₁ antihistamine daily or Topical nasal steroid and antihistamine or cromoglycate topically to eyes
If above ineffective
Refer to specialist for further investigation including: examination of the nose allergy testing systemic steroids for crisis situations possible immunotherapy

to confirm the history. Other examinations are unnecessary in uncomplicated hay fever.

Principles of treatment

Live a normal life

The quality of life can be seriously impaired in the pollen season, which is usually at the best time of the year, especially if the patient is young and the sun is shining. As effective and safe therapies are available, the goal for treatment is a normal life.

Avoidance not possible

Allergen avoidance is not possible outdoors because pollens are well mixed in the lower atmosphere. However, excessive exposure can usually be avoided by common sense. The patient should avoid close contact with wild and cultivated grass (hay), but can enjoy his or her garden, as cutting grass (by a family member) reduces pollination from the lawn. Closing the bedroom windows can be advised, and, when feasible, installation of an air conditioner can considerably increase the protection.

It can be useful to give the patient advice on how to arrange the *summer holidays*, as the season, of his or her allergen, can often be shortened by careful planning.

Pharmacotherapy

Mild disease with occasional symptoms is treated by *H₁ antihistamines* (orally or topically) or by *cromoglycate* prophylactically (Table 8.12.1).

Moderate to severe disease with daily nasal symptoms is most efficiently treated by a *steroid spray*, which is used together with *eye drops* (antihistamine or cromoglycate). Daily use of an oral antihistamine is a good first choice in patients with daily and pronounced eye symptoms.

Thus, in hay fever, both nasal steroids and antihistamines can be used as *first-line therapy* in adults and in children. The choice depends upon the frequency and severity of the symptoms and whether they are, predominantly, nasal or conjunctival.

A *short course of systemic steroid* may be added in some very sensitive patients when the pollen count is high.

Immunotherapy

Opinions about when and how often to start immunotherapy vary, but most specialists agree that: 1, drug treatment should be tried first; and 2, immunotherapy should be considered when systemic steroids are needed to control the disease. The following factors are in favour of immunotherapy: 1, *severe symptoms*; 2, a *long pollen season*; 3, *asthma* in the season; and 4, *patient's preference*.

Cheap therapy

Economy is a decisive factor in the choice of therapy in many parts of the world. The first generation antihistamines are cheaper than modern topical treatment, and prednisolone is cheaper than immunotherapy. '*Discount therapy*' for hay fever consists of a first generation antihistamine (e.g. chlorpheniramine given once daily in the evening) throughout the entire season with prednisolone tablets added at the peak.

Active death help
I die by the help of too many physicians.
Alexander the Great

8.13 Perennial rhinitis
Allergic and non-allergic

Key points
- A distinction between perennial allergic and non-allergic is made.
- Non-allergic rhinitis can be further divided into an eosinophilic and a non-eosinophilic subgroup, at least in theory.
- Sporadic symptoms are frequent, but only 2–4% of the population suffer from a real disease.
- Allergic rhinitis usually starts in childhood and non-allergic rhinitis in adult life.
- Mite allergy is the most important cause of chronic allergic symptoms and allergy to animals frequently causes intermittent symptoms.
- Ingested allergens can play a role in children, but their role is debated.
- The aetiology is unknown in most adult patients with perennial rhinitis.
- The symptoms are similar to those of hay fever, but eye itching is less frequent and nasal blockage more prominent.
- All patients with chronic symptoms react to a series of non-specific stimuli and irritants.
- A persistent, hormonal rhino-sinusitis can occur during pregnancy; it disappears promptly after delivery.

Perennial non-infectious rhinitis can be allergic or non-allergic, and a distinction is made in clinical routine. Perennial non-allergic rhinitis can be eosinophilic or non-eosinophilic, and a distinction is made only by the few specialists who do microscopy of nasal smear, but symptoms and signs can also give some information (Table 8.13.1).

Occurrence and prevalence

It is estimated that 2–4% of the general population suffer from a chronic disease with daily symptoms and need medication. The figures are uncertain because of the vague definition of the disease and the lack of epidemiological studies.

Allergic rhinitis often occurs in patients with other allergic diseases; 80% of children presenting with *asthma* and 50% with *atopic dermatitis* also suffer from allergic rhinitis. It often starts in childhood, while the first appearance of non-allergic rhinitis, as a rule, is in adult life.

Characteristics of different types of rhinitis			
	Allergic rhinitis	**Non-allergic rhinitis**	
		Eosinophilic	**Non-eosinophilic**
Age at onset	Childhood	Adult	Adult
Symptoms			
Congestion	Moderate	Marked	Slight–moderate
Sneezing	Frequent	Occasional	Rare
Itching	Usual	Occasional	Uncommon
Rhinorrhoea	Profuse	Profuse	Profuse
Anosmia	Occasional	Frequent	Rare
Physical examination			
Swollen turbinates	Moderate–marked	Marked	Moderate
Character of secretions	Watery	Mucoid	Watery
Associated findings			
Predominant cell in secretion	Eosinophil	Eosinophil	Few neutrophils
Infection	Occasional	Frequent	Rare
NSAID intolerance	Rare	Occasional	Rare
Concurrent diseases			
Conjunctivitis	Frequent	Rare	Absent
Asthma	Frequent	Frequent	Rare
Urticaria	Rare	Occasional	Rare
Sinus X-ray examination			
Mucosal thickening	Slight	Marked	Slight
Fluid	Rare	Occasional	Rare
Response to therapy			
Antihistamines	Good	Fair	Poor
Decongestants	Limited	Limited	Poor
Corticosteroids	Excellent	Excellent	Poor
Cromoglycate	Good	Poor	Poor
Ipratropium	Limited	Fair	Good

Table 8.13.1 Comparison of different types of non-infectious rhinitis

The course of the disease is capricious, but severe, persistent symptoms will usually predict a long course. Thus, perennial allergic rhinitis does not have the same favourable natural course as seasonal allergic rhinitis.

Aetiology

Aero-allergens

House dust mite
This is, world wide, the most important cause of perennial allergic rhinitis. Allergen exposure is maximal in bed, but nasal blockage is always worst in the supine position, and sneezing and rhinorrhoea are most pronounced in the hours immediately after waking in all types of rhinitis. Symptoms provoked by *making the bed* and emptying the vacuum cleaner are suggestive of mite allergy.

Animals
Allergy to mammals is *frequent* but most subjects have only *occasional symptoms*. Animal allergy can cause daily symptoms and chronic disease when: 1, a

highly sensitive patient is exposed indirectly to animal protein via others clothes; 2, a patient who, against advice, keeps his or her pet animal in the house; and 3, a patient with a low-grade allergy who does not realize that daily allergen exposure can increase the nasal reactivity without causing obvious symptoms upon contact with the animal.

Pollens
Pollen allergy is a frequent cause of perennial disease in tropical and subtropical countries.

Moulds
Mould allergy is a well-known cause of rhinitis in asthmatic children, while its role in non-asthmatic adults is probably insignificant.

Occupational allergy
Rhinitis due to an occupational allergen is usually associated with asthma (see Chapter 3.6). Allergy to flour is a common cause of rhinitis in bakers.

Foods
As a general rule, food allergy and intolerance *does not cause isolated rhinitis*. Ingested allergens only play *a minor role* as an aetiological factor in rhinitis, but their importance in children with multi-organ symptoms cannot be ignored.

Foods, and alcoholic beverages in particular, frequently precipitate symptoms by non-allergic mechanisms. Frequent use of acetylsalicylic acid or NSAIDs, and perhaps dyes and preservatives, in food might play a role in a few cases.

Unknown aetiology
As the aetiology remains obscure in patients with a negative allergy examination, it is better to tell the patient that his or her disease is 'allergy-like' but its true nature is unknown, than to claim that he or she suffers from 'allergic rhinitis' but the allergen cannot be determined. The former information will stop the patient spending time and money trying to find the offending substance in the hope that avoidance will cure him or her.

Diagnosis

Symptoms and signs
Symptoms are largely the same as those of hay fever, but *eye itching is less frequent* and *nasal blockage more prominent*.

Some patients mainly complain of sneezing and watery rhinorrhoea, '*sneezers*', while others have nasal blockage and mucoid secretion as dominant symptoms, '*blockers*'. Some patients, especially elderly gentlemen, have watery rhinorrhoea as the only symptom, '*runners*'.

The manifestations of rhinitis are largely the same both in children and in adults. Blowing the nose, however, is not the way children prefer to remove mucus: it is cleared by sniffing, snorting and other procedures annoying to parents and teachers. Most children have, in contrast to adults, obvious *signs* of the disease (see Figs 8.5.1–3).

Although not satisfactory, we have to accept a *symptom diagnosis* of perennial rhinitis as all signs can be missing and all tests can be negative. The following examinations can, however, often support the diagnosis and be of significance for correct classification and treatment.

Examinations

Rhinoscopy
This is indicated in all patients with chronic nasal symptoms. It excludes malignancy and can support the rhinitis diagnosis when the mucous membrane is *swollen*, *wet* and of a *pale-bluish colour*. However, the mucous membrane can look completely normal in a rhinitis patient and highly abnormal in a symptom-free person. The presence of nasal polyps supports the diagnosis of non-allergic eosinophilic rhinitis.

Nasal cytology
This is helpful in making a distinction between infectious and non-infectious rhinitis, and between eosinophilic rhinitis and non-eosinophilic rhinitis. However, the variation in nasal cytology is considerable, and *two to three examinations* are usually required for a reliable characterization of the disease.

Skin testing
Skin testing with a panel of allergens is routine in all patients. A positive skin test does not necessarily imply the presence of overt clinical allergy. In selected patients, it may be necessary to confirm a skin test, preferably by *RAST* or, in the rare case, by a *nasal allergen challenge test*.

Serum IgE level and blood eosinophil count
These are normal in most rhinitis patients and are of little or no diagnostic value.

Imaging of the nose and paranasal sinuses

This is indicated in selected patients. A *plain X-ray examination* can disclose involvement of ethmoidal and maxillary sinuses, often seen in non-allergic eosinophilic rhinitis, as well as a fluid level in infectious sinusitis. A *CT scan*, however, gives far more reliable and detailed anatomical information (see Fig. 8.3.2); it is the examination of choice in all chronic severe cases and in planning intranasal and sinus surgery.

Differential diagnosis

In childhood, allergic symptoms are often blamed on the 'adenoids', while adults, with a variety of nasal complaints, usually claim to be 'allergic'. Careful examination is indicated in order to make the correct diagnosis, and exclude differential diagnoses (see Table 8.3.3) and concurrent *structural abnormalities*. Unilateral symptoms, bleeding and pain are important warning signals of *malignancy*.

Chronic rhinorrhoea may be due to *cocaine* sniffing, and *rhinitis medicamentosa* is a frequent cause of nasal complaints when vasoconstrictor sprays are available over-the-counter.

Treatment

Treatment consists of environmental control, drugs, immunotherapy and surgery, or a combination of these (Fig. 8.13.1).

Allergen avoidance

Allergen avoidance is recommended in animal-allergic patients. In mite allergy, changes in the bedroom may reduce symptoms (see Chapter 9.24).

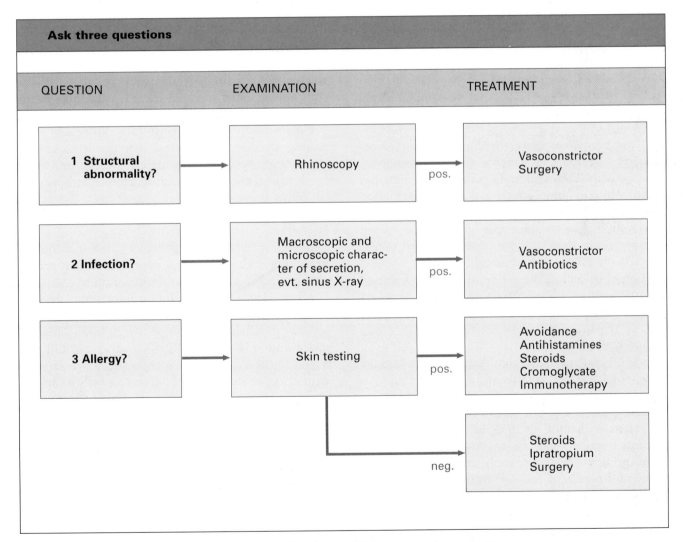

Fig. 8.13.1. A simple plan for the management of patients with chronic nasal symptoms.

Drug effect on nasal symptoms				
	Sneezing	**Rhinorrhoea**	**Blockage**	**Olfaction**
Antihistamines	+++	++	(+)	–
Oral vasoconstrictors	–	–	++	(+)
Nasal vasoconstrictors	–	–	+++	+
Cromoglycate	++	+	+	–
Intranasal steroids	+++	+++	++	+
Systemic steroids	++	++	+++	+++
Ipratropium	–	++	–	–

Table 8.13.2. Drug profile in the therapy of nasal symptoms

Elimination of foods usually fails to influence the cause of the disease, but patients with severe symptoms may want to try a diagnostic elimination diet.

Pharmacotherapy

The drugs used for rhinitis differ in their effect on specific nasal symptoms, a point of importance to remember for proper management of the disease (Table 8.13.2).

H_1 antihistamines are predominantly used for occasional symptoms in patients allergic to animals. Patients with daily symptoms will require a *steroid spray*, which is more effective than antihistamines. *Short courses of systemic steroids* may be indicated in severe adult cases to open up a blocked nose. When watery rhinorrhoea is a dominant symptom, *ipratropium* nasal spray is useful.

In children with allergic rhinitis, it is advisable to try *cromoglycate* together with an antihistamine, reserving steroid sprays for resistant cases.

Other therapies

Immunotherapy can be considered in mite-allergic patients with severe rhinitis and in selected animal-allergic patients.

Surgery plays a minor role in allergic rhinitis, but can often be helpful in non-allergic rhinitis, when medical treatment has failed. An enlarged inferior turbinate can be cauterized, preferably with a diathermy needle in the submucosa. A surgical removal of the lower edge of the turbinate, *partial turbinectomy*, is more effective and is preferable to the continuous use of a vasoconstrictor.

When the skin in the nostril becomes macerated by rhinorrhoea (vestibulitis), it can induce rhinitis symptoms via a reflex mechanism. In this case, the daily use of an *ointment* in the nostril is helpful. When secretions are viscid, repeated sniffing to remove the 'post-nasal drip' will dry the mucous membrane and worsen the condition. Patients are recommended to sniff *saline* from a spoon or use it from a spray bottle (two teaspoonfuls of salt per litre of water).

Patients with non-allergic rhinitis can benefit from regular sleeping habits, fresh air, warm socks and shoes, and avoidance of tobacco, alcohol and spicy food. It is easier to give such recommendations than to follow them.

Rhinitis and pregnancy

Perennial rhinitis may improve or deteriorate during pregnancy. When treatment is necessary, it is preferably given topically and in limited dosage.

A persistent *hormonal rhino-sinusitis* may develop in the last trimester in otherwise healthy women. Its severity parallels the blood oestrogen level. This disorder responds to topical vasoconstrictors, and perhaps topical steroids, but many women are satisfied with an assurance that the symptoms will disappear at delivery.

Treatment of boys who sneeze
Speak roughly to your little boy,
and beat him if he sneezes;
he only does it to annoy,
because he knows it teases.

Lewis Carroll
Alice in Wonderland

8.14 Nasal polyps
Fluid-filled bags

Key points
• Polyps consist of an oedematously transformed mucous membrane – the aetiology is unknown.
• Nasal polyps are pear-shaped with a stalk originating in the upper part of the nose.
• Nasal polyposis is always part of a hyperplastic rhino-sinusitis involving the ethmoidal and maxillary sinuses.
• Polyposis is often associated with perennial non-allergic eosinophilic rhinitis, non-allergic asthma and NSAID intolerance.
• Children with cystic fibrosis often have nasal polyps.
• The symptoms are nasal blockage and reduced sense of smell.
• The reduced ventilation and drainage of the nose and paranasal sinuses predispose to infection.
• Treatment consists of surgical polypectomy, short-term systemic steroids, long-term topical steroids and, in severe cases, intranasal ethmoidectomy.

Nasal polyps are protrusions of an oedematous mucous membrane (Fig. 8.14.1). A polyp is pear-shaped with a stalk; it is soft, pale-yellow and has a glistening surface (Fig. 8.14.2). Nasal polyps originate in the

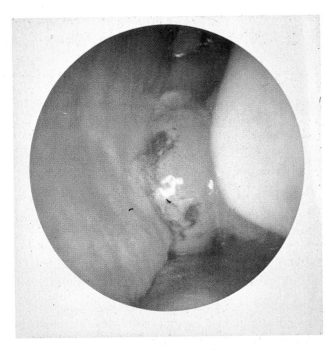

Fig. 8.14.2. Nasal polyp seen at endoscopy.

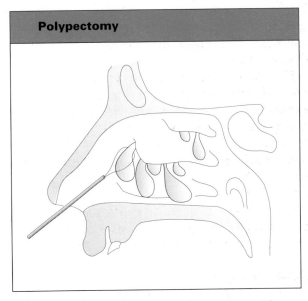

Fig. 8.14.3. Nasal polyps and a wire snare used for simple polypectomy.

upper part of the nose, around the ostia to the ethmoidal sinuses, and they protrude into the nasal cavity from the middle and superior meatus (Fig. 8.14.3). Nasal *polyposis*, consisting of recurrent multiple polyps, is always part of a *hyperplastic rhino-sinusitis*, and radiographic clouding of ethmoidal and maxillary sinuses is obligatory for diagnosis (Fig. 8.14.4).

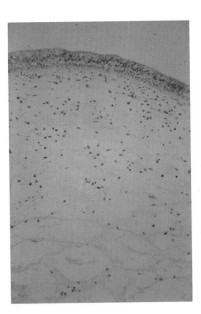

Fig. 8.14.1. Light micrograph of a nasal polyp, which mainly consists of oedema fluid.

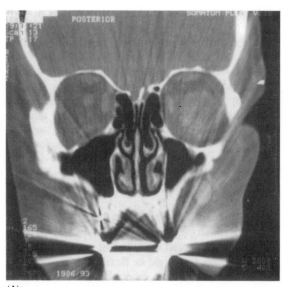

(A)

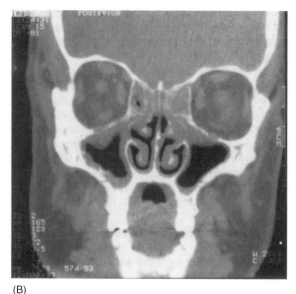

(B)

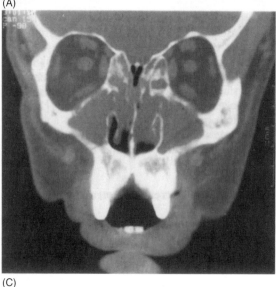

(C)

Fig. 8.14.4. Coronary CT scans in: (A) a healthy subject; (B) a patient with early-stage polyposis; and (C) a patient with advanced-stage polyposis. From Holmberg K, Karlsson G. Nasal polyps: surgery or pharmacological intervention? *Eur Respir Rev* 1994; **4**: 260–5.

Aetiology

The aetiology is unknown. As we are reluctant to expose our total ignorance to patients, we often call the polyps 'allergic', but, as skin tests to common allergens are not more frequent in patients with polyps than in the background population, this is misleading.

The formation of polyps is the result of a chronic inflammatory process in the nasal and sinus mucosa. Although polyps may be associated with any form of chronic rhino-sinusitis, they are typically seen in *perennial non-allergic eosinophilic rhinitis* and in *cystic fibrosis*.

Diagnosis

The diagnosis is easily made by rhinoscopy, prefer-

ably using an endoscope. The use of a vasoconstrictor spray, and of a probe to show motility, may be necessary. Nasal polyps are typically *multiple* and *bilateral*. Unilateral masses should alert the physician to other conditions, such as malignant tumours, invert papillomata and meningoceles, all of which may masquerade as simple polyps. For that reason, microscopy is always necessary when polyps occur for the first time.

Microscopy will show a large number of *eosinophils* in the majority of cases, but there is no tissue eosinophilia in cystic fibrosis or in a few other rare conditions (e.g. primary ciliary dyskinesia).

Children with mite allergy do not develop polyposis even though they often have markedly swollen mucous membranes in the nose. It follows that a child presenting with nasal polyps needs a sweat test more than an allergy examination.

Clinical presentation

Rhinitis

Nasal polyps, as a rule, develop in a patient who has suffered from *perennial non-allergic eosinophilic rhinitis* with sneezing and watery rhinorrhoea for some years. A sensation of 'secretion', which cannot be expelled, is often the first symptom of polyp formation. Nasal blockage gradually develops and can become complete. Impairment or loss of the *sense of smell*, and with that 'taste', due to obstruction of the upper part of the nasal airway, is characteristic. This very annoying symptom, which mars the pleasure of eating and drinking, is more pronounced, persistent and difficult to treat in rhinitis patients with polyps, than in those without.

The disease can vary in severity from a single period of nasal blockage, relieved by polypectomy, to constant daily symptoms, requiring repeated surgery and continuous medication. Nasal polyposis with hyperplastic sinusitis can be the most severe manifestation of eosinophil inflammation in the upper airways.

Sinusitis

As the nasal blockage progresses, secretions become more viscous and difficult to expel. Involvement of the *paranasal sinuses*, the mucosa of which has many goblet cells but few seromucous glands, contributes to the viscosity of the discharge.

There is a polypoid hyperplasia of the maxillary mucous membrane, and the ethmoidal cells are filled with polypous transformed mucous membrane. This increases the tendency to *bacterial infection* in the nose and paranasal sinuses, especially following a common cold.

Asthma

Severe cases, having an increased blood eosinophil count, are usually associated with *asthma*. The classical ASA triad, consisting of non-allergic Asthma, polyposis/Sinusitis and intolerance to Acetylsalicylic acid, and other NSAIDs are described in Chapter 2.2. Questioning about adverse reactions to *acetylsalicylic acid* is obligatory in patients with nasal polyps.

Principles of treatment

Therapy, which is a challenge, is a combination of: 1, simple *polypectomy*; 2, *short-term systemic treatment*; and 3, *long-term local steroid treatment*. While otologists prefer to remove large polyps (gently with good local analgesia), allergists often give systemic steroids instead. Combined use is often preferable, and it prepares the nasal cavity for topical steroid treatment. This is indicated in patients with daily rhinitis symptoms and in those who need polypectomy frequently. This basic topical treatment will both improve the rhinitis symptoms and, to some extent, prevent the growth of polyps.

Endonasal *ethmoidectomy*, with evacuation of as many ethmoidal cells as technically possible and removal of all polypoid tissue, is indicated in cases resistant to the above treatment schedule.

A problem in polyposis
For the sense of smell, almost more than any other, has the power to recall memories and it is a pity that we use it so little.

Rachel Carson

8.15 Sinusitis and otitis media
Complications of rhinitis

Key points
• Nasal blockage in rhinitis predisposes to infectious sinusitis.
• Nasal polyposis is associated with a polypoidal thickening of the sinus mucosa.
• The sinusitis symptoms in adults are persistent purulent discharge, pain and fatigue.
• In children, purulent discharge, night-time cough and sore throat are the hallmarks.
• Replacement of eosinophils with neutrophils in nasal secretions is a good indicator of an infectious complication in an allergic child.
• The diagnosis is supported by X-ray.
• Treatment consists of decongestants, antibiotics and, when necessary, sinus puncture.
• In adults with recurrent episodes, surgery is advisable.
• Allergy is not an important cause of secretory otitis media.
• Children with allergic airway disease and nasal blockage, however, have a somewhat increased risk of developing secretory otitis media.
• Allergy testing is indicated only when patients with secretory otitis media also have symptoms and signs of allergy of the airways.

Sinusitis

Causes
Sinusitis is caused by common airway pathogens (*Haemophilus influenzae* and *Streptococcus pneumonia*). It frequently affects the maxillary and ethmoidal sinuses (Figs 8.15.1–2). In most cases, it is a *common cold* that initiates an acute episode or an exacerbation of a chronic disease. A *small ostium* to the sinus and *congested nasal mucosa* are predisposing factors.

Diagnosis
The most characteristic symptoms are a *persistent purulent discharge, nasality of the voice* and a sensation of a 'stuffy head'. *Fatigue* together with *pain* over the infected sinus, which increases in intensity on bending forward, are common. Fever and malaise occur only in severe cases.

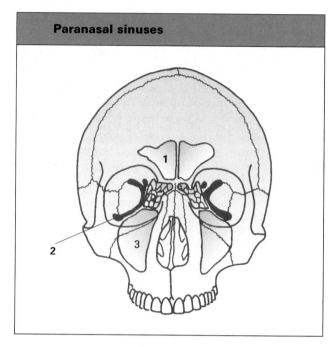

Fig. 8.15.1. Frontal projection of paranasal sinuses: 1, frontal sinuses; 2, ethmoidal cells; and 3, maxillary sinuses.

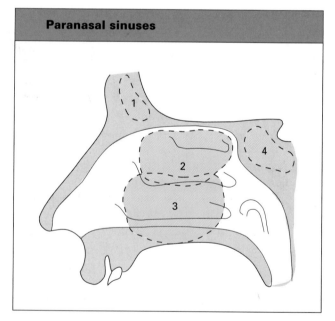

Fig. 8.15.2. Lateral projection of paranasal sinuses: 1, frontal sinus; 2, area of ethmoidal cells; 3, maxillary sinus; and 4, sphenoidal sinus.

Allergic children with chronic rhinitis/asthma have a high incidence of sinus infections, and the diagnosis is not obvious in patients who have daily airway symptoms. The hallmarks of sinusitis in children are

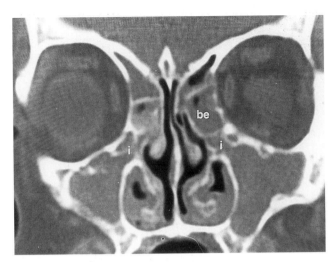

Fig. 8.15.3. CT scan of chronic rhino-sinusitis in a patient with non-allergic eosinophilic rhinitis. The diseased ethmoidal cells (be) are visible. The ethmoidal infundibulum (i) and the ostium to the maxillary sinus are blocked, and there is retention in both maxillary sinuses. Secretion can be seen on the nasal floor around the inferior turbinate. From Stammberger H. Rhinoscopy. In: Mygind N, Naclerio RM, eds. *Allergic and Non-allergic Rhinitis: Clinical Aspects* Copenhagen: Munksgaard, 1993: 51–7.

purulent nasal discharge, *pharyngeal discharge*, *night-time cough*, fatigue and irritability; pain is rare. *Asthma* may deteriorate and become more resistant to therapy.

A switch from eosinophilia to *neutrophilia in nasal secretions* is a good parameter of an infectious complication in a chronic allergic disease. The peripheral white cell count and sedimentation rate are of little value. The diagnosis is supported or confirmed by *X-ray* showing opacification, a fluid level or a marked membrane thickening (>5 mm). A CT scan, giving a much better presentation of anatomical and mucosal abnormalities, is indicated in chronic and in severe cases (Fig. 8.15.3).

Adults with nasal polyposis have a polypoid, thickened mucosa in the ethmoidal and maxillary sinuses as a parallel manifestation of the basic disease. Their 'radiographic sinusitis' *per se* needs no treatment.

It is not uncommon to mistake acute infectious ethmoiditis for conjunctivitis in a child, and this can be serious (Fig. 8.15.4).

Treatment

A correctly used *nasal decongestant* suffices in mild cases but *antibiotics* are often indicated as well. When symptoms persist or are severe, *puncture* of the maxillary sinuses and *irrigation* give immediate relief (Fig. 8.15.5).

Intranasal antrostomy (surgical window to the maxillary sinus under the inferior turbinate) will function as a means of extended drainage and is indicated in patients with recurrent sinusitis. A *Caldwell–Luc operation*, with removal of grossly pathological sinus mucosa, can be performed in adults; it should be avoided in children because of its adverse effect on unerupted teeth. Note that patients who have had this operation always have an opaque radiogram. The use of the Caldwell–Luc operation is steadily declining as more conservative and functional *endoscopic procedures*, which also deal with concomitant ethmoiditis, gain in popularity. In this context, the most important area functionally is the *ostiomeatal complex*, localized under the middle turbinate around the ostia to the sinuses.

Secretory otitis media

Since the introduction of a reliable apparatus (impedance meter) for the quick measurement of 'middle ear pressure' (acoustic compliance of the tympanic membrane), allergists have been struck by the high percentage of flat tympanometry curves in allergic children, indicating secretion in the middle ear. Otologists, on the other hand, have not reported a high frequency of allergy in their patients with secretory otitis media (otitis media with effusion).

Secretory otitis media is a very common disease in childhood, and allergy does not seem to be an important cause (Fig. 8.15.6). Children with allergic airway disease, however, may have a somewhat increased

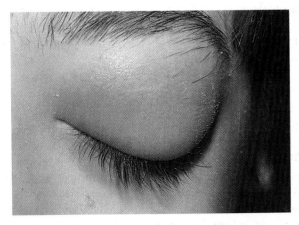

Fig. 8.15.4. This child was first treated with eye drops for 'conjunctivitis'. She has acute bacterial ethmoiditis, which in children is often complicated by orbital cellulitis.

Treatment for sinusitis

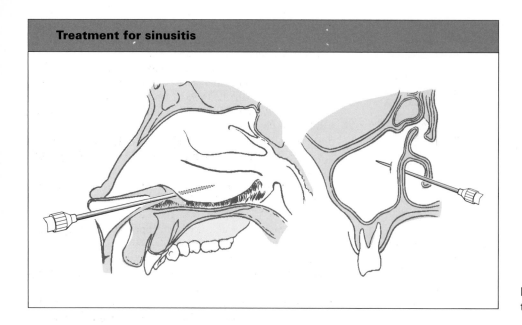

Fig. 8.15.5. Puncture of the maxillary sinus.

Otitis media and allergy

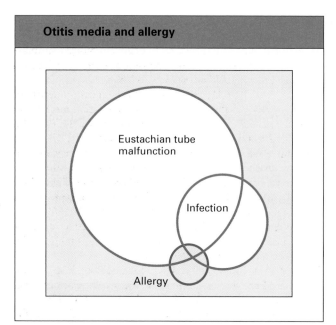

Fig. 8.15.6. Diagram to illustrate the relative importance of different aetiological factors in secretory otitis media.

adults, but other causes, especially a nasopharyngeal tumour, must be excluded.

Poor surgeons
Surgeons and anatomists see no beautiful women in all their life, but only a ghastly stack of bones with Latin names to them, and a network of nerves and muscles and tissues inflamed with disease.
Letter to the *Alta California*
San Francisco, 1867

Highway men
I have got the bill for my surgery. Now, I understand why those doctors were wearing masks.

James H Boren

risk of developing secretory otitis media, due to nasal blockage and malfunctioning of the Eustachian tube. Allergy testing is indicated only when patients with secretory otitis media also have symptoms and signs of allergy of the upper airways. Treatment consists of the insertion of ventilation tubes if the secretion persists for >3 months.

Perennial rhinitis with nasal polyposis can cause middle ear symptoms and secretory otitis media in

Further reading

Books

MYGIND N, NACLERIO RM, eds. *Allergic and Non-allergic Rhinitis. Clinical Aspects.* Copenhagen: Munksgaard, 1993: 1–199.

NASPITZ CK, TINKELMAN DG, eds. *Childhood Rhinitis and Sinusitis. Pathophysiology and Treatment.* New York: Marcel Dekker, 1990: 1–284.

SETTIPANE GA, ed. *Rhinitis 2nd ed.* Providence, Rhode Island: OceanSide Publications, 1991: 1–344.

Articles

BENTLEY AM, JACOBSON MR, CUMBERWORTH V, *et al.* Immunohistology of the nasal mucosa in seasonal allergic rhinitis: increases in activated eosinophils and epithelial mast cells. *J Allergy Clin Immunol* 1992; **89**: 877–83.

BERMAN BA. Perennial allergic rhinitis: clinical efficacy of a new antihistamine. *J Allergy Clin Immunol* 1990; **86**: 1004–8.

BORRES MP. Metachromatic cells and eosinophils in atopic children. A prospective study. *Pediatr Allergy Immunol* 1991; **2**(suppl 2): 6–24.

CAMPOLI-RICHARDS DM, BUCKLEY MM-T, FITTON A. Cetirizine: a review of its pharmacological properties and clinical potential in allergic rhinitis, pollen-induced asthma, and chronic urticaria. *Drugs* 1990; **40**: 762–81.

CHURCH M. The therapeutic index of antihistamines. *Pediatr Allergy Immunol* 1993; **4**(suppl 4): 25–32.

CLISSOLD SP, SORKIN EM, GOA KL. Loratadine: a preliminary review of its pharmacodynamic properties and therapeutic efficacy. *Drugs* 1989; **37**: 42–52.

DECHANT KL, GOA KL. Levocabastine: a review of its pharmacological properties and therapeutic potential as a topical antihistamine in allergic rhinitis and conjunctivitis. *Drugs* 1991; **41**: 202–24.

From the Food and Drug Administration. Warnings issued on nonsedating antihistamines terfenadine and astemizole. *JAMA* 1992; **268**: 705.

GRANT SM, GOA KL, FITTON A, *et al.* Ketotifen: a review of its pharmacodynamic and pharmacokinetic properties, and therapeutic use in asthma and allergic disorders. *Drugs* 1990; **40**: 412–48.

HOWARTH PH, WILSON S, LAU L, RAJAKULASINGAM K. The nasal mast cell and rhinitis. *Clin Exp Allergy* 1991; **21**(suppl 2): 3–8.

KNAPP HR. Reduced allergen-induced nasal congestion and leukotriene synthesis with an orally active 5-lipoxygenase inhibitor. *N Engl J Med* 1990; **323**: 1745–8.

LAURSEN LC, FAURSCHOU P, PALS H, SVENDSEN UG, WEEKE B. Intramuscular betamethasone dipropionate vs. oral prednisolone in hay fever patients. *Allergy* 1987; **42**: 168–172.

LUND VJ. International consensus report on the diagnosis and management of rhinitis. *Allergy* 1994; **49**(suppl 19): 1–34.

McMENAMIN P. Costs of hay fever in the United States in 1990. *Ann Allergy* 1994; **73**: 35–9.

McTAVICH D, GOA KL, FERRILL M. Terfenadine: an updated review of its pharmacological properties and therapeutic efficacy. *Drugs* 1990; **39**: 552–62.

McTAVICH D, SORKIN EM. Azelastine: a review of its pharmacodynamic and pharmacokinetic properties, and therapeutic potential. *Drugs* 1989; **38**: 778–88.

MYGIND N. Glucocorticosteroids and rhinitis. *Allergy* 1993; **48**: 476–90.

NACLERIO RM, TOGIAS AG. The nasal allergic reaction: observations on the role of histamine. *Clin Exp Allergy* 1990; **21**(suppl 2): 13–19.

RAPHAEL GD, BARANIUK JN, KALINER MA. How and why the nose runs. *J Allergy Clin Immunol* 1991; **87**: 57–67.

RICHARDS DM, BROGDEN RN, HEEL RC, *et al.* Astemizole: a review of its pharmacological properties and therapeutic efficacy. *Drugs* 1984; **28**: 38–61.

RIMMER SJ, CHURCH MK. The pharmacology and mechanisms of action of histamine H_1-antagonists. *Clin Exp Allergy* 1990; **20**(suppl 2): 3–17.

SIMONS FER. The antiallergic effects of antihistamines (H_1-receptor antagonists). *J Allergy Clin Immunol* 1992; **90**: 705–15.

SIMONS FER. The therapeutic index of newer H_1-receptor antagonists. *Clin Exp Allergy* 1994; **24**: 707–23.

SKONER DP, ASMAN B, FIREMAN P. Effect of chlorpheniramine on airway physiology and symptoms during natural pollen exposure. *Am J Rhinol* 1994; **8**: 43–8.

TERADA N, KONNO A, TOGAWA K. Biochemical properties of eosinophils and their preferential accumulation mechanism in nasal allergy. *J Allergy Clin Immunol* 1994; **94**: 629–42.

THOMAS KE, OLLIER S, FERGUSON H, DAVIES RJ. The effect of intranasal azelastine, Rhinolast, on nasal airways obstruction and sneezing following provocation testing with histamine and allergen. *Clin Exp Allergy* 1992; **22**: 642–7.

VAN WIJK RG. Nasal hyperreactivity: its pathogenesis and clinical significance. *Clin Exp Allergy* 1991; **21**: 661–7.

VAN WIJK RG. Nasal hyperreactivity and its effect on early and late sequelae of nasal challenge with house-dust mite extract. *Allergy Proc* 1993; **14**: 273–81.

VARNEY VA, JACOBSON MR, SUDDERICK RM *et al.* Immunohistology of the nasal mucosa following allergen-induced rhinitis. *Am Rev Respir Dis* 1992; **146**: 170–6.

WIHL J-Å, PEDERSEN BN, PEDERSEN LN, *et al.* Effect of the nonsedative H_1-receptor antagonist astemizole in perennial allergic and nonallergic rhinitis. *J Allergy Clin Immunol* 1985; **75**: 720–7.

Part 9 Asthma in Adults

9.1 Anatomy of the airways

An entity from nose to alveoli

Key points

• The conducting airways consist of nose, pharynx, larynx and tracheo-bronchial tree.
• The internal ostium in the nose and the area between the vocal cords are the narrowest parts of the airway.
• The mucous membrane distal to the vocal cords is loosely bound, and oedema is readily formed (angioedema).
• The trachea and main bronchi are surrounded by C-shaped cartilages, and the lumen cannot be obliterated by muscle contraction.
• Islands of cartilages support the intrathoracic bronchi, which can be completely obliterated by muscle contraction.
• Bronchioles are bronchi without cartilage.
• Gas-exchanging airways consist of respiratory bronchioles, alveolar ducts and alveolar sacs.
• The alveoli are covered by flat cells (Type I alveolar cells) and by globular cells (Type II alveolar cells).
• The typical airway epithelium is of the ciliated, pseudostratified, columnar type.
• The lining of the bronchioles consists of a single layer of cuboidal epithelial cells.
• The airways are covered by a thin layer of mucus produced by sero-mucous glands and goblet cells.
• The mucous layer is carried toward the pharynx by cilia.
• Abnormalities of airway fluids play a role in mucus plugging of the airways in asthma.

Sub-division

The airways are functionally divided into *conducting* and *gas-exchanging airways* (alveoli). The conducting airways are anatomically sub-divided into the *nose* and/or *mouth*, *pharynx*, *larynx* and the *tracheo-bronchial tree*. This complicated, branching tube system can be further sub-divided in different ways (Fig. 9.1.1). It is important not to focus exclusively on any single part of this system but to look upon the airway as an entity from the nose to alveoli. The shape of the airway lumen reflects the specialized function of that part, and the character of the wall is important in obstruction and disease (Fig. 9.1.2).

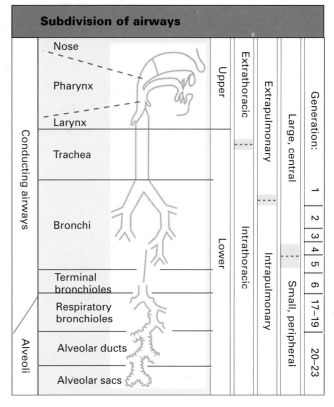

Fig. 9.1.1. Different ways of sub-dividing the airways.

Nose and mouth

The anatomy of the nose is described in Chapter 8.1.

The *mouth* can serve as a *substitute for the nose* except during the first weeks of life, when complete nasal obstruction (choanal atresia) can be fatal. Patients with rhinitis and *nasal blockage* will breathe through the mouth, especially when lying down, for the nose then becomes congested. Normal subjects breathe through the mouth *during exercise*, and air passes through the nose and mouth in approximately equal volumes. *Dyspnoeic patients* breathe through the mouth to avoid the considerable resistance in the nose, which accounts for almost half of the total resistance to airflow.

Pharynx

The pharynx contains the adenoids and tonsils, which, as immunocompetent organs, guard the entrance to the airways and the gastro-intestinal tract, respectively. Probably for that reason, they are often involved in disease. Enlargement of these tissues and slackness of the pharyngeal wall can affect respiration, especially during sleep, causing obstructive *sleep apnoea*.

Cross-sections of airways

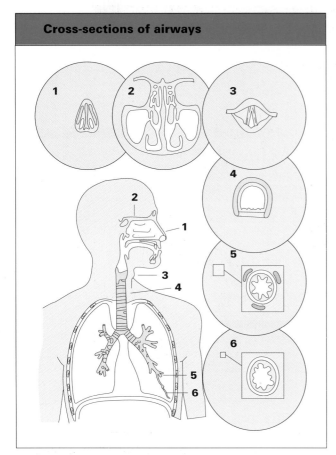

Fig. 9.1.2. Diagram and cross-sections of the airways. 1, Internal ostium of the nose; 2, nasal and paranasal cavities; 3, larynx; 4, trachea; 5, intrapulmonary bronchus; and 6, bronchiole.

Larynx

The larynx, between the vocal cords, is the second narrowest part of the airways (the anterior part of the nose is the first) (Fig. 9.1.2). The mucous membrane distal to the vocal cords is loosely bound to the supporting cartilage, so oedema fluid can readily collect. *Laryngeal oedema* leads to inspiratory dyspnoea, which is frequent in children with viral infections because of the small lumen of their airway. Allergy and complement activation can give a similar result, even in adults (angioedema). The laryngeal airway can also be obliterated when the small laryngeal muscles, normally employed for speech, are subjected to strong reflex stimulation, causing *laryngeal spasm*. Inspiratory stridor in some patients with asthma suggests that laryngeal narrowing can contribute to dyspnoea in this disease.

Trachea and main bronchi

The trachea and two main bronchi are supported by *C-shaped rings of cartilage*. Contraction of the smooth muscles, attached to the posterior ends of the cartilage, can only slightly narrow, not obliterate, the lumen (Fig. 9.1.3). The same is true of increased intrathoracic pressure, which can act on the main bronchi and part of the trachea. During coughing, the lumen of this part of the airway can be changed to a U-shaped slit by invagination of the soft posterior wall (Fig. 9.1.3).

Intrapulmonary bronchi

The intrapulmonary bronchi are supported by isolated *islands of cartilage* (Fig. 9.1.2), which gradually disappear distally. The smooth muscles are arranged in a circular layer beneath the epithelium so

Dynamics of airway lumen

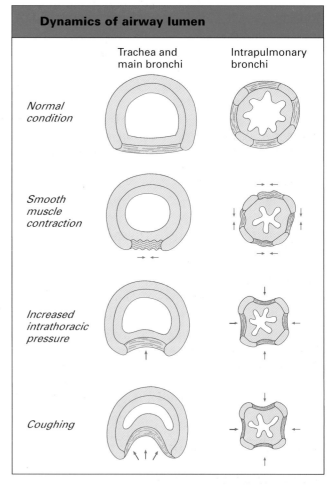

Fig. 9.1.3. Effect of smooth muscle contraction, increased intrathoracic pressure and coughing on lumen of trachea/main bronchi and intrapulmonary bronchi.

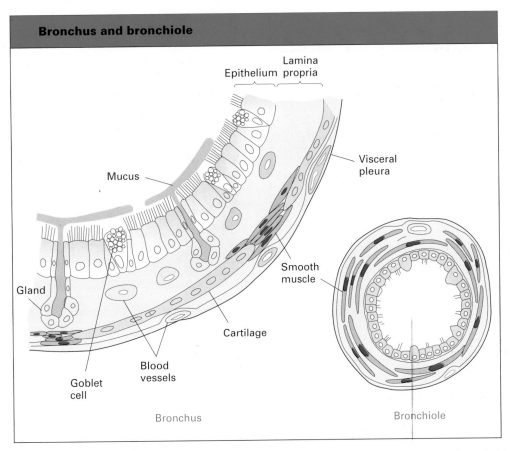

Bronchus and bronchiole

Lamina propria

Epithelium

Visceral pleura

Mucus

Smooth muscle

Gland

Cartilage

Goblet cell

Blood vessels

Bronchus

Bronchiole

Fig. 9.1.4. Diagrams of bronchial and bronchiolar structure. The bronchus has a thicker epithelium and lamina propria, together with submucosal glands and cartilage. The bronchiole has relatively more smooth muscle but no glands or cartilage. From Widdicombe J, Davies A. *Respiratory Physiology* London: Edward Arnold Ltd, 1983: 1–118.

contraction can completely obliterate the lumen (Fig. 9.1.3).

Bronchioles

Bronchioles are 'bronchi without cartilage' (Fig. 9.1.4). *Terminal bronchioles* are the last order of bronchioles without alveoli (Fig. 9.1.1). *Respiratory bronchioles* have some alveoli, and these completely occupy the *alveolar ducts and sacs*. While smooth muscle is present, even in the smallest bronchioles, the alveoli are supported only by elastic fibres (Fig. 9.1.5).

Surface epithelium

– in conducting airways

It is the task of the conducting airways to supply the alveoli with oxygen in clean, conditioned air (body temperature and fully water-saturated). The conducting airways are first covered by a squamous epithelium (anterior part of the nose), then by a *ciliated pseudostratified epithelium* (Figs 9.1.6–7) (the remainder of the nose, parts of the pharynx and larynx, the trachea and proximal bronchi), and finally by a single cuboidal epithelium, which is also ciliated (distal bronchi and bronchioles).

The *goblet cell* is the mucus-producing cell in the surface epithelium. It occurs throughout the conducting airways. In the bronchioles, it is gradually replaced by another secretory cell, the Clara cell. Goblet cells produce small amounts of viscid secretion; approximately 50 times more secretion is produced by the *sero-mucous glands*. They are distributed in the airways proximal to the bronchioles (eight glands/mm² in nose, and one gland/mm² in trachea-bronchial tree) (Fig. 9.1.8). While the

Airway cells and tissues

	Elastic fibres	Smooth muscles	Ciliated cells	Goblet cells	Glands	Cartilage
Nose						
Pharynx						
Larynx						
Trachea						
Bronchi						
Bronchioles						
Terminal bronchioles						
Respiratory bronchioles						
Alveolar ducts						
Alveolar sacs						

Fig. 9.1.5. Distribution of some cells and tissues along the airways.

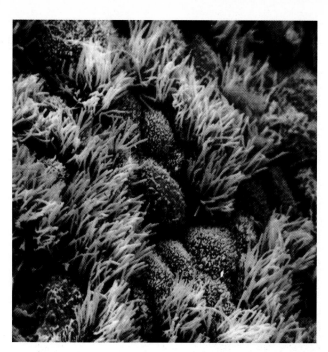

Fig. 9.1.7. Surface of a ciliated epithelium, seen in the scanning electron microscope (× 3300).

Epithelial cells

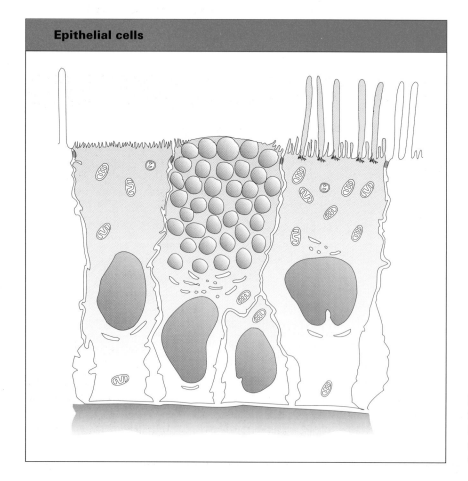

Fig. 9.1.6. The four common cell types in airway epithelium. From the left: non-ciliated columnar cell; goblet cell; basal replacement cell; and ciliated cell.

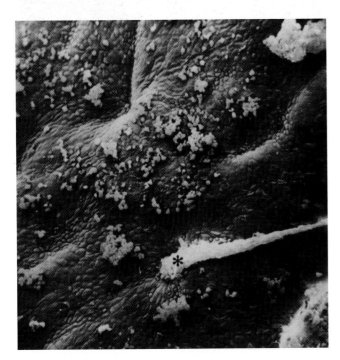

Fig. 9.1.8. Expulsion of mucus from goblet cells and glands (*) in the human airway (nose) during infection. Scanning electron micrograph (×1000). From Mygind N, Wihl J-Å. Scanning electron microscopy of a bacterial infection of the human nose. *Br J Dis Chest* 1977; **71**: 259–67.

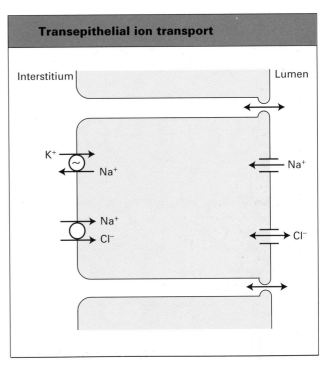

Fig. 9.1.10. Diagram of the principal ion transport pathways across epithelial cells, which are of importance for the formation and regulation of the periciliary fluid layer. On the basolateral membrane, a Na$^+$ K$^+$ pump is responsible for active transport. On the luminal membrane, there are Na$^+$ and Cl$^-$ channels, both of which are driven by passive processes.

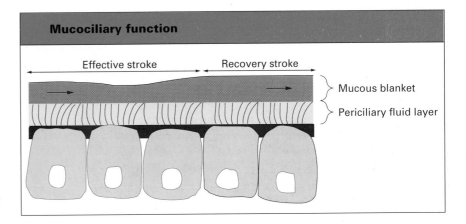

Fig. 9.1.9. Illustration of ciliary beating pattern; mucociliary transport; and the double-layer of secretion.

number of glands do not change after birth, the single gland can become hyperplastic. This occurs especially in chronic bronchitis. Glands, in contrast to goblet cells, are under the control of the autonomic nervous system. Goblet cells release mucus in response to direct stimulation by irritants and secretagogues.

The epithelial surface is covered by a *double layer of secretion*: an upper *mucous layer* (blanket) and a watery (serous) *periciliary fluid layer* (Fig. 9.1.9). The production of the periciliary layer is related to ion transport (Fig. 1.9.10). This is abnormal in *cystic fibrosis* and is the cause of mucus plugging of the airways in that disease.

Cilia have a complex ultrastructure (Fig. 9.1.11).

Cross-section of cilium

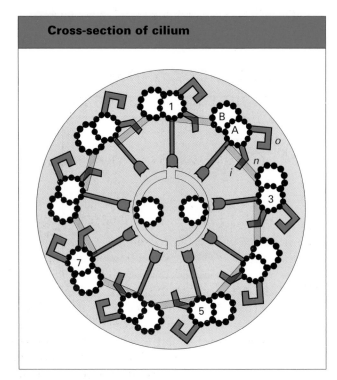

Fig. 9.1.11. Detailed diagram of components in a transverse section of a cilium. Two central single microtubules are surrounded by nine peripheral microtubule doublets, which bear outer (o) and inner (i) dynein arms. These adenosine triphosphatase-containing structures are missing in Kartagener's syndrome (primary ciliary dyskinesia). From Sleigh MA. The nature and action of respiratory tract cilia. In: Brain JD, Proctor DF, Reid LM, eds. *Respiratory Defense Mechanisms* Part 1. New York: Marcel Dekker Inc, 1977: 247–88.

Mucociliary transport

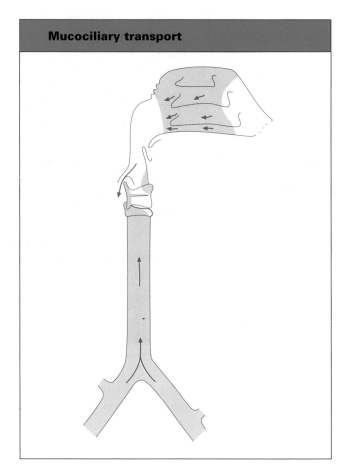

Fig. 9.1.12. Distribution of ciliated epithelium in the airways and direction of mucociliary transport.

Gas-exchanging tissue

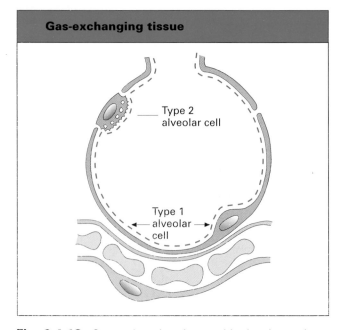

Fig. 9.1.13. Gas-exchanging tissue with alveolus and capillary. The dotted line indicates surfactant.

They beat (1000 times/min) in a highly coordinated manner, and cilia in the nose, Eustachian tube, paranasal sinuses and tracheo-bronchial tree all beat towards the pharynx (Fig. 9.1.12). The advantage of this arrangement is obvious, in that all particles trapped in the mucous layer are conveyed to the pharynx by the 'mucus escalator', swallowed and eliminated via the gastro-intestinal tract.

Active coughing is an effective substitute for mucociliary clearance. This is shown by the long-term survival of patients with *Kartagener's syndrome* (primary ciliary dyskinesia). They lack the usual mucociliary transport mechanism due to a congenital defect in ciliary ultrastructure causing a very abnormal, asynchronous pattern of beating.

– in gas-exchanging airways

There are some 100 million alveoli covering an area

of about 100 m². They are lined by flat cells, *Type I alveolar cells*, and a few globular cells, *Type II alveolar cells* (Fig. 9.1.13). The latter synthesize a phospholipid, *surfactant*, which is important for the prevention of alveolar collapse. When the alveoli are damaged, the resistant Type II cell replaces the susceptible Type I cell, resulting in fibrosis and impaired gas exchange.

A most important lung function
The lungs are the origin of the breath and the dwelling of the animal spirits or impervious soul.

Ch'i Po, 2600 BC
Minister of the Yellow Emperor

9.2 Characteristics of asthma
Episodic, wheezy and reversible breathlessness

Key points
• The characteristics of asthma are summarized in Table 9.2.1.

Short definition
Asthma is a lung disease characterized by: 1, *variable and reversible airway obstruction*; 2, *airway inflammation*; and 3, *bronchial hyper-responsiveness*.

Clinical characteristics
Asthma is clinically characterized by *episodic wheezy breathlessness*, which *varies considerably within short periods of time*, and is *reversible* (but not completely so in some patients) either spontaneously or with treatment; most important is a significant *response to beta$_2$ agonists and to corticosteroids* (Table 9.2.1).

Characteristics of asthma
1 Episodes of wheezy dyspnoea
2 Airway obstruction or narrowing: increased resistance to airflow reduced ventilatory capacity of obstructive type
3 Rapid and considerable changes in lung function (peak flow variation ⩾20%)
4 Frequent nocturnal episodes and low morning peak flow values
5 Significant reversibility with beta$_2$ agonists (⩾20%)
6 Significant reversibility with steroids (⩾20%)
7 Symptom-free periods
8 Frequent occurrence of allergy
9 Eosinophil inflammation
10 Bronchial hyper-responsiveness

Table 9.2.1. Characteristics of asthma in 10 points

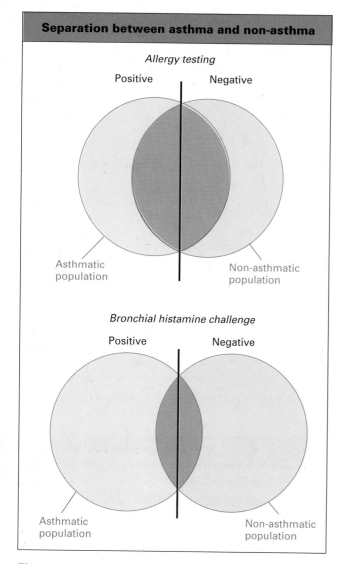

Separation between asthma and non-asthma

Allergy testing

Positive   Negative

Asthmatic population   Non-asthmatic population

Bronchial histamine challenge

Positive   Negative

Asthmatic population   Non-asthmatic population

Fig. 9.2.1. Two ways to separate an asthmatic and a non-asthmatic population.

Differential diagnostic problem

Laymen usually call any type of breathlessness at rest 'asthma', provided that they do not have a heart attack or pneumonia. The physician can also have more difficulty in making a precise diagnosis than appears from textbooks. In middle-aged and elderly smokers, the major diagnostic problem is how to differentiate between asthma and chronic bronchitis/emphysema (chronic obstructive pulmonary disease).

Allergy

Asthma is closely associated with allergy, and most asthmatic children and young adults have IgE antibodies to inhalant allergens. However, in middle-aged and elderly patients, allergy plays no or only a minor role.

Bronchial hyper-responsiveness

Asthma patients, who have frequent or daily symptoms, have bronchial hyper-responsiveness to a variety of stimuli, either alone (non-allergic or intrinsic asthma) or together with allergy (allergic or extrinsic asthma). Hyper-responsiveness is generally of greater clinical importance than allergy, as it accounts for the symptoms induced by exercise, cold air and irritants. A test for bronchial responsiveness separates a diseased and a normal population better than does allergy testing (Fig. 9.2.1). It is believed that eosinophilic inflammation is a major cause of airway hyper-responsiveness.

> **The complexity of diseases**
> The human body is like a bakery with thousands of windows. We are looking into only one window of the bakery when we are investigating one particular aspect of a disease.
>
> Bela Schick

9.3 Pathogenesis and histopathology of asthma I

Inflammation

Key points
- Inflammatory changes in the bronchi are marked in severe asthma but also occur in mild to moderate disease.
- The bronchial wall, its basement membrane and muscle layer are thickened.
- There is accumulation and activation of eosinophils.
- There is shedding of ciliated epithelium.
- The mucociliary clearance is grossly impaired.
- Extensive mucus plugging occludes the lumen.
- The lungs are hyperinflated with small atelectatic areas.

The allergic inflammation in asthma is described in detail in Part 1. Bronchoscopy studies have provided good evidence that asthma patients, even in asymptomatic periods, have pathological airways characterized by eosinophil inflammation. Airway wall thickening due to inflammation, together with contraction of bronchial smooth muscle, explains the narrowing of airways and the increased resistance to airflow in clinical asthma. The characteristic pathology of asthma is most clearly shown in autopsy specimens from asthma deaths.

Macroscopic appearance
The tragic antithesis to an isolated bronchospastic episode is death in status asthmaticus. The post-mortem picture in status asthmaticus differs markedly from that of simple smooth muscle contraction.

When the 'barrel chest' is opened at an autopsy, the *hyperinflated lungs* meet in the midline and cover the heart. They do not collapse. The surface of the lung is pale, pink-grey and with small *atelectatic areas* (Fig. 9.3.1), which correspond to regions of complete airway obstruction. The cut surface is dry with thick, prominent bronchi. Folding of the mucosa, seen in many of the lumen, indicates contraction of the prominent muscle layer. *Mucus plugging* is a constant feature (Figs 9.3.2–3), a rare exception being a patient dying of acute overwhelming bronchospasm.

Eosinophils
The most characteristic infiltrating cell is the eosinophil, and, in autopsy specimens, there is, usually, a massive *eosinophil infiltrate* in all layers of the mucous membrane. Even in mild asthma, biopsy studies have shown eosinophilia. The eosinophils show signs of activation, and there is extracellular appearance of their cytotoxic proteins (ECP and MBP).

Epithelial cell damage and shedding
Sloughing of epithelial cells is a constant feature in asthma; clusters of epithelial cells (Creola bodies) are regularly found in asthmatic sputum.

The airway epithelium is damaged or even destroyed by the combined effects of: 1, toxicity from eosinophil-derived proteins; 2, squeezing due to bronchial contraction; and 3, excessive stickiness of mucus.

Normal areas of ciliated epithelium can be difficult to find in patients dying from asthma. There is no doubt that *mucociliary clearance is grossly impaired* for some weeks after a severe asthma attack. Mucus, not moved by cilia, becomes dehydrated, sticky and difficult to cough up.

Mucus plugs
In asthma, biochemical mediators, acting as secretagogues, cause hypersecretion of mucus from goblet cells and glands. Glandular secretion is also stimulated by vagal reflexes.

The increased mucus is not moved because of epithelial damage, impaired mucociliary transport and because the hyperinflated patient cannot cough efficiently.

In autopsy specimens, the most striking features are the *intraluminal plugs* of mucus (Fig. 9.3.4). They are extensive and a major contributing factor to death. In the fulminant case, plugs completely obstruct the airways and form a cast of the bronchial tree (Fig. 9.3.5).

An asthmatic episode is often terminated by the laborious expectoration of small amounts of viscous mucus, which contains tiny casts, *Curschmann's spirals*, formed in the small airways.

Oedema
Oedema is another feature of inflammation that contributes to airway narrowing. Histamine and other pro-inflammatory mediators contract endothelial cells in the post-capillary venules, causing gap formation between the cells, and plasma exudation with

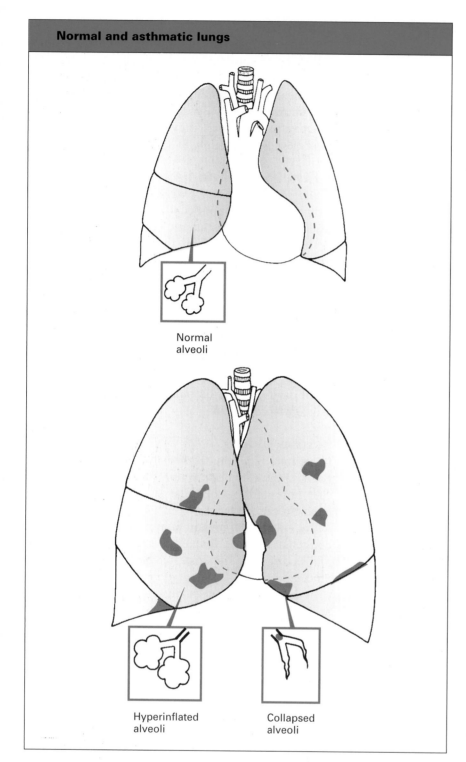

Normal and asthmatic lungs

Normal
alveoli

Hyperinflated
alveoli

Collapsed
alveoli

Fig. 9.3.1. Normal lungs (upper part), deflating to one-third when the chest is opened. Asthmatic lungs (lower part), not deflating when the chest is opened; some atelectatic areas.

oedema formation. In addition to these physical changes, exuded plasma proteins (complement factors, kallikrein and immunoglobulins) may contribute, biochemically, to asthma pathogenesis.

Bronchial thickening

Changes in the airways include *thickening of the bronchial smooth muscles* and epithelial basement membrane. This is of particular importance in the small airways.

Histopathology of asthma

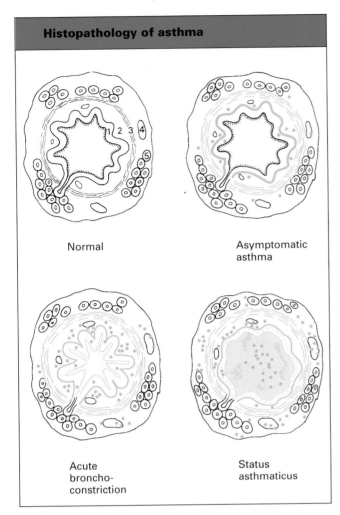

Normal

Asymptomatic asthma

Acute broncho-constriction

Status asthmaticus

Fig. 9.3.2. Cross-sections of normal and asthmatic bronchi. *Normal bronchus*: 1, ciliated epithelium; 2, epithelial basement membrane; 3, smooth muscles; 4, blood vessels; and 5, glands. *Bronchus in asthma patient free of symptoms*: thickening of basement membrane and muscle layer; scattered eosinophils. *Asthma due to acute bronchoconstriction*: folded epithelial layer with partial loss of ciliated cells; eosinophilia. *Occluded bronchus in status asthmaticus*: plug, consisting of mucus, plasma exudation and cell clusters; almost complete shedding of columnar epithelial cells; marked eosinophilia.

Pathogenesis of bronchial obstruction

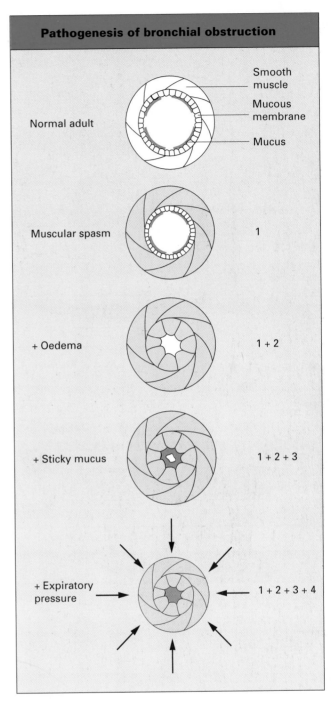

Normal adult — Smooth muscle / Mucous membrane / Mucus

Muscular spasm   1

+ Oedema   1 + 2

+ Sticky mucus   1 + 2 + 3

+ Expiratory pressure   1 + 2 + 3 + 4

Fig. 9.3.3. Pathogenic factors in asthma: 1, spasm of smooth muscle; 2, oedema of mucosa; 3, increased amount of mucus; and 4, forced expiration. From Aas K. *The Biochemical and Immunological Basis of Bronchial Asthma* Springfield: Charles C Thomas Publisher, 1972: 1–238.

Mechanisms of mucus plugging

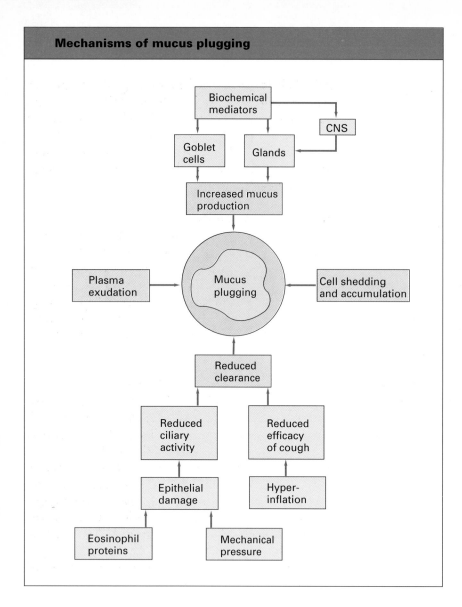

Fig. 9.3.4. Biochemical mediators and vagal reflexes stimulate the production of mucus from goblet cells and glands. Mucus is not removed from the lumen because the ciliated epithelium is damaged by cytotoxic eosinophil proteins, and by mechanical pressure during smooth muscle contraction. When mucus is not moved, it becomes more viscous, and the addition of plasma proteins and DNA, from cellular debris, further increases its viscosity. The situation is made difficult because a patient with severe asthma and hyperinflated lungs has an impaired ability to clear the airways by coughing. The vicious spiral ends in mucus plugging of the airways.

Mucus cast of bronchial tree

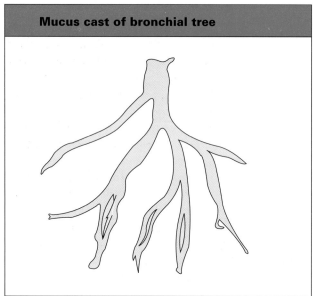

Fig. 9.3.5. Mucus cast of the airways, coughed up during an asthma attack.

Dear me, Sir Osler!
All authors agree that there is, in the majority of cases of bronchial asthma, a strong neurotic element.
Sir William B Osler
Modern Medicine, 1909

9.4 Pathogenesis and histopathology of asthma II

Bronchial smooth muscles and nervous system

Key points
• The normal function of the spiralling network of smooth muscle around the tracheo-bronchial tree is unknown.
• Contraction of bronchial smooth muscle is responsible for acute, readily-reversible asthma.
• Bronchial smooth muscles have receptors for neurotransmitters, hormones, mediators and drugs.
• Receptor activation and muscle contraction can occur as a result of allergic reactions and exposure to physical and chemical stimuli.
• A vagal reflex is an amplifier mechanism, which extends the symptoms to sites that are isolated from the stimulus.
• Stimulation of sensory C-fibres, by release of neuropeptides, causes an axon reflex and neurogenic inflammation (at least in rodents).

The rapid development of an asthma episode and its prompt relief by a bronchodilator spray provide evidence of smooth muscle contraction. The equally quick contraction induced by inhaled irritants also suggests an involvement of reflex bronchoconstriction.

This chapter deals with bronchial smooth muscles and the autonomic nervous system, which is closely associated with smooth muscle contraction. Although these tissues are important for bronchoconstriction, many studies have failed to identify abnormalities in smooth muscle or autonomic neural control as a primary cause of the increased bronchial responsiveness in asthma.

Bronchial smooth muscles
The tracheo-bronchial tree is surrounded by a spiral network of smooth muscles, extending to the most distal bronchioles. Although cells within a bundle are close, they are separated from their neighbours along most of their length by a gap. Gap junctions exist as dynamic entities. Altered formation and function may change communication and signals between cells. This may shift the behaviour of airway smooth muscles from 'single-unit' to 'multi-unit'. This means that contraction of one muscle cell will spread to other cells, resulting in increased muscular contractility. It is likely, but unproven, that this contributes to the exaggerated stimulus–response relationship, characteristic for asthma.

Intracellular calcium
The coupling between a stimulus and smooth muscle contraction depends upon the concentration of intracellular ionized *calcium*. A protein, *calmodulin*, serves as a physiological regulator and plays multiple roles in calcium-dependent systems. Calcium antagonists and calmodulin inhibitors may, in the future, be of potential benefit in the treatment of asthma.

Cyclic AMP/GMP
The cyclic nucleotides, *cyclic AMP* (adenosine monophosphate) and *cyclic GMP* (guanosine monophosphate), act as *intracellular regulators* of the cell response to extracellular stimuli. Cellular reactivity is reduced by a high cyclic AMP : GMP ratio. The formation of cyclic AMP is catalysed by the enzyme *adenylate cyclase*. This enzyme is activated and the level of cyclic AMP increased by *beta adrenoceptor stimulation*. Acetylcholine and other cholinoceptor agonists enhance the reactivity of the muscle cell by increasing cyclic GMP.

These systems are also operative in other types of cells, for example mast cells.

Smooth muscle receptors
Receptors, localized to the cell membrane, are frequently discussed in parallel with drugs, but their normal function is to sense extracellular regulatory signals, from hormones, neurotransmitters and mediator substances, and to translate them into intracellular metabolic events.

Stimulation of cell receptors in bronchial smooth muscles causes either contraction or relaxation (Table 9.4.1).

As mentioned above, the *beta$_2$ adrenoceptor* is associated with adenylate cyclase and stimulation causes marked muscle relaxation and bronchodilatation. The beta receptor is stimulated by drugs (beta$_2$ bronchodilators), by the neurotransmitter, noradrenaline, and by the hormone, adrenaline.

The neurotransmitter, acetylcholine, released by vagal reflexes, causes bronchoconstriction by stimulation of *muscarinic cholinoceptors*.

Substances with effect on bronchial smooth muscles	
Bronchoconstriction	**Bronchodilatation**
Beta antagonists (propranolol)	Beta agonists (salbutamol)
Cholinergic agonists (acetylcholine)	Cholinergic antagonists (atropine)
Histamine	(H₁ antihistamine)
Kinins	
Sulphidoleukotrienes	
PGD and PGF	PGE

Table 9.4.1. Drugs, neurotransmitters and inflammatory mediators, which contract or relax bronchial smooth muscles

Histamine, stimulating H_1 histamine receptors, is a potent bronchoconstrictor, but H_1 antihistamines have no or little effect in asthma. *Bradykinin* also contracts bronchial smooth muscles, and the *sulphidoleukotrienes* have a similar action. While PGF and PGD constrict the bronchi, PGE has the opposite effect.

Receptor characteristics
Until a decade ago, cell receptors were physiologically and pharmacologically defined, and they were thought of as 'keyholes' fitting to the specific 'keys', the agonists. Molecular biologists have now dramatically changed the situation, as they have identified and cloned the genes encoding for more than 100 receptors. The gene encoding for the asthma-relevant beta₂ receptor, for example, is localized to chromosome 5_{q31-32}! The characterization of the amino acid sequence of the receptors (Fig. 9.4.1) has created new and fascinating possibilities for modulation of receptor function, smooth muscle contraction and asthma treatment.

G proteins
The specific cell receptor, for example the beta₂ receptor, is, in the cell membrane, coupled to a G protein (guanine nucleotide-binding regulatory protein). It is the interaction between receptor and G protein that elicits a metabolic cell response. G protein genes, which belong to one large gene superfamily, have generated considerable investigative attention.

Smooth muscle contraction

Direct effect on muscle receptors
The bronchial smooth muscles possess receptors for a series of chemical mediators, which, in asthma, are released from mast cells and other inflammatory cells. These mediators can cause smooth muscle contraction by a direct action on the muscle cell (Fig. 9.4.2). The effect is confined to the area close to the site of mediator release.

Indirect effect via reflexes
Stimulation of tracheo-bronchial afferent nerves initiates a *parasympathetic reflex* resulting in bronchospasm. This vagal reflex is a potent amplifier mechanism because stimulation of nervous receptors in one part of the airway causes constriction at sites isolated from the stimulus.

Combined effects
It is currently debated as to whether the different types of triggers of bronchoconstriction act directly

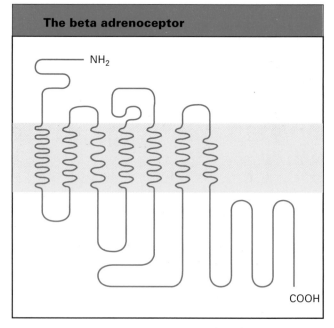

Fig. 9.4.1. Primary structure of the beta adrenoceptor. From Tota M, Candelora MR, Dixon RAF, Strader ACD. Biochemical and genetic analysis of the ligand-binding site of the β-adrenoceptor. *Am J Respir Cell Mol Biol* 1989; **1**: 82.

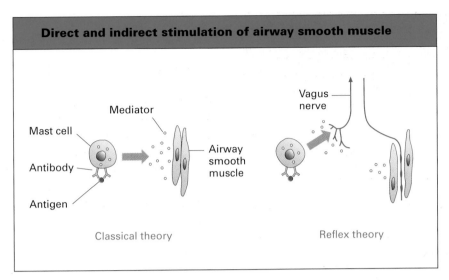

Fig. 9.4.2. The classical theory of allergen-induced asthma (left) suggests that inflammatory mediators cause direct, smooth-muscle contraction. The reflex theory (right) suggests a stimulation of sensory nerves by the mediators and reflex-induced bronchoconstriction. From Gold WM. Cholinergic pharmacology in asthma. In: Austen KF, Lichtenstein LM, eds. *Asthma: Physiology, Immunopharmacology, and Treatment* New York: Academic Press, 1973: 169–80.

or via reflexes; both mechanisms are probably at work in most situations. It follows that an allergen stimulus can be amplified twice: first, by *mast cell degranulation*, and, second, by a *vagal reflex*. Consequently, the interaction between a tiny amount of allergen and IgE can result in a vigorous clinical response.

Bronchial innervation

The autonomic nervous system consists of the sympathetic, parasympathetic, and *non-adrenergic, non-cholinergic* (NANC) nervous systems. NANC is operated by neuropeptides. It is not a specific system of nerve fibres, it uses sensory, parasympathetic and sympathetic fibres in which the neuropeptides co-exist with the classical neurotransmitters. A series of *neuropeptides*, which have potent effects on many aspects of airway function, have now been identified in human airways (Table 9.4.2). However, their physiological and pathophysiological role, in the airways, is not yet characterized.

Sensory nerves

The sensory fibres, to the larynx, tracheo-bronchial tree and alveolar wall, which run in the vagus nerve, terminate in or just beneath the surface epithelium (Fig. 9.4.3).

There are two types of sensory nerve fibres. One has myelinated epithelial endings that rapidly adapt to stimulation. These endings act as *cough receptors* in the larynx and trachea, and as *irritant receptors* in the bronchi. This receptor type, while exquisitely sensitive to mechanical stimuli, also reacts to histamine, cold air and sulphur dioxide.

The other type, the non-myelinated or *C-fibre endings*, supply the surface epithelium, blood vessels and glands. They are particularly sensitive to tobacco smoke, capsaicin (the active ingredient of chilli pepper) and bradykinin. They respond to stimulation with the release of neuropeptides (substance P and neurokinin A).

Both types of nerve fibre can form the afferent limb of a bronchoconstrictor vagal reflex (Fig. 9.4.3). In addition, C-fibre stimulation can initiate an axon reflex (running in one axon and not reaching the CNS). Axon reflexes account for the flare reaction in the skin; it has recently been proposed that they may play a role in asthma pathogenesis (see below).

Parasympathetic nerves

The vagus nerve carries the parasympathetic preganglionic fibres to the tracheo-bronchial tree; the ganglions are localized to the bronchial wall (Fig. 9.4.3). There is dense cholinergic innervation of tracheo-bronchial *smooth muscles* and *glands*, and a sparse innervation of vasculature. Parasympathetic stimulation with release of *acetylcholine* from the efferent vagus fibres results in *bronchoconstriction* and

Effects of neurotransmitters and neuropeptides

	Transmitter/Peptide	Receptor	Function
Sensory nerves	Substance P	NK$_1$ receptor NK$_2$ receptor	Microvascular leakage Goblet cell secretion Bronchoconstriction
	Neurokinin A	NK$_2$ receptor	Bronchoconstriction
	Calcitonin gene-related peptide (CGRP)	CGRP receptor	Vasodilatation
Parasympathetic nerves	Acetylcholine	Muscarinic M$_1$, M$_2$ and M$_3$ receptors	Bronchoconstriction Gland secretion Vasodilatation
	Vasoactive intestinal polypeptide (VIP)	VIP receptor	Vasodilatation Bronchodilatation
Sympathetic nerves	Noradrenaline	Adrenoceptors, beta and alpha	Bronchodilatation Vasoconstriction
	Neuropeptide Y (NPY)	NPY receptor	Vasoconstriction

Table 9.4.2. Effects of classical neurotransmitters and of neuropeptides on bronchial smooth muscles, blood vessels and mucus secretion

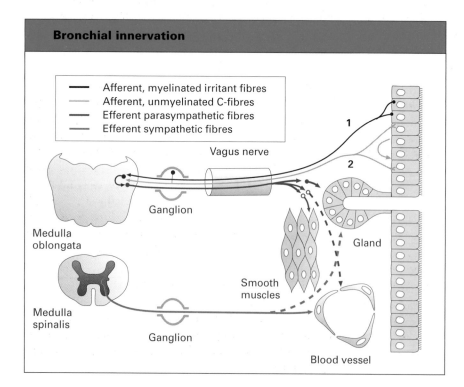

Fig. 9.4.3. Innervation of the tracheo-bronchial tree and lungs. Afferent fibres (black), running in the vagal nerve, are of two types: 1, myelinated fibres (cough and irritant receptors); and 2, unmyelinated fibres (C-fibres). Stimulation of both can initiate a vagal reflex, and stimulation of C-fibres can result in an axon reflex. Efferent fibres are parasympathetic (blue) to glands and smooth muscles (and blood vessels), and sympathetic (red) to blood vessels (and glands).

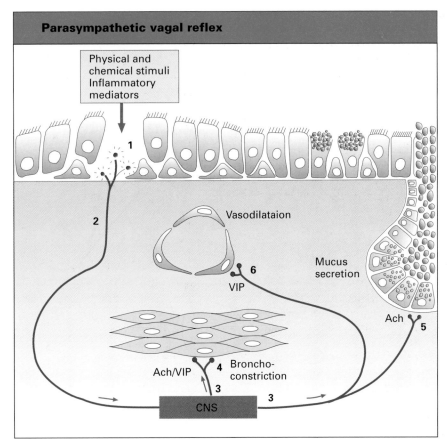

Fig. 9.4.4. Parasympathetic vagal reflexes in asthma pathogenesis. 1, Stimulation of exposed and sensitized irritant receptors and C-fibres by exogenous irritants and inflammatory mediators. 2, Activation of vagal CNS reflex. 3, Stimulation of efferent parasympathetic fibres with release of acetylcholine (Ach) and vasoactive intestinal polypeptide (VIP) from postganglionic nerve terminals. 4, Bronchial smooth muscles are contracted by acetylcholine, while VIP dilates slightly. 5, Glandular hypersecretion caused by acetylcholine. 6, Slight vasodilatation due to VIP.

glandular *hypersecretion*. This is an effect of the cholinergic muscarinic receptors of which there exist at least three subtypes (M_1, M_2 and M_3). There is co-release of acetylcholine and the neuropeptide, vasoactive intestinal polypeptide (VIP). VIP has weak bronchodilator and moderate vasodilator effects (Fig. 9.4.4).

Sympathetic nerves

The sympathetic ganglia are localized to the sympathetic trunk, while postganglionic fibres reach the lower airways largely via the pulmonary blood vessels. The sympathetic nerves appear to be *limited to the vasculature* and are not in close contact with bronchial muscle cells. Nervous release of *noradrenaline*, therefore, seems to play no or only an insignificant role in the stimulation of bronchial adrenoceptors. These receptors are predominately controlled by circulating adrenaline.

Hyperaesthesia

Damage to and the *shedding of epithelium* in asthmatic airways may expose sensory nerve endings. These endings may also be 'sensitized' by certain mediators, such as *bradykinin*, *prostaglandins* and *cytokines*. Asthma may thus be associated with hyperaesthesia (hyperalgesia) of the airways; such increased sensitivity is characteristic of inflammation at other sites in the body. It is probable that cough and chest tightness, common symptoms of asthma, are a reflection of this airway hyperaesthesia, and it may imply more easily activated reflexes.

Axon reflexes – neurogenic inflammation

Some years ago, Peter Barnes proposed a hypothesis of asthma pathogenesis involving neuropeptides, axon reflexes and so-called neurogenic inflammation (Fig. 9.4.5).

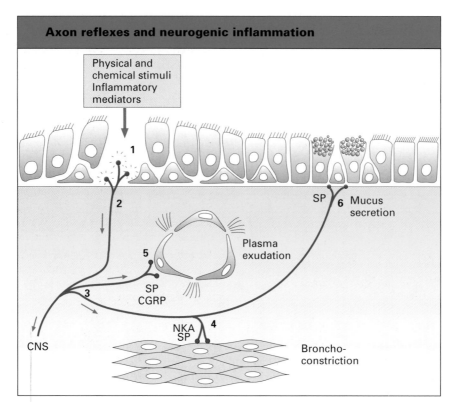

Fig. 9.4.5. Hypothesis of axon reflexes and neurogenic inflammation as mechanisms in asthma pathogenesis. 1, Stimulation of exposed and sensitized C-fibres by exogenous irritants and by inflammatory mediators. 2, Activation of afferent vagal fibres. 3, Axon reflex with antidromic impulses in sensory nerves leading to retrograde release of substance P, neurokinin A and calcitonin gene-related peptide (CGRP). 4, Bronchoconstriction (mainly neurokinin A), 5, plasma extravasation, and 6, mucus secretion (mainly substance P).

The C-fibres, exposed by epithelial shedding and sensitized by bradykinin, are stimulated by external irritants or by inflammatory mediators. This initiates an axon reflex with retrograde stimulation of other sensory C-fibres in epithelium, blood vessels and glands. The release of potent neuropeptides, especially the tachykinins (substance P and neurokinin A (NKA)) results in bronchoconstricition, mucus secretion and plasma extravasation. The microvascular leakage further contributes to inflammation by the formation of bradykinin.

Epithelial shedding may further exacerbate the condition, as the epithelium has an impaired capacity to synthesize the enzyme, neutral endopeptidase (NEP), which normally degrades and inactivates tachykinins.

While neurogenic inflammation, evidenced by plasma extravasation, occurs in rodents, it has not been definitely demonstrated in humans; whether it is relevant to human airways is not yet certain. If neurogenic inflammation is important in asthma, then drugs with an effect on tachykinins may have potential benefit in asthma therapy. Antagonists to tachykinin and to the tachykinin NK_1 receptor are currently undergoing clinical trials.

The young doctors

'The younger doctors are all the same', said Miss Marple. 'They take your blood pressure, and whatever's the matter with you, you get some kind of mass-produced variety of new pills. Pink ones, yellow ones, brown ones. Medicine nowadays is just like a supermarket – all packaged up.'

Agatha Christie
The Mirror Crack'd, Chapter 3

9.5 Pathophysiology of asthma

Obstruction, expiratory closure, hyperinflation, hyperventilation, hypocapnia and hypoxaemia

Key points

- The use of expiratory muscles is necessary to maintain adequate airflow through obstructed airways.
- The increased pressure on the bronchial wall closes the distal airways during expiration.
- This is, in part, compensated for by prolonged expiration and by chest hyperinflation.
- During an acute episode of asthma, hyperventilation results in mild respiratory alkalosis.
- In very severe asthma with respiratory failure, hypoventilation causes acute respiratory acidosis.
- Hypoxaemia is a constant feature of an asthma attack due to a ventilation/perfusion mismatch.

Airways

Airway obstruction

Smooth muscle spasm, oedema, inflammation and mucus plugging cause the prime pathophysiological disturbance in asthma: *airway narrowing* and *increased resistance to airflow*.

Asthma was formerly considered to be a process limited to the large airways, but *both large and small airways are involved*. As the condition of the patient improves following a severe attack, the large airways tend to change early, while the obstruction of the small airways, probably caused by inflammation and mucus plugging, may persist for a considerable time.

Increased alveolar pressure

A positive alveolar pressure is necessary to move air during expiration. Normally, this is accomplished by *elastic lung recoil* (Fig. 9.5.1a). In asthma, airway obstruction necessitates an increase in alveolar pressure during expiration (Fig. 9.5.1b). This cannot be obtained by elastic recoil alone; the *use of expiratory muscles* is necessary. As a consequence, the external pressure on the bronchiolar wall increases, the peripheral airways close as the lung empties, and *air is trapped* in the alveoli (Fig. 9.5.1c).

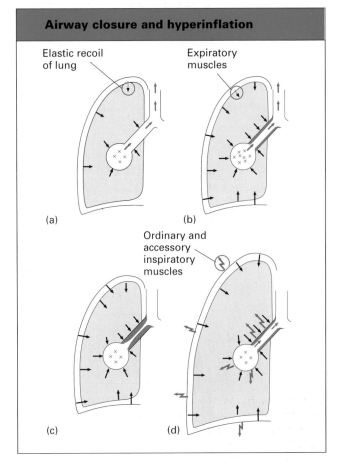

Fig. 9.5.1. Expiratory movement of air: (a) normal expiration; (b) start of asthmatic expiration; (c) end of asthmatic expiration with airway closure; and (d) compensatory hyperinflation.

Prolonged expiration and chest expansion

Air trapping is counteracted in two ways. First, by a reduction of the expiratory flow rate, giving *prolonged expiration*. Second, by *expansion of the chest*, which is accomplished by ordinary and accessory inspiratory muscles, and is transmitted to the bronchial wall (Fig. 9.5.1d). It counteracts airway closure during expiration at the expense of *increased respiratory work*, *impaired effectiveness of cough* and considerable *discomfort*.

Positive expiratory pressure

End-expiratory closure and air trapping can also be counteracted by *pursed-lip breathing*, used especially by emphysema patients, by *positive end-expiratory pressure (PEEP)*, in a respirator, and by *positive expiratory pressure (PEP)*, in a simple resistance mask (PEP mask). The latter is not used for acute asthma

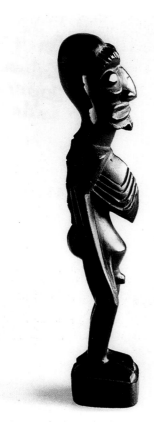

Fig. 9.5.2. Statue from the Easter Island illustrating chest hyperinflation in asthma.

but it is helpful in raising secretions in chronic obstructive pulmonary disease.

Asthma distress

The discomfort that an asthmatic patient feels during an attack can be experienced by a normal person. Make a submaximal inspiration and breathe for some minutes with the chest in this *hyperinflated state*. Then add *airway obstruction* by breathing through a partially blocked nose or through a straw (Figs 9.5.2–3). You will then experience some of the distress of an asthma patient but *fear* of suffocation is added during a real attack.

Hyperventilation

Airway obstruction can be compensated for by deep, slow breathing, but in asthma, *respiratory frequency is increased*. This is a drawback, as the functional dead space is also increased. However, the patient is unable to breathe slowly as there is an enhanced drive from the respiratory centre which results in *hyperventilation*.

Blood gases

Hypocapnia

Arterial carbon dioxide tension ($Paco_2$) is a measure of the alveolar ventilation and, as asthma patients hyperventilate during an acute episode, it follows that $Paco_2$ is reduced.

Hypoxaemia

Hypoxaemia is an *important feature of an asthma attack*. This appears to be a paradox as the patient is hyperventilating. The explanation is as follows: airway obstruction in asthma is unevenly distributed so some groups of alveoli are hyperventilated while others are hypoventilated. Unevenness or inequality of airflow and blood flow is the inevitable result (Figs 9.5.4–5).

As hyperventilation with ambient air cannot oversaturate the blood, a decreased Pao_2, due to hypoventilated alveoli, cannot be compensated for by hyperventilation of other alveoli. Consequently, the *ventilation/perfusion mismatch* in asthma results in a

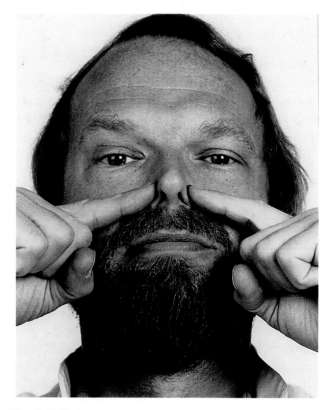

Fig. 9.5.3. This is airway obstruction. Asthma is airway obstruction. Explain the difference.

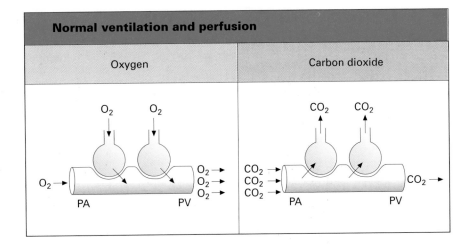

Fig. 9.5.4. Normal ventilation and perfusion. PA, pulmonary artery; PV, pulmonary vein.

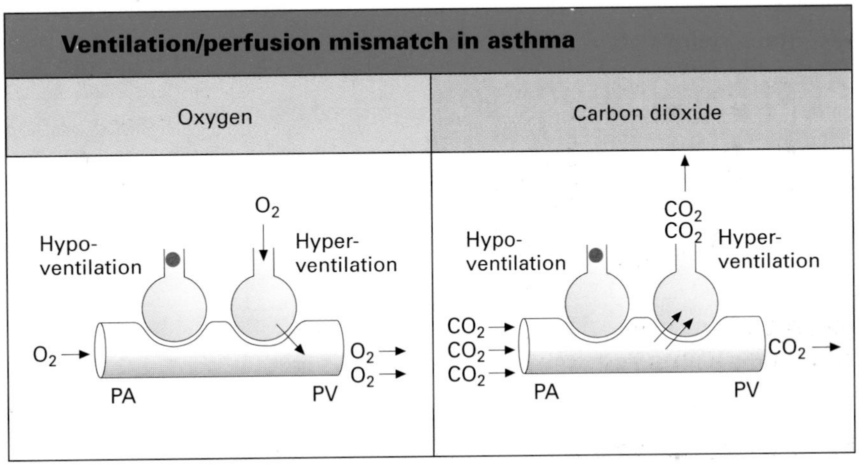

Fig. 9.5.5. Abnormal gas exchange in asthma due to unevenly blocked airways and ventilation/perfusion mismatch. Hyperventilated alveoli can compensate for hypoventilated alveoli with regard to CO_2 but not O_2, resulting in hypoxaemia. PA, pulmonary artery; PV, pulmonary vein.

hypoxaemia, which reflects the severity of the attack. It can only be corrected by increasing the concentration of oxygen in inhaled air.

A stupid patient
A doctor who treats himself has a fool as patient.
William Osler

9.6 Diagnosis of asthma I: the case history
Characteristic symptoms and triggers

Key points
- The asthma attack is typically described as an episode of chest tightness, musical wheezing and dyspnoea.
- In infants, an asthma attack is usually precipitated by an airway infection.
- Asthma, with debut in childhood, is usually allergic.
- Asthma, with debut in adulthood, is usually non-allergic.
- An asthma episode is usually precipitated by a trigger factor.
- Some triggers merely induce an acute attack (e.g. exercise).
- Other triggers also worsen the disease (e.g. allergens).
- Important points to question for evaluating disease severity are: number of nights with asthma and use of bronchodilator spray.

Diagnostic principles
Asthma is characterized by *airway narrowing*, which is 1, *variable*, 2, *reversible*, and 3, *easily triggered*. These characteristics can be identified by the typical case history, supported, as necessary, by objective examinations and quantitative tests, of which the most important is daily peak flow recordings (Table 9.6.1).

Characteristics of the asthma episode
A typical attack of asthma starts with a feeling of *chest tightness*. Audible, *musical wheezing* develops, followed by *dyspnoea*, which the patient describes as being both *expiratory and inspiratory*. The acute episode ends, usually after a few hours, with the expectoration of very *viscous sputum*. The attack is often accompanied or preceded by *dry cough*.

Cough, particularly at night or induced by exercise, cold air or laughter, can, as an *asthma equivalent*, be the only symptom of mild asthma. This is clinically important as this type of cough responds to anti-asthma therapy.

Asthma diagnosis	
Examination	**Comment**
Case history	Often typical
Physical examination	Can be normal Poor measure of severity
Lung function testing	FEV_1 can be normal when patient is examined
– with reversibility to beta$_2$ agonist	Only when lung function is reduced
Steroid reversibility test	When lung function is still reduced after beta$_2$ spray
Daily PEF recordings	Variability is important
Blood eosinophil count	Can be normal
Allergy testing	Often negative in adults
Bronchial histamine test	In selected cases
Blood gas analysis	In acute severe asthma

Table 9.6.1. Diagnosis of asthma

Triggers of asthma
Triggers that provoke an asthma episode
Cold air Hyperventilation Exercise Laughter Emotional factors Beta blockers Oesophageal reflux
Triggers that also aggravate the disease
Allergen Occupational sensitizers Viral airway infection NSAID (a few patients only) Tobacco smoke Air pollution Severe allergic rhinitis Infected sinusitis

Table 9.6.2. Trigger factors that provoke an asthma episode with or without worsening the disease

Onset of the disease

– in childhood

In infancy and early childhood, asthmatic symptoms are usually precipitated by an airway infection. The disease, at that stage, is often referred to as 'asthmatic bronchitis' or 'wheezy bronchitis', but it can be argued that it is more correct to call recurrent wheeziness 'asthma' as the condition responds to anti-asthmatic treatment. The asthma diagnosis usually becomes evident at age 3–5 years, when attacks occur without infection. Atopic dermatitis and rhinitis symptoms indicate an allergic aetiology, which is the rule when asthma starts early in life.

– in adulthood

Asthma onset in adults is usually non-allergic (intrinsic, cryptogenic or idiopathic). It is often initiated by an airway infection and thereafter becomes chronic and persistent. Although rare, allergic (extrinsic) asthma can present for the first time in adult life.

Table 9.6.3. Questions of value in the case history of asthma

Questions to an asthma patient
Do any of your parents, siblings or children have childhood eczema, asthma or hay fever?
Have you ever had eczema or hay fever?
Do you smoke/Have you smoked?
What is your occupation?
Are you in contact with animals?
Can you tolerate acetylsalicylic acid?
How old were you when the disease started?
Did the disease first start with: episodes of wheezing and breathlessness (asthma)?   daily productive cough (bronchitis)?   breathlessness on effort (emphysema)?
Is there any difference between asthma: indoors/outdoors?   at home/at place of work?   in spring/summer/autumn/winter?
What factors start or worsen your asthma?
Are you ever completely free from chest symptoms?
Have you ever been admitted to hospital for asthma?
Have you ever been treated with steroid tablets for asthma?
How often do you use your bronchodilator spray?
How many days/times per month: do you have asthma symptoms?   do you wake with asthma?   do you stay home from school/work?

Two types of triggers

Highly characteristic of asthma is increased bronchial sensitivity to a series of stimuli that can trigger an attack; patients should be encouraged to identify their specific triggers.

A trigger can either merely *provoke an attack* (triggers of bronchospasm), or it can provoke an acute episode and, at the same time, *aggravate the disease* (triggers of inflammation) (Table 9.6.2).

Inhalation of cold air, hyperventilation, *exercise* and laughter merely triggers an attack (smooth muscle contraction), which can be prevented by pre-treatment with an inhaled beta$_2$ bronchodilator. *Emotional factors* can trigger asthma by causing hyperventilation.

Allergens, occupational sensitizers and *viral airway infections*, on the other hand, not only trigger an attack but also aggravate the disease by inducing inflammation and hyper-responsiveness.

Active *allergic rhinitis* and *infected sinusitis* can, apparently, cause deterioration of the asthmatic state by increasing bronchial responsiveness.

Some patients get severe asthma from *acetylsalicylic acid* and other NSAIDs.

Only a few asthmatics have a specific sensitivity to food, but a number of patients have an unspecific reaction to histamine, histamine-releasing factors,

PEF and asthma severity
Mild
>80% predicted at baseline Variability <20% Normal after bronchodilator
Moderate
60–80% predicted at baseline Variability 20–30% Normal after bronchodilator
Severe
<60% predicted at baseline Variability >30% Below normal despite optimal therapy

Table 9.6.5. Classification of asthma severity based on lung function

sulphites and other irritants in certain types of *food and drink*.

Tobacco smoke, active and passive, as well as other types of *air pollution* can also provoke an asthma episode, as can a *beta-blocker*. Patients will often say that they are 'allergic' to these *non-specific provoking factors*.

Oesophageal reflux may, in the rare case, induce nocturnal asthma, which can be worsened by concurrent *sleep apnoea*.

Diurnal variation

Periodicity of attacks is a cardinal symptom of asthma. In addition, there is a typical diurnal variation with *nocturnal asthma* as a characteristic feature. Most patients have been woken with wheezing at night, characteristically at 3–5 a.m. Patients, who do not wake spontaneously, have a low peak flow recording on waking, '*morning dip*'. The importance of nocturnal asthma is underlined by the fact that most deaths from asthma occur in the early morning.

Questions

It will save time and enable you to make a preliminary judgement of the severity of the condition if you ask a number of specific questions. You should enquire about *trigger factors*, the *effect of medication*,

Clinical features and asthma severity
Mild
Intermittent symptoms <2 times/week Nocturnal asthma symptoms <2 times/month Asymptomatic between exacerbations
Moderate
Exacerbations >2 times/week Nocturnal asthma symptoms >2 times/month Symptoms requiring inhaled beta$_2$ agonist almost daily
Severe
Frequent exacerbations Continuous symptoms Frequent nocturnal asthma symptoms Previous life-threatening exacerbation

Table 9.6.4. Classification of asthma severity based on clinical features (one or more)

the number of *disturbed nights*, the number of *work/ school-loss days*, as well as recent *emergency calls*, *hospital admissions* and, most importantly, the *use of a bronchodilator spray* (Table 9.6.3).

Severity

Full assessment of the severity of the disease requires both a detailed *case history* and *peak flow recordings* (Tables 9.6.4–5).

Counselling
No one can give you better advice than yourself.
Cicero, 106–43 BC

Notice in British doctor's waiting room
To avoid delay, please have your symptoms ready.

9.7 Diagnosis of asthma II: physical examination
Typical signs in acute asthma

Key points
- An asthma patient sits upright with arm support.
- Wheeziness is stethoscopic and often audible at a distance.
- Speech is important for evaluation of dyspnoea.
- Respiratory frequency and pulse rate are measures of asthma severity.
- Cyanosis is a very severe but unreliable sign.
- Confusion and loss of consciousness herald death.

In acute asthma, more than in most other diseases, there are *characteristic symptoms and signs* (Fig. 9.7.1). They have formerly been the only guide to treatment; now, the additional use of objective measurements of lung function are mandatory for arriving at correct management.

Dyspnoea
Breathlessness at rest is a *subjective* measure, which, unqualified, may mean uneasy respiration as well as incapacitating dyspnoea. Physical work becomes increasingly difficult when airway obstruction is moderate and, in severe cases, dyspnoea can tie the patient to his or her chair or in a sitting position in bed. When a patient calls for help, *speech is a useful guide* (telephone assessment). Patients with moderate obstruction speak in sentences, while severe obstruction only allows single words. Ultimately, the patient may be unable to speak or call for help.

Tachypnoea
As mentioned earlier, the patient hyperventilates during an attack and *respiratory frequency* is increased; this is a good, *simple measure of asthma severity*. Make it a rule to count the respiratory frequency when examining a dyspnoeic patient. Due to tachypnoea, expiration is prolonged only in relative, and not in absolute, terms.

Wheeziness
Typically, wheeziness during the (relatively) *prolonged expiration* is *audible at a distance*, but, in mild cases, only *stethoscopic wheezes* can be heard during forced expiration or coughing. Wheeziness *correlates poorly with airway obstruction*. In extremely ill

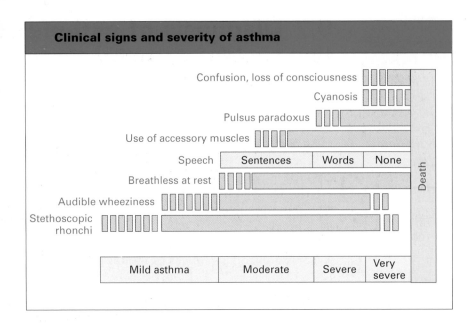

Clinical signs and severity of asthma

	Mild asthma	Moderate	Severe	Very severe
Speech	Sentences	Words	None	

Fig. 9.7.1. Clinical asthma signs related to the severity of the airway obstruction.

patients with severe hypoventilation, so little air passes through the airways that wheeziness decreases or even disappears: '*the silent chest*'.

Use of accessory muscles

A patient with acute asthma usually prefers to *sit upright*, leaning forward *using the arms* to form a fulcrum for accessory respiratory muscles, and there is visible contraction of the sternocleidomastoid muscles. Retraction of intercostal muscles and paradoxical movement of the abdomen are late and serious signs.

Pulse rate

The *pulse rate is increased* and it largely parallels the severity of the episode. The pulse rate usually exceeds 110/min during an episode of acute severe asthma. It is increased also by beta$_2$ agonists and by theophylline.

Pulsus paradoxus

Pulsus paradoxus is an abnormal *reduction in pulse volume during inspiration* due to the considerable changes in intrathoracic pressure (Fig. 9.7.2). When pulsus paradoxus can be felt easily, it is a sign of severe hyperinflation and asthma.

Fatigue

Fatigue is prominent in patients kept awake for days and nights by asthma and may herald collapse when the exhausted patient is no longer able to support the activity of his or her respiratory muscles.

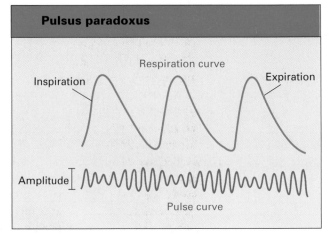

Fig. 9.7.2. Pulsus paradoxus in asthma.

Mental symptoms

Dyspnoea is associated with *distress and anxiety*. Effective bronchodilatation and a good bedside manner help to relieve these symptoms. Tranquillizers and sedatives are dangerous. *Confusion* and *loss of consciousness* are due to severe hypoxaemia (with the exception of cough syncope) and immediate action is necessary (oxygen, intubation and assisted ventilation).

Cyanosis

In asthma, in contrast to chronic bronchitis, *cyanosis is a late and unreliable sign* of respiratory failure. When it does occur, it indicates impending death.

9.8 Diagnosis of asthma III: laboratory tests
Not very useful

Key points
- Blood eosinophils are elevated in about 50% of patients with asthma, allergic and non-allergic.
- A high eosinophil count indicates steroid requirement.
- While asthmatics have eosinophils in the sputum, neutrophils dominate in bronchitics.
- Serum IgE is elevated in about 50% of patients with allergic asthma.

Blood eosinophil count
The blood eosinophil count can be helpful in *differentiating asthma from chronic bronchitis/emphysema* (Fig. 9.8.1), but a normal count is found in about 50% of asthma patients visiting an out-patient clinic.

An increased eosinophil number is *predictive for responsiveness to therapy*. The eosinophil count is a *rough measure of the severity* of the disease, allergic as well as non-allergic. Oral corticosteroids

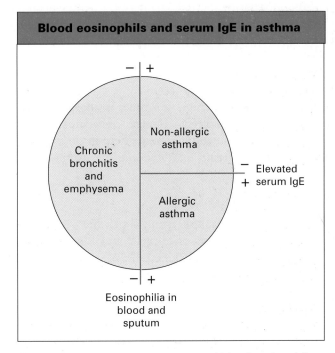

Fig. 9.8.1. Simplified presentation of blood eosinophil and serum IgE results in obstructive lung disease.

are, as a rule, required in patients with high eosino-phil counts (>1 billion/l). It is important, for correct interpretation of the blood count, to remember the eosinopenic effect of oral, and to a lesser extent in-haled, steroids.

Sputum eosinophilia

Eosinophilia in sputum (>20% of the leucocytes) may occur even when blood eosinophilia is absent. It is often associated with Charcot–Leyden crystals in the specimen (thin, colourless, pointed structures of 20–40 µm length, formed by the crystalline structures in the eosinophil granules). When patients do not expectorate, induced sputum can be sampled following an inhalation of hypertonic saline. Sputum eosinophilia is usually present in *symptomatic asthma* but, in contrast to the blood count, the number of cells in sputum correlates poorly with asthma severity. Neutrophils predominate in most sputa from chronic bronchitics and are found together with eosinophils in infective exacerbations of asthma. Methods for staining sputum are de-scribed in Chapter 8.6.

Serum IgE

The serum IgE level is a rough *measure of the number of allergies and their degree*, the highest levels being found in patients with asthma, allergic rhinitis and atopic dermatitis. Serum IgE may be within normal limits if a patient has not been exposed to allergens for months, and it must be emphasized that *a normal IgE level does not exclude allergy*.

IgE:eosinophil ratio

As this ratio may be high or normal in allergic disease and low in non-allergic disease, determination of these parameters can be of some help in *differentiat-ing between allergic and non-allergic asthma* (Fig. 9.8.1).

Chest X-ray

The radiological appearance of the lungs in asymptomatic asthma is normal, and a chest X-ray is primarily indicated to exclude other diseases. In acute severe asthma, a chest X-ray is important for the *diagnosis of complications*, such as pneu-monia, atelectasis, pneumothorax, mediastinal and subcutaneous emphysema. It will show hyper-inflation, which, incorrectly, may be diagnosed as emphysema.

Other examinations

A *sweat test* (children) and determination of *alpha₁ antitrypsin* (adults) can be considered in selected cases when chronic bronchitis/emphysema is a major component of the disease. In acute asthma, blood neutrophilia can be a sign of complicating airway infection, and determination of *serum potassium* is relevant, as beta₂ agonists, theophylline, corticoster-oids, as well as diuretics, all reduce the level. *ECG* is a routine in acute severe asthma in elderly patients.

Buy a soul!
A house without books is like a body without soul.
Marcus Tullius Cicero

9.9 Diagnosis of asthma IV: lung function tests
Important for diagnosis and assessment of severity

Key points
- Lung function tests are necessary for reliable assessment of the severity of acute asthma episodes.
- A respiratory laboratory is needed for showing the increased residual volume and total lung capacity in asthma.
- In the ward, spirometric measurement of FEV_1 is preferable to PEF.
- PEF is adequate in ambulatory settings and at home, where repeated recordings are essential.
- Repeated measurement of lung function can con-

firm the diagnosis, detect triggers, and assess the severity and response to treatment.

Residual volume and vital capacity
The *residual volume increases* considerably during an acute episode of asthma due to air trapping in the peripheral airways. Although total lung capacity also increases, the *vital capacity falls* invariably (Fig. 9.9.1). The more severe the asthma, the closer tidal breathing approaches the maximum inspiratory level and, with that, apnoea. Residual volume cannot be measured outside the *respiratory laboratory*.

Forced expiratory manoeuvres
Lung function tests with forced expiratory manoeuvres are simple and can be used at the bedside. Although they are effort dependent, the results are reproducible and provide a reliable measure of airway obstruction.

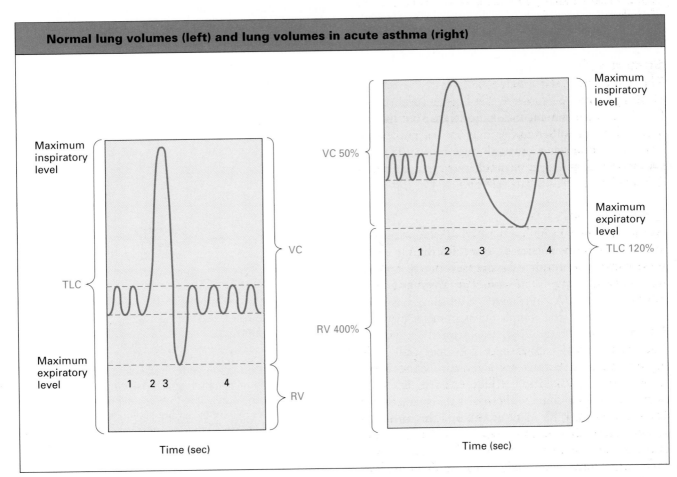

Normal lung volumes (left) and lung volumes in acute asthma (right)

Fig. 9.9.1. Spirometer curve from left to right: 1, tidal breathing; 2, maximal inspiration; 3, forced maximal expiration; and 4, tidal breathing. RV, residual volume; VC, vital capacity.

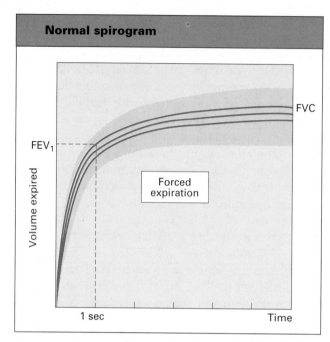

Fig. 9.9.2. Forced expiration in dry spirometer (Vitalograph). A technically acceptable result consists of three curves with less than 5% difference between the two best attempts. FEV$_1$ and FVC are read on the best curve. The normality range for the subject (height, age and sex) is indicated by the shaded area.

Repeated measurements of lung function are the most important observations that can be made in a patient with asthma. They can 1, *confirm the diagnosis*, 2, *detect trigger factors*, and be used to 3, *assess the severity* of the disease and its 4, *response to treatment*.

FEV$_1$

Forced expiratory volume in 1 second (FEV$_1$) is the single best measure for assessing severity of airflow obstruction. It can be *measured in the ward* by a dry spirometer. A spirometer recording has two advantages over the simple measurement of peak expiratory flow rate. First, the printed expiration curve can disclose lack of patient cooperation, and, second, forced vital capacity (FVC) can be measured and the FEV$_1$:FVC ratio calculated (normally >0.7) (Fig. 9.9.2). In asthma, FEV$_1$ is relatively more reduced than FVC (FEV$_1$:FVC <0.7), and this is visualized by the 'obstructive look' of the expiration curve (Fig. 9.9.3). The result of a forced expiratory manoeuvre must be *related to height, age and sex* (Fig. 9.9.4).

PEF

Measurement of peak expiratory flow (PEF) rate by a simple peak flow meter (Fig. 9.9.5) is a good substitute for spirometry, and it is especially well suited for *home monitoring*. The instrument is cheap and *repeated recordings* are essential in a disease with marked fluctuation of lung function as a cardinal symptom. A diagnosis of asthma can be strongly supported by a daily variation of ≥20% in serial measurements of PEF, often with characteristically low morning values (Table 9.9.1). The day-to-day variation, provides a reasonable index of asthma severity, as the variability correlates with bronchial hyper-responsiveness. PEF variability can be calculated from the formula:

$$\text{Daily variability} = \frac{\text{Highest PEF} - \text{Lowest PEF}}{\text{Highest PEF}} \times 100$$

Every patient with chronic asthma should have his or her own peak flow meter and use it regularly twice daily and during acute exacerbations. A PEF diary is the best way for the physician to obtain quick and precise information about the disease.

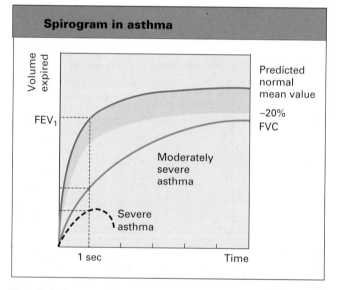

Fig. 9.9.3. During a mild to moderate attack, both FEV$_1$ and FVC are significantly reduced (i.e. 20% below the predicted mean value). Due to bronchial narrowing, it is difficult for the patient to 'empty his lungs' (reduced FVC), and especially to do so quickly (relatively more reduced FEV$_1$). Consequently, FEV$_1$:FVC <0.7. In severe asthma, only FEV$_1$ can be measured, as a full, forced expiratory manoeuvre is strenuous and induces coughing and bronchospasm.

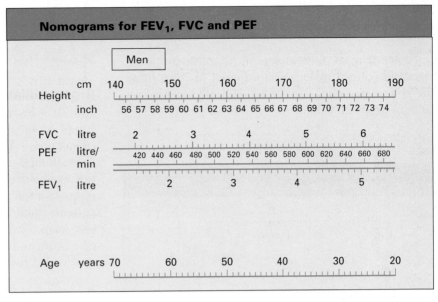

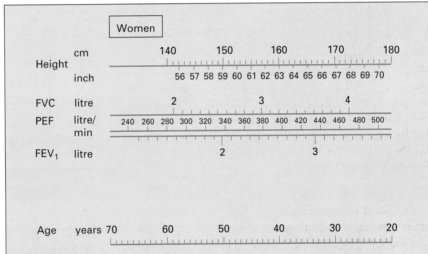

Fig. 9.9.4. Nomogram, from which normal FEV$_1$, FVC and PEF can be read by use of a ruler. Values less than the predicted mean minus 20% are abnormal.

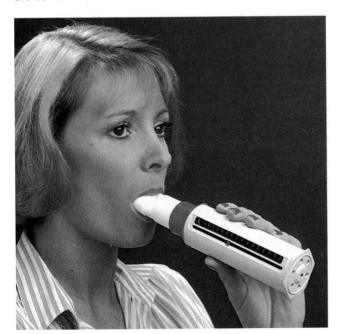

Fig. 9.9.5. Wright's mini peak flow meter.

Peak flow monitoring
Diagnosis of asthma (variation ⩾20%)
Assessment of hyper-responsiveness (variability)
Assessment of severity (lowest value)
Identification of trigger factors
Demonstration of response to bronchodilators
Demonstration of response to steroid
Improvement of patient–doctor communication
Essential for 'guided self management'

Table 9.9.1. Purposes of peak flow monitoring

The small peak flow meters show considerable instrument-to-instrument variation and, in contrast to the spirometer, they cannot be calibrated to give results in absolute values.

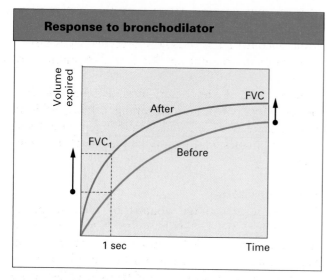

Fig. 9.9.6. Spirometric volumes in an asthmatic patient before and after inhalation of a bronchodilator. FEV₁ increases >20%.

Reversibility of airway obstruction

Bronchodilator spray

A ⩾20% increase in FEV$_1$, 10–30 minutes after the use of an inhaled beta$_2$ bronchodilator, is diagnostic of asthma (Fig. 9.9.6). But the absence of a *bronchodilator response* at a single examination does not exclude the diagnosis. The disease may be temporarily refractory to the treatment, and, in addition, patients often take bronchodilators before visiting the physician. *Daily PEF recordings*, before and after use of a bronchodilator spray, is a more sensitive way of confirming the diagnosis.

Corticosteroids

When the response to a bronchodilator spray does not result in normal lung function, the patient should be given the benefit of the doubt and a *steroid reversibility test* tried. This usually consists of a trial of oral treatment (Fig. 9.9.7).

> The importance of a normal lung function
> *Dum spiro, spero.*
> While I breathe, I hope.

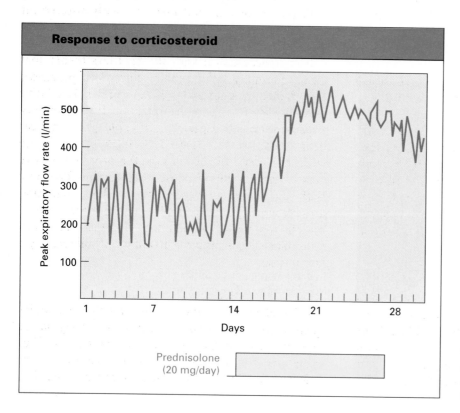

Fig. 9.9.7. Positive diagnostic corticosteroid test in an asthmatic patient shown by daily peak flow recordings. The patient is severely under-treated.

9.10 Diagnosis of asthma V: exercise test
Diagnostic for bronchial hyper-responsiveness

Key points
- Vigorous exercise provokes bronchospasm in most asthmatics.
- It is especially a problem in children.
- It is due to cooling of the bronchial mucosa, and voluntary hyperventilation with cold air provokes the same symptoms.
- Swimming is the best tolerated and free running is the most potent inducer of bronchoconstriction.
- Exercise-induced bronchoconstriction, as a measure of airway hyper-responsiveness, can be used to confirm the asthma diagnosis.
- Exercise testing requires a near-normal lung function (FEV_1 >70%).
- The test consists of running for 6 minutes, which is sufficiently hard enough to produce a pulse rate of 160–180 beats/min.
- A post-exercise fall in PEF or FEV_1 of ⩾20% is abnormal and highly suggestive of asthma.
- This is a test mainly for children and young persons.
- The bronchospasm is completely prevented and reversed by an inhaled beta$_2$ agonist.
- Exercise-induced asthma should not be confused with exertional dyspnoea in patients with considerable airway obstruction.

In most cases, asthma is easily diagnosed by the case history, physical examination, response to a bronchodilator, and daily peak flow recording. A test for bronchial responsiveness can be a useful supplement in a few cases when the case history is dubious, the patient is symptom-free and the peak flow is normal without variation (Fig. 9.10.1).

Exercise-induced asthma
Exercise-induced bronchoconstriction occurs in a large proportion of asthmatics (90%). It is so characteristic that failure to demonstrate it should lead one to reconsider the *diagnosis of asthma*. In children, it represents a restriction on daily life and a *severe handicap*. A child who coughs and wheezes at play is easily excluded from his or her peer group. Many adults are not troubled, simply because they never take exercise strenuous enough to cause asthma.

A submaximal effort of *vigorous exercise* lasting for 6 minutes is necessary. Bronchoconstriction starts shortly after cessation of exercise, is maximal after 5 minutes and returns to the resting level within 1–2 hours (Fig. 9.10.2). This *post-exercise bronchoconstriction* is usually preceded by transient bronchodilatation during the first 2–4 minutes of exercise.

Some types of exercise are more asthmagenic than others. Most potent is free running, cycling holds an intermediate position, and swimming is best tolerated. Asthmatics have won Olympic medals in swimming.

Mechanisms
With exercise, a large volume of ambient air is brought into the intrapulmonary airways where it must be heated to 37°C and be fully saturated with water vapour before it reaches the alveoli. This requires evaporation of water and transfer of heat from the bronchial mucosa.

It is the mucosal *heat and water loss* that is responsible for exercise-induced bronchoconstriction. The total quantity of heat exchange varies directly with the ventilation and inversely with inspired air temperature and water content. This explains why swimming is better tolerated than running.

It is in accordance with the heat-loss theory that exercise-induced asthma can be completely prevented by the inhalation of air at 37°C and 100% relative humidity. It is also understandable that voluntary *hyperventilation*, especially of *cold air*, induces bronchoconstriction (Fig. 9.10.3). It is not quite clear, however, how heat loss in the hyper-responsive airway triggers smooth muscle contraction. Probably both vagal reflex activity and mast cell degranulation are involved. It speaks against a significant contribution from mast cell mediators, however, that exercise-induced bronchoconstriction is not followed by a late response.

Exercise test
It is an advantage of the exercise test that the equipment required is simple: a *sidewalk or ergometer bicycle* and an inexpensive *peak flow meter*. For clinical work, an exercise test consists of free running for 6–8 minutes. The effort must be sufficiently hard to

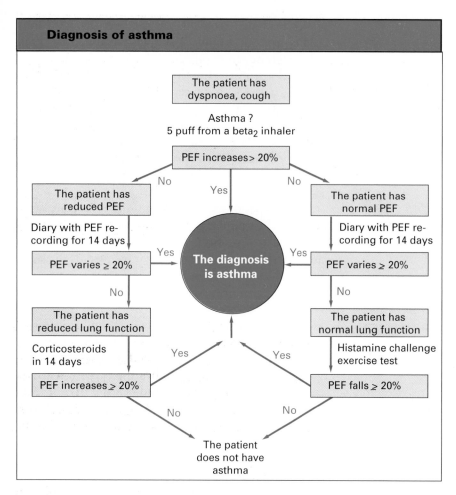

Diagnosis of asthma

The patient has dyspnoea, cough

Asthma ?
5 puff from a beta₂ inhaler

PEF increases > 20%

No   Yes   No

The patient has reduced PEF

Diary with PEF recording for 14 days

PEF varies ≥ 20%   Yes   The diagnosis is asthma   Yes   PEF varies ≥ 20%

No   No

The patient has reduced lung function

Corticosteroids in 14 days

PEF increases ≥ 20%   Yes   Yes   PEF falls ≥ 20%

No   No

The patient does not have asthma

The patient has normal PEF

Diary with PEF recording for 14 days

The patient has normal lung function

Histamine challenge exercise test

Fig. 9.10.1. A diagnosis of asthma or an exclusion of the diagnosis can be based on a combination of case history, response to a beta₂ inhaler, peak flow recording, a steroid reversibility test and histamine challenge test.

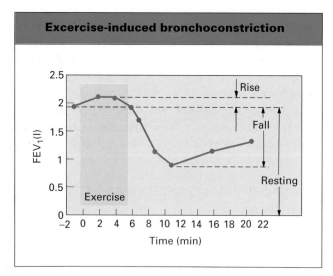

Exercise-induced bronchoconstriction

Fig. 9.10.2. Typical changes in lung function during and after 6 minutes of treadmill running in an asthmatic patient. Note that during exercise there is some improvement and that bronchoconstriction occurs only after stopping.

make the patient moderately breathless and produce a *pulse rate >160 beats/min* in adults and >180 in children. PEF or FEV_1 is measured before, and 1, 5, 10, 15, and 20 minutes after exercise. A *decrease of ≥20%* is highly suggestive of asthma. For research purposes, it is necessary to standardize exercise (treadmill), breathing pattern (nose or mouth), air temperature and humidity.

Safety

The test should not be carried out when FEV_1 is less than 70% of the predicted volume or in patients with cardiovascular disease. Exercise testing is for *children and young adults*. A lady, dressed to see her doctor in the city, is seldom motivated to take a sweat-producing run, and the test can be dangerous in middle-aged patients, who might have undiagnosed coronary disease.

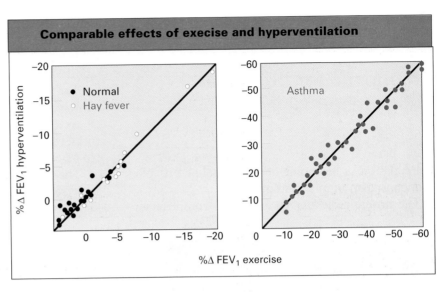

Fig. 9.10.3. Comparison of the responses of normal, hay fever, and asthmatic subjects to exercise and isocapnic hyperventilation. The diagonal lines are the lines of identity. The almost identical results suggest a similar pathogenesis. From Deal EC, McFadden ER, Ingram RH, Breslin FJ, Jaeger JJ. Airway responsiveness to cold air and hyperpnoea in normal subjects and in those with hay fever and asthma. *Am Rev Respir Dis* 1980; **121**: 621–8.

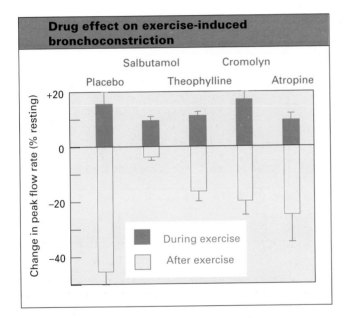

Fig. 9.10.4. Bronchodilatation during and bronchoconstriction after exercise expressed as percentage change from the resting value. Effect of pretreatment with an inhaled beta$_2$ agonist (salbutamol), oral theophylline, sodium cromoglycate (cromolyn) and a cholinoceptor antagonist (atropine). Modified after Anderson SD, Silverman M, König P, Godfrey S. Exercise-induced asthma. *Br J Dis Chest* 1975; **69**: 1–5.

Drug effect

An *inhaled beta$_2$ agonist* can both prevent and reverse exercise-induced bronchoconstriction (Fig. 9.10.4). *Oral bronchodilators* (beta$_2$ agonists and theophyl- line) can also inhibit the reaction but they are less effective. *Cholinoceptor antagonists* have an effect in some patients, suggesting that reflex mechanisms are involved. In most patients, the bronchoconstriction can be prevented, but not reversed, by *sodium cromoglycate and nedocromil sodium. Inhaled corticosteroids* have no acute, but a moderate chronic, effect.

Exertional dyspnoea

The post-exercise bronchoconstriction, provoked in an asthmatic person with normal or near-normal lung function before testing, should not be confused with another type of exercise-induced respiratory distress. This is the disabling dyspnoea, provoked by even modest physical effort, in a patient with chronic bronchitis/emphysema and considerable pre-exercise airway obstruction.

A person who complains of dyspnoea, which develops after 1–2 minutes of exercise and disappears immediately after stopping, does not suffer from exercise-induced asthma.

Exercise test
If from running, gymnastic exercise, or any other work, the breathing becomes difficult, it is called asthma . . .
Aretaeus the Cappadocian, 100 BC

Prevention of asthma
Whenever I feel the urge to exercise I lie down until it passes.
Robert Hutchins

9.11 Diagnosis of asthma VI: histamine test

Diagnostic for bronchial hyper-responsiveness

Key points
- Inhalation of histamine or methacholine provokes bronchospasm in most asthmatics.
- The histamine test given an almost complete separation between normal individuals and symptomatic asthmatics.
- Increasing histamine concentrations are inhaled until FEV_1 drops by 20%.
- The concentration, causing this fall, is called PC_{20} (low value = high sensitivity).
- As a quantitative measure of bronchial responsiveness, the test can be used to confirm the diagnosis and to assess the severity of the disease.
- The bronchospasm is completely prevented and reversed by an inhaled beta$_2$ agonist.

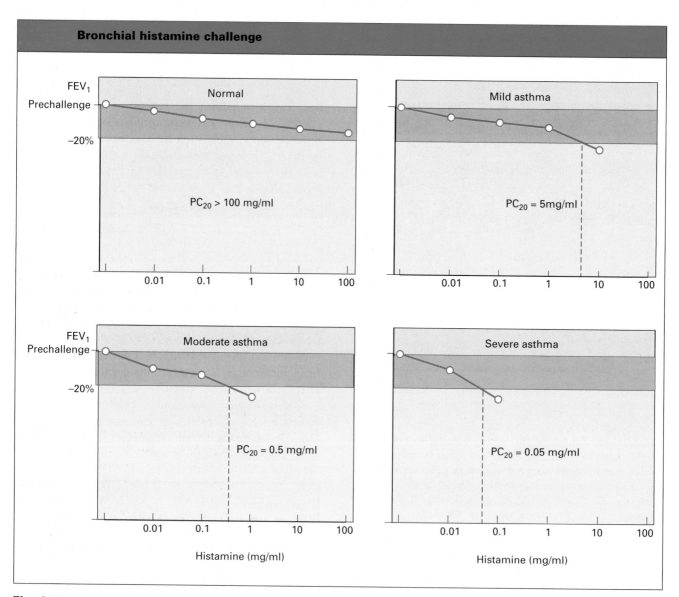

Fig. 9.11.1. Inhalation of increasing concentrations of histamine in normal persons and in patients with mild, moderate and severe asthma. The result is given as PC_{20}, which is the dose causing a 20% reduction of prechallenge FEV_1.

Airway cooling during exercise is one way of demonstrating bronchial hyper-responsiveness. Inhalation of histamine or of the acetylcholine analogue, methacholine, can do the same. An inhalation test is preferable in adults; it is somewhat more sensitive than an exercise test and the response can be quantified.

Methacholine stimulates bronchial smooth muscle directly, while *histamine* also acts via nervous irritant receptors and a vagal reflex. Nevertheless, they give similar results; in practical terms, there is little to choose between them. High doses of histamine often causes side effects (throat irritation, hoarseness, cough, flushing and headache).

Methods and results

A positive response to histamine (or methacholine) is defined as a *reduction in FEV_1 of 20%* (Fig. 9.11.1). The responsiveness can be determined by dose–response curves in one of two ways: 1, by continuous inhalation of increasing concentrations of histamine for 2 minutes during tidal breathing; the provocation concentration of histamine that causes a 20% drop in FEV_1 is termed PC_{20}; and 2, by inhalation of a timed bolus of solution at the beginning of a deep inspiration; the number of breaths and the concentration of histamine can be varied; the total provocation dose that causes a 20% drop in FEV_1 is termed PD_{20}. The second method is the quickest, but it requires a special instrument (Nebulization Dosimeter).

Similar degrees of smooth muscle shortening will cause proportionately greater reduction of airflow in constricted, compared with open, bronchi, as the rate of laminar flow in the airways is proportional to the fourth power of the radius (Fig. 9.11.2). It follows that the result of a histamine test will vary with the *baseline airway calibre* and an almost normal prechallenge FEV_1 is a requirement for comparability of the results.

For safety reasons, a bronchial provocation test should not be carried out when the FEV_1 is less than 70% of the predicted normal value. A patient with more than slight bronchoconstriction needs to have his or her bronchial lability proved the other way round, by bronchodilatation from medication.

A beta$_2$ inhaler can abolish the histamine/methacholine-induced bronchoconstriction, and it is used at the end of the test. An observation period of 1–2 hours is sufficient as patients do not get late recurrence of symptoms.

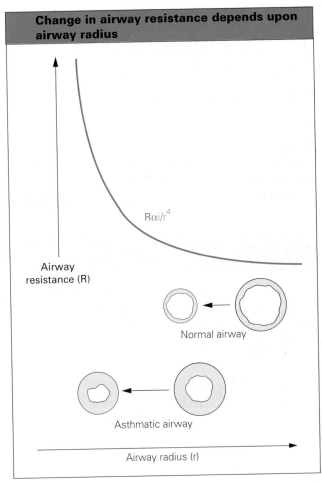

Change in airway resistance depends upon airway radius

$R \alpha i/r^4$

Airway resistance (R)

Normal airway

Asthmatic airway

Airway radius (r)

Fig. 9.11.2. When airways are thickened (in asthma and in bronchitis), they constrict disproportionally to smooth muscle contraction, as the airway resistance varies with the fourth power of the radius of the lumen. From Barnes PJ, Rodger IW, Thomson NC, eds. *Asthma. Basic Mechanisms and Clinical Management* 2nd ed. London: Academic Press, 1992: 406.

Effects of drugs

H_1 *antihistamines* block the response to histamine, but not to methacholine. Inhaled *cholinoceptor antagonists* block the response to methacholine but have less effect on the histamine response. A *beta$_2$ spray* prevents and reverses both responses. The hyper-responsiveness in asthma is reduced by long-term therapy with *inhaled corticosteroids* and, perhaps to a slight degree, with sodium cromoglycate and nedocromil sodium.

It is necessary to discontinue medication before challenge testing (Table 9.11.1), but there is little point in stopping steroid therapy as the effect is long-lasting.

Drug effect on hyper-responsiveness testing

	Exercise test	Methacholine test	Histamine test	Discontinued before challenge
H₁ antihistamine	+	−	+++	1 week*
Cromoglycate and nedocromil	++	−	−	8 hours
Inhaled beta₂ agonist (short-acting)	+++	+++	+++	8 hours
Inhaled beta₂ agonist (long-acting)	+++	+++	+++	24 hours
Oral beta₂ agonist	+	+	+	24 hours
Theophylline	+	+	+	24 hours
Inhaled steroid**	++	++	++	***
Oral steroid**	+	+	+	***
Ipratropium	+	+++	+	8 hours

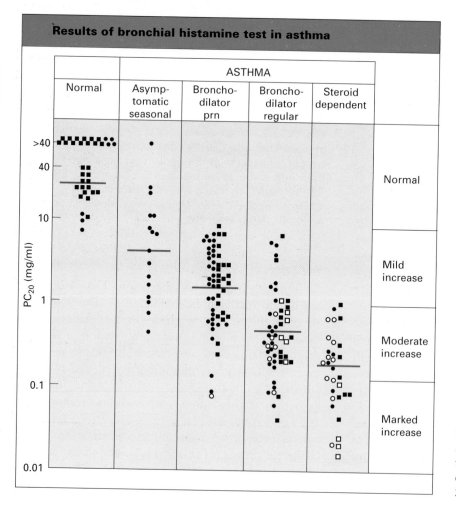

Results of bronchial histamine test in asthma

Table 9.11.1. (Above.) Effect of drugs on tests for measurement of bronchial reactivity. *1 month for astemizole; **long-term therapy; ***not possible

Fig. 9.11.3. Individual values of bronchial reactivity to histamine in normals and subgroups of asthmatics. From Cockcroft DW, Killian DN, Mellon JJA, Hargreave FE. Bronchial reactivity to inhaled histamine: a method and clinical survey. *Clin Allergy* 1977; **7**: 235–43.

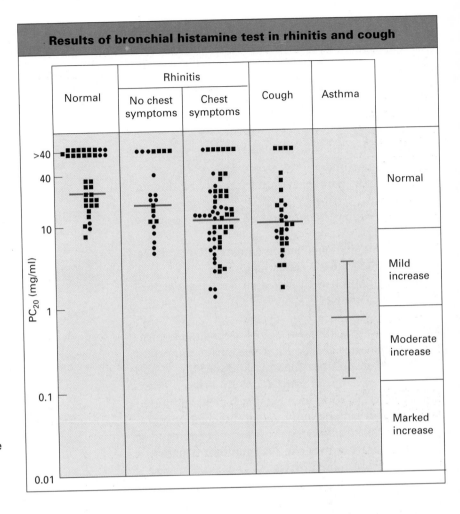

Results of bronchial histamine test in rhinitis and cough

Fig. 9.11.4. Individual values of bronchial reactivity to histamine in normals, in subjects with rhinitis, and in subjects with cough. Geometric mean ($\pm$SD) for all asthmatics is shown in column five. From Cockcroft DW, Killian DN, Mellon JJA, Hargreave FE. Bronchial reactivity to inhaled histamine: a method and clinical survey. *Clin Allergy* 1977; **7**: 235–43.

Diagnostic usefulness

A histamine test gives an almost complete separation between normal individuals and symptomatic asthmatics, who have a 10- to 1000-fold increased sensitivity to the provoking agent (Fig. 9.11.3).

The inhalation test can be used as an adjunct to making the *diagnosis of asthma* and also for *assessment of severity* of the disease (Fig. 9.11.3). It is particularly helpful when the history is atypical, when there are no signs of reversible bronchoconstriction on examination or from peak flow recordings, and when one suspects a disproportionate patient response to the symptoms.

A histamine test is the most sensitive of all diagnostic measures of asthma and the result is clinically relevant because it relates to the ease with which an attack can be triggered by non-specific stimuli. It is a test for both *latent and clinical asthma*, as hyperresponsiveness often persists for years after symptomatic recovery from the disease.

Other diseases

It is not clinical routine to test patients with *chronic obstructive bronchitis* because their lung function is usually too low. Controlled trials have indicated that a small group of these patients have airway hyperresponsiveness, although the thickened bronchial wall may, in part, account for the increased response to histamine challenge (Fig. 9.11.2).

In about half of the patients with *rhinitis and coughing*, the histamine sensitivity ranges between the normal and that of asthma (Fig. 9.11.4).

> **Do it now**
> For of all sad words of tongue or pen, the saddest are these: It might have been.
>
> Lucian

9.12 Diagnosis of asthma VII: arterial blood gases

In acute severe asthma

Key points
- Measurement of arterial blood gases is routine in acute severe asthma.
- PaO_2 falls in parallel with the severity of the episode.
- Note the biphasic configuration of the $PaCO_2$ curve (Fig. 9.12.1).
- As asthma patients hyperventilate, $PaCO_2$ is reduced in moderate–severe asthma.
- Hypoventilation with increased $PaCO_2$ is a sign of very severe asthma.

In acute severe asthma or status asthmaticus, measurement of arterial blood gas tensions is important for grading respiratory function and deciding if and *when to start artificial ventilation*. An *arterial puncture* is therefore routine in asthma patients admitted to hospital. It is done in the radial, brachial or femoral artery. *Pulse oximetry* provides measurement of oxygen saturation that can help monitor a patient's response to acute therapy.

Carbon dioxide tension
When the bronchial obstruction in asthma is moderate, $PaCO_2$ is normal or reduced due to alveolar *hyperventilation*, so a slight respiratory alkalosis is common. When the airway obstruction becomes excessive, alveolar *hypoventilation* develops, *hypercapnia replaces hypocapnia* and *acidosis replaces alkalosis*.

Due to the short duration of the asthma attack, the $PaCO_2$ changes are not compensated for by the kidneys, and arterial bicarbonate remains within normal levels. This is in contrast to chronic bronchitis/emphysema (Table 9.12.1).

When a low $PaCO_2$ returns to normal in a patient with increasing asthma symptoms and falling PaO_2, severe respiratory failure may soon develop. At this stage of acute asthma, when $PaCO_2$ and PaO_2 meet, '*the cross-over point*' (Fig. 9.12.1), hypercapnia and acidosis may develop rapidly. Remember that an *increased* $PaCO_2$ *is a very bad sign* in a patient with asthma.

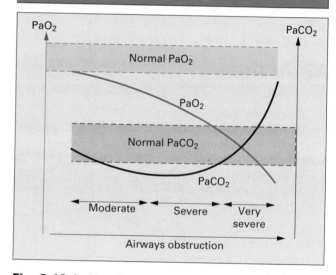

Fig. 9.12.1. Simplified presentation of the arterial blood gas tensions in acute asthma. Note the biphasic configuration of the $PaCO_2$ curve. Based on data from McFadden ER Jr, Lyons HA. Arterial blood gas tensions in asthma. *N Engl J Med* 1968; **278**: 1027–32.

Acid–base disturbancies and blood gas values					
	Acid-base disturbance	**PaO_2**	**$PaCO_2$**	**HCO_3^-**	**pH**
Moderate asthma attack	Acute respiratory alkalosis	↓	↓	–	↑
Very severe asthma attack	Acute respiratory acidosis	↓↓	↑	–	↓
Exacerbation of COPD	Compensated respiratory acidosis	↓↓↓	↑↑	↑↑	–

Table 9.12.1. Acid–base disturbancies and blood gas changes in asthma and chronic bronchitis. COPD, chronic obstructive pulmonary disease; HCO_3^-, the bicarbonate radical

Oxygen tension

In a moderately severe asthma attack, hypoxaemia is caused by a ventilation/perfusion mismatch, while alveolar hypoventilation contributes in the very severe stage. A level below 8 kPa indicates severe asthma. The lowest level reached in uncomplicated asthma is about 6 kPa, while patients with chronic bronchitis/emphysema can survive even lower levels.

As a measure of hypoventilated alveoli, Pao_2 *is the best parameter of asthma severity*. In acute asthma, there is a rough linear *correlation between* Pao_2 *and* FEV_1.

Oxygen treatment of asthma versus chronic bronchitis

While an asthma patient will only have increased $Paco_2$ for hours in connection with a very severe attack, a patient with *chronic bronchitis/emphysema*, on the other hand, can sustain hypoventilation with CO_2-retention for prolonged periods. In popular terms, the ventilation-regulating chemoreceptors become desensitized to hypercapnia in chronic bronchitis and the respiratory centre is stimulated instead by the low oxygen tension. If Pao_2 is suddenly raised by a high oxygen concentration in the inhaled air, progressive hypoventilation with severe hypercapnia and CO_2 narcosis can follow. Thus, while *oxygen* must be given with caution in chronic bronchitis, it *is safe in asthma* – and very important.

The method of learning
I hear and I forget.
I see and I remember.
I do and I understand.

Chinese proverb

Experience
Experience is a marvellous thing. It enables you to recognize a mistake whenever you make it again.

Franklin P Jones

9.13 Diagnosis of asthma VIII: differential diagnosis

Is it asthma, chronic bronchitis or both?

Key points
- Asthma is characterized by episodes of wheezy dyspnoea at rest.
- Chronic obstructive bronchitis and emphysema (COPD) are characterized by productive cough and dyspnoea and exertion.
- While asthma often starts in childhood or adolescence, COPD begins in middle-aged and elderly smokers.
- Daily peak flow recordings are important in making a correct diagnosis.
- In asthma, the airway obstruction is reversible, while in COPD it is mainly irreversible.
- In uncomplicated asthma, normal lung function can be obtained, while this is not the case in COPD.
- The response to beta$_2$ agonists is good in asthma and varying in COPD.
- The response to steroid is good in asthma and poor in COPD.
- In elderly smokers with chronic disease, it is often difficult to make a clear distinction between asthma and COPD.

Paroxysmal wheezing is more prominent in asthma, productive cough in chronic bronchitis, and dyspnoea on exertion in emphysema, but the diseases commonly overlap. The diagnosis is identified by: 1, clinical history; 2, sputum cytology; 3, repeated peak flow recodings; 4, response to bronchodilator inhalation and steroid treatment; and 5, arterial blood gases in advanced cases.

Obstructive lung diseases

Asthma
Asthma is a disease characterized by: 1, *paroxysmal wheezy dyspnoea*; 2, considerable *changes in airway resistance* to airflow over a short time, spontaneously or in response to therapy; and 3, *bronchial hyperresponsiveness*.

Chronic bronchitis

Chronic bronchitis is defined as *cough with expectoration* on most days, for at least 3 months of the year in at least 2 consecutive years. *Smoking* is responsible for the basic abnormality: excessive production of mucus from hyperplastic glands; chronic bronchitis is virtually confined to smokers. Some of them merely develop non-obstructive bronchitis, while, in others, the disease continues in *obstructive bronchitis*.

Breathlessness on exertion can start after years of productive cough. Airway infections, as a rule, will induce *acute exacerbations* accompanied by wheezy breathlessness at rest, which the patients usually call 'asthma'. The airway obstruction is due to intraluminal mucus and pus, thickening of the mucous membrane with hyperplastic glands, and damage to lung tissue.

The disease worsens gradually and, in severe cases, *respiratory failure* (hypoxaemia and hypercapnia) develops with polycythaemia, cyanosis, pulmonary hypertension and cor pulmonale.

Emphysema

Emphysema is characterized by an increased size of the distal air spaces, arising from *destruction of the alveolar septa*. This results in loss of elastic recoil, which is the major cause of obstruction to airflow. The main symptom is *progressive breathlessness on exertion*. The clinical diagnosis is based on a history of tobacco smoking, exertional dyspnoea, and a constantly hyperinflated chest. It can be supported by measurement of the diffusion capacity for carbon monoxide (CO test) and by a CT scan, but emphysema is a histological diagnosis, which only can be made with certainty at autopsy.

COPD

In most patients, chronic obstructive bronchitis and emphysema occur together, and these two terms are now, in modern parlance, being replaced by *chronic obstructive pulmonary disease* or simply *COPD*, or COLD or COAD (scientists love acronyms – but patients still call it bronchitis).

Differential diagnosis

Asthma can easily be separated from COPD in the typical case (Table 9.13.1). In middle-aged smokers and elderly patients, however, there is a considerable overlap, and the diagnosis in these patients is more often 'both' than 'either/or'. This is because airway obstruction is often both reversible and irreversible in the two diseases. It is usually said that asthma does

Table 9.13.1. Differential diagnosis between asthma and COPD

Is it asthma or COPD?	Asthma	COPD
Age at start of disease	Child, adolescent	Middle age, elderly
Smoking	Occasionally	Nearly always
Allergy	Frequent	Rare
Eosinophilia	Frequent	Rare
Dyspnoea at start of disease	Episodes at rest	Exertional dyspnoea
Symptom-free periods	Yes	No
Nocturnal dyspnoea	Yes	No
Normal PEF	Occasionally	Never
PEF variation	$\geq 20\%$	$<20\%$
Response to beta$_2$ agonist	Good	Moderate and varying
Response to steroid	Good	Poor or none

not lead to irreversible airway obstruction, but recent studies indicate that patients with chronic persistent asthma have an accelerated decline in lung function with age (Fig. 9.13.1).

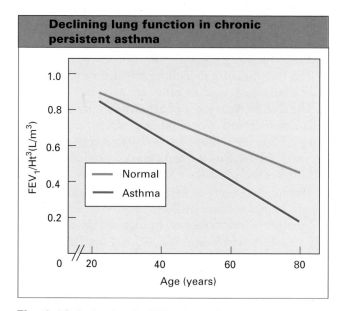

Fig. 9.13.1. Decline in FEV_1 with age in normal and asthmatic subjects. From Peat JK, Woolcock AJ, Cullen K. Rate of decline of lung function in subjects with asthma. *Eur J Respir Dis* 1987; **70**: 171–9.

PEF

Daily peak flow recordings typically show more, larger and quicker changes in asthma patients than in COPD, and, in addition, asthmatics have a characteristic dip in the morning with frequent attacks of nocturnal dyspnoea.

Pao_2 and $Paco_2$

In *COPD*, *hypoxaemia* is more severe than in asthma; in addition, it is frequently accompanied by persistent *hypercapnia*. The finding of hypercapnia in a stable, moderately ill patient points at COPD as does a raised serum bicarbonate (compensated respiratory acidosis).

Therapeutic response

The different responses to therapy are most important for distinguishing between *reversible* airway obstruction (asthma) and *irreversible* airway obstruction (COPD). The demonstration of a striking increase ($\geq 20\%$) in FEV_1 or PEF after use of a *bronchodilator spray* is usual in asthma, but some response (5–15%) is common in COPD. Repeated daily recordings of PEF, before and after use of a bronchodilator spray, is the most reliable way of evaluating the reversibility of the disease.

Little change is to be expected from corticosteroids

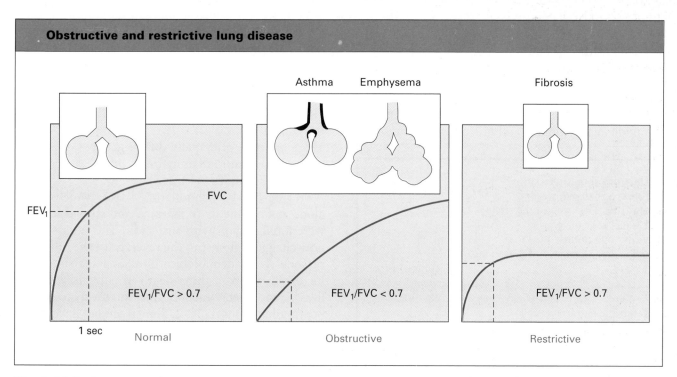

Fig. 9.13.2. Spirometry of obstructive and restrictive airway disease.

in patients with clear-cut COPD. It is therefore un-likely that a patient will respond to therapy if none of the findings suggesting asthma are present (Table 9.13.1). However, a few patients with 'typical COPD' will benefit from steroid therapy and, in case of doubt, the patient should be given a *steroid reversibility test* (see Chapter 9.16).

Restrictive lung diseases

A restrictive lung disease, such as pulmonary fibrosis, can be distinguished from obstructive lung disease by the spirometric determination of the $FEV_1:FVC$ *ratio* (Fig. 9.13.2). In addition, a *CO test*, which is normal in asthma, shows reduced values in fibrosis. The *chest X-ray* will usually be abnormal.

In a severe, chronic, persisting obstructive disease (asthma or COPD), there can be a component of restrictive lung disease due to sequelae after airway infections, pneumonia, bronchiectasis, and mucus impaction with atelectasis.

Cardio-vascular diseases

Pulmonary embolism and cardiac decompensation with pulmonary stasis can induce some wheeziness in patients with asthma and hyper-responsive airways. Patients with severe COPD will often have pulmonary hypertension and develop right- and left-sided cardiac decompensation, which worsens their dyspnoea.

Mixed diagnosis

It follows from the discussion above that the clinical picture seen in the emergency room often is more complex and less simple than described in textbooks. This applies, in particular, to chronic, severe disease in middle-aged smokers and in elderly patients.

The truth about tobacco
Tobacco is an evil weed.
It was the Devil sowed the seed.
It stains your fingers,
burns your clothes
and makes a chimney of your nose.

Tobias Venner
Voa Recta Advitam Longam

Reversible and irreversible
My diseases are asthma and dropsy, and what is less curable, 75.

Samuel Johnson, 1709–84

9.14 Therapeutic principles
Anti-inflammatory and topical therapy

Key points
- The first measure in asthma management is avoidance of allergens and of other triggers.
- The second measure is pharmacotherapy with anti-inflammatory and bronchodilator drugs.
- In all but the mildest cases, basic therapy consists of anti-inflammatory medication; bronchodilators are used when needed.
- The inhaled route is preferred to oral medication, due to higher efficacy and fewer adverse effects.
- Inhaled treatment is given by metered-dose inhalers, dry powder systems and wet aerosol nebulizers.

There is general agreement that *avoidance of allergens* and of other triggers of asthma is the first measure to consider in asthma (see Chapter 9.28). The role of *immunotherapy* in asthma is still controversial (see Chapter 9.33).

Since World War II, a number of new drugs have become available for the treatment of asthma, but it is amazing to realize the marked differences in their use between countries (Table 9.14.1). Maybe the recent 'International Consensus Report on Diagnosis and Management of Asthma' will render asthma management more uniform world wide.

Bronchodilators versus anti-inflammatory drugs

There are two, principally different, types of asthma medication: anti-inflammatory drugs and bronchodilators (Tables 9.14.2–3).

Previously, bronchodilators were widely used alone as first-line daily therapy, and steroid inhalers were looked upon with suspicion. The situation has now changed, almost to the reverse, for the following reasons. 1, Epidemiological studies have shown an increased risk of asthma death in patients who rely heavily upon beta$_2$ inhalers and who use a large number of inhalations daily. 2, Similar studies have found a reduced risk in patients who are on inhaled steroids. 3, Twenty years of experience has shown that inhaled steroid treatment is safe and not associated with any significant risk of serious adverse effects. 4, Histologi-

Table 9.14.1. Sales of anti-asthma medications, 1989 (expressed as per cent of total). From Clark TJH. International variations of asthma therapy. In: Miyamoto T, Okuda M, eds. *Progress in Allergy and Clinical Immunology* volume 2. Seattle: Hogrefe & Huber Publishers, 1992: 251–5

Percentage of sales of anti-asthma medications, 1989				
	UK	**USA**	**Japan**	**Global**
Beta$_2$ agonist inhaled	32	33	7	27
Theophylline	8	31	17	23
Anti-allergics	9	4	49	16
Inhaled steroids	39	9	2	15
Beta$_2$ agonist oral	4	13	25	12
Others	7	11	1	9

Table 9.14.2. Some anti-inflammatory drugs currently used in the treatment of asthma in Europe and the USA

Anti-inflammatory drugs used for asthma		
Class of drug	**Generic name**	**Trade name**
Systemic steroids	Hydrocortisone (i.v.) Prednisolone (oral) Prednisone (oral) Methylprednisolone (i.v.) Methylprednisolone (oral)	Solu-Cortef Prednisolone Prednisone Solu-Medro Medro
Inhaled steroids	Beclomethasone dipropionate Budesonide Flunisolide Triamcinolone acetonide Fluticasone propionate	Becotide/Becloforte Vanceril Pulmicort/Spirocort Aerobid/Flutide Azmacort Flixotide
Non-steroids	Sodium cromoglycate Nedocromil sodium	Intal/Lomudal Tilade

Table 9.14.3. Some bronchodilators currently used in the treatment of asthma in Europe and the USA

Bronchodilators used for asthma		
Class of drug	**Generic name**	**Trade name**
Short-acting beta$_2$ agonists	Salbutamol/albuterol Terbutaline Fenoterol Pirbuterol Bitolterol	Vertolin Bricanyl Berotec Maxair Tornalate
Long-acting beta$_2$ agonists	Salmeterol Formoterol	Serevent Foradil
Theophylline	Theophylline	Theo-Dur/Nuelin/others
Anti-cholinergics	Ipratropium bromide Oxitropium bromide	Atrovent Oxivent

cal studies have shown inflammation, even in mild asthma, and this contributes to airway hyper-responsiveness. 5, It is now realized that chronic asthma often results in the development of irreversibly reduced lung function and it is possible, but not proven, that this can be inhibited by the early introduction of inhaled steroids. 6, The 'International Consensus Report' recommends anti-inflammatory therapy even in mild asthma and takes a cautious attitude to regular bronchodilator treatment.

Oral versus topical treatment

Local medication by the inhaled route has three fundamental advantages over oral administration. 1, The onset of action is quicker (important for bronchodilators in acute asthma). 2, The effect is more pronounced due to higher drug concentration in target tissue (e.g. an inhaled beta$_2$ agonist is highly effective in exercise-induced bronchoconstriction, while, orally, its effectiveness is poor). 3, The risk of systemic adverse effects can be minimized (essential for steroids).

It is often argued that oral drug administration is more convenient for the patient but, since the introduction of modern powder inhalers, this is generally incorrect.

Drug delivery systems

Metered-dose inhalers

In a metered-dose inhaler (MDI), the pressurized canister contains the drug suspended in liquid chlorofluorocarbon (CFC) gas. This evaporates when the canister is actuated, releasing the drug as a *micronized powder* (Fig. 9.14.1). Although the particle size of 2–5 µm favours peripheral deposition in the lungs, only some 10% enters the bronchi. The other 90% is swallowed as most of the particles strike the pharyngeal wall (Fig. 9.14.2). This is due to the high velocity of the aerosol, which, at the actuator orifice, is similar to that of a train. A *proper inhalation technique* is essential for deposition of the remaining 10% in the lungs (Fig. 9.14.3) and frequent checks of patient usage must be undertaken. If only written instructions are relied upon, 50% will use the inhaler incorrectly. This type of inhaler contains lubricants that can *irritate sensitive airways*, and a frequent use can produce bronchospasm.

Due to the well-known, CFC-induced depletion of the ozone layer in the stratosphere, the *CFC gases*

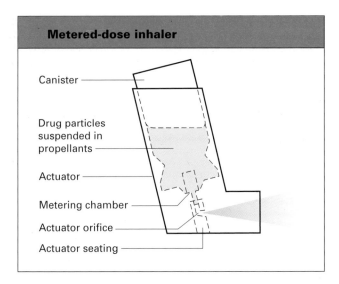

Metered-dose inhaler

Canister

Drug particles suspended in propellants

Actuator

Metering chamber

Actuator orifice

Actuator seating

Fig. 9.14.1. In a MDI, the drug, as a fine powder, is suspended in liquid freon propellants. A surface active agent is added to minimize conglomeration of the drug particles. By courtesy of Stephen P Newman, Royal Free Hospital, London.

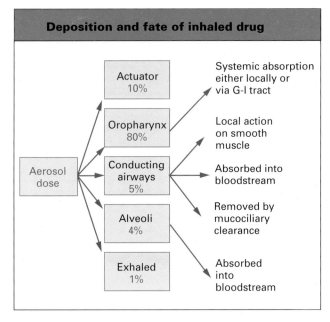

Deposition and fate of inhaled drug

Aerosol dose

Actuator 10%

Oropharynx 80%

Conducting airways 5%

Alveoli 4%

Exhaled 1%

Systemic absorption either locally or via G-I tract

Local action on smooth muscle

Absorbed into bloodstream

Removed by mucociliary clearance

Absorbed into bloodstream

Fig. 9.14.2. Deposition and fate of a bronchodilator aerosol delivered from a MDI. By courtesy of Stephen P Newman, Royal Free Hospital, London.

will soon be replaced by ozone-friendly gases. The task is not easy, however, as wide toxicity testing programmes are required, and the formerly used lubricants are not directly soluble in the new gases.

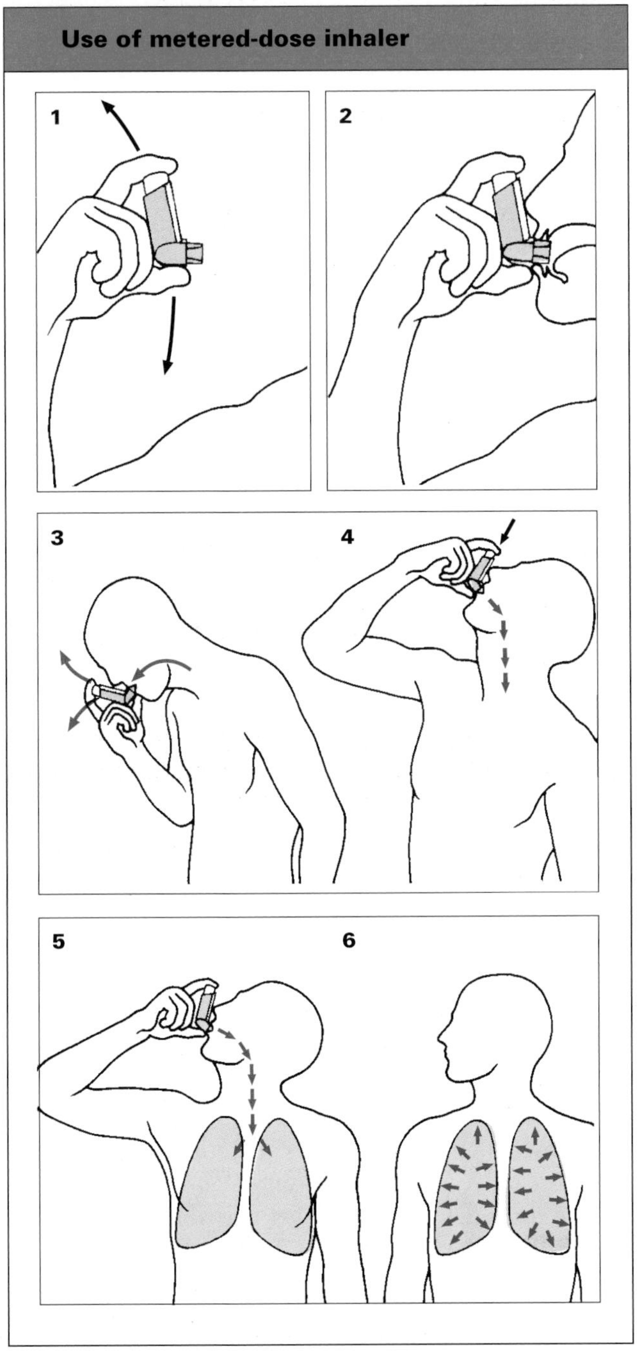

Use of metered-dose inhaler

Fig. 9.14.3. Instruction in use of a MDI.
1 Shake the inhaler.
2 Place the mouthpiece between the teeth and close the lips around it.
3 Breath out slowly until no more air can be expelled.
4 Bend the head backwards, start inhaling and actuate the canister.
5 Continue a full slow inhalation, lasting about 2 seconds.
6 Hold the breath for 10 seconds.
7 Repeat the inhalation after a few minutes.

Spacers

Some patients cannot coordinate actuation of the MDI with inhalation. They can still benefit from inhalation therapy by using a *large volume spacer device* attached to the MDI (Fig. 9.14.4). The spacer allows the patient to *use his or her bronchodilator spray when asthma is severe* as he or she can simply breathe naturally through the spacer. Oral and pharyngeal drug deposition is largely avoided with the spacer, and this *reduces the local adverse effects of steroid inhalers*.

When there is a lag between spraying and inhalation, electrostatic forces can cause adsorption and loss of aerosolized drug to the spacer surface. This problem varies with the type of spacer and drug used.

Dry-powder inhalers

In dry-powder inhalers (DPIs), the drug is provided as a fine powder, in large aggregates, either alone or in combination with some carrier substance (Figs 9.14.5–6). The turbulent airstream created in the inhaler during inhalation causes the aggregates to break up into particles sufficiently small to be carried to the lower airways. A very low inspiratory flow rate will generally move the dose from the inhaler to the patient's mouth, with very little deposition in the intrapulmonary airways. The pattern of deposition depends on inspiratory airflow and varies from one inhaler to another. While optimal drug distribution is obtained with a slow (1–2 seconds) inhalation from a MDI, a *quick inspiration* is necessary with a DPI in order to break down the aggregates and render the powder respirable.

Spacer

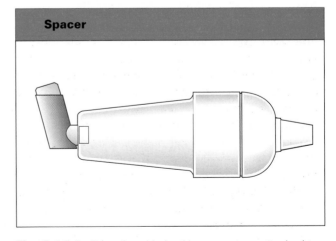

Fig. 9.14.4. Pear-shaped plastic cone spacer attached to a MDI.

Multi-dose dry-powder inhaler

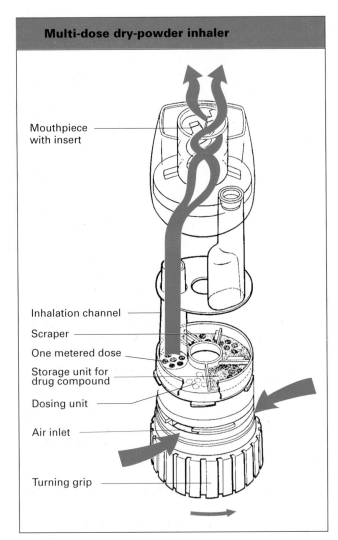

- Mouthpiece with insert
- Inhalation channel
- Scraper
- One metered dose
- Storage unit for drug compound
- Dosing unit
- Air inlet
- Turning grip

Fig. 9.14.5. A powder inhaler is a simple and physiological way to deliver drugs to the bronchi. This device (Turbuhaler), shown in a sectional diagram (airflow visualized), has two advantages. First, it contains only the active drug without any additives. Second, it is a multi-dose device with 200 doses.

The advantage of DPIs is that the *patient does not need to coordinate* actuation of the inhaler with inhalation. DPIs are as effective as MDIs and they are gaining in popularity because they do not contain freon gases or lubricants.

Nebulized wet aerosols

A bronchodilator can be delivered as an aqueous aerosol from an electric nebulizer and this is now the first choice of therapy for *acute severe asthma*. Patients often like to inhale the mist, which moistens their dry mucous membranes and does not require

Diskus inhaler

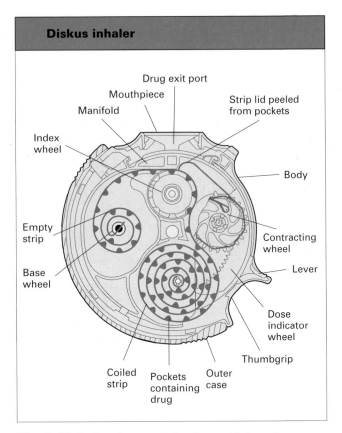

- Drug exit port
- Mouthpiece
- Manifold
- Index wheel
- Strip lid peeled from pockets
- Body
- Empty strip
- Contracting wheel
- Base wheel
- Lever
- Dose indicator wheel
- Thumbgrip
- Coiled strip
- Pockets containing drug
- Outer case

Fig. 9.14.6. Another example of a multi-dose dry powder inhaler is the Diskus inhaler. It contains 60 doses of drug suspended in lactose, individually foil-blister packaged.

them to change their respiration pattern during medication. The wet aerosol has a clear advantage over a MDI, when the latter causes irritation and cough in hyper-reactive and infected airways.

The dose delivered as a wet aerosol is many times larger than that given by a MDI and a DPI. It is a disadvantage that the dosing is imprecise because the amount of nebulized drug reaching the lower airways depends upon the size of the aerosol particles. This varies considerably from apparatus to apparatus and also depends on whether a mouthpiece or a face mask, with partial nasal deposition, is used. The electric nebulizer pump and the solution required are expensive, and the inhalation takes time.

Patient compliance?
Good medicine always has a bitter taste.

Japanese proverb

9.15 Steroids in asthma I
Modes of action

Key points
- Corticosteroids have a broad anti-inflammatory action, which is the main reason for their beneficial effect in asthma.
- This action is based on a change of cellular protein synthesis, induced by a steroid–receptor complex.
- An example is the synthesis of the protein, lipocortin, which inhibits the generation of arachidonic acid metabolites (PGs and LTs).
- Steroids reduce the number of circulating eosinophils, basophils, monocytes and, to a lesser degree, CD4+ T helper cells.
- Steroids inhibit the function of macrophages, Langerhans' cells and, in particular, T cells, including Th2 cell production of IL-3, IL-4 and IL-5.
- Steroids have little or no direct effect on degranulation of mast cells and eosinophils or mediator release.
- Secondary to an effect on T cells and adhesion molecules, steroids markedly reduce eosinophil accumulation and activation.
- While steroids have a marked effect on the late bronchial response to allergen challenge, they have less effect on the early response.
- Long-term inhaled therapy reduces non-specific bronchial responsiveness.

The natural corticosteroid, cortisol (hydrocortisone), has equal *glucocorticoid* and *mineralocorticoid* effects. The glucocorticoid effect is intimately connected to an anti-inflammatory activity, and steroid molecules, having this effect, are therefore referred to as *glucocorticosteroids*, *glucocorticoids*, or simply *steroids*.

Glucocorticoid receptor
Corticosteroids exert their effects via a specific *cytoplasmatic receptor* (Fig. 9.15.1). The potency of the various synthetic glucocorticoids correlates with their affinity for this glucocorticoid receptor. The receptor–hormone complex modifies gene transcription and induces a *change of protein synthesis* in the cell; this is responsible for the tissue effects. Consequently, the clinical response to treatment is delayed for some hours (Fig. 9.15.2).

As glucocorticoid receptors are found in most cells and are of one subtype, it follows that topical appli-

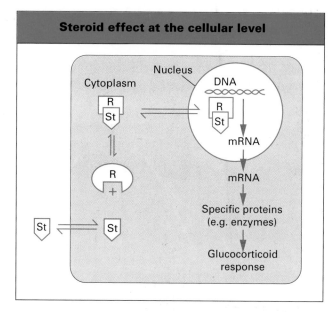

Fig. 9.15.1. The steroid molecule (St) penetrates the cell membrane and binds to a cytoplasmic glucocorticoid receptor (R). The receptor–hormone complex moves to the cell nucleus, binds to a specific sequence of the DNA (glucocorticoid responsive element), and interacts with gene transcription. This can be increased or decreased. The DNA sequence is, via messenger RNA, translated into an amino acid sequence in a protein molecule. The enhanced (or reduced) protein synthesis is considered to be responsible for most steroid effects.

cation of glucocorticoids is the only means of limiting the effects to a desired target organ.

The number of glucocorticoid receptors can, in both patients and healthy subjects, be reduced by glucocorticoid administration. However, clinical studies have not indicated any development of tolerance to therapy in asthma.

Effect on inflammatory cells
(Table 9.15.1)

Circulating cell numbers
Systemic administration of glucocorticoids causes marked changes in circulating leucocyte numbers. Most striking of these changes is a fall in the number of *eosinophils, basophils and monocytes* to approximately 20% of normal. Recirculating lymphocyte numbers also fall but not so dramatically. Among T cells, steroids cause a fall in helper (CD4+) but not cytotoxic (CD8+) cell numbers.

Macrophages and Langerhans' cells
Macrophages/monocytes are *highly sensitive* to

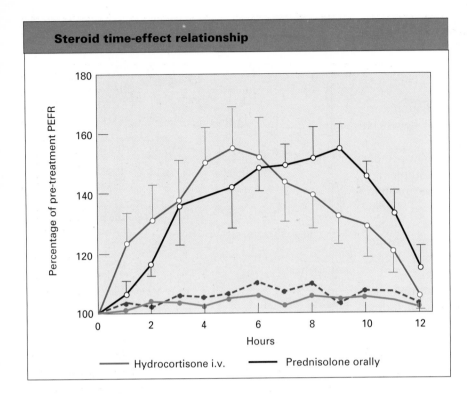

Steroid time-effect relationship

Hydrocortisone i.v.   Prednisolone orally

Fig. 9.15.2. Time course of response to 200 mg hydrocortisone intravenously, 40 mg prednisolone orally, and placebo in eight patients with stable asthma (mean ± SEM). The curve for inhaled steroid is in an intermediary position. From Ellul-Michalef R. The acute effects of corticosteroids in bronchial asthma. *Eur J Respir Dis* 1982; **63**(suppl 122): 118–25.

Table 9.15.1. Effects of glucocorticoids on inflammatory cells

Steroid effects on inflammatory cells

Cell	Effects of glucocorticoid
Macrophage	Marked inhibition of generation of inflammatory mediators and cytokines
T cell	Marked inhibition of proliferation and cytokine generation
Mast cell	No effect on IgE-mediated degranulation Topical therapy reduces the number of epithelial mast cells
Eosinophil	Minimal effect on degranulation and secretion Inhibition of cytokine effects on eosinophils Markedly reduced number in airways and blood
Neutrophil	Generally minimal effects Treatment with oral steroids results in modest neutrophilia
Endothelial cell	Reduced microvascular leakage

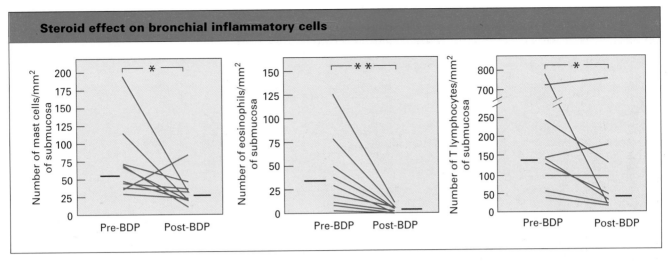

Steroid effect on bronchial inflammatory cells

Fig. 9.15.3. The effect of inhaled beclomethasone dipropionate (BDP) on mast cell, eosinophil and T lymphocyte numbers in the submucosa of atopic asthmatic individuals (*$p < 0.05$; **$p < 0.01$). From Djukanovic K. Bronchial biopsies. In: Busse WW, Holgate ST, eds. *Asthma and Rhinitis* Oxford: Blackwell Science, 1995: 118–29.

steroids, which reduce the number of cells, and inhibit their phagocytic capability and their synthesis of mediators and secretory response. An important consequence of the inhibition of macrophage function (and synthesis of IL-1) may be a switching off of T cell activation. Steroids reduce the number of Langerhans' cells.

T cells

T cells are also *very sensitive* to glucocorticoids, which inhibit T cell proliferation partly by reducing the production of the T-cell growth factor, IL-2. Recent evidence indicates that steroid treatment in the human airways *inhibits the activation of Th2 cells* and their synthesis of IL-3, IL-4 and IL-5.

Mast cells

Many studies have shown that glucocorticoids do not inhibit the IgE-dependent release of mediators from mast cells. Prolonged topical treatment in the airways, however, results in a *reduced number* of cells at the epithelial surface. This may be part of the explanation as to why inhaled steroids reduce the early response to allergen challenge.

Eosinophils

Glucocorticoids have little effect on eosinophil degranulation and secretion, but they have a *marked effect on the number* of eosinophils in blood and tissue (Fig. 9.15.3). The eosinophil response to steroids is likely to be indirect, by a reduced release of Th2 cytokines.

Endothelial cells

Many of the inflammatory mediators, including histamine, leukotrienes, PAF and substance P, implicated in asthma, cause airway microvascular leakage and submucosal oedema. A reduction in the level of these mediators is probably the reason why steroid treatment *reduces microvascular leakage*.

Allergen challenge

A single dose of a steroid has no effect on the *early response* to allergen, but the effect of the allergen will be reduced by treatment lasting for days or weeks (Fig. 9.15.4). The *late response* is *inhibited very efficiently* by a single dose of steroid.

It is in accordance with the modern concept of asthma as an inflammatory disease that the clinically highly efficient, anti-inflammatory steroids have a relatively poor effect on the early spasmodic response and a pronounced effect on the late inflammatory response.

Non-specific responsiveness

Clinical experience indicates that non-specific bronchial reactivity can be reduced by glucocorticoid treatment. This has been confirmed by exercise testing and histamine/methacholine provocation tests (Fig. 9.15.5). Treatment for some months is necessary to obtain maximal effect. At conventional therapeutic dosage, inhaled steroids can reduce bronchial hyper-responsiveness to a greater extent than can oral treatment.

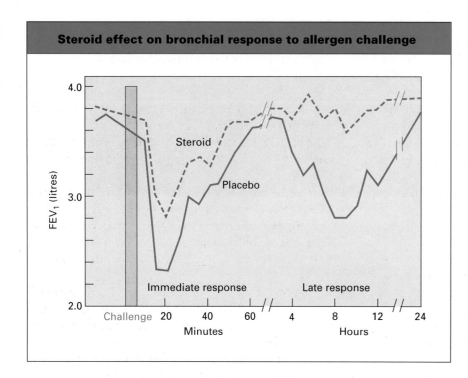

Fig. 9.15.4. Bronchial response to allergen inhalation challenge after inhaled steroid and placebo pretreatment for 2 weeks.

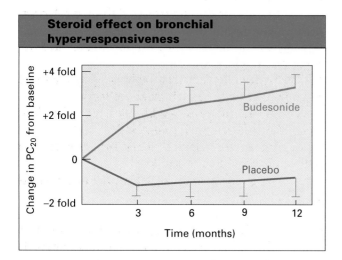

Fig. 9.15.5. Changes in PC_{20} methacholine at 3, 6, 9 and 12 months in patients with mild asthma treated with either inhaled budesonide 400 µg/day or placebo. From Juniper EF, Kline PA, Vanzieleghem MA, *et al.* Effect of long-term treatment with an inhaled corticosteroid (budesonide) on airway hyperresponsiveness and clinical asthma in nonsteroid dependent asthmatics. *Am Rev Respir Dis* 1990; **142**: 832–6.

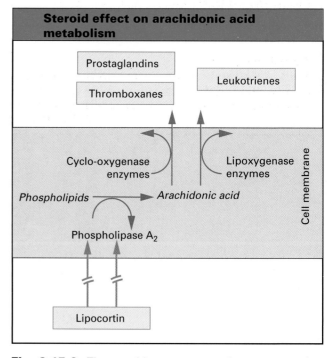

Fig. 9.15.6. The steroid–receptor complex generates the formation of a protein, lipocortin, which inhibits the enzyme phospholipase A_2 and thereby the formation of membrane-derived mediators.

Secretions
Clinical experience indicates that steroids are of importance for expectoration of the viscous mucus in asthma. A reduced quantity of mediators, which act as secretagogues, is probably part of the explanation.

Lipocortin
The steroid–receptor complex induces the synthesis of lipocortin, which, by an anti-phospholipase effect, prevents the synthesis of arachidonic acid and its metabolites, *prostaglandins and leukotrienes* (Fig. 9.15.6).

Permissive effect
Steroids have no direct effect on airway smooth muscles. They may, however, be important in maintaining a normal response to beta$_2$ adrenergic stimulation. They prevent the drug-induced down-regulation of pulmonary beta$_2$ receptors. Probably, this 'permissive effect' of steroids is beneficial in status asthmaticus.

Postgraduate education
I didn't start to learn anything until I had finished my studies.

Anatole France

The retired teacher
The teacher's life should have three periods, study until 25, investigation until 40, profession until 60, at which age I would have him retired on a double allowance.

William Osler

9.16 Steroids in asthma II
Systemic administration

Key points
- Prednisolone is preferable for oral use and methyl-prednisolone for intravenous use.
- A steroid reversibility test can be used to show steroid responsiveness and to define the patient's best lung function.
- Objective measurements of lung function are absolutely necessary to demonstrate the effect.
- Long-term therapy is always associated with adverse effects and it is used as the last resort.
- It can be given once daily or as alternate-day therapy.
- Short-term therapy (2 weeks), carrying a very small risk of adverse effects, can abort acute severe asthma.
- Short-term, in contrast to long-term, therapy can be used liberally.
- Early use of systemic steroids is an important part of management of acute severe asthma.
- In children, inhibition of growth is the most serious adverse effect.
- In adults, it is osteoporosis with painful compression fractures.
- Weight gain and Cushingoid appearance are frequent and unpleasant.
- Development of diabetes mellitus, glaucoma and cataract are also potential adverse effects.
- Steroids do not cause peptic ulcer complications unless they are given with an NSAID.
- Suppression of the hypothalamo-pituitary–adrenal (HPA) axis is seldom a problem.
- Knowledge of 'steroid withdrawal symptoms' is important.

Glucocorticoids are four-ring, 21-carbon molecules (Fig. 9.16.1). Their detailed structure determines: 1, the ratio between glucocorticoid and mineralocorticoid effects; 2, their affinity for the glucocorticoid receptor; and 3, their metabolism, of particular importance for the separation between topical and systemic activities.

Preparations
Systemic administration can be oral, intravenous or a depot-injection, but it is generally agreed that the latter should not be used for asthma. A number of preparations are available (Table 9.16.1).
Prednisolone and prednisone are the most fre-

quently used oral preparations; they are cheap and have little mineralocorticoid effect. Prednisolone is, in principle, preferable to prednisone, which needs to be metabolized in the liver to the active prednisolone. When large intravenous doses are used, *methylprednisolone*, which has virtually no mineralocorticoid effect, is preferable to hydrocortisone as the latter has equal glycocorticoid and mineralocorticoid effects.

Use of systemic steroids

Different types of regimens can be used (Fig. 9.16.2). It is important to realize that while *long-term therapy* is always associated with a considerable risk of serious adverse effects, *short-term therapy* can be given almost without risk.

Steroid reversibility test

A steroid reversibility test is indicated in a patient with chronic airway obstruction when normal lung function cannot be attained with a bronchodilator. It serves two purposes: 1, to demonstrate steroid responsiveness; and 2, to define the patient's optimal lung function, which is the goal for subsequent treatment.

Test medication usually consists of oral prednisolone, for example 20 mg/day for 2 weeks. As oral steroids usually give *a feeling of well-being*, measurement of lung function is necessary in order to avoid a false positive result. *Spirometry*, including beta$_2$ reversibility, is carried out before and after treatment. *PEF is measured daily* during therapy, for 1 week before and for 1 week after.

Continuous corticosteroid therapy should only be given when a significant ($\geq$20%) increase in lung function can be demonstrated.

It is important to start the trial with the patient *in a stable period*. A 'steroid reversibility test', started in hospital during recovery from a recent exacerbation, cannot be relied upon, as improvement of

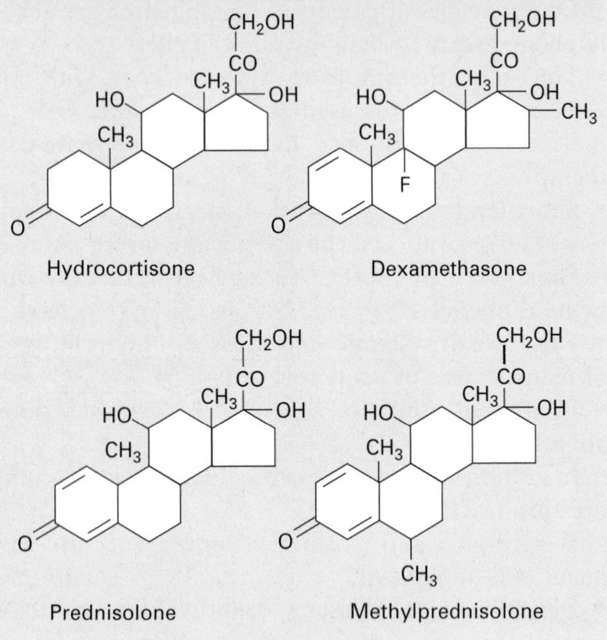

Fig. 9.16.1. Chemical structure of some glucocorticoids for systemic use.

Characteristics of some corticosteroids			
Preparation	**Equivalent dose* (mg)**	**Sodium retaining potency**	**Plasma half-life (min)**
Hydrocortisone	20	1	90
Prednisone	5	0.8	90
Prednisolone	5	0.8	200
Methylprednisolone	4	0.25	200
Triamcinolone	4	(0)	200
Dexamethasone	0.75	(0)	300
Betamethasone	0.6	(0)	300

Table 9.16.1. Characteristics of some commonly used corticosteroids. *Refers to anti-inflammatory activity

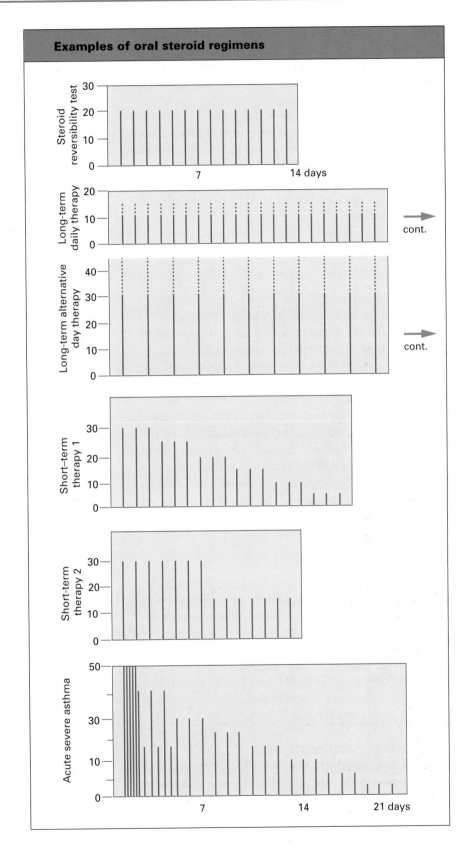

Fig. 9.16.2. Different regimens for oral steroid administration (see text).

lung function can be expected even without steroid treatment.

Patients who clinically have *asthma* will respond to glucocorticoids with the exception of some 1% who appear to be steroid-resistant.

When uncertain as to whether the patient has *asthma or COPD*, the following points are indicative of a positive response to steroid: 1, no history of tobacco smoking; 2, marked PEF variation; 3, a clear response ($\geq 20\%$) to a beta$_2$ agonist; 4, positive skin prick test to aero-allergens; and 5, eosinophilia in blood or sputum.

Long-term therapy

Indications

Oral steroids are considered when normal lung function cannot be maintained by any other means. It is not clear why some patients with severe disease need oral steroids in addition to high-dose inhaled therapy. It is a theoretical possibility that peribronchial inflammation is counteracted by systemic and not by inhaled treatment.

While steroids are best used initially in high rather than low dosage, the maintenance dose should be the lowest possible that can *control the disease*. Both patient and doctor should realize that the dose must follow the changing severity of the disease and be *reduced whenever possible*. The potential benefit of oral treatment must always be carefully balanced against the risk of adverse effects.

Daily corticosteroids

Most asthma patients, who need prednisolone, can be controlled by 10–15 mg daily. A few patients will require higher doses and they need close contact with a specialist unit.

The frequency of medication is kept low in order to minimize the effect on the hypothalamo-pituitary–adrenal (HPA) axis. This adverse effect is least when the drug is given as a single dose *in the morning* rather than in the evening.

Alternate-day corticosteroids

Some adverse reactions, that is, HPA suppression and growth inhibition, are significantly reduced when oral steroids are given in the morning on alternate days only. The total dose needs to be about 50% higher than in daily therapy. In some patients with stable asthma, alternate-day administration of prednisolone may improve the ratio between anti-asth-

matic and adverse effects, but it is unsatisfactory in patients with unstable disease. Daily medication is generally used in Europe and alternate-day treatment in the USA.

Short-term therapy

While long-term oral treatment always carries a risk of adverse effects, this risk is very small when short-term treatment (2 weeks) is given no more than six times a year. Many asthmatics know when their disease is going to deteriorate (e.g. during a cold), and the prompt use of oral steroids can often abort a severe attack. The patient can, for example, start on 30 mg prednisolone a day with 5 mg reduction every third day, or use 30 mg/day until control is obtained and then 15 mg/day for a similar number of days. There is less risk in allowing patients to start their own steroid treatment, getting it confirmed by their doctor the next day, than in not making steroids available to them until the attack is severe enough to bring them to the hospital.

Acute severe asthma

Use of systemic corticosteroids is considered to be essential for the management of status asthmaticus. There are, however, no precise guidelines for the dosage and route of administration. At present, it is common practice to give intravenously either 200 mg hydrocortisone (3 mg/kg body weight), or preferably, *40 mg methylprednisolone every 6–8 hours.*

Once a satisfactory response is obtained, usually after 1–2 days, the intravenous medication is changed to *oral prednisolone, 40–60 mg daily*. These high daily doses are preferably given in two divided doses, although an evening dose may disturb the sleep. Depending on the patient's condition, the treatment can be *tapered off over 2–4 weeks*. The introduction of high-dose inhaled steroids, started as early as possible, reduces the length of prednisolone treatment.

Adverse effects

As the glucocorticoid receptor is present in most cells, systemic therapy is inevitably associated with a risk of adverse effects (Figs 9.16.3–4). The following discussion will deal with 10–15 mg prednisolone/day or less, which is the dosage used by most steroid-requiring asthmatics.

Cushingoid appearance

Skin changes and *changed appearance*, consisting of 'moon face', 'buffalo hump', central obesity, striae,

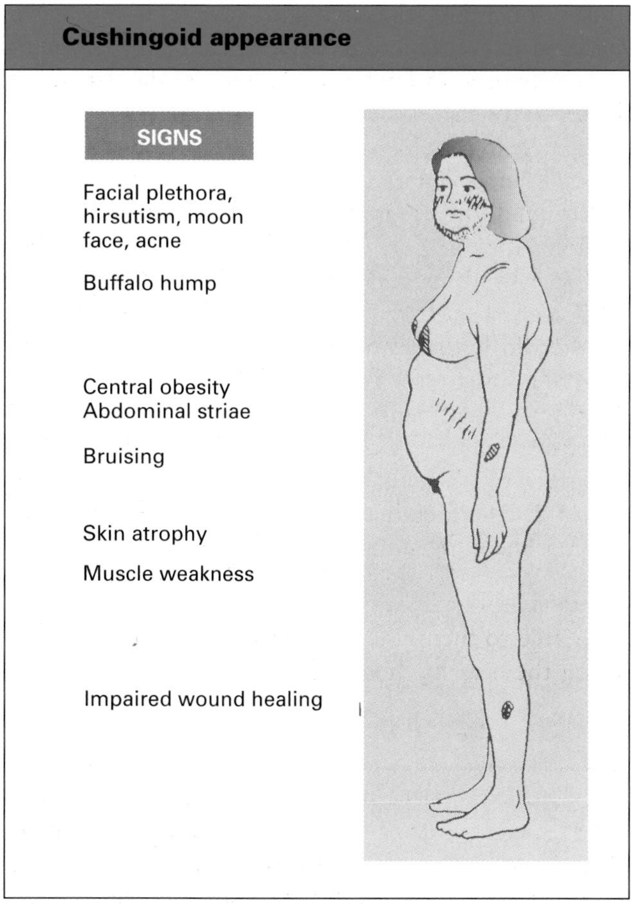

Cushingoid appearance

SIGNS

Facial plethora,
hirsutism, moon
face, acne

Buffalo hump

Central obesity
Abdominal striae

Bruising

Skin atrophy

Muscle weakness

Impaired wound healing

Fig. 9.16.3. Signs of glucocorticoid excess. Idea by Robert P Schleimer, Johns Hopkins University.

ecchymoses, acne and hirsutism, are well-known side effects.

Weight gain

Increase in weight is *the most common adverse effect*. Patients must be warned of the increase in appetite before treatment is started and be encouraged to avoid increasing their caloric intake.

Growth inhibition

Inhibition of growth will occur when children are continuously treated with systemic steroids. Growth inhibition is partly avoided by alternate-day steroids (and completely by inhaled steroids).

Osteoporosis

This is a frequent and often troublesome adverse effect from long-term therapy. It is particularly so in *post-menopausal women*, who often get very painful *compression fractures of the vertebrae*, even from small doses of oral steroid.

Diabetes mellitus

Glucocorticoids have an *anti-insulin action*. Transient glucosuria can occur in non-diabetic subjects and latent diabetes can become manifest. Insulin requirement will increase in diabetic patients, and prednisolone weaning is complicated by frequent changes of insulin dosage.

Fig. 9.16.4. Comparison of incidence of adverse effects in steroid-treated and control groups. 2HPPBS, 2-hour postprandial blood sugar. From Lieberman P, Patterson R, Kunske R. Complications of long-term steroid therapy for asthma. *J Allergy Clin Immunol* 1972; **49**: 329–36.

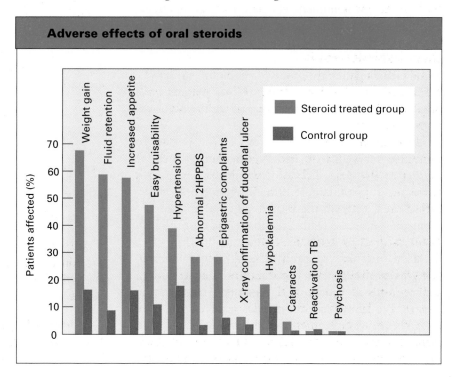

Adverse effects of oral steroids

Eye diseases

Steroid-induced *glaucoma*, *cataract* and reactivation of *herpes keratitis* can occur. Glaucoma is a risk even after short-term therapy in predisposed subjects. Cataract, of the posterior subcapsular type, develops after years of treatment as the risk is proportional to the total consumption of steroid.

Mental changes

Mental changes can occur during steroid therapy but they are reversible. In predisposed patients, steroid therapy can even provoke *psychotic episodes*. *Sleeplessness* is often a problem when an evening dose is given.

Hypertension and oedema

Prednisolone in low doses has little effect on blood pressure and tissue fluid.

Peptic ulcer

Epigastric complaints can occur during oral steroid therapy. The frequency of peptic ulcer is doubled but *only in patients on NSAIDs*. The usual asthma dosage can *mask the symptoms* of perforation. An H$_2$-blocker is recommended when predisposed patients are treated with oral steroids.

Reactivation of tuberculosis

The balance between host defence and tubercle bacteria is negatively influenced by steroids, and patients who have had tuberculosis should be checked at regular intervals. The risk of reactivation is, however, very small, and it is rarely necessary to give prophylactic isoniazid therapy.

Prednisolone, 10–15 mg/day, has no demonstrable adverse effects on other bacterial or viral infections.

Suppression of the HPA axis

Any exogenous glucocorticoid dosage will *reduce the endogenous release* of corticotrophin-releasing factor from the hypothalamus, adrenocorticotrophic hormone (ACTH) from the pituitary gland and cortisol from the adrenals. Daily treatment for more than *2 months* can also result in significant impairment of the HPA *response to stress*. The suppression of the HPA axis is reversible, but it can take up to a year before normal function is regained. During that period exogenous corticosteroids can, in the rare case, be necessary in stress situations (e.g. fever, accidents and surgery). After treatment with high doses for years, the changes may, in a few cases, become irreversible due to *atrophy of the adrenals*.

Steroid withdrawal symptoms

Oral steroid therapy will often, initially, give a feeling of well-being, mentally and physically. When therapy is stopped the opposite symptoms occur: malaise, fatigue, mental depression, myalgia and arthralgia. These symptoms can last for some weeks and it is important to inform the patient about the existence of 'steroid withdrawal symptoms'.

While short-term therapy can be stopped abruptly, long-term treatment should be discontinued gradually over some weeks. The problems during steroid weaning of an asthmatic are: 1, withdrawal symptoms; 2, a serious deterioration of the bronchial disease; 3, the unmasking of rhinitis and dermatitis; and, in the very rare case, 4, the risk of an Addisonian crisis. When patients have used prednisolone for years, weaning must be very slow under 10 mg/day, as this dose is equivalent to the normal production of cortisol.

Prednisolone for chronic bronchitis
Every hospital should have a plaque in the physicians' entrance: There are some patients whom we cannot help – there are none whom we cannot harm.

Arthur L Bloomfield

9.17 Steroids in asthma III
Inhaled treatment

Key points
- Inhaled beclomethasone dipropionate, budesonide, fluticasone propionate and others separate anti-asthmatic from systemic activity.
- This is because they have high affinity for the glucocorticoid receptor and are subjected to first-pass hepatic deactivation.
- They can be delivered from DPIs and from MDIs with a spacer attached.
- Low-dose therapy, 0.2–1 mg/day, carries no significant risk of systemic adverse effects.
- High-dose therapy, 1.2–2 mg/day, carries a small risk.
- Treatment is highly effective and inhalation of 1 mg equals about 40 mg prednisolone.
- It may take 3 months before full efficacy, for example inhibition of exercise-induced asthma, is attained.
- Oral candidiasis and horseness are local side effects, prevented by mouthwash and use of a spacer.
- Preventive therapy with inhaled steroids is now considered to be the most important part of asthma management.

Early attempts to use corticosteroids topically in the airways failed. Hydrocortisone and prednisolone were ineffective, and dexamethasone had equal local and systemic activity. The situation changed fundamentally when *beclomethasone dipropionate* was introduced as an aerosol in 1972 (Fig. 9.17.1).

Two qualities are responsible for the success of beclomethasone dipropionate: 1, in contrast to hydrocortisone and prednisolone, it has a *high affinity for the glucocorticoid receptor* and, consequently, a high anti-inflammatory potency, necessary when a small inhaled dose is distributed over a large surface; 2, in contrast to dexamethasone, the portion swallowed (80–90% of the inhaled dose) is subjected to *first-pass deactivation* in the liver before reaching the systemic circulation.

Thus, in comparison with the earlier steroid molecules, inhaled beclomethasone dipropionate *separates anti-asthmatic and unwanted systemic activities*. A convincing evidence for this is the reactivation of rhinitis and dermatitis in some asthma patients when they were transferred from oral to inhaled therapy. Evidence, based on more precise and quantitative data, has been provided for another topical steroid, budesonide. Inhaled budesonide, 1 mg/day, has the same systemic activity as oral prednisolone, 4 mg/day, but an anti-asthma effect equal to that of 40 mg.

Compounds
Beclomethasone dipropionate has now been used world wide for more than 20 years. The next steroid introduced was *budesonide*, which is a non-halogenated glucocorticoid molecule. It is slightly more potent than beclomethasone dipropionate and is more completely metabolized in the liver. The systemic activity of an equipotent dose is reduced by about one-third. This drug is not yet on the market in the USA where *triamcinolone acetonide* and *flunisolide* have been introduced. More recently, *fluticasone propionate* became available. It is twice as potent as beclomethasone dipropionate and has significantly less systemic activity.

Delivery systems
The steroid is traditionally delivered as an *aerosol* from a MDI. A *spacer*, attached to the MDI (see Fig. 9.14.5), has the advantage of less steroid being deposited in the mouth and throat. *Dry-powder inhalers* are now available for most steroid molecules, and they are increasingly used. A DPI has the advantage, as with the spacer device, that it can be used by patients who fail to coordinate actuation and inhalation.

Dosage
Low-dose therapy twice, 0.2–1 mg/day in adults and half the dose in children, is given *twice daily*. Even once daily may suffice when 0.2–0.4 mg/day is used for mild asthma. It is an advantage that the inhaler can be kept at home and, preferably, be used in the bathroom immediately before toothbrushing. Gargling and spitting immediately after the inhalation will reduce the amount of steroid swallowed and absorbed.

High-dose therapy (1.2–2.0 mg/day) is used in patients with moderate–severe disease, as there exists a log–dose–response relationship (Fig. 9.17.2). It is highly effective and can, in most patients, completely replace oral steroids. High–dose therapy should always be given from a spacer, or as a DPI, in order to reduce local side effects. While twice-daily inhalation

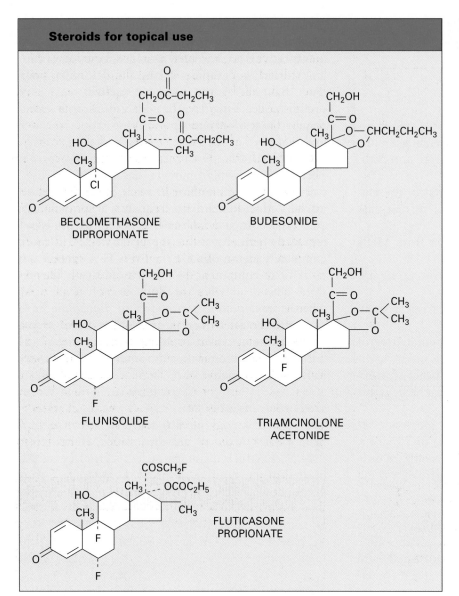

Steroids for topical use

BECLOMETHASONE DIPROPIONATE

BUDESONIDE

FLUNISOLIDE

TRIAMCINOLONE ACETONIDE

FLUTICASONE PROPIONATE

Fig. 9.17.1. Chemical structure of glucocorticoids for topical application. They are 16α-, 17α- or 17α-, 21α-ester derivatives of hydrocortisone. The ester side chains are readily cleaved in the liver following absorption and this dramatically reduces systemic effects.

is sufficient in stable asthma, it may be beneficial to use the inhaler three to four times a day in unstable periods.

Efficacy

Inhaled steroids are the most reliable anti-inflammatory agents for the treatment of asthma, and they are predictably effective. It is important for both the patient and the doctor to realize the effectiveness, potency and protection offered by the inhaler. Abrupt discontinuation of high-dose inhaled treatment can be dangerous as asthma control may then be lost.

The effects of inhaled steroids can be summarized as follows: 1, reduction of daily and nocturnal asthma symptoms, starting after a few days and developing further over months (Fig. 9.17.3); 2, improvement of lung function and peak flow recordings; 3, reduced hyper-responsiveness and increased tolerance to exercise and other non-specific, as well as specific, stimuli (see Fig. 9.15.5); 4, reduced risk of exacerbation, acute severe asthma and death; 5, reduction or elimination of the excessive dependence on inhaled beta$_2$ agonists; and 6, reduced need for regular or intermittent oral steroid therapy.

Additional use of systemic steroids

Patients on inhaled steroids may need short courses

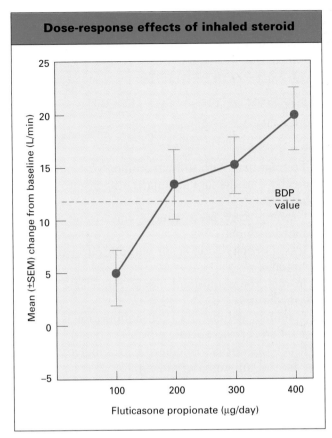

Fig. 9.17.2. Change of morning PEF from baseline (mean ± SEM) for groups of asthma patients (*n* = 125–133) treated with fluticasone propionate, 100–800 μg/day for 4 weeks, and compared with the mean value for those treated with beclomethasone dipropionate (BDP), 400 μg/day for 4 weeks. From Dahl R, Lundbäck B, Malo J-L, *et al.* A dose-ranging study of fluticasone propionate in adult patients with moderate asthma. *Chest* 1993; **104**: 1352–8.

of systemic steroids during acute exacerbations. They should have prednisolone tablets, which are to be taken if severe bronchoconstriction or infection with excessive coughing may compromise proper inhalation of the steroid.

In acute severe asthma, the penetration and effect of inhaled steroids is uncertain, but treatment should not be discontinued while oral steroids are given.

Side effects

Immediate *cough and irritation* can occur in patients with sensitive mucous membranes. It can be reduced by use of a DPI instead of a freon-propelled MDI containing irritating lubricants.

Candidiasis in the mouth and throat will occur in at least 10% of the patients when a MDI is used directly in the mouth. The risk increases with the daily dosage and with the frequency of spraying. The infection can be prevented by regular mouthwashing immediately after spraying and the risk is considerably reduced by the use of a spacer or a DPI. Candidiasis is easily treated with a local antimycotic. It may be necessary, temporarily, to reduce the steroid dosage, but it is unnecessary and dangerous to stop inhaled steroid treatment as asthma control may then be lost.

Hoarseness is, like thrush, a side effect that relates to the steroid dose and the frequency of spraying. It is not caused by candidiasis but is due to a steroid-induced myopathy of the laryngeal muscles. It can be prevented by use of a DPI but not by a spacer; it is usually intermittent and it is not progressive. Chronic voice stress and colds are contributing factors; treatment is voice rest.

Concern is often expressed about the risk of serious damage to lung tissue from long-term therapy. There are some cogent counter arguments: 1, patients with Cushing's syndrome have damage to the skin and other tissues but not of the lungs; 2, human biopsy studies have not disclosed any significant changes in bronchial histology after some years' treatment; 3, the airway mucosa of the nose, which, compared to

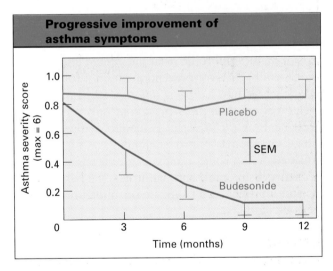

Fig. 9.17.3. Changes in the asthma severity score (assessed from patient questionnaire) at 3, 6, 9 and 12 months. By 12 months, symptoms were reduced to near-zero in the budesonide-treated group. From Juniper EF, Kline PA, Vanzieleghem MA, *et al.* Effect of long-term treatment with an inhaled corticosteroid (budesonide) on airway hyperresponsiveness and clinical asthma in nonsteroid dependent asthmatics. *Am Rev Respir Dis* 1990; **142**: 832–6.

that of the bronchi, receives a much higher dose of steroid, shows no obvious signs of damage following nasal steroid medication; and 4, the most convincing counter argument is that inhaled steroids have now been used for many million patient-years without reports of serious adverse effects.

No data or observations indicate that inhaled steroid treatment increases the risk or the severity of airway infections with viruses, bacteria or fungi, and treatment should not be stopped during acute infections.

Systemic side effects may occur during high-dose therapy but they are usually mild. Thinning of the skin, increased prevalence of bruising and skin bleedings have been observed. It is difficult, with certainty, to say that there is no risk of osteoporosis in elderly patients, but it has definitely not been the clinical problem that it has been with oral steroid. When the indication for use of inhaled steroids in a high dose is correct and the lowest effective dose is given, then there is little doubt that the benefit for the patient by far outweighs the small risk of systemic side effects. If, on the other hand, for example, a little, elderly, cigarette-smoking lady with COPD received high-dose inhaled steroid therapy for years, the negative aspects of treatment may very well outweigh the positive aspects (which may be non-existent).

Patient instruction

It is of major importance that the patient understands that the inhaler is for prevention and not for immediate relief. While a *bronchodilator spray* is for the treatment of *symptoms*, a *steroid spray* is for the treatment of the *disease*. Although symptoms and lung function may improve after days or a few weeks, it usually takes some months before bronchial hypersensitivity is reduced and, with that, the risk of acute episodes provoked by exercise or inhalation of allergens or irritants.

> **True for asthma**
> Stop it at the start, it is late for medicine to be prepared when disease has grown strong enough through long delays.
>
> Ovid, 43 BC–AD 17
> *Remedia Amoris*

9.18 Cromoglycate in asthma
Non-steroidal anti-inflammatory treatment

Key points
- Pretreatment with sodium cromoglycate attenuates the early and the late asthmatic response to allergen inhalation.
- Cromoglycate pretreatment ameliorates exercise-induced asthma.
- It is a prophylactic agent without effect on actual symptoms.
- In rats, the compound blocks the release of mast cell mediators.
- In human asthma, mast cell stabilization is unlikely to explain the therapeutic efficacy.
- It is more correct to consider cromoglycate as being an anti-inflammatory agent.
- Cromoglycate is inhaled as a powder, from a MDI, or as a nebulized solution.
- It can be used either occasionally before allergen exposure and exercise, or on a regular basis four times daily.
- It is usually clinically effective in young allergic patients with mild to moderate asthma.
- The effect is poor in non-allergic asthma and in chronic severe asthma.
- Cromoglycate is very safe, but it is clearly less effective than inhaled steroids.
- A new compound, nedocromil sodium also seems to be effective in some non-allergic, middle-aged patients.
- Other so-called 'anti-allergic compounds' (ketotifen and tranilast) are widely used in some countries.

Sodium cromoglycate (cromoglycate, cromolyn in the USA) was first shown to *inhibit the allergen-induced asthmatic response*. It was then discovered, in *in vivo* experiments in rats (passive cutaneous anaphylaxis), that the compound *blocks the release of mast cell mediators*.

However, mast cell stabilization is unlikely to explain the therapeutic efficacy of cromoglycate in the treatment of asthma because: 1, cromoglycate-induced stabilization of mast cells has not convincingly been shown in humans; 2, a series of compounds that are far more potent as mast cell stabilizers have failed to show therapeutic usefulness; and 3, cromoglycate has clinical effects that are probably independent of an action on mast cells − for example, the ability to inhibit bronchospasm induced by irritants, such as SO_2 and bradykinin, which are thought to act at the level of airway nerves.

It was subsequently shown that cromoglycate has an *inhibitory effect on sensory nerves*. Recent experiments have shown that the drug causes a dose-dependent inhibition of substance P, and neurokinin B-induced oedema in the human skin. It is therefore a reasonable hypothesis that cromoglycate possesses anti-inflammatory activity by acting as a tachykinin antagonist.

When cromoglycate was introduced in the 1960s, to provide a new principle for the *prophylactic treatment* of asthma, it was introduced as a *mast cell stabilizing agent*. Probably, it is now more correct to consider cromoglycate as being an *anti-inflammatory agent*.

Pharmacology and preparations

Cromoglycate (Fig. 9.18.1) does not pass cell membranes, is *poorly absorbed* from the gastro-intestinal tract and must be given by the inhaled route. It can be given in a *powder form* (20 mg four times daily), from a *metered-dose inhaler*, and as an aqueous solution delivered by a power-driven nebulizer; the latter is especially used for young children.

Allergen-induced asthma

Pretreatment with cromoglycate can attenuate both the *early* and the *late asthmatic response* to allergen inhalation (Fig. 9.18.2). It is sufficient to inhale the drug a few minutes *before* the challenge, the effect is maximal for 1–2 hours and has disappeared within 4–6 hours.

The clinical effect of cromoglycate in patients naturally exposed to aero-allergens in their environment is similar to that obtained under controlled laboratory conditions. This is convincingly shown by dander-allergic patients occasionally exposed to animals. Pretreatment will enable them to stay longer, with less symptoms, in a house with the animal in question. Dose and frequency of medication has to be adjusted to the individual need; a high degree of sensitivity and exposure necessitates frequent medication. Cromoglycate also provides protection against allergen exposure in the pollen season.

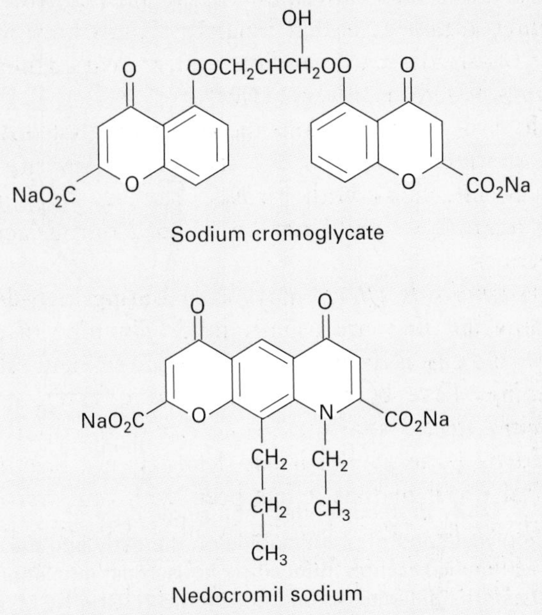

Fig. 9.18.1. Sodium cromoglycate and nedocromil sodium.

Exercise-induced asthma

Cromoglycate pretreatment ameliorates exercise-induced asthma. The onset of action is rapid, but the protective effect of the drug is short, and inhalation 15–30 minutes before exercise is necessary for maximum protection.

As exercise induces bronchoconstriction by cooling the bronchial mucosa, *hyperventilation with cold air* can be used as a precise means of simulating exercise. This thermal model has shown that cromoglycate produces a shift to the right in the stimulus–response curve, which means that, as the stimulus for bronchoconstriction increases, the protective effect of the drug can be overcome. Hence, a treatment schedule that permits a person with asthma to walk briskly on a cold winter day can become ineffective in protecting him or her from the consequences of exercise requiring higher ventilation, such as ice hockey or cross-country skiing. These activities usually necessitate the added use of a beta$_2$ inhaler.

Bronchial hyper-responsiveness

Cromoglycate may reduce the allergen-induced increase in non-specific bronchial responsiveness, for

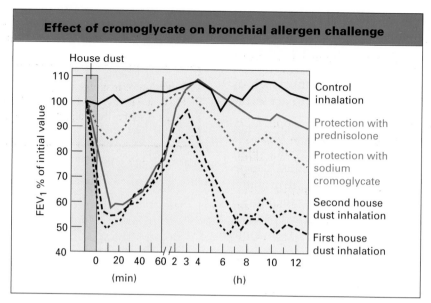

Fig. 9.18.2. Protective effect of a single dose of cromoglycate and of prednisolone on the early and the late asthmatic reaction induced by house dust inhalation in 10 asthma patients. From Booij-Noord H, Orie NGM, de Vries K. Immediate and late bronchial obstructive reactions to inhalation of house dust and protective effects of disodium cromoglycate and prednisolone. *J Allergy Clin Immunol* 1971; **48**: 344–8.

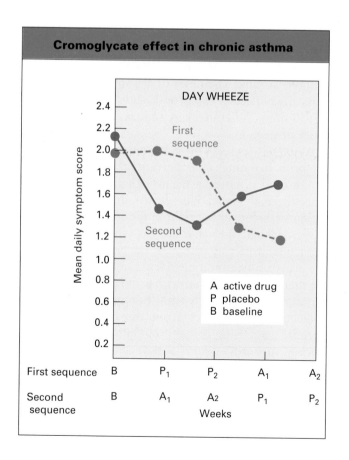

Fig. 9.18.3. Clinical effect of regular use of inhaled cromoglycate in 252 asthmatic patients. From Bernstein IL, Siegel SC, Brandon ML, *et al.* A controlled study of cromolyn sodium sponsored by the Drug Committee of the American Academy of Allergy. *J Allergy Clin Immunol* 1972; **50**: 235–45.

example during the pollen season. There is no evidence, however, that cromoglycate can reduce an already existing bronchial hyper-responsiveness as do inhaled corticosteroids.

Clinical use

Cromoglycate is used as a *first-line prophylactic agent*, either occasionally *before allergen exposure and exercise*, or on a regular basis four times daily. It has no or only a *poor effect in non-allergic asthma*, and it is of little help in chronic severe asthma. Usually, cromoglycate is effective in *young patients* with strong evidence of *allergy* and with *mild–moderate asthma*, but it is advisable always to *test the efficacy of the drug* in the individual patient.

Even in responders the effect on symptoms is merely moderate (Fig. 9.18.3), and cromoglycate is clearly less effective than inhaled steroids. As time has shown inhaled steroids, in low dosage, to be very safe, it is, in fact, difficult to define a place for cromoglycate in the management of chronic asthma. It is mainly used by those paediatricians who still have concern about the safety of inhaled steroids. It is unclear whether cromoglycate has a place in the treatment of patients with severe allergic disease, by limiting steroid dosage and thereby the risk of adverse effects.

The drug is *very safe*. It is usually poor patient compliance (due to low efficacy, high price, no immediate effect and medication four times daily) that is the objection to therapy.

New compounds

The mast cell stabilizing effect of cromoglycate, first demonstrated in rat skin, was later found to be both species and tissue specific. The drug has no effect in the guinea-pig, for example, or in human skin on connective tissue mast cells (MC_{TC}) or basophil leucocytes.

A new compound, *nedocromil sodium* (nedocromil), seems to act on both mast cell subsets (MT_T and MC_{TC}) and to have a better experimental effect than cromoglycate, for example on bradykinin-induced bronchoconstriction. This drug has equal efficacy in allergic and non-allergic asthma, but the degree of efficacy is similar to that obtained with cromoglycate.

So-called 'anti-allergic compounds' are widely used in some parts of the world: *tranilast* in Japan, and *ketotifen*, which also has antihistamine properties, in southern Europe and South America. Their precise mode of action remains uncertain.

Definition of man
The desire to take medicine is perhaps the greatest feature which distinguishes man from animals.

William Osler

9.19 Adrenoceptors and sympathomimetic bronchodilators
Alpha and beta$_2$ effects

Key points
- Alpha receptors dominate in vasculature and beta$_2$ receptors in bronchial smooth muscles.
- The predominant effect of alpha stimulation is vasoconstriction.
- Stimulation of beta$_1$ receptors, localized to the heart, increases the rate and force of contraction and the risk of arrhythmias.
- Beta$_2$ stimulation results in relaxation of bronchial smooth muscle, which is important in asthma.
- It also causes tremor and a shift of potassium from the extra- to the intracellular compartment.
- Adrenaline has equal alpha and beta effects, useful in anaphylactic shock and asthma.
- Modern asthma treatment requires beta$_2$ selective bronchodilators.
- Short-acting beta$_2$ agonists (salbutamol and terbutaline) can be given by any route.
- They are used as p.r.n. medication and for acute severe asthma, preferably by the inhaled route.
- The new long-acting beta$_2$ agonist inhalers (salmeterol and formoterol) are very efficient bronchodilators.

There are alpha and beta$_2$ adrenergic receptors in the smooth muscles surrounding blood vessels and the bronchial lumen. Alpha receptors dominate in vasculature and beta$_2$ receptors in bronchial smooth muscles. Stimulation of the adrenoceptor may be humoral, nervous or drug-induced (Fig. 9.19.1). Bronchial, in contrast to vascular, muscle possesses little or no sympathetic innervation, and the normal function of bronchial adrenoceptors is unknown.

Alpha adrenoceptors
Stimulation of alpha receptors, of which there now are seven subtypes, results in smooth muscle contraction. The predominant effect of alpha stimulation is vasoconstriction, so alpha agonists are used to treat *anaphylactic shock*, *angioedema* and *nasal obstruction*. Alpha stimulants do not play a significant role in asthma.

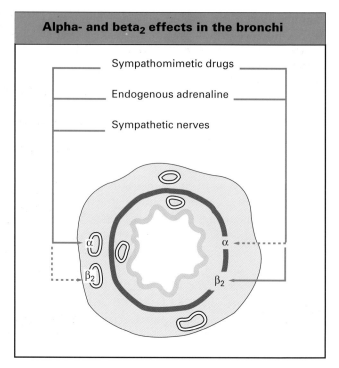

Alpha- and beta$_2$ effects in the bronchi

Sympathomimetic drugs

Endogenous adrenaline

Sympathetic nerves

Fig. 9.19.1. Stimulation of bronchial adrenoceptors. Beta$_2$ receptors, predominant in bronchial muscles, have a relaxing effect, while alpha receptors, predominant in vasculature, have a constricting effect.

Beta adrenoceptors

Beta$_1$
Beta$_1$ adrenoceptors are localized to *the heart*. Stimulation increases the rate and force of contraction and the risk of arrhythmias.

Beta$_2$
As described in Chapter 9.4, molecular biologists have, in the last decade, made considerable progress in the study of cell membrane receptors. The beta$_2$ receptor has been studied in great detail and its 415 amino acids have been sequenced. As this knowledge, so far, has not given clinical results, the description of the beta$_2$ receptor below will be overly simplistic.

The beta$_2$ receptor is part of the adenylate cyclase system, stimulation of which increases cyclic AMP. Relaxation of *bronchial smooth muscle* is the important result in asthma. There is experimental evidence that beta$_2$ agonists have other effects in the airways but they are probably of little clinical significance (Table 9.19.1).

Beta$_2$ agonists *dilate blood vessels*, so a high oral or parenteral dosage often results in a small fall in blood

Table 9.19.1. Effects of adrenoceptor stimulation related to the treatment of asthma. Parentheses indicate effects of little or unknown clinical significance

Adrenoceptor effects			
	Alpha	**Beta₁**	**Beta₂**
Bronchial muscles	(Contraction)	0	Relaxation
Cardiac muscle	0	Stimulation	0
Blood vessels	Contraction	0	Dilation
Extravasation	Inhibition	0	(Inhibition)
Skeletal muscle tremor	0	0	Increase
Mast cell degranulation	(Increase)	0	(Decrease)
Mucociliary clearance	0	0	(Increase)

Table 9.19.2. Effects of sympathomimetic agents

Alpha and beta effects of adrenoceptor agonists				
	Alpha stimulation	**Beta₁ stimulation**	**Beta₂ stimulation**	**Duration of effect**
Noradrenaline	++	+	+	Very short
Adrenaline	++	++	++	Very short
Ephedrine	+	+	+	Very short
Isoprenaline	(−)	++	++	Very short
Salbutamol	−	(−)	++	Short
Terbutaline	−	(−)	++	Short
Fenoterol	−	(−)	++	Short
Salmeterol	−	(−)	++	Long
Formoterol	−	(−)	++	Long

pressure. A reflex *increase in heart rate* mimics beta₁ stimulation; this has been the accepted explanation of the tachycardia induced by beta₂ bronchodilators. However, recent studies have indicated that cardiac muscle cells also have some beta₂ receptors.

Skeletal muscles possess beta₂ receptors. Tremor of the hands and cramps of the legs are common side effects from systemic treatment.

Beta₂ agonists stimulate glycogenolysis and slightly increase blood sugar. Clinically more important is a beta₂-induced shift of potassium from the extra- to the intracellular compartment. This results in a fall in plasma potassium of 0.5–1 mmol/l during intravenous and intensive inhalation therapy.

Noradrenaline

Adrenoceptor agonists are also called sympathomimetic agents, because their effects simulate those of the sympathetic nervous system. Noradrenaline (norepinephrine), which is the postganglionic transmitter substance in the sympathetic nervous system, has *weak beta* and *strong alpha effects* (Table 9.19.2). Consequently, it has little bronchodilating effect.

Adrenaline

Adrenaline (epinephrine), which is the major hormone of the adrenal medulla, has *equal alpha and beta effects*. It contracts blood vessels in the skin, stimulates the heart and dilates the bronchi. Adrenaline is very short-acting due to enzymatic breakdown.

Its *alpha*-stimulating action makes it the drug of choice for *anaphylactic shock*. The *beta* action of adrenaline has, in the past, made it a useful drug in *asthma* therapy.

Ephedrine

Ephedrine acts primarily by *releasing noradrenaline*. It activates both alpha and beta receptors, and stimulates the CNS. Given as a spray, it is a useful *nasal vasoconstrictor*. Ephedrine tablets give brief relief from mild asthma.

Isoprenaline

Isoprenaline (isoproteronol) has powerful *beta$_1$ and beta$_2$* effects but virtually no alpha effect. Inhaled from an MDI, it causes prompt bronchodilatation but it has a very short duration of action (1–2 hours). Inhalation of an ordinary dosage causes tachycardia and heavy overdosing can result in arrhythmias.

Beta$_2$ selective bronchodilators

Short-acting

Short-acting beta$_2$ selective agonists (salbutamol and terbutaline) are potent, safe and, by and large, equivalent bronchodilators, which have minimal beta$_1$ effects (Fig. 9.19.2). They have now replaced adrenaline, ephedrine and isoprenaline.

They can be given *by any route* of administration. The route chosen determines the onset and duration of action and the frequency of adverse effects (Fig. 9.19.2). The risk of serious adverse effects is very small, even when therapy is aggressive. These drugs are widely used in their inhaled form for *episodes of asthma* and for *severe acute asthma*.

Long-acting

Long-acting beta$_2$ selective molecules (salmeterol and formoterol) have recently been marketed. As very potent and long-acting bronchodilators, they are particularly effective in the *prevention of nocturnal asthma*. They can very considerably reduce the need of short-acting beta$_2$ inhalers and they can *replace oral bronchodilators*.

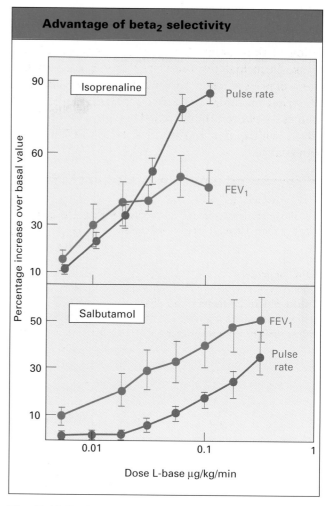

Fig. 9.19.2. Comparison between bronchodilating effect and adverse effects from intravenous isoprenaline (beta$_1$ and beta$_2$) and salbutamol (beta$_2$). The dose–response curves show similar bronchodilating effects, but less increase in pulse rate on salbutamol therapy, demonstrating the beta$_2$ selectivity of this drug. From Thiringer G, Svedmyr N. A comparison of the effects of isoprenaline and salbutamol on different beta-receptors in asthmatic patients. *Postgrad Med J* 1970; (suppl 47): 44–6.

Development of tolerance?

When asthma worsens, the response to inhaled beta$_2$ bronchodilators declines. At first, this can be compensated for by increasing the dosage but, later, the response will decrease. The fact that nebulized beta$_2$ agonists are the most effective treatment of acute severe asthma shows that the *clinical tolerance* to beta$_2$ agonists is not due to any marked down-regulation of beta receptors. This partial tolerance is mainly *a pathophysiological phenomenon* caused by inflammation and mucus plugging.

Recently, some studies of limited numbers of asthma patients have indicated that regular inhalation of short-acting beta$_2$ agonists may slightly increase bronchial responsiveness. Some concern has been expressed that this might increase the risk of serious asthma exacerbations and death. Most studies, however, have failed to identify such an effect, which, if it exists, may be of little clinical significance.

The easy way to knowledge
A single conversation across the table with a wise man is better than 10 years' study of books.
Chinese proverb

Bon appetite!
Some books are to be tasted, others to be swallowed, and some few to be chewed and digested.
Francis Bacon, 1561–1626

9.20 Inhaled beta$_2$ adrenoceptor agonists
For symptoms only

Key points
- An inhaled beta$_2$ agonist has a higher therapeutic index than medication given by any other route.
- Inhaled short-acting beta$_2$ agonists produce bronchodilatation within 5 minutes; it peaks after 30–90 minutes and lasts for 4–6 hours.
- Long-acting beta$_2$ agonist inhalers (salmeterol and formoterol) bronchodilate for more than 12 hours.
- They are particularly useful in patients with nocturnal asthma.
- Inhaled treatment can be given by a MDI or preferably by a DPI.
- When a spacer is attached to a MDI, the patient can use his or her bronchodilator even when asthma is severe.
- A nebulized wet aerosol is the treatment of choice for acute severe asthma in hospital.
- Patients who are on regular bronchodilator treatment also need an inhaled steroid.

Favourable therapeutic index
Inhaled beta$_2$ agonists have a wide safety margin. Moderate over-use causes the same side effects as oral treatment, and only excessive abuse carries a risk of serious adverse effects. It has repeatedly been proven that an inhaled beta$_2$ agonist has a higher therapeutic index than medication given by any other route (Fig. 9.20.1), and inhalation therapy plays a key role in asthma.

Short-acting beta$_2$ agonists

Duration of effect
Inhaled short-acting beta$_2$ bronchodilators (Fig. 9.20.2) produce marked bronchodilatation *within 5 minutes*. The effect is at a peak after 30–90 minutes and a clinically apparent effect *persists for 4–6 hours*. The duration of action increases with dosage and decreases with the severity of the attack.

Inhalers
The, formerly, so popular MDIs are now being replaced by *dry powder inhalers (DPIs), which have the following advantages*: 1, no effect from CFC gases on the atmospheric ozone layer; 2, no need for the

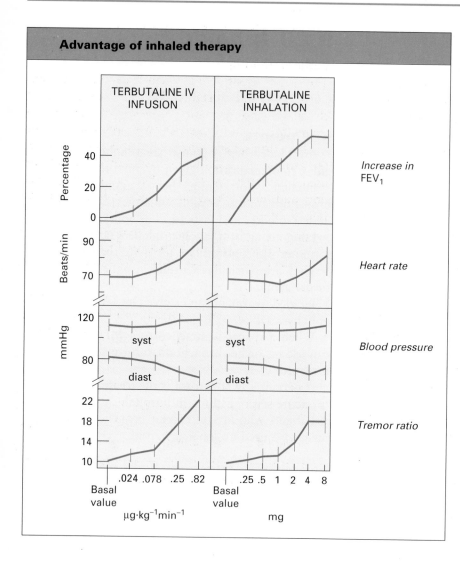

Advantage of inhaled therapy

Fig. 9.20.1. Bronchodilating effect and adverse effects from a beta$_2$ stimulant, given intravenously and by inhalation. It is obvious that a certain increase of FEV$_1$ (40%) is associated with far less side effects when terbutaline is inhaled as compared with intravenous infusion. It is remarkable that 32 puffs merely increased the pulse rate by 16 beats/min. From Thiringer G, Svedmyr N. Comparison of infused and inhaled terbutaline in patients with asthma. *Scand J Respir Dis* 1976; **57**: 17–24.

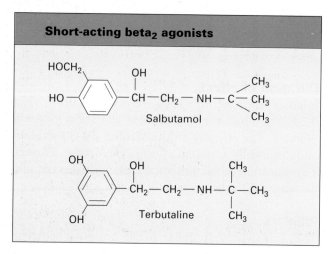

Short-acting beta$_2$ agonists

Fig. 9.20.2. Salbutamol and terbutaline.

patient to coordinate activation of inhaler with inhalation; and 3, no irritant effect in the airways from the carrier gas or lubricant.

When *a spacer* is attached to a MDI, the patient can use his or her bronchodilator even *when asthma is severe.* He or she can then take a puff of a beta$_2$ agonist in the spacer and inhale it without changing his or her breathing pattern. This can be repeated as often as necessary.

The small inhaled dose of a beta$_2$ agonist is rarely associated with side effects, and only a few patients experience mild tremor.

Nebulized wet aerosols

An aqueous aerosol of salbutamol or terbutaline (5–10 mg) from a nebulizer, preferably driven by pressurized oxygen, is now the first choice of treatment for *acute severe asthma* in emergency rooms and hospital wards.

A wet aerosol, driven by compressed air, can also be used for domiciliary treatment of severe chronic asthma. Although lung function tests often fail to demonstrate an advantage of the wet aerosol over a simple inhaler, it is preferred by some patients. The cost of nebulized treatment, however, is considerably higher than that of simple inhalers.

New principle for usage

A short-acting beta₂ inhaler is the medication of choice for treatment of acute exacerbations of asthma and for the pretreatment of exercise-induced bronchoconstriction. While these inhalers were, formerly, widely used for the daily management of asthma, it is now recommended, in International Consensus Reports, that regularly scheduled treatment with short-acting beta₂ inhalers should be kept to a minimum. Their use is now confined to an as-needed basis. *When there is a need for regular daily bronchodilator treatment, a steroid inhaler should be prescribed!*

It is important to emphasize to the patient that a large number of inhalations, while not dangerous in themselves, are a warning signal that the control of the disease is deteriorating. There is a danger that patients with worsening asthma continue inhalation therapy at home instead of seeking medical help. A warning must be clearly communicated – *if the inhalation does not produce relief, lasting for 3 hours, medical help must be sought!*

Long-acting beta₂ agonists

Clinical efficacy

The new long-acting beta₂ agonist inhalers, salmeterol and formoterol (Fig. 9.20.3), bronchodilate and *prevent bronchoconstriction*, for example induced by exercise *for more than 12 hours*.

These drugs, used twice daily, offer markedly better asthma control than salbutamol or terbutaline used four times daily. The effect on morning peak flow and *nocturnal asthma* is particularly improved (Fig. 9.20.4).

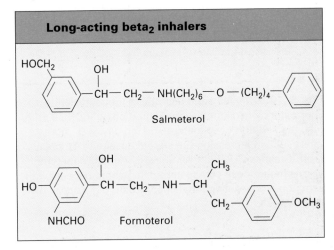

Fig. 9.20.3. Salmeterol and formoterol.

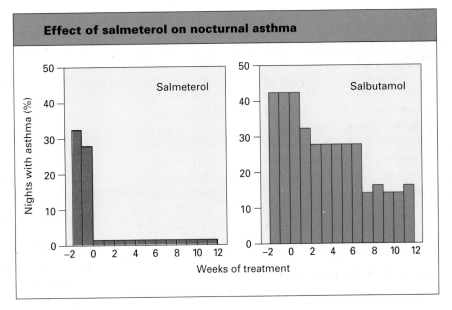

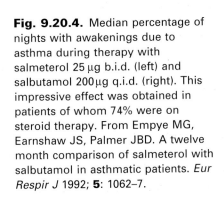

Fig. 9.20.4. Median percentage of nights with awakenings due to asthma during therapy with salmeterol 25 µg b.i.d. (left) and salbutamol 200 µg q.i.d. (right). This impressive effect was obtained in patients of whom 74% were on steroid therapy. From Empye MG, Earnshaw JS, Palmer JBD. A twelve month comparison of salmeterol with salbutamol in asthmatic patients. *Eur Respir J* 1992; **5**: 1062–7.

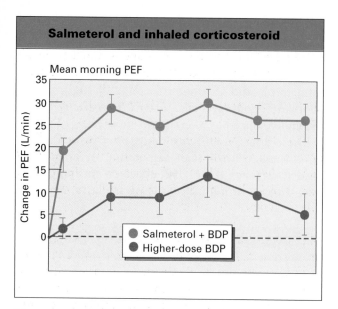

Salmeterol and inhaled corticosteroid

Mean morning PEF

Salmeterol + BDP
Higher-dose BDP

Fig. 9.20.5. In 429 adult asthmatics, not sufficiently controlled by beclomethasone dipropionate (BDP), 0.4 mg/day, the addition of salmeterol, 0.1 mg/day, was more effective than increasing the steroid dosage to 1 mg/day. From Greening AP, Ind PW, Shaw G. Added salmeterol versus higher-dose corticosteroid in asthma patients with symptoms on existing inhaled corticosteroid. *Lancet* 1994; **344**: 219–24.

The onset of action of formoterol is similar to that of salbutamol, while that of salmeterol is slower. This is not so important, however, because these drugs are to be used regularly and not on a p.r.n. basis. Patients still need to have a short-acting beta₂ agonist that can serve as rescue medication for acute attacks, but it is rarely needed due to the high efficacy of the long-acting inhalers.

Pros and cons

The following *concern*, mainly based on theoretical considerations, has been expressed about the use of the new long-acting beta₂ agonists: 1, patients who experience the pronounced bronchodilating effect of these new inhalers may tend exclusively to rely upon them and to discontinue the use of inhaled anti-inflammatory therapy; 2, treatment may result in down-regulation of beta₂ receptors, and reduced responsiveness of bronchial smooth muscles and of mast cells to beta₂ agonists; 3, regular use of inhaled beta₂ agonist may increase bronchial responsiveness and, ultimately, the risk of asthma death; and 4, allergic patients, who are so efficiently protected against bronchoconstriction, may increase their exposure to allergens.

The following arguments speak *in favour* of the treatment: 1, even patients on inhaled steroid get less nocturnal asthma and higher morning peak flow when they are treated with one of the new long-acting beta₂ inhalers; 2, avoiding nocturnal asthma improves the quality of life considerably; 3, significant bronchoconstriction may itself contribute to inflammation by epithelial damage and impaired muco-ciliary transport; and 4, studies of thousands of patients on these new inhalers have, so far, shown no evidence of a clinical relevance of the above points of concern.

Conclusions

The new long-acting beta₂ inhalers are very potent bronchodilators, which should always be used in conjunction with adequate anti-inflammatory medication (Fig 9.20.5).

A dangerous aerosol
Flattery never hurts a man unless he inhales.
Harry Emerson Fosdick

9.21 Oral and parenteral beta$_2$ adrenoceptor agonists

Tremor and tachycardia as side effects

Key points
- A slow-release beta$_2$ tablet, given twice daily, produces a 24-hour lasting moderate bronchodilatation.
- It is usually at the expense of adverse effects (tremor and cramps).
- Oral treatment has less effect on exercise-induced asthma than has inhaled beta$_2$ agonists, which definitely have a higher therapeutic ratio.
- Oral beta$_2$ agonists can now be replaced by long-acting inhalers in all patients who can master the inhalation technique.
- In acute asthma, a subcutaneous or intramuscular injection can be given when inhaled therapy is not available.
- In acute severe asthma, intravenous treatment can be used as an additive to inhalation of nebulized beta$_2$ agonist.
- Intravenous infusion of salbutamol or terbutaline is preferable to theophylline.
- Tremor, tachycardia and a reduction in plasma potassium are adverse effects.

Oral treatment
An oral dosage of a beta$_2$ agonist (salbutamol or terbutaline) produces bronchodilatation in about 20–30 minutes and lasts for 4–6 hours. A liquid formulation can be given to infants and children. Plain tablets have generally now been replaced by *sustained-release formulations* (5–10 mg twice daily). They are useful when night attacks and 'morning dips' are a problem.

In theory, oral treatment has the advantage over inhaled therapy in that it can reach all parts of the airways in spite of obstruction to the lumen. In practice, this theory is largely incorrect. Inhaled bronchodilators are more efficient than tablets in preventing exercise- and allergen-induced bronchoconstriction.

Oral treatment with beta$_2$ agonists is associated with *tremor* in most patients, but some tolerance to this side effect usually develops. Many patients develop *cramps* in the legs. Oral beta$_2$ agonists can now be replaced by the new long-acting inhalers in all patients who can master the inhalation technique.

Subcutaneous and intramuscular injection
Subcutaneous or intramuscular injection can relieve bronchospasm within 10–20 minutes. *Salbutamol* and *terbutaline* (0.25–0.5 mg) are preferable to adrenaline, which has been widely used for the treatment of childhood asthma.

Intravenous injection and infusion
Intravenous salbutamol or terbutaline can replace, or be used in addition to, intravenous aminophylline for *acute severe asthma*. A bolus dose of 250 µg is as effective as 250 mg aminophylline, and is more rapid in action and less prone to cause side effects. The beta$_2$ agonists can be given intravenously over a period of 1–2 minutes, which is an advantage over the >15 minutes required for the safe administration of aminophylline. The duration of action of intravenous injection is short so a continuous infusion of 5–10 (max. 20) µg/min (7.5–15 mg/day) is used in acute severe asthma.

Tremor and *tachycardia* will occur after injection and infusion. A reduction in *plasma potassium* (0.5–1 mmol/l) occurs quickly; this is due to a shift of potassium from the extracellular to the intracellular phase. This may imply a potential risk of cardiac arrhythmia in patients with a pre-existing low plasma potassium (diuretics).

An imperial view on pharmacotherapy
Medicine is only fit for old people. Take a single dose of medicine once, and in all probability you will be obliged to take an additional hundred afterwards.

Napoleon Bonaparte

9.22 Cholinoceptor antagonists

Only together with beta₂ agonists

Key points
- The anti-cholinergic agent, ipratropium bromide, given by the inhaled route, has a high therapeutic index.
- It increases the lung function significantly for about 4–6 hours but it has a slow onset of effect.
- Mouth dryness seems to be the only significant side effect.
- An inhaled beta₂ agonist is more effective than ipratropium in asthma, but the two types of drugs seem to be equally effective in COPD.
- If full relief of bronchospasm cannot be attained with an inhaled beta₂ agonist due to adverse effects, inhaled ipratropium can be added.
- In acute severe asthma, nebulized ipratropium is a useful addition to a beta₂ agonist.

The inhalation of atropine-like agents (cholinoceptor antagonists, anti-cholinergics or parasympatholytics) for the treatment of asthma has a long history; it was mentioned in Yoga literature in the seventeenth century AD. The earliest use in Europe dates back to 1802 when Dr Sims, in Britain, recorded the beneficial effect from inhalation of the dried and pulverized roots of the Indian plant, datura. The alkaloid of *Datura stramonium* (Devil's apple) was later identified as being similar to atropine, also known from *Atropa belladonna* (deadly nightshade), a plant frequently used in the Middle Ages by professional poisoners. Stramonium and belladonna have been widely used for inhalation therapy in asthma, throughout Europe and the USA, as burning powder and in the form of cigarettes and cigars.

Rationale
Cholinoceptors (cholinergic receptors) are involved in a series of functions in the respiratory system. Stimulation by the parasympathetic neurotransmitter, *acetylcholine*, dilates blood vessels and, more importantly, stimulates glandular secretion and *contracts bronchial smooth muscles*. Clinical experience suggests that only the latter is significantly affected by

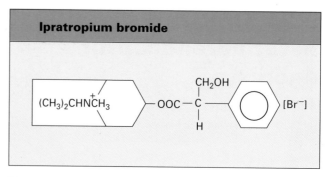

Fig. 9.22.1. Ipratropium bromide.

cholinoceptor antagonists; blood vessels are largely atropine-resistant.

Airway obstruction in asthma is due to contraction of smooth muscles and inflammation. A part of the muscular spasm is caused by a *vagal reflex* with stimulation of the smooth muscle cholinoceptor. As this is the only pathway blocked by anti-cholinergic agents, it follows that these drugs cannot counteract all asthmatic symptoms.

Drugs
The best known cholinoceptor antagonist is *atropine sulphate* (atropine), which is absorbed rapidly from the gastro-intestinal tract and penetrates the blood–brain barrier. The *quaternary anti-cholinergics*, on the other hand, are poorly absorbed from the gastro-intestinal tract and pass the blood–brain barrier with difficulty. One of them, *ipratropium bromide* (ipratropium) (Fig. 9.22.1), when given by the inhaled route, has a high therapeutic index as a bronchodilator.

Ipratropium can be given from a metered-dose inhaler, from a powder inhaler and as a wet aerosol from a nebulizer.

Experimental models
In experimental work, the effect of a cholinoceptor antagonist is taken as an indicator of the role played by cholinergic mechanisms (Fig. 9.22.2). Ipratropium has a marked protective effect on bronchospasm induced by *methacholine* challenge, while the effect on *exercise*-, *histamine*- and *allergen*-induced bronchospasm (early response) is poor and variable.

Clinical effect
In asthma, inhaled beta₂ agonists are more effective than ipratropium, while the two types of drugs seem to be equally effective in *COPD* (Fig. 9.22.3). Inhaled

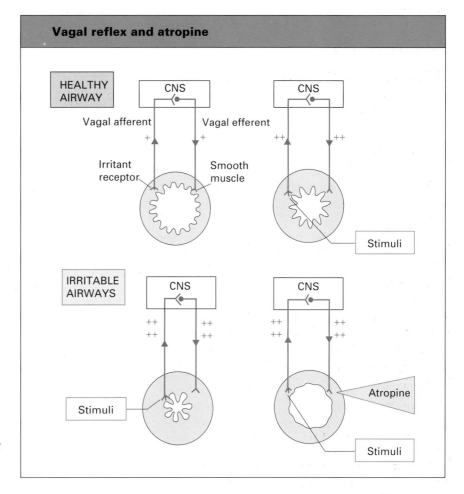

Vagal reflex and atropine

Fig. 9.22.2. Reflex-induced bronchoconstriction and effect of atropine. A series of stimuli initiate a vagal reflex via irritant receptors. The bronchoconstrictory response, more marked in patients with irritable airways than in normal subjects, is blocked by atropine by producing an effect on the efferent limb of the reflex arc. From Nadel JA. Neurophysiologic aspects of asthma. In: Austen KF, Lichtenstein LM, eds. *Asthma: Physiology, Immunopharmacology, and Treatment* New York: Academic Press, 1973: 29–38.

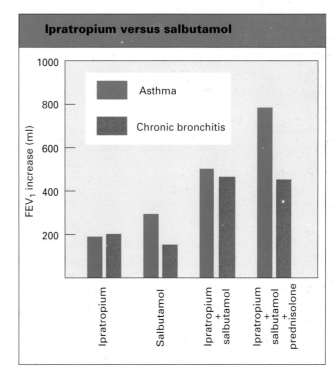

Ipratropium versus salbutamol

Fig. 9.22.3. This figure shows that: 1, a beta$_2$ agonist (inhaled salbutamol, 200 µg, four times daily) is more effective in asthma than an anti-cholinergic agent (inhaled ipratropium, 40 µg, four times daily); 2, they are equally effective in chronic bronchitis; 3, the effects are additive; and 4, steroids (prednisolone, 10 mg, three times daily) are effective in asthma, not in bronchitis. From Lightbody IM, Ingram CG, Legge JS, Johnson RN. Ipratropium bromide, salbutamol and prednisolone in bronchial asthma and chronic bronchitis. *Br J Dis Chest* 1978; **72**: 181–6.

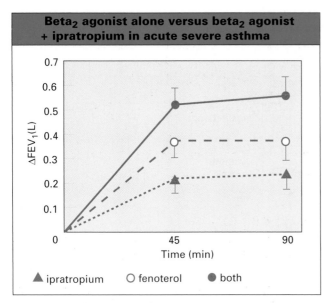

Fig. 9.22.4. Increase in FEV$_1$ (mean ± SEM) after inhalation of nebulized ipratropium solution 0.5 mg (triangles), a beta$_2$ agonist (fenoterol 1.25 mg) (open circles) or the combination (solid circles) in 148 patients with status asthmaticus. From Rebuck AS, Chapman KR, Abboud R, *et al.* Nebulized anti-cholinergic and sympathomimetic treatment of chronic obstructive airways disease in the emergency room. *Am J Med* 1987; **82**: 59–65.

ipratropium increases the lung function parameters significantly for about 4–6 hours but it has a *slow onset* of maximum effect (about 1–2 hours).

Combined treatment

Sympathetic stimulation together with parasympathic blockade seems a logical approach, but human studies have merely shown an added effect from ipratropium and then only when a submaximal dose of a beta$_2$ agonist has been given. While ipratropium has a very limited place in management of chronic asthma, it is increasingly used for acute severe asthma.

Chronic asthma

When full relief of bronchospasm, in the rare case, cannot be attained with an inhaled beta$_2$ agonist due to adverse effects, inhaled ipratropium can be added. The drug is then used on a regular basis as its slow onset of action makes it unsuitable for p.r.n. use. As the response of patients to ipratropium varies, an initial trial with the drug is recommended before long-term therapy is started.

Acute severe asthma

While ipratropium is not suitable for monotherapy, it can, in its nebulized form (0.25–0.5 mg), be a useful addition to a beta$_2$ agonist in the initial treatment of acute severe asthma (Fig. 9.22.4). It improves bronchodilatation without contributing to the side effects induced by the beta$_2$ agonist.

Adverse effects

Inhaled ipratropium, in ordinary doses (20–80 μg, three to four times daily), implies no risk of the well-known systemic atropine effects (tachycardia, blurred vision, difficulty in urination, flushing and CNS symptoms). Drying of the airway mucous membrane with inspissation of secretions has not been observed. The safety of higher nebulized doses (0.25–0.5 mg), used in acute severe asthma, has been less well studied, but clinical experience has not indicated any serious adverse effects. Mouth dryness seems to be the only significant side effect.

Postsynaptic blockade

If I were to express what appears to me to be the peculiar excellence of belladonna as a sedative in asthma, I should say that it consisted in its power of diminishing reflex irritability.

Dr HH Salter
Lancet, 1869

9.23 Theophylline
A bronchodilator with a low therapeutic index

Key points
- Theophylline stimulates the heart, the CNS and relaxes bronchial muscles.
- Theophylline, as sustained-release preparations, is suitable for oral use, but absorption is influenced by food.
- As theophylline is poorly soluble in water, aminophylline is used for intravenous infusion.
- The plasma level is important as it correlates directly with therapeutic and toxic effects.
- There is a high inter-subject variation in the rate of hepatic metabolism of theophylline and in drug requirement.
- Metabolism is reduced by liver disease, heart failure and drug interaction.
- Mild adverse effects are frequent: headache, flushing, restlessness, insomnia, nausea and vomiting.
- High plasma levels imply a risk of serious toxic effects, convulsions, cardiac arrhythmias and deaths.
- A maximum bronchodilator effect cannot be obtained with theophylline owing to the risk of severe adverse effects.
- The maintenance dose is individual and varies largely.
- High-dose therapy requires check of the plasma level.
- Low-dose therapy in combination with a beta$_2$ agonist gives added effects but not added side effects.
- Better bronchodilatation with fewer side effects can now be obtained with the new long-acting beta$_2$ inhalers.
- In hospitalized patients with acute severe asthma, intravenous theophylline is occasionally used.
- A loading dose is followed by an accurately calculated maintenance dose.
- Beta$_2$ agonists, inhaled and intravenous, offer maximum efficacy with less adverse effects.
- The use of theophylline can therefore be questioned.

Theophylline (Fig. 9.23.1) stimulates the heart, the CNS and is a diuretic similar to other xanthine alkaloids (caffeine and theobromine). It also relaxes smooth muscles resulting in *vasodilatation* and, importantly, *bronchial dilatation*.

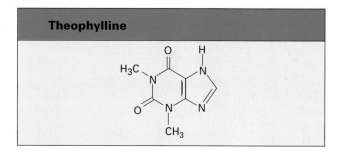

Fig. 9.23.1. Theophylline.

Mode of action
Theophylline increases intracellular cyclic AMP levels *in vitro* via phosphodiesterase inhibition, but only at concentrations that are many times higher than the therapeutic plasma level. It is not clear whether its bronchodilating effect is caused by phosphodiesterase inhibitor activity.

Preparations
Theophylline is suitable for *oral use*, as it is readily absorbed from the gut, but absorption is influenced by food.

Plain tablets will not give a constant plasma level so reliable *sustained-release preparations*, 12 hourly, are preferred. These preparations have the advantage of maintaining plasma theophylline levels during the night, thus preventing early morning asthma. A few quick metabolizers (see below) may need medication 8 hourly.

Rectal suppositories are popular but absorption is erratic and often incomplete. Deaths have occurred because mothers in a panic have heavily overdosed children with acute asthma.

As theophylline is poorly soluble in water, *aminophylline* (theophylline solubilized by the addition of ethylenediamine) is used for *intravenous* infusion (Fig. 9.23.2).

Metabolism and plasma level
The plasma level is important as it correlates directly with therapeutic and toxic effects. To obtain a certain plasma concentration, individual dosing is necessary because of a genetically determined, *variable* rate of metabolic *inactivation in the liver*. This results in a high inter-subject variation in plasma half-life (4–12 hours); the variation is high (2–24 hours) when the determinants below are included.

Most important is the slow metabolism and, with that, the risk of toxicity in patients with *liver disease*

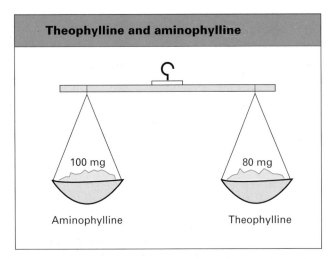

Theophylline and aminophylline

100 mg

80 mg

Aminophylline

Theophylline

Fig. 9.23.2. Equipotent doses of theophylline (the active compound; for oral use) and aminophylline (for intravenous use).

Factors affecting theophylline metabolism
Reduced metabolism (risk of toxicity)
Liver disease
Congestive heart failure
Febrile illnesses
Old age
Liver enzyme inhibition: cimetidine erythromycin oral contraceptives propranolol allupurinol
Increased metabolism (lack of efficacy)
Childhood
Smoking
Liver enzyme induction: phenytoin rifampicin carbamazepine phenobarbital

Table 9.23.1. Drugs and other factors that influence theophylline metabolism

and with *congestive heart failure* (Table 9.23.1). The metabolism is also reduced by *febrile infections* and by the intake of *drugs* that *inhibit microsomal enzymes* in the liver (e.g. cimetidine or erythromycin).

Microsomal enzyme induction in the liver, for example by phenytoin and phenobarbital, increases theophylline metabolism. *Cigarette smokers* have a more rapid metabolism than non-smokers. Plasma half-life also depends upon *age*, and metabolism is rapid in children. In the absence of the above factors, theophylline metabolism remains fairly constant over prolonged periods.

Adverse effects

A single tablet can cause *gastric irritation* but, as a rule, adverse effects relate to the plasma level. Theophylline-induced vasodilatation can cause *headache* and *flushing* (Table 9.23.2). CNS stimulation causes *restlessness*, *insomnia* (theophylline minus one methyl group = caffeine), *nausea* and *vomiting*.

When the plasma level exceeds 20 mg/l (110 µmol/l) there is a serious risk of toxic effects; *convulsion* (in children) and *cardiac arrhythmias* (in adults) may occur without warning and the risk of death is considerable at levels higher than 40 mg/l. As the plasma theophylline level, recommended for high-dose therapy, is 10–20 mg/l (55–110 µmol/l), it follows that the therapeutic index is very low. To illustrate the danger in using high-dose therapy without close control, it can be mentioned that cimetidine reduces theophylline metabolism by 50%. To give cimetidine to a patient with a plasma level in the high therapeutic range without reducing the oral dose can cause life-threatening toxicity.

Dose–response relationship

There is a linear log–dose–response relationship for theophylline over the plasma concentration range 5–20 mg/l (Fig. 9.23.3). A maximum bronchodilator effect cannot be obtained with this type of drug owing to the risk of severe adverse effects when the plasma level exceeds 20 mg/l.

Oral theophylline

While many doctors in the USA accept a therapeutic theophylline level of 10–20 mg/l as a compromise between efficacy and toxicity, their European colleagues, in general, will accept these levels only in selected patients with severe chronic disease, which is inadequately controlled by the less toxic sympathomimetics (and inhaled steroids).

Table 9.23.2. Pharmacological effects of theophylline — beneficial and toxic. *Plasma level 10–20 mg/l; **≥20 mg/l; ***>>20 mg/l

Theophylline effects	
Pharmacological effect	**Symptom/Sign**
Relaxation of bronchial smooth muscle	Bronchodilatation
Relaxation of vascular smooth muscle	Flushing, headache and hypotension
Increase of urinary excretion of potassium	Hypokalaemia
Stimulation of CNS	Restlessness and insomnia* Nausea, vomiting and haematemesis** Convulsion, coma and death***
Stimulation of heart	Palpitation and tachycardia* Arrhythmia** Cardiac arrest and death***

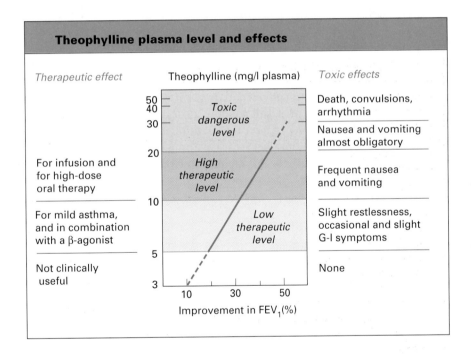

Fig. 9.23.3. Relationship between plasma theophylline concentration and onset of therapeutic and toxic effects.

High-dose therapy

High-dose therapy, aiming at a plasma concentration of 10–20 mg/l (55–110 μmol/l), should only be used by experienced specialists who can check the plasma level at frequent intervals, have a close doctor–patient relationship and have organized, good patient education. It should not be employed in the elderly or in patients with heart or liver disease.

The maintenance dose is *individual* and varies largely (usually 800–1200 mg/day in adults). It is determined by measurement of the *plasma theophylline level*, which must be checked at least every 6–12 months.

Low-dose, combined therapy

When inhaled bronchodilator therapy cannot be given, the combined use of oral theophylline and beta₂ agonist, each in a suboptimal dose, can be advantageous because the therapeutic effects, but not the side effects, are additive. Low-dose theophylline treatment can be given without measurement of the plasma level. It consists of about 300 mg twice daily, in a 70-kg adult, which gives a plasma level of about 5–10 mg/l.

Better bronchodilatation with less side effects can now be obtained with the new long-acting beta$_2$ inhalers, but oral treatment is still extensively used world wide.

Intravenous therapy

Loading and maintenance dose
Hospitalized patients, with acute severe asthma, who have not taken theophylline preparations in the last 24 hours, can be given a loading dose of aminophylline, 6 mg/kg (max. 440 mg) over 15–30 minutes. This is followed by infusion of a maintenance dose, 0.6 mg/kg/hour (lean weight). This regimen will result in a plasma theophylline concentration of about 10 mg/l.

If patients on adequate *oral theophylline* cannot continue oral medication, the intravenous *loading dose* should be omitted, while the maintenance dose is unchanged. Patients with *congestive cardiac disease* or *liver failure* can receive a full loading dose, but it is necessary to at least halve the *maintenance dose*. Patients with ischaemic heart disease must be treated with caution due to an increased risk of arrhythmia.

Safety
Aggressive therapy has resulted in *severe intoxication and death*, mainly in patients with coexisting diseases. This was a common risk some years ago when it was frequent practice to give a higher maintenance dose (0.9 mg/kg/hour) than is now recommended. Repeated *plasma theophylline estimations* will add to the safety of the therapy and a plasma analysis is mandatory when treatment lasts for more than 24 hours.

When patients with acute severe asthma are treated with a beta$_2$ agonist, both by the inhaled and by the intravenous route, theophylline will not give further bronchodilatation. In many departments, theophylline has been *discarded* or reserved for rare or very severe cases.

Theophylline minus one CH$_3$ group
One of the commonest and best-reputed remedies of asthma, one that is almost sure to have been tried in any case that may come under our observation, and one that in many cases is more efficacious than any other, is strong coffee.

Dr HH Salter
Edinb Med J, 1859; 4: 1109

9.24 Management of chronic asthma I
Environmental control

Key points

• Avoidance of allergens and of non-specific irritants is the first measure to be recommended in allergic airway disease.
• A home visit by a health professional can provide important information for improvement of the environment.
• It may not be possible to avoid outdoor pollutants, but avoid exercising in heavily polluted areas.
• Indoor pollutants, such as wood smoke and cooking oils, should be avoided when possible.
• Tobacco smoking should not be allowed in the house of an asthma patient but even some asthmatics smoke.
• Exposure to house dust mites can be diminished by following measures given in Table 9.24.1, especially that of using non-permeable covers.
• Reducing a high indoor humidity, although difficult to effectuate, is efficient in decreasing the number of mites.
• The indoor number of pollens can be reduced by using air conditioners and by closing the windows and doors.
• Avoidance of animals is easy – at least in principle.
• It may take some months after an animal has been removed for the full benefit to be perceived.
• Indirect exposure from animal protein in others' clothes can usually not be avoided.

There is general agreement that avoidance of allergens and of non-specific irritants is *the first measure* to be recommended in the case of allergic airway disease. It can, however, be difficult to convince a patient about the necessity of the proposed changes if they interfere with his/her ordinary lifestyle, and it can be impossible for the patient completely to avoid the offending allergen.

Specific recommendations about allergen avoidance are given to *patients with specific allergies*, and also to *highly atopic children*, in order to avoid development of new allergies. Obviously, it is bad advice to tell a dog-allergic patient to replace the dog with a cat, or to tell the parents of a child with atopic dermatitis that they can have a guinea-pig in the house.

Air pollution

Ozone and *sulphur dioxide* are important outdoor pollutants, especially in cities with heavy traffic. Outdoor exercise should be avoided on high pollution days as the combination of smog and exertion are particularly asthmagenic.

Formaldehyde, evaporated from urea glue, used in chipboard and other building materials, can be of significance as an indoor pollutant especially in new houses. *Wood smoke*, household sprays and volatile organic compounds (e.g. cooking oils and polishes) are other important indoor pollutants.

Tobacco smoke

Smoke provokes symptoms in the majority of asthma patients. *No smoking* should be allowed in the house, but, unfortunately, it is still difficult to avoid tobacco smoke in social life and in public places. This thoughtlessness of smokers is a limiting factor in the daily activities of many asthma patients. Although passive inhalation of smoke increases asthma symptoms and, in children, increases the frequency of respiratory infections, it is often difficult to persuade the parents to give up smoking. Astonishingly, even a number of asthma sufferers smoke.

House dust mites

House dust mites cannot be completely avoided, but the degree of exposure can be diminished. As the mites mainly live in beds and as one-third of a patient's life is spent in the same place, anti-mite precautions are largely limited to *the bedroom* (Figs 9.24.1–3).

All materials in the bed should be *washable* or *easy to clean*. Bare floors are best, with washable throw rugs if necessary.

Old mattresses, which can be giant graveyards for mites, should be replaced. Water matresses make ideal beds for mite-allergic asthmatics but not for mites. Other mattresses can be encased in an allergen *non-permeable cover*. Feather pillows are replaced with *washable foam pillows*; these are less hospitable for the mites and can be encased or washed regularly.

The recommendations in Table 9.24.1 are given to adult asthmatics with mite allergy and to all children with asthma; if they are not mite-allergic, these changes will reduce their risk of developing mite allergy.

A *home visit* by a health professional can provide important information for improvement of the

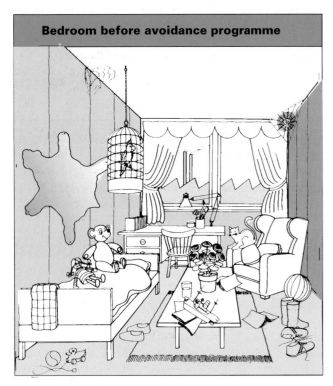

Fig. 9.24.1. Example of bedroom before allergen avoidance programme.

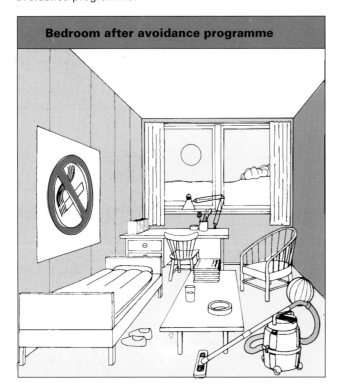

Fig. 9.24.2. Bedroom after allergen avoidance programme. By courtesy of Jørgen Bent Andersen, Department of Paediatric Allergy, Hillerød Hospital, Denmark.

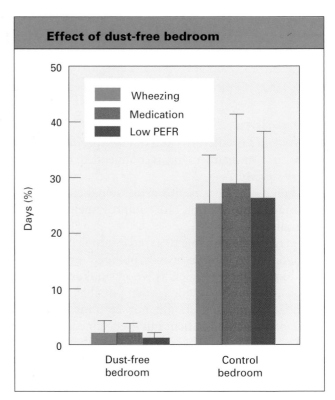

Fig. 9.24.3. Percentage of days on which wheezing was noticed, medication was given, and abnormally low PEF rate was recorded during a 4-week study period with dust-free bedroom or control bedroom. From Murray AB, Ferguson AC. Dust-free bedrooms in the treatment of asthmatic children with house dust or dust-mite allergy: a controlled trial. *Paediatrics* 1983; **71**: 418–22.

environment, especially in the allergic patient with poorly controlled symptoms.

Moving to another house or climate can be successful. If a move of this kind is anticipated, a trial period should be attempted and, ideally, the concentration of mite allergen measured.

Air humidity and ventilation

A bed provides the house dust mites with food (1 gram skin scales/day, feeding 200 000 mites) and a high humidity. The *bed humidity* during the day largely depends upon the *indoor air humidity*, which is the essential factor determining the size of a mite population. A high correlation between indoor humidity and the occurrence of house dust mites exists, especially in the cold winter season. The indoor humidity depends upon human activities (e.g. in kitchen, bathroom and washroom), water leakages in the building and the *external humidity*. The amount of water vapour in the outdoor air differs according to climate and altitude. The tropics are a

Table 9.24.1. House dust mite control measures in the bedroom

Allergen avoidance in bedroom
Let the patient have his or her own bedroom, which is used for no other activity
Ban animals and smoking in the room
Accept only a linoleum or wooden floor, which is smooth and easy to clean
Avoid all unnecessary dust-collecting items
Only allow simple furniture and washable drapes
Replace an old box-spring mattress with a new mattress and encase it in an allergen non-permeable cover; alternatively, a water bed is suitable
Replace old feather pillows with new ones made of a synthetic foam material and encase them or wash them regularly
Replace old quilts with new ones and wash regularly (>55°C or 130°F)
Replace old eiderdowns with new ones and encase them
Clean, vacuum and change bed linen regularly

paradise for mites, while they dislike high altitudes and dry deserts. Mite allergy is rarely a problem at altitudes >1000 metres and are not found above 1700 metres.

Ventilation of the rooms reduces internal humidity, which increases with the degree of insulation of the house. In temperate climate zones, energy-saving measures have led to draught-free houses, with very little ventilation, and subsequently an increase in indoor humidity and the mite population.

Other allergens

Pollens in the outdoor air cannot be avoided, but indoor exposure can be reduced by using air conditioners and by closing the windows and doors during peak pollen seasons. *Mould spores* are impossible to avoid completely, but the contribution to the spore count from indoor sources should be sought for and eliminated.

Animal dander is eliminated, by avoidance of animals, which is easy – at least in principle. When pets are asthmagenic, they must be excluded from the house or, at the very least, the bedroom. It may take several weeks or months after the animal has been removed for the full benefit to be perceived. Indirect exposure from animal dander in clothes can be a problem for highly sensitive patients.

> An intriguing question
> Who shall decide when doctors disagree?
> Alexander Pope, 1688–1744

9.25 Management of chronic asthma II
Stepwise pharmacotherapy and action plan

Key points
- Initially, the goal for management, including the patient's best PEF, is defined.
- Asthma severity is currently assessed in order to attain the treatment goal.
- Asthma severity is judged by symptoms, PEF and use of beta$_2$ inhaler.
- A self-management plan, consisting of a stepwise approach to daily treatment and an action plan for acute exacerbations, is issued to each patient.
- The stepwise approach to the daily treatment allows it to be currently adjusted to the requirement.
- It is preferable to start on a high step, get full control of the disease, and then step down.
- Step 1: short-acting beta$_2$ inhaler p.r.n.
- Step 2: low-dose inhaled steroid ($\leqslant$1 mg/day).
- Step 3: high-dose inhaled steroid (>1 mg/day) and regular use of a bronchodilator (long-acting beta$_2$ inhaler).
- Step 4: regular oral steroid.
- Short-term oral steroid therapy may be needed at any level of disease severity.
- A written action plan for acute exacerbations is important (Tables 9.25.3–4).

The following programme can be used for the effective management of asthma: 1, definition of the goal for treatment; 2, patient education and active participation; 3, daily assessment of lung function and symptoms; 4, avoidance of allergens and irritants (see Chapter 9.24); 5, a *self-management plan*, consisting of a stepwise plan for daily pharmacotherapy and an action plan for management of acute exacerbations; and 6, regular follow-up and revision of plans.

Treatment goals
It is important, together with the patient, to define the goal for treatment. The goal described in Table 9.25.1 is realistic for patients with mild to moderate, but not severe, asthma.

Patient education
Developing a patient–doctor partnership, by educat-

Goals for asthma treatment
Normal lung function (>80%)
Lung function without variability (<20%)
Minimal symptoms and no nocturnal asthma
No acute severe asthma and risk of death
Near normal life and lifestyle
No adverse effects from medication

Table 9.25.1. Goals for asthma treatment, realistic for patients with mild and moderate disease

ing the patients, is important, as it enables them to alter their own treatment without constantly referring to their physician. Education also leads to improved control of asthma and a reduction in the number of attacks, particularly those that are life-threatening.

Assessment of asthma severity
Asthma severity is judged by: 1, symptoms; 2, medication requirements; and 3, objective measurement of lung function.

Symptoms and use of beta$_2$ inhaler
A diary of symptoms and medication use, to be kept by the patient for at least 2 weeks prior to a follow-up consultation, is recommended. The requirement for a short-acting beta$_2$ inhaler mirrors the degree of disease control. Increasing usage is a warning of deterioration of the disease, as is failure to achieve a quick and sustained response to the inhaler during an exacerbation. Obviously, direct questioning by the physician also helps to evaluate the condition (Table 9.25.2).

Peak flow monitoring
Measurement of PEF is essential for assessing the severity of asthma, and it can be accomplished by all patients over 5 years of age. Most patients can be motivated to record measurements of lung function daily when they are told that it will enable attainment of the goals of therapy with the least possible medication.

PEF variability provides an indirect assessment of airway inflammation and hyper-responsiveness, which correlates with the patient's tendency to bronchoconstrict.

Patients with chronic asthma will tend to underestimate the severity of their disease unless they regularly measure PEF. These home measurements will enable the patients to assess their condition precisely and change therapy accordingly, analogous to the fine control diabetics maintain of their therapy.

The patient's best lung function is defined by repeated recordings, if necessary after short-term prednisolone therapy. The personal best value becomes the target for therapy.

Drug therapy is prescribed with the aim of keeping the patient well, with lung function close to the defined target each day. It follows that there is no alternative to home-monitoring of PEF.

A stepwise plan for daily therapy

As asthma is a dynamic as well as chronic condition, the goal for treatment can best be achieved using a stepwise approach to therapy.

Using stepwise therapy does not imply that patients need to start on a low step and then increase step by step. It is preferable to *start on a high step*, get full control of the disease, and then step down. Patients with moderately severe asthma, for example, can start with a high dose of inhaled steroid and then have the dose adjusted after 3 months when full effect is achieved. In severe asthma, the initial addition of 2 weeks prednisolone treatment to their therapy can be recommended.

Progression from one step to the next is indicated when control cannot be achieved and there is assurance that the patient is using the medication correctly.

Obviously, the steps suggested below are guidelines only (Fig. 9.25.1). In every single case the choice of treatment for asthma must be based on a *cost–risk–*

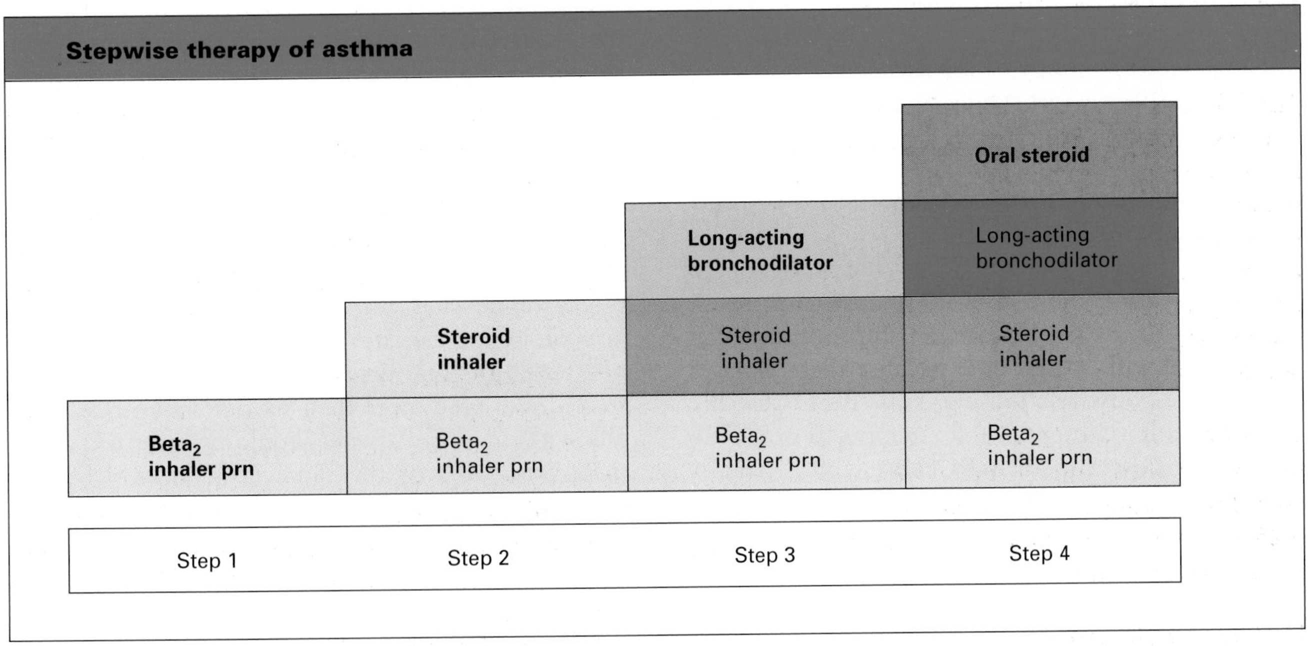

Questions for assessment of asthma severity
Have your activities (e.g. work, social life and sport) been restricted due to asthma?
Has there been any cough, wheezing and breathlessness, and, if so, how many days a month?
How many nights have you woken up with asthma during the last month?
How often do you use your bronchodilator inhaler?
Have you used prednisolone tablets since the last visit?
Have you made any emergency calls?

Table 9.25.2. Questions that can guide the physician to prescribe adequate anti-asthmatic medication

Fig. 9.25.1. Stepwise therapy of chronic asthma. There are four steps and four drugs.

benefit analysis, and on the patient's ability to understand, accept and follow instructions – patient compliance. Consequently, treatment must always be individualized and the guidelines, given below, have to be adapted according to patient, doctor and country. In many parts of the world, patients cannot afford modern asthma medicine.

Step 1: short-acting beta₂ inhaler p.r.n.

A short-acting *beta₂ inhaler* can be used for treatment of occasional attacks and before exercise. In patients with normal lung function who have only infrequent symptoms and no sleep disturbance, this may be the only treatment required.

Cromoglycate can be used before known exposure to allergen and, together with a beta₂ inhaler, before exercise.

Proceed to Step 2 if the patient needs to use his or her bronchodilator more than three times a week (pre-exercise use not included), or the goals for asthma control are not achieved (Table 9.25.1).

Step 2: low-dose inhaled steroid/cromoglycate

The primary therapy is inhaled anti-inflammatory medication, taken on a daily basis. Usually, a *steroid inhaler* (0.2–1 mg/day of beclomethasone dipropionate, or the equivalent) is preferred in *adults* because of its high success rate, but some doctors prefer to begin with *a trial of cromoglycate in youngsters*. If this is not sufficient, it is withdrawn and a steroid spray prescribed.

The patients continue to use their beta₂ inhaler as needed for the relief of symptoms, but it should not be used on a regular daily basis.

Step 3: high-dose inhaled steroid and regular use of bronchodilators

High-dose inhaled steroid. When initial treatment with inhaled steroids in a low dose not result in full control of the disease, an improvement can be expected with a high dose because there exists a log–dose–response relationship. Full effect is usually achieved within 3 months and attempts to gradually reduce the dose can then be considered. There is not the same impetus to reduce the dose of inhaled steroids as there is for oral steroids, but high-dose therapy should not be maintained 'as a routine'.

Regular use of bronchodilator. Patients who need high-dose inhaled steroids for prolonged periods usually have a high degree of bronchial responsiveness. They bronchoconstrict easily in response to exercise, inhalation of irritants, and allergens, and at night. If a steroid inhaler, used in a high dosage for 3 months, has not abolished these symptoms, the patients will benefit from added use of a bronchodilator on a regular basis. It is, however, important to stress that the bronchodilator, acting on bronchoconstriction only, must not replace an otherwise necessary dose of inhaled steroid, which counteracts the disease more fundamentally. The best choice for regular bronchodilator therapy is a *long-acting beta₂ inhaler*. When combined oral beta₂ agonist and theophylline are used instead, the efficacy is lower and the side effects more frequent.

Step 4: regular long-term oral steroid therapy

A few patients cannot be controlled on Step 3 treatment and need oral steroid on a regular basis. Complete control of asthma, as defined in Table 9.25.1, will not be possible for these patients, and the goal of treatment is to achieve a suboptimal control of the disease with as good a quality of life as possible and as low a dosage of prednisolone as possible. If the patient can be kept relatively symptom-free without serious asthma episodes on a small dose of prednisolone, the benefits may well outweigh the adverse effects, but the decision as to when to start long-term oral treatment is always difficult.

Regular daily use of an oral steroid is *an additive treatment and not a substitute* for other drugs, which should all be given in maximum doses. Repeated attempts to reduce prednisolone dosage and stop treatment should be made by a specialist.

Short-term oral steroid therapy

While regular oral therapy definitely is the final step in maintenance treatment, short courses of prednisolone (1–2 weeks) can be necessary at any level of disease severity when inhaled medication cannot penetrate the airways. A short course of oral steroid, not used more than six times a year, is virtually without risk. Patients should be informed about these two faces of the same drug, to which most of them, as well as their doctors, have a hate–love relationship.

Action plan for acute exacerbations

It is part of patient education and patient–doctor partnership that an action plan for management of

Action plan		
	Peak flow	**Action**
Green zone	>80%	Continue therapy
Yellow zone	40–80%	Increase inhaled steroid Short course of oral steroid Contact your doctor
Red zone	<40%	Go directly to hospital

Table 9.25.3. Self-management plan for asthma

Situations when patient should call ambulance
Patient is too distressed to measure PEF
PEF is less than 40% of personal best (or predicted) in spite of bronchodilator treatment
Asthma ties patient to the chair
Patient can only speak single words
There has been temporary confusion or loss of consciousness

Table 9.25.4. Situations with an acute need for medical attention

acute exacerbations is made. It must include guidelines for when the patient: 1, can change medication; 2, should contact the doctor; and 3, should directly to hospital. A green–yellow–red zone system, adapted to a traffic-light system, is easy for most patients to use and remember (Tables 9.25.3–4).

Green zone (all clear)

PEF is >80% of personal best or predicted, and the variability is <20%. There are minimal daily symptoms and no nocturnal symptoms.

Yellow zone (warning)

PEF is 40–80% and the variability 20–30%. There is frequent coughing, wheezing, chest tightness, decreased activity and nocturnal asthma. Daily use of a short-acting beta$_2$ inhaler is needed.

In this situation, the dosage of inhaled steroid is increased (doubled if possible), and eventually a short burst of oral steroids is given, and tapered off as soon as PEF and symptoms return to green zone.

Red zone (medical emergency)

PEF <40% and remains there despite repeated use of a beta$_2$ inhaler. The patient needs immediate medical care, and, while awaiting the ambulance, he or she should continue to use his or her inhaler at short intervals, preferably from a spacer.

If this text isn't clear
Nobody has the right to speak more clearly than he thinks.

AN Whitehead

If you learn from this book
Wise men learn more from fools than fools from wise men.

Marcus Porcius Cato

9.26 Management of acute severe asthma I
A life-threatening medical emergency

Key points
• Acute severe asthma is usually preceded by deterioration over some days, but severe bronchoconstriction can develop within minutes.
• As a potentially fatal condition, acute severe asthma must be treated aggressively and observation must be intensive.
• The wheezing patient sits upright, fixing his or her shoulder girdle; he or she cannot speak a full sentence; there is tachypnoea and tachycardia.
• PEF is <40% of the personal best or predicted.
• Pao_2 is reduced according to the severity of the attack (<8 kPa in severe asthma).
• Additionally, $Paco_2$ is reduced, and a raised $Paco_2$ is a very serious sign in asthma.
• Oxygen must be given without hesitation (≥4 l/min).
• Inhalation of a beta$_2$ agonist, repeated and in a high dose, preferably from a oxygen-driven nebulizer, is the cornerstone of therapy.
• Ipratropium bromide may be added initially.
• If an inhaled beta$_2$ bronchodilator is given optimally, intravenous medication will add little to the effect.
• Initial use of two routes of administration, however, can, in some situations, add to the security of drug administration.
• Theophylline adds but little to the correct use of a beta$_2$ agonist, but it can be tried in very severe cases.
• Systemic steroids are obligatory and should be started early.
• Inhaled high-dose steroid therapy is started as early as possible.

The term *status asthmaticus* was earlier used to describe a prolonged episode of severe asthma temporarily refractory to the patient's usual medication. Today, the term *acute severe asthma* is used instead, and it is defined by peak flow recordings together with clinical characteristics (Table 9.26.1).

In most cases, a severe episode is preceded by a deterioration of the condition over some days, but, in a few cases of extreme bronchial hyper-responsiveness, bronchoconstriction can develop within minutes; '*brittle asthma*'.

As a potentially fatal condition, treatment of patients with acute severe asthma must be aggressive and observation must be intensive. The condition demands that patients be treated in a respiratory unit with close collaboration between respiratory specialist, anaesthetist and experienced nurses.

Clinical examination
For the experienced clinician, one educated look is almost enough to diagnose acute severe asthma. The air-hungry patient *sits upright*, fixing his or her shoulder girdle to enhance the effectiveness of his or her accessory respiratory muscles; he or she is *wheezing*, *expiration is prolonged* (relatively) and he or she *cannot speak a full sentence*, perhaps only a few words at a time. There is *tachypnoea* (≥25/min) and *tachycardia* (≥110/min).

A brief history of the development of the attack, provoking factors (e.g. infection, allergen exposure and pollutants), concurrent diseases (e.g. COPD, cardio-vascular disease or liver disease), previous hospital admissions and the recent use of prednisolone and/or theophylline is taken from the patient or his or her companion.

Lung function tests
Recording of peak flow is a must, but a patient who can only manage single words may be too dis-

Characteristics of acute severe asthma
Severe dyspnoea at rest
Speech in single words or broken sentences
Relatively prolonged expiration
Stethoscopic wheezes
Tachypnoea ≥25
Tachycardia ≥110
Peak flow <40%
Pao_2 <8 kPa
$Paco_2$ low or normal

Table 9.26.1. Characteristics of acute severe asthma

tressed to make the expiratory effort, which can worsen the condition. *PEF is <40% of the personal best or predicted in spite of inhaled bronchodilator therapy* (e.g. <160 l/min in a 170-cm, 30-year-old female).

Blood gases

Arterial blood should be taken and blood gases estimated immediately. *PaO_2 is reduced* according to the severity of the attack (<8 kPa in severe asthma). Additionally, *$PaCO_2$ is reduced* in the hyperventilating patient, and a *raised $PaCO_2$ is a very serious sign* in asthma (not necessarily in COPD). Increased HCO_3^- and positive base excess suggests a diagnosis of COPD.

Give oxygen

Oxygen must be given without hesitation. Initially, the flow must be high, at least 4 l/min (or 50%); it can be reduced as the patient responds to treatment. In asthma, in contrast to COPD, there is no risk of oxygen therapy causing CO_2-retention and narcosis.

Nebulized bronchodilators

Inhalation of a *beta$_2$ agonist*, *repeated* and in a *high dose* by any means, is the cornerstone of acute asthma therapy. It is started immediately after admission and is preferably given as a wet aerosol, delivered from an *oxygen-driven nebulizer*. Nebulized salbutamol or terbutaline (5 mg or 10 mg initially) is inhaled over 5 minutes. It can be repeated as required in the acute situation (e.g. every 20 minutes for 1 hour) and, when the condition is improving, it can be given every 4 hours. *Ipratropium* (0.5 mg) can be added initially in order to get further bronchodilatation.

Intravenous beta$_2$ agonist

An intravenous line is set up in all patients for drug administration and because intubation can become necessary quickly.

If an inhaled bronchodilator is given optimally, intravenous medication will add little to the effect. Initial use of two routes of administration, however, can, in some situations, add to the security of drug administration.

A bolus dose of salbutamol or terbutaline is followed by a maintenance dose (Table 9.26.2). Treatment results in tachycardia, tremor and a fall in plasma potassium.

Quick check-list in acute severe asthma
Rapid clinical examination
Peak flow measurement
Arterial sample
Oxygen at high flow (at least 4 l/min)
Nebulized salbutamol or terbutaline 5 mg; repeat as necessary, and later, every 4 hours; add ipratropium 0.5 mg initially
Intravenous salbutamol or terbutaline 0.25 mg; continue with 10 µg/min (10 mg/l, 60 ml/h)
Intravenous aminophylline* 6 mg/kg over 30 minutes; continue with 0.6 mg/kg/h
Intravenous methylprednisolone 40 mg; repeat every 6–8 hours
Re-assess the condition every 2–4 hours (PEF, blood gases, pulse rate and respiratory rate)

Table 9.26.2. Examination and treatment of acute severe asthma. *In very severe cases

Theophylline

Theophylline adds but little to the correct use of a beta$_2$ agonist. It can be tried in selected and in very severe cases.

If theophylline has not been taken, in any form, for the last 24 hours, a full loading dose is given followed by a maintenance dose (Table 9.26.2). No loading dose is given to patients on full oral therapy. The maintenance dose is reduced by at least 50% in patients with cardiac or hepatic disease. Plasma–theophylline must be checked after 24 hours and dosage be adjusted accordingly.

Steroids

Steroids are obligatory and should be started early, preferably with an intravenous bolus injection of 40 mg methylprednisolone, followed by injections every 6–8 hours. It is soon replaced by oral prednisolone, as described in Chapter 9.16. High-dose therapy with inhaled steroids is started as early as possible.

Differential diagnosis

In the emergency situation, it is often difficult to say whether a patient, who presents with acute airway

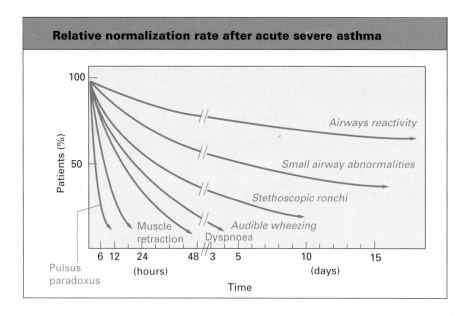

Fig. 9.26.1. Diagram to illustrate the different speeds of recovery of various parameters following status asthmaticus.

obstruction, suffers from reversible asthma or from partly reversible COPD. The patient should benefit from the doubt and receive full asthma treatment. When the correct diagnosis is COPD, glucocorticoid therapy should be stopped abruptly.

Warning

In patients with severe dyspnoea, *sedatives and tranquillizers are dangerous* and contra-indicated unless mechanical ventilation can be started quickly, if needed.

Chest X-ray

When the initial emergency measures have been completed, a chest X-ray is necessary to exclude pneumonia, atelectasis and pneumothorax.

Electrolytes

Serum electrolytes are examined as beta$_2$ agonists lower the plasma level temporarily by potassium transport to the intracellular compartment. When high doses are inhaled or injected, the fall will be 0.5–1.0 mmol/l or even more. This may imply a risk of cardiac arrhythmias in patients on digitalis and diuretics.

Examination for bronchial infection

Chest X-ray, blood leucocyte count, body temperature, and examination of the first sample of sputum for neutrophils and bacteria will indicate whether the patient needs antibiotic treatment. It should not be given as a routine.

Re-assessment

The regimen for any patient with acute severe asthma should be organized into periods with planned re-assessment every 2–4 hours. Most important are peak flow recordings. Initially, blood gases are part of the assessment but they become unnecessary when the patient's condition improves. Pulse rate and respiration frequency are valuable as simple and reliable parameters of asthma severity.

Recovery

After 24–72 hours, intravenous bronchodilators can usually be replaced by oral drugs, wet aerosols can be replaced by an ordinary inhaler, and the steroid can be administered by mouth. Inhaled steroid, in a high dosage, is started as early as possible.

Patients can usually be dismissed after approximately 1 week, when PEF is >70%, diurnal variation of PEF is <30%, and there is no nocturnal asthma. It is important to realize, however, that it can take several weeks after a severe episode before all disease parameters have reached their pre-episode baseline (Fig. 9.26.1).

Not recommendable for asthma
If you intend to give a sick man medicine, let him get very ill first, so that he may see the benefit of your medicine.
African (Nupe) proverb

9.27 Management of acute severe asthma II
Intubation and assisted ventilation

Key points
- Mechanical ventilation is life-saving in about 1% of patients with acute severe asthma.
- Intubation and ventilation should be considered when a patient has reduced consciousness, cyanosis, a silent chest, or is exhausted.
- In asthma, in contrast to COPD, even a slightly raised Pa_{CO_2} is a very serious sign.
- Of the same serious import is an increasing Pa_{CO_2} in a patient who is deteriorating clinically with falling Pa_{O_2} and PEF.
- Otherwise, the decision is based on close clinical observation (pulse rate and respiration rate) and consecutive measurements of blood gases and PEF.
- A planned and unhurried intubation is much safer than an emergency one in an arrested patient.

Mechanical ventilation is life-saving in about 1% of patients with severe acute asthma. These are the patients who develop respiratory arrest, usually soon after admission to hospital, and who develop progressive respiratory failure in spite of treatment.

When to intubate and ventilate
(Table 9.27.1)
Cardiac or respiratory arrest is, of course, an absolute indication for intubation and mechanical ventilation.

Indications for intubation
Cardiac or respiratory arrest
Reduced consciousness, cyanosis and silent chest
Patient speechless due to dyspnoea
Exhausted patient
Hypercapnia (even the slightest degree)
Increasing Pa_{CO_2}, with decreasing Pa_{O_2} and PEF

Table 9.27.1. Call anaesthetist immediately and consider intubation with artificial ventilation in these cases

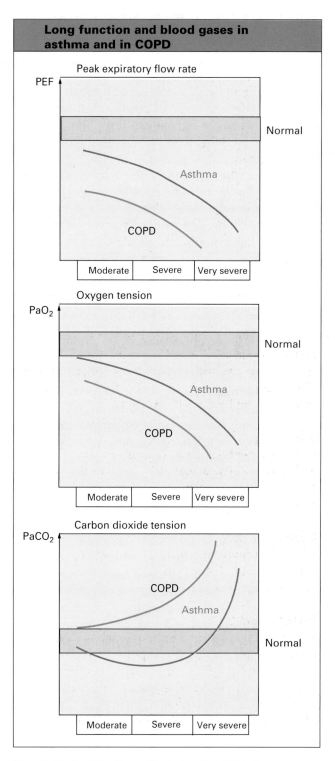

Fig. 9.27.1. This figure illustrates that PEF, Pa_{O_2} and Pa_{CO_2} relate differently to the severity of disease in asthma and in COPD.

When an asthma patient has reduced consciousness, central cyanosis, or a silent chest, arrest is close at hand and immediate action must be taken.

An exhausted patient who has been awake for days, fighting to breathe, should be intubated before he or she is on the verge of collapse. An unhurried intubation when the patient can just cope on his or her own is far safer than an emergency one in an arrested patient.

Otherwise, the decision is based on close clinical observation (pulse rate and respiration rate) and consecutive measurements of blood gases and PEF.

Serious warning signals are hypercapnia, and an increase in $Paco_2$ associated with a decrease in Pao_2, together with a clinical deterioration. If the 'crossover point' of equal $Paco_2$ and Pao_2 values is reached, death can occur without warning.

When a patient has had severe asthma for hours in spite of aggressive medical treatment, mechanical ventilation must be considered.

Assisted ventilation

Oxygen is the main requirement for respiratory arrest in asthma; ventilation with pure oxygen, by any means at hand, is the essential emergency treatment. Ventilation of unintubated patients is very difficult, because a high inspiratory pressure is needed to overcome the increased airway resistance.

Mechanical ventilation of intubated patients carries a risk of *complications*: machine failure, arrhythmias, infection and pneumothorax. The latter can quickly develop into a pressure pneumothorax during intermittent positive pressure respiration.

Neither oxygen therapy nor assisted respiration treat the basic abnormalities: bronchoconstriction, inflammation and mucus plugging. Continuous *pharmacological treatment* and attempts to remove secretions are therefore mandatory throughout the whole course of the acute episode.

Asthma versus COPD

It is important for the clinician to know that the interpretation of clinical signs, peak flow and blood gas values, differs in asthma and COPD (Fig. 9.27.1). An asthma patient with peripheral cyanosis, Pao_2 6 kPa and $Paco_2$ 9 kPa, is dying, while a chronic bronchitic patient with similar symptoms and signs can watch television in the living-room.

Discuss allergy
Great minds discuss ideas, average minds discuss events, little minds discuss people.

9.28 Death in asthma
Can it be avoided?

Key points
- The asthma death-rate is low at about 5/100 000 persons/year, and most deaths occur in elderly patients.
- About half of all deaths occur at home or before admission to hospital.
- Such deaths appear sudden and unexpected, but patients have usually had severely compromised lung function for a considerable time.
- The severity of the airway obstruction has been misjudged, and inadequate therapy has been prescribed or taken.
- In the rare case, a patient dies suddenly within minutes due to overwhelming bronchoconstriction, or pressure pneumothorax.
- Death in fulminant status asthmaticus can occur in hospital but it is rare.
- During the first 1–2 weeks following acute severe asthma, there is an increased risk of death associated with a marked PEF variation.
- Patients with deteriorating asthma use an increasing number of doses from their beta$_2$ inhaler, and this is an important warning signal.
- While asthma death correlates positively with the number of puffs from a beta$_2$ inhaler, it correlates negatively with the use of an inhaled steroid.
- Use of sedatives in acute severe asthma implies a risk of death and is contra-indicated.
- Theophylline is the only anti-asthma drug that is known to have caused a number of deaths.
- Asthma deaths may be prevented by early use of inhaled steroids, regular measurement of PEF, and identification of high-risk patients.

The old adage that asthmatics never die in the acute attack is not true but the overall *death rate is low* at about 5/100 000/year. Most deaths occur in elderly patients (Fig. 9.28.1).

Death associated with insufficient therapy
About half of all asthma deaths occur at home or before admission to hospital. These deaths are often considered to be 'sudden and unexpected'. As a rule, however, analysis of the case report shows that the severity of the airway obstruction was misjudged and inadequate therapy was prescribed or taken. The

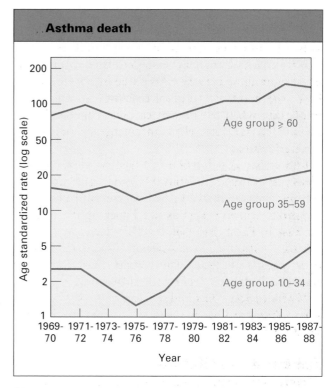

Fig. 9.28.1. Death from asthma in Denmark related to age of patient and to year of study. From Juel K, Pedersen PA. Increasing asthma mortality in Denmark 1969–88 not a result of changed coding practice. *Ann Allergy* 1992; **68**: 180–2.

patients have often had severely compromised lung function for a considerable time but appear and consider themselves well. It is a trap that patients who do not employ measurements of peak flow fall into.

Sudden, unexpected death
In the rare case, a patient dies suddenly, perhaps within minutes of the onset of an acute attack, which has not been preceded by days of impaired lung function. The cause of death is *overwhelming bronchoconstriction* (or pressure pneumothorax). Such patients have often had marked variation of PEF ('brittle asthma').

Death in fulminant status asthmaticus
Even with the best hospital care, acute severe asthma has a mortality rate, but it is low: <1%. The patients who die usually have non-allergic asthma. Death is due to progressive respiratory failure, cardiac arrhythmias, or complications from mechanical ventilation.

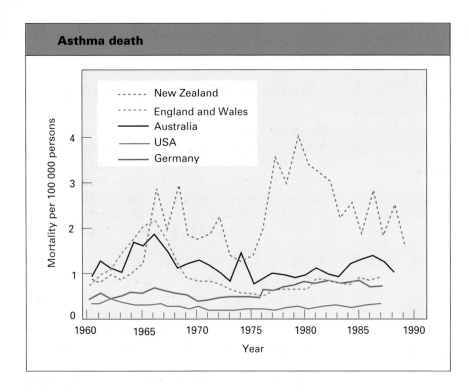

Fig. 9.28.2. Asthma deaths in different countries between 1960 and 1990 in individuals aged 5–34 years. Note the epidemics in the 1960s in the UK, and in the 1980s in New Zealand. From Jackson R, Sears MR, Beaglehole R, *et al.* International trends in asthma mortality: 1970 to 1985. *Chest* 1988; **94**: 914–18.

Death in the convalescent period

Attention has been drawn to a number of deaths occurring during the convalescent period. They appear to be related to a *marked diurnal variation* of airway obstruction. This should be looked for and, if found, considered a danger signal. The first 1–2 weeks following acute severe asthma always constitutes a danger period.

Asthma death and beta$_2$ sprays

There was a significant increase in the number of asthma deaths in the UK in the 1960s (Fig. 9.28.2), associated in time with the introduction of a high-dose isoprenaline spray. Excessive dosing may have contributed to cardiac arrhythmias in some cases, but *lack of patient instruction* is the most likely explanation for the majority of deaths. Having experienced the marked, immediate relief in their 'good periods', patients thought that 'bad periods' could be treated with a higher dosage without reference to their physician. What was needed was not more bronchodilators but steroids to combat the inflammation. Only half of these patients had ever received corticosteroids.

A more recent increase in asthma deaths in New Zealand has been attributed to excessive daily use of inhaled beta$_2$ agonists, which, without concomitant steroid therapy, have suppressed the symptoms but not the inflammation and the hyper-responsiveness. A Canadian study has found a positive correlation between asthma death and the number of puffs from a beta$_2$ inhaler, and a negative correlation between death and use of inhaled steroid. This is an important reason why inhaled steroids have now acquired a place early in asthma therapy, while inhaled beta$_2$ agonists are used mainly on an as-needed basis. Their use then serves as a warning signal of uncontrolled disease.

Sedatives and hypoventilation

Earlier in this century, asthma was considered to be a psychosomatic disease; sedatives, often barbiturates and narcotics, were the common treatment. Death from respiratory depression and hypoventilation was a not uncommon occurrence. Such drugs are now recognized as being *contra-indicated* in patients with acute severe asthma, unless they can be intubated and ventilated quickly if needed.

Drug toxicity

Severe asthma requires aggressive therapy and the risk of this therapy must be balanced against the severity of the disease. Even high-dosage systemic steroid treatment carries little risk provided its duration is limited to some days. Adrenaline and isoprenaline can now be replaced by drugs with far

High risk of asthma death
'Brittle asthma' with large PEF variation
Low PC_{20} with steep dose–response curve
Previous life-threatening attack
Previous attacks induced by food
Prior intubation for asthma
Lack of compliance with therapy
Drug and alcohol abuse

Table 9.28.1. Characteristics of patients with a high risk of asthma death

less cardio-toxicity. *Theophylline*, which has been pushed to near-toxic levels in severe asthma, has, unfortunately, caused a number of deaths.

It is possible, but has never been documented, that the sudden and considerable fall in plasma potassium during intravenous treatment with beta$_2$ agonists can result in arrhythmias in patients with cardiac diasease, especially when they use diuretics and digitalis.

Prevention
Asthma mortality and morbidity is unacceptably high. The following recommendations may reduce the risk of death: 1, greater use of inhaled anti-inflammatory steroids, even in patients with mild asthma; 2, objective monitoring of the condition based on the patient's own measurements of PEF; 3, greater participation of the patient in the management of the condition; and 4, the identification of patients with a high risk of asthma death, who should have an open line to a specialist ward (Table 9.28.1).

Fear of dying
Personally, I am not afraid of dying. I just don't want to be there when it happens.
Woody Allen

9.29 Pregnancy and asthma
Hypoxaemia the real danger

Key points
- Sexual intercourse can provoke asthma and pre-treatment with a beta$_2$ inhaler is helpful.
- During pregnancy, asthma may become worse, become less severe, or remain unchanged.
- Pregnant asthmatics are concerned about the possible effect of their asthma medication on the fetus.
- Inform them that ordinary anti-asthma therapy does not imply a risk for the fetus.
- The greatest risk for fetus and mother is severe asthma and hypoxaemia.
- Acute severe asthma must be avoided at all costs and, if it does occur, the usual intensive regimen is applied.
- The patient should be followed closely during pregnancy.
- In acute asthma, oxygen should be freely available.
- The ordinary anti-asthma treatment is given throughout pregnancy, preferably by the inhaled route.
- Oral vasoconstrictors may cause spasm of the uterine vessels and are best avoided.

Love affair
An asthmatic woman is handicapped from the very start of a love affair, which often takes place in a restaurant or similar place associated with dancing, drinking and smoking. Sexual intercourse is quite a severe exercise and, as such, may provoke broncho-constriction. This problem is seldom brought to the notice of the physician and a tactful enquiry may be relevant. Pretreatment with a bronchodilator aerosol is helpful as may be cromoglycate, although there is but one brief report in the literature. Most important is a loving understanding and a patient attitude on the part of her partner. This will prevent aggravation of the bronchoconstriction from fear and emotional stress.

Change of asthma during pregnancy
During pregnancy, asthma may become worse, become less severe, or remain unchanged in approximately equal numbers of women. The change is usually consistent from pregnancy to pregnancy.

Medication

It is understandable that pregnant asthmatics are concerned about the possible effect of their asthma medication on the fetus. Detailed information on this point is necessary, and it is preferably given before the pregnancy.

Prefer topical therapy

The ideal medication for the pregnant asthmatic would be topical, non-absorbable and effective. Inhaled beta$_2$ agonists, cromoglycate, and inhaled steroids approach this ideal and are preferable to oral medication. Systemic preparations may have unpredictable effects on the fetus but, in practice, both beta$_2$ agonists and theophylline appear to be safe. The former, however, may delay labour and the latter can aggravate the nausea and vomiting of pregnancy.

Avoid systemic vasoconstrictors

Injected adrenaline and oral alpha adrenoceptor agonists, including common cold remedies, may cause spasm of the uterine vessels and are best avoided in pregnancy. Vasoconstrictor nasal sprays, in usual dosage, are safe.

Oral corticosteroids

Cleft palate and placental insufficiency can occur in steroid-treated animals but evidence in humans is less clear. Clinical experience has indicated that prednisolone in ordinary anti-asthma doses apparently has little, if any, effect on the developing fetus. Continuous daily corticosteroids from conception to delivery may be associated with increased fetal wastage but the severe steroid-requiring disease itself is a more likely explanation than the drug.

Risk of hypoxaemia

Management of the pregnant asthmatic is a balance between the risk to the fetus from medication and from maternal hypoxaemia. The risk to the fetus is theoretical for the present anti-asthmatic drugs, but the risk from hypoxaemia is real. The fetus has little tolerance to maternal hypoxaeia, because Pao_2 in the fetal vessels is lower than maternal Pao_2.

Prevent severe asthma

The patient's lung function must be carefully monitored throughout the pregnancy; allergen and other precipitating factors should be avoided as far as possible.

In spite of any concern for drug effects on the fetus, the usual anti-asthmatic therapy must be given both for prevention and for treatment of acute exacerbations. It is not in the interest of mother or fetus to withhold either high-dose inhaled steroids or prednisolone, when this treatment is otherwise indicated.

Acute severe asthma must be avoided at all costs, and, if it does occur, the usual intensive regimen is applied. *Hypoxaemia is a known and potent teratogen*, and it is dangerous for the mother. *Oxygen should be freely available* during an acute asthma attack.

Love and life
Love while you've got love to give.
Live while you've got life to live.

Piet Hein

Further reading

Books

BARNES P, RODGER IW, THOMPSON, NC, eds. *Asthma. Basic Mechanisms and Clinical, Management* 2nd ed. New York: Academic Press, 1992: 1–782.

BUSSE, WW, HOLGATE ST, eds. *Asthma and Rhinitis* Oxford: Blackwell Science, 1995: 1–1488.

CLARK TJH, GODFREY S, LEE TH eds. *Asthma* 3rd ed. London: Chapman & Hall Medical, 1992: 1–622.

HOLGATE ST, AUSTEN KF, LICHTENSTEIN LM, KAY AB, eds. *Asthma. Physiology, Immunopharmacology, and Treatment* London: Academic Press, 1993: 1–443.

MIDDLETON E, REED CE, ELLIS E, *et al.*, eds. *Allergy. Principles and Practice* 4th ed. ST Louis: The CV Mosby Company, 1993: 1–1793.

SCHATZ M, ZEIGER RS, eds. *Asthma and Allergy in Pregnancy and Early Infancy* New York: Marcel Dekker, Inc, 1993: 1–636.

WEISS EB, STEIN M, eds. *Bronchial Asthma. Mechanisms and Therapeutics* 3rd ed. Boston: Little, Brown & Co, 1993: 1–1259.

Articles

ANONYMOUS. Beta$_2$ agonists in asthma: relief, prevention, morbidity. *Lancet* 1990; **336**: 1411–12.

AZZAWI M, ASSOUFI B, COLLINS JV, *et al.* Identification of activated T-lymphocytes and eosinophils in bronchial biopsies in stable atopic asthma. *Am Rev Respir Dis* 1990; **142**: 1407–13.

AZZAWI M, JOHNSTON PW, MAJUNDAR S, KAY AB, JEFFERY PK. T lymphocytes and activated eosinophils in airway mucosa in fatal asthma and cystic fibrosis. *Am Rev Respir Dis* 1992; **145**: 1477–82.

BARNES NC. Effects of corticosteroids in acute severe asthma. *Thorax* 1992; **47**: 582–3.

BARNES PJ. A new approach to the treatment of asthma. *N Engl J Med* 1989; **321**: 1517–27.

BARNES PJ, Neural control of airway function: new perspectives. *Mol Aspects Med* 1990; **11**: 351–423.

BARNES PJ, BARANIUK J, BELVISI MG. Neuropeptides in the respiratory tract. *Am Rev Respir Dis* 1991; **144**: 1289–314.

BARNES PJ, PEDERSEN S. Efficacy and safety of inhaled corticosteroids in asthma. *Am Rev Respir Dis* 1993; **148**: S1–26.

BENTLEY AM, MENZ G, STORZ CHR, *et al.* Identification of T lymphocytes, macrophages and activated eosinophils in the bronchial mucosa in intrinsic asthma. *Am Rev Respir Dis* 1992; **146**: 500–6.

BOUSQUET J, BURNEY P. Evidence for an increase in atopic disease and possible causes. *Clin Exp Allergy* 1993; **23**: 484–92.

BOUSQUET J, CHANEZ P, LACOSTE JY, *et al.* Eosinophilic inflammation in asthma. *N Engl J Med* 1990; **323**: 1033–1039.

BOWLER SD, MITCHELL CA, ARMSTRONG JG. Corticosteroids in acute severe asthma: effectiveness of low doses. *Thorax* 1992; **47**: 582–3.

British Thoracic Society. Guidelines on the management of asthma. *Thorax* 1993; **48**(suppl): S1–24.

BURNEY PGJ, CHINN S, RONA RJ. Has the prevalence of asthma changed? Evidence from the national study of health and growth. *Br Med J* 1990; **300**: 1306–10.

CASTLE W, FULLER R, HALL J, PALMER J. Serevent nationwide surveillance study: comparison of salmeterol with salbutamol in asthmatic patients who require regular bronchodilator treatment. *Br J Med* 1993; **306**: 1034–7.

CHAN-YEUNG M. Occupational asthma. *Chest* 1990; **98**(suppl): 148S.

COCKROFT DW, HARGREAVE FE. Airway hyperresponsiveness: relevance of random population data to clinical usefulness. *Am Rev Respir Dis* 1990; **142**: 497–502.

COLLOFF MJ, AYRES J, CARSWELL F, *et al.* The control of allergens of dust mites and domestic pets: a position paper. *Clin Exp Allergy* 1992; **22**(suppl 2): 1–28.

CYPCAR D, BUSSE WW. Steroid-resistant asthma. *J Allergy Clin Immunol* 1993; **92**: 362–72.

DAHL R, HAAHTELA T. Prophylactic pharmacologic treatment of asthma. *Allergy* 1992; **47**: 588–93.

DOLOVICH J, O'BYRNE P, HARGREAVE FE. Airway hyperresponsiveness: mechanisms and relevance. *Pediatr Allergy Immunol* 1992; **3**: 163–70.

DOUGLAS NJ. Nocturnal asthma. *Thorax* 1993; **48**: 100–2.

ENGEL T, HEINIG JH. Glucocorticosteroid therapy in acute severe asthma — a critical review. *Eur Respir J* 1991; **4**: 881–9.

HAAHTELA T, JÄRVINEN M, KAVA T, KOSKINEN S, LEHTONEN K. Comparison of a β$_2$-agonist terbutaline with an inhaled steroid in newly detected asthma. *N Engl J Med* 1991; **325**: 388–92.

HARGREAVE FE, DOLOVICH J, NEWHOUSE MT. The assessment and treatment of athma: a conference report. *J Allergy Clin Immunol* 1989; **85**: 1098–102.

HOLT PG, SCHON-HEGRAD MA, MCMENAMIN PG. Dendritic cells in the respiratory tract. *Int Rev Immunol* 1990; **6**: 139–149.

HUMMEL S, LEHTONEN L. Comparison of oral steroid sparing by high-dose and low-dose inhaled steroid in maintenance treatment of severe asthma. *Lancet* 1992; **340**: 1483–7.

IDRIS AH, MCDERMOTT MF, RAUCCI JC, *et al.* Emergency department treatment of severe asthma. Metered-dose inhalers plus holding chamber is equivalent in effectiveness to nebulizers. *Chest* 1993; **103**: 665–72.

International Consensus Report on Diagnosis and Management of Asthma. *Allergy* 1992; **47**(suppl 13): 1–61.

JUNIPER EF, KLINE PA, VANZIELEGHEM MA, HARGREAVE FE. Reduction of budesonide after a year of increased use: a randomized controlled trial to evaluate whether improvement in airway responsiveness and clinical asthma are maintained. *J Allergy Clin Immunol* 1991; **87**: 483–9.

KAMM RD, DRAZEN JM. Airway hyperresponsiveness and airway wall thickening in asthma. *Am Rev Respir Dis* 1992; **145**: 1249–56.

LAITINEN LA, LAITINEN A, HAATELA T. A comparative study of the effects of an inhaled corticosteroid, budesonide, and a beta$_2$ agonist, terbutaline, on airway inflammation in newly diagnosed asthma. *J Allergy Clin Immunol* 1992; **90**: 32–42.

LENFANT C, BOSCO LA, SANDER N, *et al.* Management of asthma during pregnancy. *J Allergy Clin Immunol* 1994; **93**: 139–62.

MCFADDEN JR ER. Dosages of corticosteroids in asthma. *Am Rev Respir Dis* 1993; **147**:1306–10.

MCFADDEN JR ER, GILBERT IA. Asthma. *N Engl J Med* 1992; **327**: 1928–37.

MALO JL, L'ARCHEVEQUE J, TRUDEAU C, D'AQUINO C, CARTIER A. Should we monitor peak expiratory flow rates or record symptoms with a simple diary in the management of asthma? *J Allergy Clin Immunol* 1993; **91**: 702–9.

MONTEFORT S, HERBERT CA, ROBINSON C, HOLGATE ST. The bronchial epithelium as a target for inflammatory attack in asthma. *Clin Exp Allergy* 1992; **22**: 511–20.

MULLEN M, MULLEN B, CAREY M. The association between β-agonist use and death from asthma. *JAMA* 1993; **270**: 1842–5.

O'DRISCOLL BR, KALRA S, WILSON M, *et al.* A double-blind trial of steroid tapering in acute asthma. *Lancet* 1993; **341**: 324–7.

PAGE C. Sodium cromoglycate, a tachykinin antagonist? *Lancet* 1994; **343**: 70–6.

PARKER SR, MELLINS RB, SOGN DD. Asthma education: a national strategy. NHLBI workshop summary. *Am Rev Respir Dis* 1990; **149**: 848–53.

PERLMAN DS, CHERVINSKY P, LAFORCE C, *et al.* A comparison of salmeterol with albuterol in the treatment of mild-to-moderate asthma. *N Engl J Med* 1992; **327**: 1402–5.

PIPER JM, WAYNE AR, DAUGHERTY JR, GRIFFIN MR. Corticosteroid use and peptic ulcer disease: role of nonsteroidal anti-inflammatory drugs. *Ann Intern Med* 1991; **114**: 735–740.

ROBINSON DS, HAMID Q, YING S, *et al.* Predominant Th2 type bronchoalveolar lavage T-lymphocyte population in atopic asthma. *N Engl J Med* 1992; **326**: 298–304.

ROCHE WR, BEASLEY R, WILLIAMS JH, HOLGATE ST. Subepithelial fibrosis in the bronchi of asthmatics. *Lancet* 1989; **1**: 520–4.

SCHATZ M. Asthma during pregnancy: interrelationships and management. *Ann Allergy* 1992; **68**: 123–33.

SEARS MR, TAYLOR DR, PRINT CG, *et al.* Increased inhaled bronchodilator vs. increased inhaled corticosteroid in the control of moderate asthma. *Chest* 1992; **102**: 1709–1715.

SHEFFER AL. Global strategy for asthma management and prevention. *NHLBI/WHO Workshop Report. NIH Publication No. 95–3659.* 1995: 1–176.

SLY RM. Asthma mortality, East and West. *Ann Allergy* 1992; **69**: 81–4.

SLY RM. Changing asthma mortality. *Ann Allergy* 1994; **73**: 259–68.

SPITZER WO, SUISSA S, ERNST P, *et al.* The use of β-agonists and the risk of death and near death from asthma. *N Engl J Med* 1992; **326**: 501–6.

SPORIK R, HOLGATE ST, PLATTS-MILLS TAE, COGSWELL JJ. Exposure to house dust mite allergen (*Der p* i) and the development of asthma in childhood. A prospective study. *N Engl J Med* 1990; **323**: 502–7.

STEIN LM, COLE RP. Early administration of corticosteroids in emergency room treatment of acute asthma. *Ann Intern Med* 1990; **112**: 822–7.

TAYLOR IK, SHAW RJ. The mechanisms of action of corticosteroids in asthma. *Respir Med* 1993; **87**: 261–77.

TOOGOOD HJ. High dose inhaled steroid therapy in asthma. *J Allergy Clin Immunol* 1989; **83**: 528–36.

TOOGOOD JH. Effects of inhaled and oral corticosteroids on bone. *Ann Allergy* 1991; **67**: 87–90.

TOOGOOD JH, BASKERVILLE J, JENNINGS B, LEFCOE NM, JOGANSSON S-Å. Bioequivalent doses of budesonide and prednisone in moderate and severe asthma. *J Allergy Clin Immunol* 1989; **84**: 688–700.

ULRIK CS, BACKER V, DIRKSEN A. A 10-year follow-up of 180 adults with bronchial asthma: factors important for the decline in lung function. *Thorax* 1992; **47**: 14–18.

WARDLAW AJ. Air pollution and asthma. *Clin Exp Allergy* 1993; **23**: 81–106.

WARDLAW AJ, GEDDES DM. Allergic bronchopulmonary aspergillosis: a review. *J Roy Soc Med* 1992; **85**: 747–51.

WARNER JO, GÖTZ M, LANDAU LI, *et al.* Management of asthma: a consensus statement. *Arch Dis Child* 1989; **64**: 1065–79.

WOOD RA, CHAPMAN MD, ADKINSON NF JR, EGGLESTON PA. The effect of cat removal on allergen content in house-dust samples. *J Allergy Clin Immunol* 1989; **83**: 730–734.

Part 10 Asthma in Childhood

10.1 Diagnosis
– and special features

Key points
- Asthma ranks as one of the most important causes of ill health in children in the western world.
- Children, especially young children, are at increased risk of airway obstruction for a number of reasons.
- They have disproportionally small peripheral airways and cross-sectional airway area.
- A relative lack of elastic recoil in the chest wall predisposes to early airway closure.
- Together with a soft bronchial wall, it produces ventilation–perfusion mismatch and low oxygen tension.
- Undeveloped channels between alveoli and collateral ventilation predispose to segmental collapse and atelectasis.
- A horizontal insertion of the diaphragm makes it less efficient and less suitable to cope with prolonged increased workloads.
- Therefore, young children readily develop respiratory failure during acute episodes of asthma.
- Children need simple, direct and specific questions, not 'How is your asthma?'.
- They often consider their state of chronic invalidism as 'normal'.
- Parents may be unaware of important details; they interpret their observations and often dislike regular medication.
- Night-time cough, recurrent cough after colds, or unwillingness to participate in sports may be the only symptoms of asthma.
- In the individual child, PEF in per cent of personal best after a period of aggressive treatment is more informative than PEF in per cent of predicted normal.
- PEF can be measured by most children ⩾5 years.
- PEF variability and drug reversibility are useful as in adult asthma.
- An exercise test is often valuable in children.
- Wheezing in the lower airways is extremely common in infants.
- A viral infection is the most important trigger factor and parental smoking is predisposing.
- In 65%, wheezing is not associated with atopic allergic diseases.
- In 35%, it is an early manifestation of asthma.
- In the first group, symptoms disappear before the age of 3 years, while they often persist into adult life in the second group.
- Chronic asthma in childhood may result in irreversible airway obstruction.
- Children with severe chronic asthma show growth retardation and delayed onset of puberty but achieve normal final height.

Children are not small adults
Asthma in children ranks as *one of the most important causes of ill health* in the western world, creating a myriad of physical, emotional, economical and social problems for the child and the family.

Although childhood asthma and adult asthma share the same underlying pathophysiological mechanisms, there are important anatomical, physiological, social, emotional and developmental, age-related differences. Therefore, it is necessary to consider the diagnosis and management of this age group in its own right and not merely extrapolate from experience with adults.

Within the childhood population, it is appropriate to make a distinction between *older children* and *infants or young children <3 years*, as these two age groups show clinically important differences.

Anatomical and physiological factors
There are many reasons why children, and especially young children, are at *increased risk of airway obstruction* and at times do not respond so well to treatment. Compared to adult airways, young children have disproportionally smaller peripheral airways and smaller cross-sectional airway area, rendering them *more easily obstructed* by oedema, secretions, cellular debris and smooth muscle contractions. The chest wall of an infant is more compliant than in later life, but there is a relative *lack of elastic recoil* predisposing to early airway closure even during tidal breathing. This, in combination with *less rigid walls* of the bronchi, produces ventilation–perfusion mismatching, and *lower oxygen tensions* than in adults.

The collateral channels between the alveoli (pores of Kohn) and the bronchoalveolar communications (Lambert's canals) are reduced in number and size. Therefore, *collateral ventilation is less developed*, and airway obstruction is more prone to cause *segmental collapse and atelectasis* than in older subjects.

Finally, the angle of insertion of the *diaphragm is more horizontal* than in adults. This means that

History taking
Family history
General medical history
Atopic history
Environmental history
Specific symptoms
Frequency and severity of symptoms
Description of typical attack
Precipitating factors
Impact of disease on child and family
Physical exercise (play and sport)
School attendance and performance
Psychosocial evaluation
Previous and current therapy

Table 10.1.1. The history in childhood asthma taken from child and parents

during inspiration the infant's diaphragm tends to cause *retraction of the compliant rib-cage* rather than elevation and increased diameter. This makes the diaphragm less efficient and, due to few fatigue-resistant muscle fibres, less suitable to cope with prolonged increased workloads. Therefore, young children *more readily develop respiratory failure* during acute episodes of asthma.

History taking

The history should describe the specific symptoms, their severity and impact on child and family, the child's school attendance and performance, the environment, and include a psychosocial evaluation (Table 10.1.1).

– from parents

Most of the important information is usually obtained by questioning the parents, and that complicates the matter. Many parents are *unaware of important details*, and they *interpret their observations* and present an 'edited version'. For example,

the majority of children find parental smoking a problem for their asthma, but less than 10% of smoking parents realize that. A question about whether or not the child participates in sport activities is rarely answered by a simple yes or no but with a more plausible explaining answer, such as 'he/she is not interested in sport', emphasizing that the problem is not that the child is sick. Furthermore, their description of the child's symptoms may be influenced by their *dislike of regular medication*, which they fear has side effects and which daily reminds them that they have a sick child.

– from the child

Communicating directly with the child is often more useful but not without problems either: 1, children have a limited vocabulary; 2, they do not readily open themselves to the physician; 3, they are influenced by their parents' opinion; and 4, they do not want to disappoint or bother the doctor.

Most children with chronic asthma have had their symptoms since early childhood. Consequently, they have gradually adjusted their life-style to the condition, and they have come to *accept a state of chronic invalidism as 'normal'.*

Children require some time for their answers and therefore are frequently interrupted by their parents. Inaccurate and unspecific questions such as 'How is your asthma?' are useless, as the answer will be 'Fine' or 'OK' from nine out of 10 children in whom subsequent, careful and *specific questioning* may reveal important problems interfering with an unrestricted daily life.

Other symptoms

It is often anticipated that asthma is easy to diagnose in older children and wheeze is always present, but *cough* (often at night) may be the only symptom. Typically, the child coughs for some weeks every time it has had a common cold, and that is not normal. *Recurrent colds, chest infection or 'bronchitis'* may be the way the parents' describe asthma symptoms, so always ask about the specific symptoms. *Unwillingness to participate in sports and other physical activities* may also be the only complaint.

Diary recordings and symptom scores

Standardized questionnaires and diary recordings with specific questions about cough, wheeze, physical activities, wake-ups at night are useful. However, they may not disclose to what extent the child has adapted its life-style to avoid symptoms. In other words, a low symptom score does not necessarily mean that there is no problem.

Lung function

Per cent of personal best
Most *children ≥5 years* are able to do reproducible PEF measurements and should do this at home for some weeks when establishing the asthma diagnosis. However, it is important to realize that, in children, PEF and FEV_1 can be normal in the presence of quite marked small airway obstruction and hyperinflation.

Measured pulmonary function values are often expressed in per cent of predicted normal. However, there is a substantial inter-individual variation in lung function values in children. A pulmonary function of 85% of predicted normal may be quite good in one child whereas is may be unacceptable in another whose best pulmonary function, after aggressive treatment, is 125% of the predicted. Therefore, a *lung function in per cent of personal best after a period of aggressive treatment is very useful* in children.

Variability and daily PEF
Repeated measurements at home, morning (as soon as the child gets out of bed) and evening, are very useful in assessing the magnitude of the variation. This can be supplemented by measurements before and after inhalation of a beta$_2$ agonist.

A ≥15–20% variation in lung function over a short period of time is usually considered diagnostic for asthma. However, in some young children with a PEF around 150 l/min, such a variation may be close to the error of measurement.

Beta$_2$ reversibility
Measurements of lung function, at hospital, before and after four to six doses of an inhaled beta$_2$ agonist, can also be used to demonstrate reversibility. An insignificant increase in lung function, however, does not exclude the diagnosis.

Steroid reversibility
A trial of 4–6 weeks' treatment with inhaled corticosteroids in a fairly high dose (400–800 µg/day) is very useful in establishing the diagnosis and defining the personal best lung function. If it increases ≥15–20% during treatment, an asthma diagnosis can be made with confidence. If symptoms improve but lung function only changes <15%, the asthma diagnosis is likely but it should be confirmed by recurrence of symptoms when the treatment is stopped and by renewed amelioration when it is reintroduced.

Exercise test
A standardized exercise test is a clinically very useful test in order to assess bronchial responsiveness (see Chapter 9.10). A fall in PEF or FEV_1 ≥15–20% strongly suggests the presence of hyper-responsiveness and of asthma. Generally, methacholine or histamine provocation tests are not clinically helpful in children.

Wheezing illnesses in young children
Wheezing-associated lower respiratory tract illnesses in infants or young children (<3 years) are *extremely common* in the western world, with estimates of its cumulative prevalence *ranging between 30% and 50%*. Parental tobacco smoke is a predisposing factor and the most common trigger is a viral infection.

The past few years have increased our understanding of wheezing disorders in early childhood, and it has been recognized that there are *two major groups of recurrent wheezers in early life*. From a clinical point of view, it is difficult to distinguish between these two groups during the first few years of life. In addition, other rare causes of wheezing must be excluded (Tables 10.1.2–3).

Early manifestation of asthma
This group constitutes 35% of the wheezy children. They have often a family history of atopy, allergic markers, and signs of bronchial hyper-responsiveness with symptoms between the episodes of severe wheeze (Table 10.1.4). Without any treatment, a significant *deterioration in lung function* during the first 6 years of life is seen in this group, and they usually *continue to have symptoms* later in life.

Transient infant wheezers
In this group (65%), wheezing is associated with *small airway calibre*, which is present from birth. These children, who do not have the characteristics of the patients in the asthma group, to not develop reduced lung function. They have *a good prognosis,*

Other causes of wheezing in young children
Bronchial stenosis
Bronchopulmonary dysplasia
Cardiac disease
Congenital obstructive emphysema
Cystic fibrosis
Cysts
Foreign body
Gastro-oesophageal reflux
Immunodeficiency
Mediastinal mass
Primary ciliary dyskinesia
Recurrent infections
Pulmonary sequester
Tracheomalacia
Tuberculosis
Vascular ring

Table 10.1.2. Rare diseases in childhood that can cause wheezing

the vast majority growing out of their symptoms before the age of 3 years.

Other important issues in childhood asthma

Irreversible airway obstruction

For years it was taken for granted that childhood asthma does not lead to lung damage even though some children obviously developed chest deformities. However, recent findings strongly indicate that chronic asthma in childhood, as in adulthood, may result in irreversible airway obstruction. It seems that it can be prevented or reduced by early treatment with inhaled steroids.

Natural history

It is often anticipated that childhood asthma is a self-

Symptoms and signs of alternative diagnosis
History
Neonatal onset of symptoms
Neonatal history of ventilatory support
Intractable wheeze unresponsive to bronchodilators or steroids
Wheeze associated with feeding or vomiting
Sudden onset (coughing/choking)
Steatorrhoea
Physical signs
Failure to thrive
Clubbing
Cardiac murmur
Stridor
Focal lung signs
Investigations
No reversibility with therapy
Persistent chest radiographic finding

Table 10.1.3. Unusual clinical features in children with wheeze that suggest an alternative diagnosis

Features favouring asthma
Atopic family history
Atopic dermatitis
Symptoms from other organs
Positive allergy test
Symptoms between acute episodes

Table 10.1.4. Features favouring the asthma diagnosis in young children with wheezing illness

limiting disorder, which will improve spontaneously during adolescence. This is an over-simplification that mainly applies to children with mild, episodic symptoms. The majority of children with persistent symptoms in childhood will continue to wheeze and have reduced pulmonary function into adult life, though many tend to improve. Furthermore, a large proportion of children with remission in early adolescence will have recurrence of their symptoms when they grow older. Finally, the term 'outgrowing the asthma' may be somewhat misleading as recent studies indicate that many patients, who consider themselves symptom-free, still have reduced pulmonary function and increased bronchial reactivity to specific and non-specific agents.

Growth

Many children with moderate and severe chronic asthma show *growth retardation* and *delayed onset of puberty*. Generally, these children tend to grow for a longer period of time than their peers so that before the age of 20 they will achieve *normal final height*. By contrast, growth retardation caused by daily and alternate-day administration of systemic corticosteroids may be permanent.

The deviant growth pattern complicates the interpretation of results from studies comparing the heights of asthmatic children treated with inhaled steroids with the heights of normal children. Furthermore, it means that case reports of apparently reduced growth in association with an asthma treatment should not lead to conclusions about cause–effect relationships.

Often, one of the aims of the management of childhood asthma is to ensure a normal growth. If normality, in this respect, means a growth pattern like a non-asthmatic child, this aim cannot be achieved in one-third of the asthmatic childhood population.

Lack of objective
If you don't know where you are going, you will probably end up somewhere else.

Søren Pedersen

10.2 Daily management I
General measures

Key points
- The treatment objectives are: freedom from symptoms, a normal lung function, prevention of lung damage and a minimum risk of death.
- The child should be able to live an unrestricted life without avoidance of physical exercise.
- Though these objectives are achievable in the majority of children, they are not fulfilled in many patients.
- Environmental control consists of removal of important allergens and irritants, such as cigarette smoking.
- Such measures, however, may have considerable psychological consequences in the family.
- Giving information and advice rather than ordering various measures is likely to preserve a good physician–patient/family relationship.
- Young children in day-care institutions often get viral airway infections and asthma exacerbations.
- Advice to stay away from day-care centres may be considered in severe cases.
- Participation in sport and play is important for normal growth and psychosocial development of the child.
- Consequently, exercise-induced asthma is a bigger problem in children than in adults.
- Children with asthma should be encouraged to participate in all physical activities and play.
- They may benefit from a physical training programme.
- Immunotherapy may be considered in children $\geqslant 5$ who cannot avoid an allergen of major importance for the disease.
- However, the role of immunotherapy in the treatment of childhood asthma still remains controversial.

Objectives of treatment
Before treatment of an asthma child is decided, it is important to *define the objectives of the management* (Table 10.2.1). As in adults, the objectives imply symptom freedom, a normal lung function, prevention of lung damage, and a minimum risk of deaths. In a child, *freedom from symptoms* means more than simple absence of wheeze and cough at rest. It implies that the child can *live an unrestricted life* without

Objectives of asthma management
Freedom from symptoms
An unrestricted life with normal physical activity
Normal lung function at the child's personal best
Prevention of irreversible airway obstruction
Prevention of asthma-related psychosocial problems
No or few acute hospital admissions
No mortality

Table 10.2.1. Objectives of asthma management in children

avoidance of symptom-provoking situations and, in particular, of *physical exercise*. Asthma management in children also aims at preventing the development of psychosocial problems, associated with chronic illnesses in childhood.

Though these objectives are probably agreed upon by most physicians and they are achievable in the majority of children, clinical experience and the literature suggests that *the objectives are not fulfilled in many children* (the majority?). There is a number of reasons for this, including variations in the perception and definition of the terms 'symptom-free' and 'normal lung function' (as discussed in Chapter 10.1). Furthermore, insufficient knowledge about the problems associated with the management of childhood asthma and about optimal choice of inhalers, drugs and doses in the various age groups is also important in this respect.

Achievement of the goals for asthma management usually require a combination of *general supportive measures* and a *positive attitude to active pharmacotherapy* (see Chapters 10.3–5).

Environmental control

Removal of important *allergens* and irritants, such as *cigarette smoking*, is a very important requisite for good management of childhood asthma. Removal of, for example, an offending pet is even *more important in children* than in adults. This topic is discussed in Chapter 9.24.

When recommendations of avoidance measures are given, it is wise always to have considered their *psychological consequences*. The asthmatic child is an integral part of a family and the suggested measures may have an important impact upon the family relations, as the restrictions often involve subjects who are not sick. Removal of the father's sporting dog, banning cigarette smoking or moving the asthmatic child to a sibling's room because it has a better indoor climate, may create negative tensions. Therefore, the physician should supply the family with knowledge and discuss the problems rather than just ordering various measures. Such policy is more likely to preserve a good physician–patient relationship.

Young children in *day-care institutions* get *viral upper airway infections* much more frequently than their peers. This increases the likelihood of wheeze, and it may be tempting to advise these children to stay away from the crowded day-care centres. Though likely to be beneficial, such an intervention can have a heavy impact not only upon the child's social development but also upon the life of the parents, who may not be able to work full-time if the child has to be isolated from contact with other children. Therefore, such advice should be reserved for the severe cases who cannot be controlled on regular therapy with bronchodilators and inhaled corticosteroids.

Exercise

Participation in sport and play is important for a normal growth and psychosocial development of children. Therefore, exercise-induced asthma is a much *bigger problem in children* than in adults, and children with asthma should be *encouraged to participate in all physical activities* and play. Much effort should be put into stimulating enjoyable, balanced physical activities to build up fitness and self-confidence in the child's own environment. Many asthmatic children are physically unfit and therefore may require a short *physical training programme* to break the vicious circle of exercise-induced asthma and unfitness. Such a programme does not have any direct effect upon the asthma, but it is likely to improve physical fitness, exercise tolerance, the child's ability to cope with the asthma, neuromuscular coordination and *self-confidence*, all of which are important for a normal integration of the child with his or her peers. It is important that this aspect of asthma management is not forgotten. Often a 6–8 weeks' training course is sufficient.

Immunotherapy

This issue is discussed in detail in Part 11. Therefore,

only some considerations particular for childhood asthma will be mentioned. A subcommittee of the European Academy of Allergology and Clinical Immunology recently recommended that immunotherapy should *not be used in children <5 years.* Furthermore, it should only be initiated when *a relevant allergen has been identified* by proper allergy testing, when it is considered to be *of major importance* for the daily symptoms, and when it *cannot be avoided.*

Immunotherapy seems most beneficial in children with *mild and moderate asthma*, a condition that is normally safely and effectively treated with sodium cromoglycate or low-dose inhaled corticosteroids. Furthermore, these groups of children seem to have the best prognosis for outgrowing their asthma. Once initiated, immunotherapy must be continued for as long as any other form of prophylactic treatment. For these reasons, its role in the treatment of childhood asthma still remains *controversial.*

Freud about asthma
Our sense of identity is rooted in our physical being.
                                                    Sigmund Freud

---

10.3 Daily management II
Pharmacotherapy

Key points
- Pharmacotherapy, given by the inhaled route, is the mainstay in asthma therapy.
- Oral bronchodilator therapy plays a limited role.
- Generally, our knowledge of pharmacokinetics and pharmacodynamics in children is sparse.
- Theophylline is the drug that has been most studied with regard to pharmacokinetics in children.
- In general, children metabolize theophylline, as well as other drugs, more rapidly than adults.
- Children also show considerable inter-individual variation in metabolism and drug half-life.
- Consequently, children require high and individually adjusted doses.
- The rapid clearance of drugs means that children may need more frequent dosing than adults.
- Slow-release preparations are preferable but absorption may be influenced by food.
- The bioavailability of slow-release beta$_2$ agonists is lower than that of plain tablets and syrup (30% dose increase).
- Optimal use of oral beta$_2$ agonists should be based on individual dose titration.

Route of administration
Asthma in children is rewarding to treat as the life of the child can usually be radically altered. We still have no cure for asthma, so pharmacotherapy is likely to remain the cornerstone of asthma management in children for the next decade.

As in adults, the various drugs can be given either systemically or by inhalation. *Much speaks in favour of the inhaled route.* The medication is deposited directly at the receptors in the airways, allowing a rapid onset of action. The administered therapeutic dose is small, and, hence, the incidence of side effects for a given clinical effect is low. Exercise-induced bronchoconstriction can only be effectively blocked by inhaled therapy, and the drugs available for a safe, effective long-term treatment of the inflammatory component of the disease can only be given by the inhaled route. For these reasons, *inhaled therapy should be the mainstay of treatment* of childhood asthma.

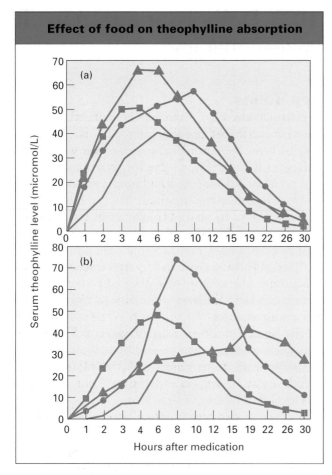

Fig. 10.3.1. Mean serum levels of theophylline in children with asthma taking a single dose of four different brands of slow-release preparations while (a) fasting and (b) after a standardized breakfast. From Pedersen S. Effect of food on the absorption of theophylline in children. *J Allergy Clin Immunol* 1986; **78**: 704–9.

Pharmacokinetics and pharmacodynamics

Theophylline

Only the pharmacokinetics of theophylline have been studied to a satisfactory extent in all age groups of children. It appears, however, that *children metabolize drugs more rapidly* than adults and that the clearance of drug varies from age group to age group and from patient to patient. Therefore, children often require quite *high and individually adjusted doses* of oral drugs to achieve a satisfactory effect. This is not always appreciated and, consequently, many drugs are used in suboptimal or ineffective doses in children. Furthermore, the tablet sizes available often do not allow the dose to be related accurately to the size of the child. This may also contribute to *suboptimal therapy.*

The *rapid clearance* of drugs means that children must *take oral drugs at short intervals* or *slow-release preparations* two (to three) times a day. The latter is preferable due to an improved compliance with twice-daily dosing. However, the advantages of slow-release products may sometimes be outweighed by inconsistent absorption characteristics of these products when taken in combination with *food* (Fig. 10.3.1). As the various products are influenced in different and unpredictable ways, children should only be treated with slow-release preparations whose absorption characteristics have been found reliable in the presence of food.

The dose recommendations given for theophylline (see Table 10.6.1) are based on lean body weight, and they aim at plasma theophylline levels between 55 and 110 μmol/l (10–20 mg/l), which may be too high. Within each age group, the *inter-individual variations* in theophylline half-life may be up to 10-fold, and, in addition, *other drugs* including beta$_2$ agonists (increase clearance) and *viral infections* (reduce clearance) may also *affect the metabolism.* Therefore, the theophylline dose must always be individualized and, if high doses are used, plasma levels must be measured. When dose adjustments are made on the basis of plasma theophylline determinations, it is important to remember that theophylline often shows dose-dependent kinetics so that the per cent change in plasma concentration is about 50% greater than the per cent change in dose.

Oral beta$_2$ agonists

Generally, the bioavailability of *slow-release* beta$_2$ agonists is lower than that of *plain tablets* and syrup. Therefore, the dose should normally be increased by 30% or more when switching from plain oral beta$_2$ therapy to slow-release therapy. *Food* also reduces the bioavailability and, if the product is normally taken with the meals, the dose should be further increased by an additional 30%.

Dosing with a beta$_2$ agonist should be *individualized* under the monitoring of the therapeutic response and the occurrence of side effects. Only few dose–response studies have been conducted, so that optimal dose regimen is not known. A rational approach would be to start at a low dose (around 0.2 mg/kg/day) and then gradually increase the dose until a sufficient clinical effect or systemic side effects occur. Studies doing so indicate that higher than the normally recommended oral doses of terbutaline (around 0.5 mg/kg/day) are required by many children to produce significant clinical effects. This emphasizes the importance of *individual dose titration*.

In the day-to-day management, sparse knowledge about pharmacokinetics and pharmacodynamics of the various drugs may, to some extent, be compensated for by careful monitoring of the effect, plasma drug measurement (theophylline) and repeated adjustment of dose. This is time-consuming but mandatory for successful therapy with oral medication.

The advantage of a handbook
Knowledge is of two kinds; we know the subject ourselves, or we know where we can find information upon it.

Samuel Johnson

– but it helps
It is not necessary to understand things in order to argue about them.

De Beaumarchais

10.4 Daily management III
Inhaled therapy

Key points
- Inhalation therapy is the mainstay of asthma treatment, but there are problems and pitfalls.
- Children have considerable difficulties with MDIs and thorough tuition is necessary.
- Conventional MDIs cannot be recommended when alternative devices are available.
- A breath-actuated MDI abolishes the coordination difficulties and it can be used by children older than 6–7 years.
- Actuation during the first part of a deep, slow inhalation, followed by a breath-holding before exhalation, produces the best effect of a MDI.
- Even when used optimally, a MDI results in a high oropharyngeal deposition and hence a low therapeutic ratio.
- Attachment of a spacer to a MDI leads to reduced oropharyngeal deposition of drug and increased therapeutic ratio.
- Spacers are easy to use particularly when they have a valve system.
- All school children can learn to use a spacer and also use it effectively during acute attacks.
- Most preschool children can use a spacer for prophylactic medication, but they may not be able to use it efficiently during acute attacks.
- Multi-dose DPIs are easier to use and more convenient than single-dose inhalers.
- With a DPI, there is no need for exhalation before the inhalation or breath-holding afterwards.
- The effect of DPIs increases with the inspiratory flow rate.
- Children should be taught to inhale rapidly through these inhalers.
- DPIs cannot be used by most children <5 years.
- Some older children, ≥5 years, on powder inhaler therapy, may need a spacer inhaler during severe acute wheeze.
- Nebulizers are expensive and inconvenient delivery systems.
- For daily treatment, they can usually be replaced by an alternative delivery system.
- A common exception is children ≤2–3 years.
- A nebulizer is the delivery system of choice for the in-hospital treatment of acute severe asthma.
- Simple inhaler strategy would be: 1, daily

treatment, $\leq$5 years, with a spacer; 2, >5 years, with a DPI or spacer, for steroids with a high gastro-intestinal bioavailability; and 3, acute severe asthma, with a nebulizer.

Inhalation therapy is the *mainstay of treatment* of asthma in children, but there are *problems and pitfalls*. Accurate knowledge about the nature and magnitude of these problems and pitfalls and about which age groups can normally use the various inhalation devices correctly is a precondition for an effective inhaled therapy in children. Therefore, the most widely used inhalers and their advantages, disadvantages and limitations will be discussed in some detail with special attention to two important factors: 1, Which inhaler is the most simple and *easiest to use optimally*? 2, Which inhaler has the *best therapeutic ratio*?

The *systemic effect* of an inhaled drug depends upon the amount of drug absorbed from airways and the amount absorbed from the gastro-intestinal tract. The *clinical effect* only depends upon the intrapulmonary deposition. Consequently, the therapeutic ratio increases with the proportion of the drug that is deposited in the intrapulmonary airways. This is most important for a drug with high oral bioavailability.

Metered-dose inhalers

Ease of use and optimal use

Children have *considerable difficulties* with MDIs: 1, poor coordination of actuation and inhalation; 2, inhalation stops when the cold aerosol hits the soft palate; 3, actuation of the aerosol into the mouth followed by inhalation through the nose; and 4, a too rapid inhalation.

All prescriptions of a MDI should be accompanied by repeated, *thorough tuition* of correct inhaler use followed by the child's demonstration of inhalation technique. Such instruction may take 10–20 minutes. Even when this is done, about 50% of children can be expected to gain reduced benefit from the prescribed medication, and most preschool children will not be able to learn effective MDI use. Therefore, *conventional MDIs cannot be recommended for children if alternative devices are available*.

Use of a *breath-actuated MDI* (Autohaler) will reduce tuition time and abolish the coordination difficulties. The remaining problems are unaffected,

however, and this inhaler should be reserved for children older than 6–7 years.

Actuation during the first part of a deep, *slow inhalation*, followed by a *breath-holding* before exhalation, produces the best effect of a MDI.

Therapeutic ratio

Even when used optimally, a MDI results in a *high oropharyngeal deposition* and hence a relatively low therapeutic ratio for most drugs. This is even more pronounced for children than for adults.

MDI with spacer

Attachment of a spacer to the mouthpiece of a MDI (see Fig. 9.14.5) leads to reduced impaction on the posterior wall of the pharynx and a *reduced oropharyngeal deposition* of drug.

The optimal *volume of a spacer* depends upon the child's tidal volume, and it is therefore assumed that a low-volume spacer is advantageous for young children, but further studies are needed to assess this.

Ease of use and optimal use

Spacers are *easy to use*, particularly if they have a valve system (Nebuhaler, Volumatic, Babyhaler and Aerochamber). Virtually *all school children* can learn to use these devices and also use them effectively *during acute attacks*. It is also possible to train *most preschool children* to use a spacer with a valve system and a face mask *for prophylactic medication*. During episodes of acute wheeze, however, many young children may not be able to open or close the valve system properly. This can be compensated for by using a higher dose.

Only one dose should be fired into the spacer at a time, as multiple actuations reduce the output of respirable particles. This phenomenon is more pronounced for low-volume devices. *Slow tidal breathing*, starting immediately after actuation, produces a maximum effect.

For low-volume devices there should not be any delay between actuation and inhalation. When a large-volume spacer is used, delaying the inhalation for a few seconds is not associated with a reduced effect. However, a long delay (>5 seconds) between actuation and inhalation will reduce the effect.

Due to their many advantages a variety of *new spacer systems* is being launched every year. Though deceptively similar in appearance, there may be marked differences in the amount of drug retained in them and hence their clinical effect. Therefore, use of a new spacer device cannot be recommended until its value has been documented in controlled trials.

The problem with spacers is that they are *bulky and difficult to carry* about, although this problem is small when they are used for prophylactic treatment given at home morning and evening.

Therapeutic ratio

Because a spacer reduces the oropharyngeal deposition of drug, the gastro-intestinal bioavailability is markedly diminished. As intrapulmonary deposition in not reduced, a spacer has a *high therapeutic ratio*, and it is often considered the device of choice for delivery of inhaled steroids.

Dry-powder inhalers

Ease of use and optimal use

For many years, DPIs have been *single-dose inhalers* and therefore less convenient than the MDIs. Furthermore, some children have difficulties with correct loading and splitting of the capsules when using the single-dose inhalers, particularly during episodes of acute wheeze. Several recent studies have shown that the new *multi-dose inhalers* are easier to use and more convenient, so these inhalers are to be preferred.

The effect of DPIs increases with the inspiratory flow rate. Therefore, children should be taught to *inhale rapidly* through these inhalers. Many young children and some older children with severe wheeze cannot generate a sufficient inspiratory flow rate to benefit optimally from a powder inhaler. Therefore, *DPIs should not be routinely prescribed for children younger than 5 years*, just as a few older children on powder inhaler therapy may need a spacer inhaler during episodes of severe acute wheeze.

Apart from a rapid inspiration, DPIs can be used with a very *simple inhalation technique*. There is *no need for exhalation before* the inhalation *or breath-holding afterwards*. This is advantageous as *tuition becomes easy*. It should be emphasized that exhaling through the inhaler after it has been loaded is deleterious for its effect.

Therapeutic ratio

Generally, DPIs have a *low therapeutic ratio* and therefore may not be the delivery system of choice for

inhaled steroids, at least in principle. However, recent findings with the Turbuhaler DPI show that this inhaler delivers a higher dose to the intrapulmonary airways than other DPIs. As a consequence, the therapeutic ratio of *budesonide* delivered *from Turbuhaler* is quite similar to that of a spacer. Furthermore, because of the low oral bioavailability of *fluticasone propionate*, this drug also has a high therapeutic ratio when delivered *from a Diskhaler*.

Nebulizers

For many years, wet nebulizers have been extremely *popular* among paediatric patients and were therefore widely used. In 1995, such widespread use is not justified as *alternative devices can be used* with the same efficacy. Compared with other devices, nebulizers are *expensive, bulky, inconvenient, time-consuming* delivery systems. Therefore, *their use should be limited* to children who cannot be trained in the correct use of another device. In clinical practice, this means *children younger than 2–3 years*, mentally retarded older children and *children with acute severe asthma* who require a high dose of inhaled beta$_2$ agonist. The vast majority of school children who claim that they use a nebulizer for home treatment are under-treated with anti-inflammatory drugs, and, once their asthma treatment has become optimized, the requirement of a nebulizer disappears.

Ease of use and optimal use

Our knowledge about optimal use of nebulizers and dose requirement for the young age groups is limited. It is still not known which nebulizer or which various drugs used for nebulization are best for young children. Some drugs, such as beclomethasone dipropionate, may not be effective at all after nebulization.

Remarkably few controlled nebulizer studies have been carried out in the age groups that require this treatment. So, at present, nebulized therapy of young children is based on a few controlled studies, clinical experience and extrapolation from studies in adults.

Young children's inhalation technique, tidal volume and anatomy of the upper airways are different from those in older children and adults, and the dose these children actually inhale to the intrapulmonary airways is lower than that inhaled by the older age groups.

Quiet tidal breathing through a tightly fitting face mask is normally recommended. Removing the face

Simple inhaler strategy		
Age	**Day-to-day use**	**Acute severe asthma**
≤5 years	MDI with spacer	Nebulizer
>5 years	Multi-dose DPI	Nebulizer

Table 10.4.1. Simple strategy for choice of inhaled therapy for asthma in childhood

mask 2–3 cm from the face of the child will reduce the inhaled dose by about 50%, so this is dissuaded.

Therapeutic ratio

We have little knowledge about the therapeutic ratio for the various nebulizer systems, but *presumably it is low*. Nasal breathing through a face mask will filter off a large proportion of the inhaled particles. The drug retained in the nose is likely to be absorbed from the nasal mucosa or the gastro-intestinal tract. In this way, it may cause systemic effects without adding to the beneficial effect.

Inhaler strategy

Based on the above considerations, a simple, yet rational, inhaler strategy in children can be outlined (Table 10.4.1).

Children ≤5 years can use a *spacer* with a valve system and a face mask for the delivery of all drugs except when they are severely obstructed, in which case they may need a *nebulizer*. If the child cannot be taught correct use of a spacer, a nebulizer should be prescribed.

Children >5 years can be prescribed a *multi-dose DPI* (if not available, a single-dose DPI may be used) or a breath-actuated MDI for beta$_2$ agonists or sodium cromoglycate and a large volume spacer for the administration of inhaled corticosteroids with high gastro-intestinal bioavailability. If these alternatives are not available, a conventional MDI can be used in these age groups provided that careful tuition is given.

Nebulizers are mainly used for *severe acute attacks* of bronchoconstriction and for *children <2–3 years* who cannot be taught correct use of any other device.

With this approach, children can be taught effective inhaler use with a minimum of instruction time. Finally, it is important to remember always to consider the child's wishes, as prescription of an inhaler, which the physician but not the child likes, is likely to reduce compliance.

10.5 Daily management IV
Treatment strategy

Key points

- The correct way to treat a child requiring daily medication is still a matter of debate.
- In principle, there are two strategies: the conservative 'step-up strategy' and the aggressive 'step-down strategy'.
- Supporters of the step-up strategy are concerned about the risk of side effects of inhaled steroids.
- In such a strategy, therapy is gradually increased using inhaled beta$_2$ agonists, cromoglycate, oral theophylline and oral beta$_2$ agonist.
- In the step-up strategy, inhaled steroid is introduced in about 10% as the last resort.
- In the step-down strategy, inhaled steroids are used early to establish optimal control and the child's personal best lung function.
- Typically, a 6–8-week treatment period with high-dose inhaled steroid (800–1000 µg/day) is given.
- After this initial period, the treatment is stepped-down every 6–8 weeks.
- With this approach, the majority of children end up on continuous treatment with inhaled steroids.
- Early treatment with inhaled steroids may prevent the development of irreversible structural changes in the airways.
- Low-dose therapy (≤400 µg/day), used for 20 years, seems to be as safe as other treatments.
- As our experience with high-dose therapy (>400 µg/day) is limited, such treatment is reserved for otherwise uncontrolled and severe cases.
- Self-management plans, written and illustrated, need to be tailored individually to each patient.
- As there are few controlled studies in young children <3 years, the best treatment strategy in this age group is not known.

The correct way to treat a child requiring daily medication is often discussed among paediatricians, and important differences in strategy exist between specialists and between countries. Simplified, there exist two different strategies: the conservative '*step-up strategy*' and the more aggressive (and progressive?) '*step-down strategy*'.

The step-up strategy
Treatment is gradually built up, typically starting with inhaled beta$_2$ agonists (Fig. 10.5.1). If the effect is insufficient, sodium cromoglycate, oral theophylline, oral beta$_2$ agonist, and perhaps a long-acting inhaled beta$_2$ agonist are added stepwise in varying order of succession and combination. Finally, if added *multi-drug therapy* is inadequate, inhaled steroid is given as the last resort before daily or alternate-day oral steroid medication.

In practice, the clinician assesses asthma severity at the first visit, decides which combined treatment should be given, and then builds up treatment from that point.

It is a major point in this strategy that *inhaled steroids are used late* and are reserved for the severe cases. As only a minority of the children (about 10%) will receive steroids, it implies that the child's personal best lung function is not regularly established.

Due to the problems with severity assessment and estimation of optimal control in children, this strategy implies a substantial *risk of ending up at a suboptimal treatment level*. One of the reasons for this is that, with this approach, the clinical condition after initiation of treatment is always compared with the situation when no or less treatment was given and not with personal best control. Having had a fourth non-steroidal drug prescribed, patient and parents may be tempted to believe that they have now attained what the doctor can offer (and what they can afford).

The step-down strategy
It is the major principle of this strategy that all children with chronic asthma *are initially treated aggressively* in order to *define their best lung function* and their optimal clinical condition. Typically, a 6–8-week treatment period with high-dose inhaled steroid (800–1000 µg/day), in combination with an inhaled beta$_2$ agonist, is given (Fig. 10.5.2).

Early use of inhaled steroids allows both the asthmatic child, his or her family and the physician to experience how the child's life may be during optimal treatment, and that offers a good basis for defining the objectives of treatment, deciding the final therapy, and assessing whether it attains the goal.

After the initial treatment period, the lowest amount of medication needed to maintain optimal control is determined by gradual reduction of the dose of inhaled steroid every 6–8 weeks.

In addition to improvements in quality of life and a reduced morbidity, the step-down strategy also

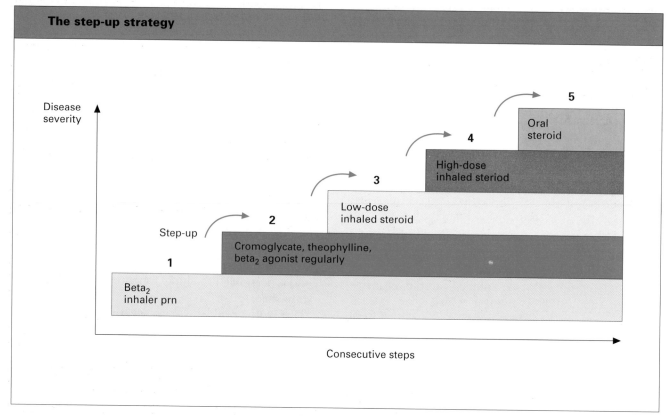

The step-up strategy

Disease severity

5

Oral steroid

4

High-dose inhaled steriod

3

Low-dose inhaled steroid

2

Step-up

Cromoglycate, theophylline, beta₂ agonist regularly

1

Beta₂ inhaler prn

Consecutive steps

Fig. 10.5.1. With the step-up strategy, the first treatment level is chosen based on the initial assessment of asthma severity. If the clinical result of the treatment is assessed as being satisfactory, the child continues on the first treatment level without having his or her personal best control and lung function established. If control is not satisfactory, the treatment is gradually built up until control is assessed as being satisfactory.

reduces the numbers of acute admissions, increases lung function and *reduces the risk of under-treatment*.

With this approach, a majority of the children end up on continuous treatment with inhaled steroids.

Inhaled steroids: pros and cons

Beneficial effects

The main argument for the step-down theory and an early introduction of inhaled steroids is the *extraordinary clinical efficacy* of this type of therapy. In a low dose ($\leq 400\,\mu g$/day), inhaled steroid is at least as effective as other therapies, and, in a high dose ($>400\,\mu g$/day), it is definitely more effective (Fig. 10.5.3).

Use of inhaled steroids also has the advantages of *good patient compliance* (twice-daily dosing and avoidance of multi-drug therapy).

Obviously, steroids cannot cure the disease, and children with severe asthma may require treatment for the rest of their life. However, recent studies have provided evidence that early treatment with inhaled steroids may *prevent the development of irreversible airway obstruction*, and this effect is more pronounced when the treatment is initiated early after the onset of symptoms than when it is started some years after the onset of asthma.

Potential adverse effects

Supporters of the step-up strategy are still concerned about the risk of side effects of inhaled steroids.

Low-dose therapy. The majority of children with moderate asthma can be optimally controlled on daily doses of $400\,\mu g$ or less, together with an inhaled beta₂ agonist p.r.n. Doses of inhaled steroids in that dose range have been used in children for more than 20 years and studied in prospective continuous

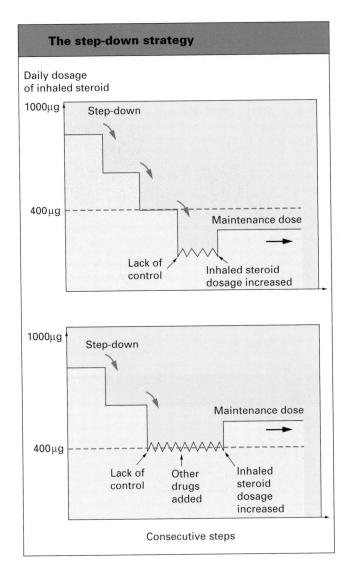

Fig. 10.5.2. With the step-down strategy, treatment is started with inhaled steroid in a high dose (800–1000 µg/day) in order to achieve optimal control and define personal best lung function. The dose is gradually reduced at 6–8-week intervals until optimal control is no longer maintained. The steroid dose is then increased to the previous level, and the treatment is continued on that dose if it is ≤400 µg/day. If the required maintenance dose is >400 µg/day, treatment with other drugs is added. Only if that is not sufficient is the dose of inhaled steroid increased.

treatment for 5 years. So far, there are no controlled data indicating that long-term use is associated with any serious side effects. In contrast, the vast majority of studies suggest that such treatment is *as safe as other treatments*. The safety of no other drug has been evaluated prospectively over such time periods.

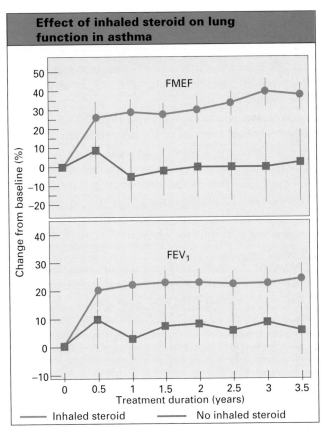

Fig. 10.5.3. Changes in lung function in 216 children treated with inhaled budesonide (mean daily dose decreasing from 710 to 430 µg) (bullets) and in 62 children (squares) who received other asthma treatment but not corticosteroids (mean and 95% confidence values). From Agertoft L, Pedersen S. Effect of long-term treatment with an inhaled corticosteroid on growth and pulmonary function in asthmatic children. *Resp Med* 1994; **88**: 373–81.

High-dose therapy. High doses of inhaled steroids is the most effective treatment available for children with severe asthma, and such treatment cannot be replaced by any other drug except oral prednisolone. However, as the *experience with long-term, high-dose therapy is limited*, such treatment should be reserved for patients who are not controlled on lower doses in combination with oral bronchodilators or inhaled long-acting beta₂ agonists (salmeterol or formoterol).

Self-management plan

Patients and parents have to be educated in preventing and controlling symptoms. When the treatment level has been decided, each child should be supplied with a *written, personal management plan* for early treatment of exacerbations. This plan should include; 1, criteria to introduce or increase a treatment; 2, criteria to reduce the increased treatment to the normal level; and 3, criteria that indicate when the patient should contact the physician or an emergency department.

As no two children are alike, the criteria and the action to be taken need to be *tailored individually to each patient*. Addition of an oral bronchodilator, increase in the dose of inhaled steroid, addition of oral steroids, or combinations of these, are valuable alternatives. It is important that the instructions are simple and in writing, preferably with illustrations, otherwise the risk of misunderstandings is too high.

No matter which strategy and drugs that have been chosen, it is important that both the child and the family are involved in the therapeutic decisions, otherwise *compliance* is likely to become poor. Scrutiny and strict control will not improve compliance, only collaboration with the child and the parents will do so.

Exercise-induced asthma

Prophylactic medication with *inhaled beta₂ agonists* and/or *cromoglycate* just prior to exercise is the most widely recommended treatment. However, many children do not know beforehand when they are going to be physically active. Furthermore, experience shows that many children are reluctant or forget to take their medication before exercise. Instead, they choose not to participate wholeheartedly in the physical activity. Therefore, for maximum effectiveness, it is often better to treat this socially disabling symptom with drugs that do not require premedication immediately prior to the exercise. In this respect, continuous treatment with *inhaled steroids* and/or *long-acting beta₂ agonists* is very effective. Exercise-induced asthma is often a reflection of bronchial hyper-responsiveness and should therefore be treated accordingly.

Special problems in infants

There are few controlled studies in children younger than 3 years, and therefore the best treatment strategy is not known.

Oral beta₂ agonists are widely used but their effectiveness is often disappointing. It is not known whether this is due to the use of insufficient doses or whether it is because young children may be poorly responsive to beta₂ agonists. It is the author's experi-

ence that oral terbutaline in doses around 0.5 mg/kg/day may sometimes be beneficial.

In contrast, controlled studies with spacers have convincingly shown that *inhaled beta₂ agonists* produce significant bronchodilatation in most children in this age group. Furthermore, such therapy may also have a prophylactic role, as it offers significant protection against bronchoconstriction induced by various challenges, including exercise.

Nebulized *ipratropium bromide* has been shown to relieve bronchial obstruction in some young wheezers. However, clinical trials evaluating its value in the day-to-day management have been disappointing, so the role of ipratropium bromide is still debated.

The same is the case for *ketotifen*, which is widely used in young children in many parts of the world. Most controlled studies have failed to justify such use.

As for most other drugs, the clinical documenta-

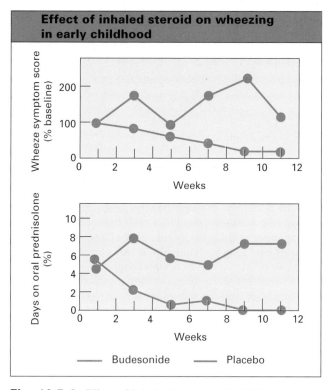

Fig. 10.5.4. Effect of inhaled budesonide (400 µg twice-daily from a spacer) (red circles) compared with placebo (blue circles) in 77 young children (11–36 months) with recurrent wheezing. *Upper part*: wheeze symptom score. *Lower part*: days on oral prednisolone. From Bisgaard H, Munck SL, Nielsen JP, Petersen W, Ohlsson SV. Inhaled budesonide for treatment of recurrent wheezing in early childhood. *Lancet* 1990; **336**: 649–51.

tion for *cromoclycate* in young children is more sparse than in school children. Some trials have not been able to demonstrate any effect, whereas others have found an effect but no reduction in hospital admission rates or severe wheeze after viral respiratory tract infection. So far, nedocromil sodium has not been studied in young children.

In contrast to other therapies, *inhaled steroids* have been found very effective in young children when administered from a spacer or as nebulized budesonide (Fig. 10.5.4). Such treatment reduces both morbidity and number of acute admissions. At present, the safety of long-term treatment still remains to be settled in children younger than 3 years, and, until that has been done, it should be reserved for severe cases.

It is the author's experience that it often takes longer (8–10 weeks) to achieve a maximum effect with inhaled steroids in younger children than in older children. If a quicker effect is desirable, the inhaled therapy has to be combined with oral prednisolone during the first 10 days of treatment.

Prescribe H$_2$O
Pure water is the world's first and foremost medicine.
Slovakian proverb

A simple advice
Learn simplicity, then be doubtful.
Whitehead

10.6 Acute asthma I
Drugs and doses

Key points
• An inhaled beta$_2$ agonist is superior to treatment with other bronchodilators.
• Nebulizers are the delivery system of choice in all age groups of hospitalized children.
• However, in school children, the same results can be obtained with other inhalation systems.
• Spacers require lower doses than do nebulizers to produce the same response.
• Frequent administration from a spacer of terbutaline/salbutamol (total 0.1 mg/kg) is highly efficient.
• DPIs should not be used for acute asthma in children ≤5 years.
• Conventional MDIs are used only when another delivery system is not available.
• Systemic administration of a beta$_2$ agonist causes side effects but they are not serious.
• Adrenaline should be used only when modern beta$_2$ agonists are not available.
• In contrast to common belief, infants do have bronchial beta$_2$ receptors and respond to beta$_2$ agonists.
• Systemic steroids are beneficial in the management of acute severe asthma.
• Usually, steroid is given orally as prednisolone (1–2 mg/kg/day).
• Started early during a viral airway infection, oral steroid may prevent an exacerbation.
• Theophylline has been used frequently for acute asthma in children but the documentation is not convincing.
• An intravenous bolus of 6 mg/kg lean body weight can be given to children who are not on oral theophylline.
• Continued theophylline infusion must be calculated precisely and plasma levels measured.
• Theophylline can add little to the effect of frequent inhalations of beta$_2$ agonists.
• Its role in acute asthma can be questioned.
• Side effects from theophylline are numerous and potentially lethal if overdosed.
• Ipratropium bromide, delivered from a nebulizer, has a role as an adjunct to a beta$_2$ agonist.

In the last decades, there have been an *increasing number of hospitalizations* due to acute asthma in children. This is probably because of an increase in asthma prevalence and severity, but other factors, including poor patient understanding, inadequate recognition and under-treatment, may also have contributed.

An acute severe attack of asthma is a *potentially life-threatening* event, which should always be treated effectively without delay. The principles and modalities of the treatment are the same as in adults. However, there are differences in dosages of medication and in clinical assessment.

Beta$_2$ agonists

The value of beta$_2$ agonists in the treatment of acute asthma in school- and preschool-children has been demonstrated in several controlled trials. Such treatment works within minutes and is *superior to treatment with other bronchodilators.* The *inhaled route* provides a better clinical effect-to-side effect ratio than systemic administration. Furthermore, inhaled therapy is less affected by the pretreatment given prior to admission.

It is always dangerous to give dose recommendations for acute severe asthma. This is because *the dose required depends upon the response.* The correct strategy is to administer enough drug for each individual patient under guidance of careful monitoring for adverse effects and measurement of the clinical response.

Inhalation systems and doses

Nebulizers. They are simple to use, and, in the acute situation, it is advantageous that oxygen can be administered through the nebulizer at the same time as the drug. Therefore, *nebulizers are the delivery system of choice in the treatment of acute severe asthma in all age groups of hospitalized children,* even though most studies show that, in school children, the same results can be obtained with other inhalation systems.

The optimal dose of a nebulized beta$_2$ agonist for acute asthma not only depends upon the nebulizer brand but also upon volume fill; more drug will be delivered if the same amount of drug is given in 4 ml rather than in 2 ml in the chamber. *High doses* of salbutamol (0.30 mg/kg) have been found to be better than low doses (0.15 mg/kg) when given at 3-hourly intervals. Furthermore, *continuous nebulization*

produces better results than the same dose nebulized intermittently.

Inhalation of high dose of beta$_2$ agonists causes significant systemic absorption so that, after some inhalations, plasma drug levels are in the same range as after continuous systemic administration. As a consequence, the same side effects may occur.

Spacers. Generally lower doses are required from spacers to produce the same response as a nebulizer. Doses from 2 to 6 mg or about 0.1 mg/kg have been used without unacceptable side effects. In agreement with the nebulizer studies, *frequent administration* seems to be better than a single high dose.

Dry-powder inhalers. A fast inhalation and a minimum inspiratory flow rate are required to produce a maximum effect from DPIs. Many preschool children cannot generate sufficiently high inspiratory flow rates during acute episodes of asthma, and therefore *DPIs should not be used for acute asthma in children ≤5 years.*

Metered-dose inhalers. The same is true for *conventional MDIs,* which can normally only be used effectively in school children after careful tuition but often not during episodes of acute wheeze.

Systemic administration

There is a significant correlation between plasma drug level and bronchodilating effect after systemic administration of a beta$_2$ agonist. An *intravenous loading dose* of terbutaline 2–5 µg/kg followed by a *continuous infusion* of 5 µg/kg/h has been found to be suitable for the majority of children. However, *considerable inter-individual variations* exist in plasma levels obtained after a given dose. Therefore, standard doses are not feasible for effective therapy. *Dosing should be individualized* under the monitoring of the therapeutic response and the occurrence of side effects.

Similarly, a *subcutaneous or intramuscular injection* of doses around 5–10 µg/kg of terbutaline or salbutamol produce significant clinical effect without unacceptable side effects.

It is sometimes suggested that *adrenaline,* with its alpha adrenoceptor activity, would be better than other drugs for decreasing bronchial oedema. However, controlled clinical trials have failed to demonstrate any advantages over the modern beta$_2$ selective drugs in relieving airway obstruction in children, and it causes more side effects.

Side effects

Generally, treatment of children with beta$_2$ agonists is *very safe*. The occurrence of side effects is directly proportional to the plasma concentrations and, therefore, mainly *depends on route of administration*. Skeletal muscle *tremor, palpitations* and some agitation are the most common complaints when high doses are used. After systemic administration, the occurrence of side effects can be used as an indication that the top of the bronchodilatory dose–response curve has been reached.

A small drop in blood pressure and a compensatory *increase in pulse rate* is seen after systemic use or administration of high inhaled doses. Furthermore, *hypokalaemia*, hyperglycaemia and an increase in free fatty acids are common. The clinical importance of this remains to be elucidated.

A *slight fall in* Pao$_2$ may occur, but it is usually without any clinical importance.

Special considerations in infants

Several early studies failed to demonstrate a bronchodilator response to nebulized beta$_2$ agonists in infants, and, for many years, it was believed that these drugs were ineffective in young children. However, recent controlled studies have demonstrated significant bronchodilator effects, protective effects against bronchoconstrictor agents and clinical improvement in infants treated with beta$_2$ agonists. Thus, *infants have functioning beta$_2$ receptors from birth, and receptor stimulation produces bronchodilatation*. However, the response is often rather small and shows considerable inter-individual variation.

Steroids

The beneficial effect of systemic steroids in the management of acute severe asthma has been shown in several controlled trials in all age groups, although studies in infants are few. When treatment is started early on during the exacerbation, it has been shown to reduce the severity of virus-induced asthma attacks and hospital admissions. The optimal doses of steroid and route of administration have not been carefully evaluated, so the following recommendations are largely empirical.

Oral prednisolone is rapidly and reliably absorbed and therefore usually sufficient in the majority of children, especially when used early on during the exacerbation.

The *recommended dose* of steroid, having produced significant effects in controlled trials, is prednisolone, 1–2 mg/kg/day (maximum 60 mg), divided into twice-daily doses.

Some patients with a very severe attack or with gastro-intestinal problems may need *intravenous* hydrocortisone, or preferably *methylprednisolone*, given 6 hourly (see Table 10.6.1).

High doses of *inhaled corticosteroids* are sometimes recommended for the treatment of exacerbations. However, at present, there are no studies to support this except for a recent study that did find a significant additional effect of nebulized budesonide in acute wheeze in children up to 18 months of age. It seems, however, that, if given early to children with asthma provoked by viral upper airway infection, such treatment can reduce the severity of asthma.

Theophylline

Theophylline, often administered intravenously as aminophylline, has been used for many years in the treatment of acute severe asthma in children. It has been demonstrated that a bolus dose of theophylline causes significant increases in lung function in school children with acute wheeze, but, otherwise, the number of placebo-controlled studies assessing the acute effect is sparse. Theophylline has not been thoroughly studied in preschool children and infants with wheeze.

It is usually recommended to aim at plasma levels between 55 and 110 μmol/l (10–20 mg/l), which can be achieved in all age groups by giving an *intravenous bolus of 6 mg/kg* lean body weight and then by continuing with theophylline infusion rates or oral therapy as shown in Table 10.6.1. If the child is already receiving treatment with theophylline, additional medication should only be given under the guidance of plasma theophylline monitoring. *Gastro-intestinal and rectal absorption* of an aqueous solution is almost complete with peak plasma theophylline levels being measured within 1 hour after the administration. Somewhat higher loading doses are required when these administration forms are used (8–9 mg/kg).

Though significant bronchodilating effects have been demonstrated in children, *the role of*

Drug dosing in acute childhood asthma	
Beta₂ agonists	
Nebulizer	Salbutamol 0.2 mg or terbutaline 0.4 mg/kg May be repeated at frequent intervals
Spacer or other inhaler	One puff every minute until satisfactory response Maximum dose: salbutamol 50 μg or terbutaline 100 μg/kg
Subcutaneous or intramuscular	Salbutamol or terbutaline 10 μg/kg
Intravenous	Loading dose: salbutamol or terbutaline 2–5 μg/kg Continuous: salbutamol or terbutaline 5 μg/kg/h
Ipratropium bromide	
Nebulizer	250 μg to all age groups May be repeated 4–6 hourly
Corticosteroids	
Oral prednisolone	Loading dose: 1–2 mg/kg (max. 60 mg) Continuous: 2 mg/kg/day divided into two doses
Intravenous methylprednisolone	Loading dose: 1–2 mg/kg Continuous: 1 mg/kg 6 hourly
Intravenous hydrocortisone	Loading dose: 10 mg/kg Continuous: 5 mg/kg 6 hourly
Theophylline*	
Intravenous	Loading dose: 6 mg/kg lean body weight over 15 minutes
Oral or rectal	Loading dose: 9 mg/kg lean body weight
Continuous treatment** (oral or intravenous)	<1 year: 0.3 × age in weeks + 8 mg/kg/24 h 1–9 years: 24 mg/kg/24 h 9–12 years: 20 mg/kg/24 h 12–16 years: 18 mg/kg/24 h >16 years: 14 mg/kg/24 h

Table 10.6.1. Recommended average doses of the various drugs used to treat acute severe asthma in all age groups of children. *For patients not receiving theophylline prior to treatment; **measurement of serum theophylline required

theophylline in the acute management of asthma has been questioned on the basis of a recent controlled study, which did not find any additional benefit of theophylline in children treated with frequent inhalations of beta$_2$ agonists, probably because theophylline is a weaker bronchodilator than inhaled beta$_2$ agonists.

Side effects

Theophylline has a low therapeutic index and *potentially lethal side effects* when overdosed. During the last decade, 63 deaths have been reported in studies with theophylline. The most common side effects are *anorexia, nausea, vomiting and headache.* These symptoms are quite common. Mild *central nervous stimulation, tachycardia, arrhythmias, abdominal pain, diarrhoea* and, rarely, gastric bleeding may also occur.

The most serious toxicity is the risk of *seizures*, which have been associated with a 50% mortality rate. However, seizures appear to be rare at serum levels <220 µmol/l. Theophylline-induced seizures are treated with benzodiazepines, and higher than usual doses should be used, as theophylline antagonizes the benzodiazepine effect in the brain.

Ipratropium bromide

Anticholinergics result in less bronchodilatation than do inhaled beta$_2$ agonists, and, administered alone, these drugs have no role in the management of acute severe asthma in school children. However, controlled studies have found that the *combination of a beta$_2$ agonist and an anti-cholinergic agent* produces somewhat better results than either drug alone *without an increase in side effects.* Though statistically highly significant, the advantages of the combination therapy is rather small in most studies.

These data suggest that ipratropium bromide has a role as an adjunct to inhaled beta$_2$ agonists in the treatment of acute asthma in children older than 1 year.

Side effects

Paradoxical bronchoconstriction has occurred after inhalation of nebulized ipratropium bromide, which was formerly preserved with benzalkonium chloride. Otherwise, dryness of the mouth in some patients seems to be the only problem.

> **If you don't pass the examine**
> To a man of strong character misfortune may do him more good than harm.
>
> Roger Bacon

10.7 Acute asthma II
Assessment of severity

Key points
- The asthma severity is often underestimated by patient, parents and physician.
- Objective measurements are necessary for a correct assessment.
- Composed symptoms and signs correlate weakly with lung function and oxygen saturation.
- A quiet chest on auscultation, inability to talk, cyanosis, paradoxical thoraco-abdominal movement and confusion strongly suggest very severe asthma.
- Measurement of blood gases is a reliable way of assessing asthma severity in children.
- Pa_{CO_2} can be reliably measured in capillary blood and is very useful, particularly in young children.
- Pa_{CO_2} is low due to hyperventilation during an asthma episode.
- A normal or elevated Pa_{CO_2} value should be considered a sign of danger.
- An oxygen saturation ≤91% is predictive of a severe condition, and 92–93% of moderate and ≥94% of a mild attack.
- As the best measurement of airway obstruction, PEF should be measured whenever possible.
- Generally, infants are more severely obstructed than older children and are at increased risk.

The asthma *severity is often underestimated* by patient, parents and physician. Even in the presence of wheeze, many children still want to participate in other children's activities. The child may appear deceptively well and yet suffer from quite marked airway obstruction. Even trained doctors may not be good at predicting a patient's lung function. *Objective measurements are necessary for a correct assessment.* Table 10.7.1 provides some parameters, which are normally used in the assessment. As these are guidelines only, all features in one category need not be present. When in doubt as to whether the condition should be categorized as moderate or severe, it is usually severe.

History
History should always include likely triggers (e.g. infection, allergy or lack of compliance), duration of symptoms and treatment prior to admission.

Objective findings
Composed scores of *auscultatory findings, respiratory rate, pulse rate, patient distress, and retractions* have been used to assess the severity of disease. These objective findings correlate weakly with lung function and oxygen saturation, and they cannot be used as the single criterion to predict outcome.

Findings of *a quiet chest* on auscultation, *inability to talk* and *cyanosis* strongly suggest hypercapnia and very severe bronchoconstriction. Respiratory muscle fatigue may result in slowing of the respiratory rate, disappearance of retractions and appearance of *paradoxical thoraco-abdominal movement*. Remember that anxiety and *confusion* may be due to hypoxaemia and therefore never treat with sedatives.

Blood gases
Measurement of blood gases is a reliable way of assessing asthma severity in children.

Pa_{CO_2}
Pa_{CO_2} can be reliably measured on capillary blood, which makes this parameter very useful, particularly in young children. It may also be monitored transcutaneously together with Pa_{O_2}. Usually, Pa_{CO_2} is low due to hyperventilation during an asthma episode. When airway obstruction becomes excessive, the low Pa_{CO_2} returns to normal and severe respiratory failure may soon develop. Therefore, *normal or elevated Pa_{CO_2} values should be considered a sign of danger*. A high value, which increases in spite of aggressive treatment, is one of the indications for assisted ventilation.

Pa_{O_2} and oxygen saturation
In a child with acute asthma symptoms, an oxygen saturation ≤91% is predictive of a severe condition, and 92–93% of moderate and ≥94% of a mild attack.

Lung function
Most children ≥5 years can make reproducible PEF measurements. However, forced expiratory manoeuvres will increase bronchoconstriction when the airways are highly hyper-responsive, and, in the acute situation, it is better to treat the child than to use the time training him or her in lung function measurements.

Lung function, however, is the best measurement of the degree of airway obstruction, and there is a

Table 10.7.1. Assessment of severity of asthma exacerbations in children

Assessment of asthma severity in children			
	Mild	**Moderate**	**Severe**
Treatment place	Home	Home/outpatient	Hospital
Wheeze	Only end-expiratory	Loud	Loud or absent
Breathlessness: infant older child	Crying Playing	Difficult feeding Walking	Stops feeding Talks in single words
Accessory muscles, retractions	Usually not	Moderate	Marked
Respiratory rate: <3 months 3–12 months 1–6 years >6 years	<60 <50 <40 <30	60–70 50–60 40–50 30–40	>70 >60 >50 >40
Pulse rate: <1 year 1–2 year >2 years	<150 <120 <110	150–170 120–140 110–130	>170 >140 >130
PEF	>70%	50–70%	<50%
Pa_{CO_2}	<4.9 kPa	<5.6 kPa	>5.6 kPa
Sa_{O_2} (on air)	>94%	92–94%	<92%

highly significant association between PEF rate, PEF response to beta$_2$ inhalers, and the need for intensive treatment. Therefore, *PEF should be measured whenever possible*. These measurements are the most valuable of all parameters in assessing the response to treatment and for deciding when to step down treatment or discharge the patient.

Chest X-rays

Chest X-rays are reserved for cases where the initial progression in clinical improvement is poor, or objective findings or history suggest that complicating factors or differential diagnoses may be important.

Who should be admitted?

Absolute criteria for admission to hospital is difficult to formulate and depends upon several factors, including past history, availability of treatment, social circumstances (parental understanding and capability

High-risk patients
Young children*
Recent withdrawal of oral steroid
Hospitalization for asthma in past year
Earlier catastrophic attack
Psychiatric disease/psychosocial problems
Poor compliance

Table 10.7.2. Characteristics of high-risk patients who require a low admission threshold. *Develop respiratory failure more readily and are difficult to assess

of accurate monitoring), geographic isolation and, of course, objective findings (Table 10.7.2).

Special considerations in infants

Differences in lung anatomy and physiology and a poorer response to treatment place infants *at greater risk* than older children. Marked hyperinflation is often prevalent in young children with wheeze. As a consequence, respiratory work is increased and these age groups are prone to develop hypercapnia and respiratory failure more readily than older children. It is *common to underestimate severity in infants*, and, generally, young children are more severely obstructed and have higher Pa_{CO_2} than older children. Therefore, measurement of time trends in Pa_{O_2} and Pa_{CO_2} or oxygen saturation is usually indicated in severe wheeze in young children.

$n = 5$; $p < 0.01$
There are three types of lies: ordinary lies, damned lies, and statistics.

10.8 Acute asthma III
Treatment and monitoring

Key points
- A child with acute asthma should be seen without delay.
- Outside the hospital, a beta$_2$ agonist is administered, preferably by a MDI with a spacer.
- Give one puff every minute until satisfactory improvement occurs.
- Following a mild attack, inhaled steroid is added until the condition has been stable for 1 week.
- Following a moderate attack, a short course of prednisolone is also given.
- A child with a severe attack is admitted to hospital without delay.
- In hospital, the initial treatment consists of oxygen and nebulized beta$_2$ agonist followed by prednisolone.
- When the response to initial treatment is poor, nebulized ipratropium bromide and intravenous beta$_2$ agonist or theophylline can be added.
- Assisted ventilation is started when indicated by the clinical condition and repeated blood gas measurements.
- The patient is discharged when PEF >75% of personal best and diurnal variation of PEF <25%.
- Further acute attacks may be prevented by a written, self-management plan.

There is more than one way to manage an acute asthma exacerbation in a child. No two patients or situations are alike, and many excellent reviews have suggested various management plans. The following is the author's suggestion of a protocol for treating acute asthma in various age groups. It is based upon controlled studies, personal experience and the fact that the primary factors leading to obstruction are bronchoconstriction, inflammation, mucus plugging and oedema.

Management outside hospital
The child should be *seen without delay*. In order to get an accurate perception of the severity, it is necessary to *assess the child both before, during and after treatment*. When treatment is started, it is important that the parents are instructed in monitoring procedures and encouraged to call the doctor again if the

resolution of the exacerbation is not progressing satisfactorily.

Immediate treatment

In all cases, a *beta₂ agonist* is administered, *preferably by a MDI with a spacer* and, in preschool children, a face mask. If a spacer is not available, use any other inhaler. Give one puff every minute until satisfactory improvement occurs, that is, the clinical condition is changed into mild severity (see Table 10.7.1). *Maximum dose* is equivalent to $50\,\mu g$ salbutamol/kg or $100\,\mu g$ terbutaline/kg.

If inhaled treatment cannot for some reason be given or taken by the child, salbutamol or terbutaline 6–$10\,\mu g$/kg can be administered subcutaneously or intramuscularly.

Subsequent treatment

Mild attack. Continue with regular inhaled beta₂ agonist (every 3–6 hours) as long as it is required, and double the normally taken dose and add *high-dose inhaled steroid* ($800\,\mu g$/day) until the condition has been stable for 1 week.

Moderate attack. As for mild attacks, plus add a *short course of prednisolone* 1–2 mg/kg/day (maximum dose 60 mg) divided into two doses per day for 3–5 days.

Severe attack. Admission to hospital without delay after the initial treatment. When possible, give oxygen *en route* and prednisolone.

Hospital management

Immediate treatment

1, *Oxygen* (5–10 l/min) via a face mask or nasal cannula. 2, *Salbutamol/terbutaline* 0.2/0.4 mg/kg (see Table 10.6.1) in a volume fill of 4 ml via *oxygen-driven nebulizer*. 3, *Prednisolone* 1–2 mg/kg orally, or, in the critically ill child, intravenous methyl-prednisolone.

Subsequent treatment

In many children, the immediate treatment produces significant and marked improvement. Subsequent management in these cases may only require repeated *nebulized beta₂ agonist 2–4 hourly* and continued treatment with oral *prednisolone* 2 mg/kg/day.

In those with a poor response to the initial treatment, the following should be tried in addition to repeated beta₂ inhalation and continued prednisolone. 1, Addition of nebulized *ipratropium*

Life-threatening features
PEF <40% of best
Cyanosis
Bradycardia
Fatigue/exhaustion
Reduced consciousness
Silent chest
Paradoxical thoraco-abdominal movement
Disappearance of retractions without concomitant clinical improvement

Table 10.8.1. Life-threatening features in childhood asthma requiring urgent anaesthesiological assistance

bromide, 0.25 mg every 4–6 hours. 2, *Intravenous beta₂ agonist or theophylline*.

Additional treatment

Supplemental *oxygen* is given to maintain saturation above 90%. The need for *intravenous fluid* is assessed but the patient should not be overhydrated. *Antibiotics* should not be given routinely but only to patients suspected of bacterial pneumonia or other bacterial infections.

Useless or dangerous treatments

Cough medicine is useless and never indicated in acute severe asthma. *Sedatives are dangerous* and may induce respiratory failure or apnoea. Therefore, these drugs should only be given at the intensive care unit when facilities for intubation and assisted ventilation are available and ready.

Intensive care and assisted ventilation

Children with acute severe asthma require intensive monitoring by experienced staff, and all patients with life-threatening features (Table 10.8.1) not responding convincingly to treatment require intensive care.

Not all children admitted to the intensive care unit need ventilation, but it may be necessary in a small number of patients as a life-saving procedure. In general, it is accepted that this procedure is necessary in those patients who fulfil the following criteria: 1, $Paco_2$ >8.6 kPa and rising; 2, Pao_2 <6.6 kPa and falling; 3, pH ≤7.25 and falling; 4, apnoea; and 5, cardio-respiratory arrest.

Recovery and discharge

When the condition has been stable for 12 hours, the intensive *treatment can be gradually reduced*, starting with intravenous bronchodilators. Nebulized $beta_2$ inhalations are given less frequently and the patient is switched to inhaled therapy with the inhaler that is going to be used at home. High-dose inhaled steroid is introduced as early as possible in order to make the prednisolone treatment period as short as possible. It is usually 1–2 weeks depending upon the severity of the attack and the response. Inhaled steroid, on the other hand, should continue for at least 6–8 weeks, because the child after recovery remains vulnerable with hyper-responsive airways and compromised small airway function.

The patient should not be *discharged* until: 1, symptoms have disappeared; 2, PEF >75% of personal best or predicted normal; 3, diurnal variation of PEF <25%; 4, a maintenance treatment, including high-dose inhaled steroid, is established; and 5, it is ensured that the child is able to comply with the regimen. Otherwise, there is a 20–30% risk of relapse within a few weeks.

Prevention of further acute attacks

In order to prevent new episodes, it is useful to *investigate the circumstances of admission*. 1, Was there an avoidable precipitating factor? 2, Was this a catastrophic sudden attack or was there a period of recognizable deterioration before the 'acute' attack? 3, Did the patient and relatives react appropriately when the asthma got worse? 4, Was the patient complying with regular treatment? 5, Was medical management appropriate? 6, Was the acute episode predictable, for example by a high number of $beta_2$ inhalations, which, as in adults, is a marker of uncontrolled asthma.

All patients should have a written, *self-management plan* informing them at what PEF values or level of symptoms they should increase their treatment, how treatment should be increased and for how long, and when to call the doctor, or remit themselves to hospital without delay.

The admission to hospital provides an opportunity to educate the patients about their asthma and train them to respond to changes in symptoms and PEF.

Children ≥5 years should have a peak flow meter and PEF should be recorded and brought at the planned *follow-up visit*.

Informed consent

Remember, no one can make you feel inferior without your consent.

Eleanor Roosevelt

Further reading

Books

Silverman M, ed. *Childhood Asthma and Other Wheezing Disorders*. London: Chapman and Hall, 1995.

Articles

Agertoft L, Pedersen S. The importance of delivery system for the effect of budesonide. *Arch Dis Child* 1993; **69**: 130–133.

Agertoft L, Pedersen S. Effects of longterm treatment with an inhaled corticosteroid on growth and pulmonary function in asthmatic children. *Respir Med* 1994; **88**: 373–381.

Agertoft L, Pedersen S. Influence of spacer device on drug delivery to young children with asthma. *Arch Dis Child* 1994; **71**: 217–20.

Henriksen JM, Agertoft L, Pedersen S. Protective effect of action of inhaled formoterol and salmeterol on exercise-induced asthma in children. *J Allergy Clin Immunol* 1992; **89**: 1176–82.

Henry RL, Robertson CF, Asher I, *et al.* Management of acute asthma. *J Pediatr Child Health* 1993; **29**: 101–3.

Ilangovan P, Pedersen S, Godfrey S, *et al.* Treatment of severe steroid dependent preschool asthma with nebulised budesonide suspension. *Arch Dis Child* 1993; **68**: 356–9.

Merkus PJFM, van Essen-Zandvliet EEM, Duiverman EJ, *et al.* Long-term effect of inhaled corticosteroids on growth rate in adolescents with asthma. *Pediatrics* 1993; **6**: 1121–1126.

Murphy S, Kelly HW. Management of acute asthma. *Paediatrician* 1991; **18**: 287–300.

Noble V, Ruggins NR, Everard ML, Milner AD. Inhaled budesonide for chronic wheezing under 18 months of age. *Arch Dis Child* 1992; **67**: 285–8.

Pedersen S. Choice of inhalation therapy in paediatrics. *Eur Respir Rev* 1994; **4**: 85–8.

Pedersen S. Safety aspects of corticosteroids in children. *Eur Respir Rev* 1994; **4**: 33–43.

Rachelefsky GS, Warner JO. International consensus on the management of pediatric asthma: a summary statement. *Pediatr Pulmonol* 1993; **15**: 125–7.

Silberman M, Taussig L. Early childhood asthma: what are the questions? *Am Rev Respir Crit Care Med* 1995; **151**(2): 1–42.

Warner JO, Götz M, Landau LI, *et al.* Management of asthma: a consensus statement. *Arch Dis Child* 1989; **64**: 1065–79.

Wolthers O, Pedersen S. A controlled study of linear growth in asthmatic children during treatment with inhaled corticosteroids. *Pediatrics* 1992; **89**: 839–42.

Wolthers O, Pedersen S. Short term growth during treatment with fluticasone propionate and beclomethasone dipropionate. *Arch Dis Child* 1993; **68**: 673–6.

Part 11 Immunotherapy for Rhinitis and Asthma

11.1 Immunotherapy I

Is it effective?

Key points
- Immunotherapy for allergic rhino-conjunctivitis and asthma consists of a series of subcutaneous allergen injections.
- The treatment is controversial for it was introduced on an empirical basis and has been considerably misused.
- A series of placebo-controlled studies have now shown efficacy of immunotherapy with pollen, mite and animal extracts.
- It is still an open question as to whether the therapy can alter the natural history of allergic diseases.
- Therefore, it is difficult to give precise guidelines for the use of immunotherapy.
- Form your own opinion based on the abstracts below.

Specific allergen immunotherapy (hyposensitization) consists of a series of subcutaneous *injections of allergen extract* with the aim of reducing the patient's sensitivity to the allergen in question and, with that, the allergic *symptoms in the conjunctiva, nose and bronchi* (immunotherapy with venoms is discussed in Chapter 13.3).

Immunotherapy is *controversial*. Some doctors never use this treatment, while others use it in most patients with allergic rhino-conjunctivitis and asthma. Immunotherapy is rarely used in some countries (e.g. the UK) and often in others (e.g. the USA).

It is still an *open question* as to whether immunotherapy can *alter the natural history* of the disease. It is claimed that it is efficacious for years after the injections are stopped, and that it can prevent the development of new allergies, the progression of rhinitis to asthma and the development of irreversible lung damage in chronic asthma. But, at present, these claims are based on theoretical thinking supported by thin experimental evidence.

As such fundamental questions remain unanswered, it is difficult to give precise indications for the use of immunotherapy. It is essential for all who deal with allergic diseases that they *form their own opinion*, based on placebo-controlled studies and unbiased reviews. A series of the more significant contributions to the literature is abstracted below and referred to in *Further reading*.

Abstracts

11.1.1 FRANKLAND AW, AUGUSTIN R. Prophylaxis of summer hay fever and asthma. *Lancet* 1954; **1**: 1055–7. In a study of 200 patients with hay fever, with and without asthma, the authors found excellent or good result in 79% treated with a preseasonal series of injections of an aqueous grass pollen extract, while only 33% of placebo-treated patients responded ($p = 0.001$). The corresponding figures for pollen asthma were 94% and 30% ($p < 0.002$). *This is the first double-blind, placebo-controlled study of the efficacy of immunotherapy. It did not apear until 43 years after the introduction of this form of therapy.*

11.1.2 VARNEY VA, GAGA M, FREW AJ, et al. Usefulness of immunotherapy in patients with severe summer hay fever uncontrolled by antiallergic drugs. *Br Med J* 1991; **302**: 265–9. Forty adults with a history of severe grass pollen allergy were randomized to receive either a biologically standardized depot grass pollen extract or placebo. Treatment started 1.5 months before and continued throughout the pollen season. There was a highly significant difference in symptom score and drug use between the two groups ($p = 0.001$) (Fig. 11.1.1), and treatment was assessed positively by all actively treated patients. The sensitivity to allergen in conjunctiva and skin was reduced in the actively treated group ($p < 0.001$). *This study demonstrates a remarkable efficacy in patients with severe hay fever.*

11.1.3 WARNER JO, PRICE JF, SOOTHILL JF, HEY EN. Controlled trial of hyposensitization to *Dermatophagoides pteronyssinus* in children with asthma. *Lancet* 1978; **2**: 913–15. Fifty-six mite-allergic children with moderate to severe asthma and allergic rhinitis were enrolled in the study. They were allocated at random to a placebo group or a group treated for 1 year with tyrosine-adsorbed *Dermatophagoides pteronyssinus* extract. In the active group, asthma improved in 85% and rhinitis in 60%, while the corresponding percentages in the placebo group were 50% ($p < 0.01$) and 23% ($p < 0.05$). Additional medication was significantly less in the active treatment group. *This study supports earlier reports in showing efficacy of immunotherapy with mite extract in children.*

11.1.4 GADDIE J, SKINNER C, PALMER KNV. Hyposensitization with house dust mite vaccine in bronchial asthma. *Br Med J* 1976; **2**: 561–2. Fifty-five adult patients with asthma and mite allergy were randomized to either treatment with a tyrosine-adsorbed extract of *Dermatophagoides pteronyssinus* for 12 months or placebo. At the end of the study period, there was no difference between the two groups. *This is one of the few completely negative results with immunotherapy, but, in general, studies of adults with mite allergy and asthma have been disappointing.*

11.1.5 SUNDIN B, LILJA G, GRAFF-LOMMEVIG V, et al. Immunotherapy with partially purified and standardized animal dander extracts. *J Allergy Clin Immunol* 1986; **77**: 478–87. Thirty-two patients with cat-induced asthma were

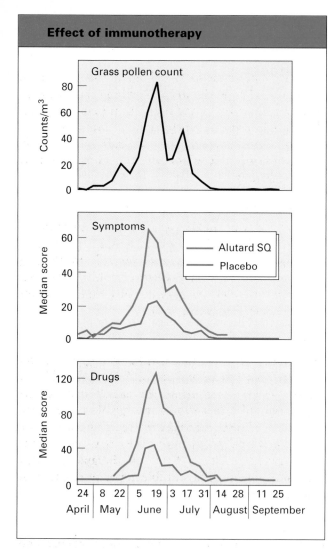

Effect of immunotherapy

Grass pollen count

Counts/m³

Symptoms

Median score

— Alutard SQ
— Placebo

Drugs

Median score

24 | 8 22 | 5 19 | 3 17 31 | 14 28 | 11 25
April | May | June | July | August | September

Fig. 11.1.1. Average weekly grass pollen count, and symptom and medication scores for allergen and placebo groups. From Varney VA, Gaga M, Frew AJ, *et al.* Usefulness of immunotherapy in patients with severe summer hay fever uncontrolled by antiallergic drugs. *Br Med J* 1991; **302**: 265–9.

treated with cat dander extract or placebo for 1 year by use of a double-blind protocol. In the treated group, the bronchial sensitivity toward cat was reduced (*p* < 0.001), and these patients also demonstrated a tendency toward less pronounced symptoms after exposure to cat. *This study shows that it is possible to reduce the sensitivity to cat allergen by a factor of 10, which probably is of clinical significance in some patients.*

11.1.6   Committee on Safety of Medicine. Desensitizing vaccines. *Br Med J* 1986; **293**: 948. 'Desensitizing vaccines have the potential to induce severe bronchospasm and anaphylaxis, and these reactions have (in the UK) resulted in 26 deaths since 1957, five in the past 18 months.' 'It is essential, therefore, that physicians carefully weigh the potential ben-

efits of the vaccines against their known risks before embarking on treatment in any patient. In view of the appreciable risks incurred during treatment, these agents should be used only where facilities for full cardiorespiratory resuscitation are immediately available, and patients should be kept under medical observation for at least 2 hours after treatment.' *A timely comment on safety, but an observation period of 2 hours is unrealistic and not well motivated, as almost all severe allergic reactions occur within 30 minutes.*

11.1.7   GRANT IWB. Does immunotherapy have a role in the treatment of asthma? *Clin Allergy* 1986; **16**: 7–10. 'Senior physicians may recall with cynicism the financially profitable cult of hyposensitization with haphazard mixtures of numerous allergens practised by unscrupulous self-styled allergists.' 'In its present form, it is an unreliable, inconvenient, expensive and potentially dangerous method of treating asthma.' *All the arguments against – in colourful expressions.*

11.1.8   COLEMAN JW, DAVIES RJ, DURHAM SR, *et al.* Position paper on allergen immunotherapy. Report of a BSACI working party. *Clin Exp Allergy* 1993; **23**(suppl 1): 1–44. The recommendations of the British Society of Allergy and Clinical Immunology. 'Immunotherapy is recommended only for pollen rhino-conjunctivitis uncontrolled by drugs and only in patients without asthma.' 'The effectiveness of allergen specific immunotherapy in asthma has not been compared to conventional management with avoidance measures and pharmacological treatment. Without such comparisons, it is not possible to assess the risk–benefit ratio of immunotherapy with other treatments. Until such studies are undertaken, specific allergen immunotherapy in asthma should be regarded as an experimental form of treatment.' *A competent review with a negative bias.*

11.1.9   MALLING H-J, WEEKE B. EAACI immunotherapy position paper. The recommendations of the European Academy of Allergy and Clinical Immunology. *Allergy* 1993; **48**(suppl 14): 9–36. 'We recommend that immunotherapy begin early in the disease process in order to prevent the further development of severe disease.' 'The indication for immunotherapy should be considered to be equivalent to that of prophylactic drug treatment, and immunotherapy (for allergic rhinitis and asthma) should be started on the same disease severity. Patients who need daily pharmacotherapy should be offered supplementary immunotherapy.' *A competent review with a positive bias.*

Indication for immunotherapy?
Bias in both physician and patient colour the opinion of success of treatment. The patient may be moved to defend the wisdom of his decision to undergo the expense and discomfort of injection treatment, whereas the physician would like to consider himself engaged in something useful as well as profitable.

FC Lowell, W Franklind
N Engl J Med, 1965; **273**: 675

11.2 Immunotherapy II

Indications

Key points
- Immunotherapy can be effective in allergic rhino-conjunctivitis and asthma.
- But proven efficacy does not necessarily mean clinical indication; the question is when and how often to start immunotherapy.
- The specific diagnosis must be correct, and allergen exposure must be the major cause of symptoms.
- Immunotherapy is a treatment for children and young adults, not for the elderly.
- The ideal patient suffers from severe rhino-conjunctivitis and mild asthma.
- The major indication for immunotherapy is pollen allergy.
- A long pollen season, a high degree of allergy and heavy pollen exposure all speak in favour of immunotherapy.
- The role of immunotherapy in mite allergy is unsettled as is the question as to whether or not it can change the natural history of the disease.
- Studies have shown efficacy in children with mite allergy, while the results in adults are less impressive.
- Immunotherapy may be tried in children and youngsters with mild to moderate symptoms in spite of a mite avoidance programme.
- Immunotherapy may be tried in selected patients, with allergy to cats and dogs, when avoidance has been unsuccessful.
- Immunotherapy should not be used instead of avoidance.

There is ample evidence that immunotherapy can be effective in allergic rhinitis and asthma (Fig. 11.2.1). However, proven efficacy does not necessarily mean clinical indication, as efficacious and safe pharmacotherapy is also available. The difficult and currently debated question is *when and how often* to start immunotherapy.

Prerequisites for therapy
It is absolutely necessary for a positive result that: 1, the specific *diagnosis is certain*; and 2, exposure to *the allergen plays a predominant role* in eliciting symptoms and in the overall severity of the disease. Treatment of a positive skin test of little importance to the patient's disease is futile.

Age
Immunotherapy is a treatment for *young adults and children*, aged 5 years and above. It is not suitable for the treatment of asthma in the elderly because the importance of IgE-mediated allergy decreases with age, and because anaphylactic reactions are more severe in elderly people, who may have concurrent cardio-vascular disease. Thus, the therapeutic index is considerably more favourable in youngsters than in mature adults.

Symptoms
Obviously, a patient with mild pollen allergy and occasional rhino-conjunctivitis symptoms does not

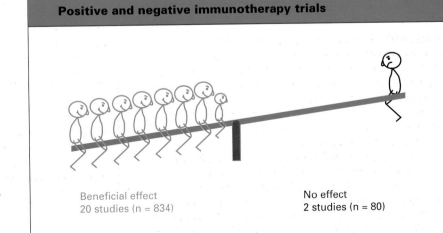

Fig. 11.2.1. Results of 22 placebo-controlled studies of the effect of immunotherapy in rhinitis and asthma. Since this figure was made by Kjell Aas in 1977, a number of new studies have been published, but the ratio between success and failure is unchanged.

Positive and negative immunotherapy trials

Beneficial effect
20 studies (n = 834)

No effect
2 studies (n = 80)

require immunotherapy, while it has a clear role in patients with severe symptoms not controlled by pharmacotherapy (see Fig. 11.1.1).

Not only the *severity of the symptoms* but also the *length of the pollen season* is of importance. The pollen season is long in Southern Europe, California and South Africa, and pollen allergy is perennial in tropical zones. Such patients are less satisfied with daily drug therapy than are their colleagues in temperate zones. The indication for immunotherapy is widened with the length of the season.

If immunotherapy is attempted in a mite-allergic patient with severe asthma, the treatment is unlikely to cause any significant clinical benefit, while the risk of provoking a serious asthma attack is considerable.

It follows from the above description that the ideal patient for immunotherapy is a young person, who suffers from *severe rhinitis* and *mild asthma*.

Mono- and poly-sensitized patients

Some data suggest that mono-allergic patients respond better to immunotherapy than those who are allergic to a series of allergens.

Pollen

Controlled studies have shown that immunotherapy with pollen allergen, *grass, ragweed, birch, mugwort and mountain cedar* has a clear effect on *rhino-conjunctivitis* and *asthma* symptoms, while a single study has failed to show an effect on the oral allergy syndrome.

While modern pharmacotherapy can control symptoms in mild to moderate disease, patients with a *high degree of allergy* that are *heavily exposed* to allergen will merely experience a reduction of symptoms. These patients may benefit from the *added use of pharmacotherapy and immunotherapy*, and the same applies to patients with asthma in the pollen season.

Few patients will be completely free of symptoms when treated with immunotherapy alone, and it should not be started as the first choice of treatment 'in order to prevent the development of perennial asthma'. This risk is only increased two to three times in seasonal allergic rhinitis, and there is no proof that it can be reduced by pollen immunotherapy.

Immunotherapy with *a single grass pollen species* (rye grass or orchard grass) is as effective as treatment with four or five species.

House dust mite

The *indications* of immunotherapy with mite allergen are *not well defined*, as it is not yet known whether the treatment can *change the natural history* of the disease. As immunotherapy has not been compared with pharmacotherapy, it is not possible to carry out a proper cost–risk–benefit analysis.

Controlled studies have shown clinically significant effects of immunotherapy on asthma and rhinitis symptoms in children, while the results in adults have been less impressive.

In children with mite allergy and perennial rhinitis and/or asthma, immunotherapy may be considered if: 1, a mite avoidance programme has been carried out; and 2, nasal and/or bronchial symptoms cannot be controlled by ordinary drug therapy.

In adult patients, a mite avoidance programme is advised, supported by topical steroids in nose and bronchi. If this regimen fails in controlling the symptoms, immunotherapy may be considered *in a few*

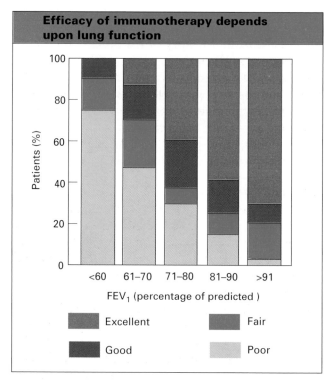

Fig. 11.2.2. Efficacy of immunotherapy with *Dermatophagoides pteronyssinus* extract related to lung function. From Bousquet J, Hejjaoui A, Clauzel AM, *et al.* Specific immunotherapy with a standardized *Dermatophagoides pteronyssinus* extract. II. Prediction of efficacy of immunotherapy. *J Allergy Clin Immunol* 1988; **82**: 971–7.

Contra-indications for immunotherapy
Significant medical or immunological disease
Concurrent use of beta blocker (increased risk of death from anaphylaxis)
Coronary disease and hypertension (increased risk of death from anaphylaxis)
Poor patient compliance
FEV_1 persistently below 70%
Severe and uncontrolled asthma
Pregnancy*

Table 11.2.1. Contra-indications for immunotherapy.
*The Position Paper of The European Academy of Allergology and Clinical Immunology states that 'treatment should not be started during pregnancy but maintenance treatment may be continued if pregnancy occurs'

young patients in whom mite exposure is the dominant cause of asthma.

Immunotherapy is not indicated in adults with mite allergy when: 1, this allergy is only part of the asthma aetiology; 2, the patient has a significant irreversible component (FEV_1 <70%) (Fig. 11.2.2); or 3, the disease is severe with daily symptoms (risk of serious allergen-induced asthma attack).

Animal proteins
Controlled studies have shown that immunotherapy with cat (and dog) proteins reduces the sensitivity of the airways to allergen challenge, but there is no definite proof that immunotherapy can control asthma symptoms when allergen exposure continues.

Immunotherapy with animal proteins may be considered in: 1, *occupational allergies* (veterinarians, farmers, laboratory workers); and 2, *highly allergic children* who cannot attend ordinary school education due to animal protein in schoolmates' clothes.

It is a poor allergist who, for instance, tells his patient that he may keep his pet while he is being 'cured' for his allergy by a series of injections. Cure cannot be promised, but it is likely that immunotherapy will reduce the sensitivity, which may be of clinical benefit for the patient but *never a substitute for allergen avoidance.*

Moulds
Mould extracts are occasionally used for asthma apparently with some success. As the efficacy has not been definitely proven, and there is a lack of standardized, high-quality extracts, this therapy is, at present, *confined to controlled trials.*

Contra-indications
Immunotherapy is a treatment for otherwise healthy young persons with good compliance to therapy. Abuse of alcohol or drugs, significant concurrent disease, fixed airway obstruction and severe asthma are contra-indications (Table 11.2.1). The latter are contra-indications because the expected benefit is small and the risk of serious reactions is considerable.

> **Profitable for the doctor**
> God heals, and the doctor takes the fees.

11.3 Immunotherapy III
Possible modes of action

Key points
- The mechanism(s) by which immunotherapy exerts its beneficial effect is still unclear.
- It induces a series of immunological changes, which may be responsible for symptom relief or epiphenomena.
- Circulating IgG-blocking antibodies, synthesized during therapy, may prevent the interaction between allergen and cell-bound IgE.
- The blocking activity, probably of importance in venom immunotherapy, seems to be of little significance in airway disease.
- Immunotherapy results initially in an increased synthesis of IgE antibody.
- Subsequently, IgE decreases with time, but long-term treatment is required to return it to pretreatment level, or lower.
- The lymphocyte response to allergen is increased in allergic patients, and immunotherapy tends to return it towards normal.
- Importantly, it reduces the number of infiltrating T cells and seems to induce a switch from Th2 to Th1 cells.
- Immunotherapy reduces the number of mast cells in airway epithelium and their release of mediators.
- It also prevents the increase in the number of activated eosinophils in the airways.
- Immunotherapy reduces allergen-induced histamine release from basophils.
- Successful therapy is associated with a reduced allergen sensitivity in skin and airways.
- Possibly, immunotherapy in the future may consist of the injection of allergenic peptides with specificity for T-cell epitopes.

A variety of immunological changes are described during immunotherapy, but it remains uncertain as to whether they are responsible for relief of symptoms, or epiphenomena. The mechanism(s) by which immunotherapy exerts its beneficial effect is still unclear.

Blocking antibody
It was shown many years ago, using the Prausnitz–Küstner reaction, that immunotherapy results in the formation of antibodies, which are able to inhibit the allergic reaction. These blocking antibodies, belonging to the *IgG* class, may combine with free allergen, thereby preventing its interaction with cell-bound IgE. The blocking activity is probably of relevance in the protective effect of *venom immunotherapy*, but it is unlikely to be a major mechanism with inhaled allergens.

IgE antibody
Both natural allergen exposure and allergen injections stimulate the formation of IgE antibody. Consequently, immunotherapy results initially in an *increased level of IgE antibody*. It decreases with time, but long-term treatment is required to return it to pretreatment level, or lower (Fig. 11.3.1). It follows that a reduced synthesis of IgE antibody does not contribute to the clinical efficacy of immunotherapy, which occurs in the majority of patients within the first year.

Lymphocyte response
The lymphocyte response to allergen, demonstrated *in vitro* by, for example, lymphocyte transformation

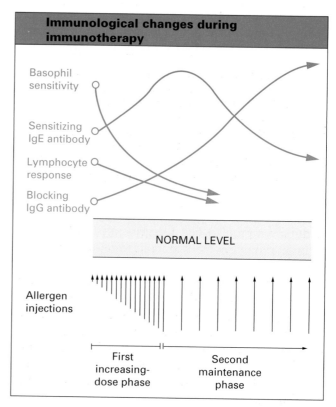

Fig. 11.3.1. Immunological changes during immunotherapy.

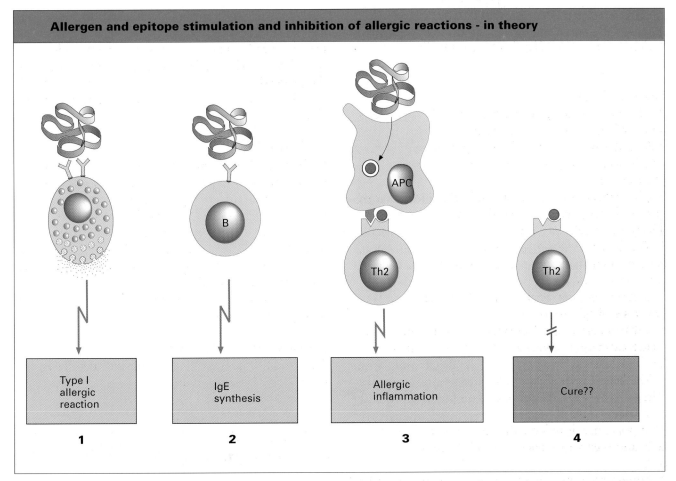

Fig. 11.3.2. How allergens and epitopes, in theory, may stimulate and inhibit allergic sensitization and inflammation. 1, An allergen (the full protein molecule) interacts with mast cell-fixed IgE and elicits a Type I allergic reaction. 2, The allergen interacts with cell membrane-bound IgE on a B cell and stimulates the synthesis of IgE. 3, The allergen is processed by an APC, and a peptide fragment (an epitope) is, together with a MHC class II molecule, presented for the T-cell receptor of a CD4+ Th2 cell. The Th2 cell becomes stimulated and contributes to the allergic inflammation. 4, Injected alone, the epitope reacts directly with the T-cell receptor of the Th2 cell, which is inhibited, resulting in a turn-off of IgE synthesis and allergic inflammation. The safe immunotherapy for the future?

or cytokine production, is increased in allergic patients, and immunotherapy tends to return it towards normal.

Immunotherapy *reduces the number of infiltrating CD4+ T lymphocytes* during the late-phase response to allergen, and recent results indicate a *switch from Th2 cells to Th1 cells*. As described in Chapter 1.6, Th2 cells synthesize cytokines, which promote IgE formation (IL-4), as well as infiltration and activation of mast cells (IL-3), and of eosinophils (IL-3 and IL-5).

Mast cells and eosinophils

Immunotherapy *reduces the number of mast cells* in airway epithelium and also their allergen-induced *release of mediators*. It also prevents the increase in the *number of activated eosinophils* in the airways following allergen challenge and exposure.

Basophil leucocytes

Basophil leucocytes from allergic individuals release histamine when they are challenged *in vitro* with the allergen. An early effect of immunotherapy is a *reduced basophil sensitivity*, which occurs in some, but not all, patients.

Skin and airway sensitivity

Successful immunotherapy is associated with a *reduced allergen sensitivity* in skin and airways, with inhibition of both early- and late-phase responses to allergen challenge. The increase in bronchial responsiveness to unspecific stimuli during the pollen season is also reduced.

Immunotherapy for the future?

T and B cell epitopes

T cells and B cells recognize different epitopes on the same antigenic molecule. B cells (and antibodies) are capable of direct reaction with the protein molecule. T cells, on the other hand, need the presentation of a peptide fragment by an antigen-presenting cell (see Chapter 1.5).

Importance of T cell epitopes

The recognition that B cell production of IgE antibodies depends on T cell regulation led to the consideration of how to alter T cell stimulation of B cells. Further, the T cells that appear to play a direct role in allergic inflammation are probably the same cells (Th2 cells) that are involved in IgE class switching. Down-regulation of these Th2 cells could, at the same time, reduce IgE synthesis and limit inflammatory responses to allergen.

Characteristics of T-cell epitopes

The identification of T-cell epitopes on allergens is now progressing rapidly. A number of major allergens have been cloned, sequenced and expressed. Epitope mapping with knowledge of the full peptide sequence of an allergen allows the synthesis of a series of peptides that can be used as test materials for T cell-specific treatment.

Treatment without risk?

In vitro experiments have indicated that T cells are down-regulated and made tolerant when they are treated with peptides representing T-cell epitopes without a co-stimulatory signal from APCs. Human studies have now started with the injection of T-cell epitopes of the major cat allergen. Ideally, this therapy may render Th2 cells tolerant with a subsequent inhibition of IgE synthesis, and of mast cell activation and eosinophil accumulation, without concurrent reaction with

B cells and IgE antibody attached to mast cells (Fig. 11.3.2).

Any questions?
Ah! Don't say that you agree with me. When people agree with me, I always feel that I must be wrong.
Oscar Wilde

11.4 Immunotherapy IV
Technique and safety

Key points
- It is important always to use high-quality, standardized allergen extracts for immunotherapy.
- Aqueous allergen extracts have a short shelf-life and require many injections, and systemic reactions are relatively frequent.
- When extracts are physically modified by aluminium hydroxide, or tyrosine, allergen absorption is delayed.
- Such depot extracts are usually preferred as they require fewer injections and the risk of systemic reactions is reduced.
- Immunotherapy consists of an increasing-dose phase and a maintenance phase.
- The increasing-dose phase can follow an ordinary schedule, a rush regimen or a clustered regimen (only aqueous extracts).
- The maintenance therapy is given at regular intervals (6–8 weeks for depot preparations).
- Pollen immunotherapy can be given as preseasonal and as perennial therapy.
- The duration of therapy is usually 3–5 years.
- Even a perfectly undertaken course of immunotherapy is associated with a risk of severe allergic reactions.
- Therapy is only justified if all possible attempts are made to reduce this risk to zero.

Centres starting this type of therapy are recommended to adhere to strict protocols for performance and especially safety (e.g. according to Abstract 11.1.9).

Choice of allergen(s)
It is advisable to *select one or two* allergens based on the result of allergy testing, knowledge of allergen occurrence in the patient's environment and the possibilities of allergen avoidance. Allergen mixtures cannot be recommended, with the exception of related allergens with marked immunological identity (e.g. different grasses).

Allergen extracts

Standardization
The ideal extract contains all allergens and epitopes of relevance for the individual patient and no other proteins. In practice, a good extract of the allergen source material contains all major and most minor allergens of relevance for a group of patients who have individually varying patterns of epitope sensitivity. Obviously, the single patient will receive relevant as well as irrelevant proteins.

The ideal extract has an identical composition and concentration of allergens from batch to batch. In practice, biologically produced material can never be manufactured and standardized so precisely. A realistic standardization goal for high-quality extracts can be attained by the methods described in Table 11.4.1.

Aqueous extracts
Aqueous extracts were first introduced in 1911 and are still widely used. Their *advantages* are: 1, exactly the same extract can be used for diagnosis and therapy; 2, the immediate local reaction to an injection is a useful guide for selection of the next dose; and 3, aqueous extracts can be used for rush- and cluster-immunotherapy. Their *disadvantages* are: 1, poor stability and short shelf-life; 2, proteins adhere to the surface of the glass, so the allergen concentration falls

Methods for standardization of allergen extracts

Determination of extract composition
    e.g. by crossed immunoelectophoresis, using a
    broad poly-specific rabbit antibody

Quantitation of content of specific major allergens
    e.g. by an ELISA technique, using murine
    monoclonal antibody

Quantitation of total allergenic activity by *in vitro* methods
    e.g. by RAST inhibition, using a well-characterized
    reference extract and pooled sera containing IgE
    antibodies to the extract

Quantitation of total allergenic activity by *in vivo* methods
    e.g. by skin testing at least 20 allergic patients with
    the extract in question

Table 11.4.1. Methods for standardization of allergen extracts. Adapted from Ipsen H, Klysner SS, Larsen JN, *et al.* Allergenic extracts. In: Middleton E, Reed CE, Ellis EE, *et al.*, eds. *Allergy. Principles and Practice* 4th ed. St Louis: Mosby, 1993: 529–53

with the contents in the bottle, and thus a reduction in dose is necessary when changing to a new bottle; 3, many injections are necessary; and 4, systemic allergic reactions are relatively frequent.

Physically modified extracts—depot extracts

Aluminium hydroxide or tyrosine added to the extract, will adsorb and precipitate the allergen; thus, systemic absorption from the injection site is delayed.

Depot preparations are as efficacious as aqueous extracts (Fig. 11.4.1). There is a *reduced risk* of systemic allergic reactions, although they can occur and may be delayed. An additional advantage of depot preparations is that they require *fewer injections* than is needed for aqueous extracts. In general, depot extracts are preferable, with the exception of rush- and cluster-immunotherapy.

Chemically modified extracts

Treatment of allergen extracts with *formaldehyde* and with *glutaraldehyde* has been tried in the hope that the allergenicity (ability to elicit histamine release and allergic reaction) is reduced, while the immunogenicity (ability to stimulate the immune system) is retained.

So far, this type of extract has not shown any definite advantage over the extracts already on the market, and they have been difficult to standardize.

Ordinary rush- or cluster-immunotherapy?

Immunotherapy consists of two phases: the *increasing-dose phase* and the *maintenance phase*.

When a depot preparation is used, weekly injections are given in the first phase; this interval is increased to 6–8 weeks in the second phase.

For aqueous extracts the *ordinary schedule* is two to three injections per week in the first phase, increasing the interval to 3–4 weeks in the second. The entire first phase can be completed within 1 week as a *rushed regimen* in a hospitalized patient by administering two to six daily injections of aqueous extract. The risk of generalized reaction is high, but so is the readiness in the specialized ward to treat such reactions. A *clustered regimen*, in which two to four injections are given in a day and repeated after 1–2 weeks, can also be used.

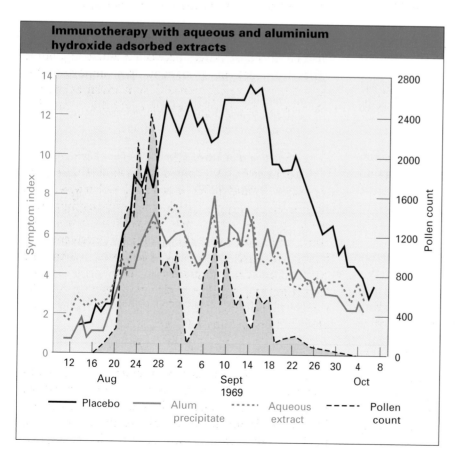

Immunotherapy with aqueous and aluminium hydroxide adsorbed extracts

Placebo — Alum precipitate ····· Aqueous extract ----- Pollen count

Fig. 11.4.1. Average daily symptom scores of ragweed hay fever in patients treated as indicated. Immunotherapy diminished the symptoms by one-half. The data also illustrate that treatment with aqueous extract and with aluminium hydroxide-adsorbed extract gave similar degrees of symptom amelioration. From Norman PS, Lichtenstein LM, March DG. Studies on allergoids from naturally occurring allergens. IV. Efficacy and safety of long-term allergoid treatment of ragweed hay fever. *J Allergy Clin Immunol* 1981; **68**: 460–70.

Preseasonal or perennial immunotherapy?

Preseasonal therapy is started 3–4 months before the pollen season; increasing doses are given until the maintenance dose is attained. Treatment is discontinued during the season and resumed the following year.

In *perennial* therapy, the maintenance dose is administered all year round with some reduction during the season.

The efficacy of the two treatment protocols is similar. Perennial therapy requires the lowest number of injections and it is therefore preferable.

Choice of dose

The initial dose must be low. It is often a standard dose, tolerated by all patients, but some allergists prefer to determine the starting point by skin testing. The initial dose is then determined as 0.1 ml of the highest concentration giving a negative intracutaneous test. During the increasing-dose phase, the dose is, for example, doubled at each injection, but only when the preceding injection has not caused a large local or any systemic reaction (Table 11.4.2).

The maintenance dose is, in principle, the highest tolerated dose not eliciting side effects, that is, the optimal dose. Based on the content of purified major

Reasons for not increasing the allergen dose

Large local reaction:
    immediate >5 cm (read after 30 minutes)
    maximum >8 cm (read by patient)

Generalized reaction: rhinitis, asthma, urticaria and anaphylaxis

Too long an interval between injections:
    50% prolongation = give 75% dose
    100% prolongation = give 50% dose
    200% prolongation = start over again

Pronounced allergen exposure (pollen season)
Manifest asthma (peak flow <70%)
Airway infection (only for asthmatics)
Change to a new bottle (only for aqueous extracts)

Table 11.4.2. Reasons for not increasing or for reducing the allergen dose in immunotherapy

Precautions in immunotherapy
Check name of patient, allergen extract, and dose and concentration, and always tell the patient the dose given
Make a quick examination with regard to *respiratory status*, including PEF in asthmatics
Ask about local and systemic reactions following the *preceding injection*
Never give an injection without having a syringe containing *adrenaline* on hand
Always be prepared to treat an *anaphylactic reaction* and *severe asthma*
Always attempt *aspiration* of the syringe before and during an allergen injection
Have the patient under *observation* for at least 30 minutes
Give injections at *regular intervals*

Table 11.4.3. Precautions in immunotherapy

allergen, this dose ranges between 5 and 20 μg, but it varies from patient to patient. It is important for safety that the maintenance dose is given at regular intervals and the rules in Tables 11.4.2–3 are followed.

Duration of therapy

If the patient has not improved after 1–2 years, the treatment should be reconsidered. Otherwise, it is continued, usually for a period of *3–5 years*, but there are no firm rules for when to stop immunotherapy. Some textbooks make the optimistic statement that immunotherapy can be discontinued when the patient has been symptom-free for at least 1 year. Unfortunately, freedom from symptoms is not the rule, but it is likely that the effects last for some years after immunotherapy has been stopped.

Precautions

Even a perfectly undertaken course of immunotherapy is associated with a *risk of severe generalized allergic reactions*. Fortunately, the risk is very small, but therapy is only justified if all possible attempts are made to reduce it to zero. It is of particular importance that the injection is given by a trained specialist in a location where *facilities for cardio-vascular resuscitation* are available and that strict safety rules are followed (Table 11.4.3).

Necessitates a new edition

Scientific truth which is formerly thought of as fixed, as though it could be weighed and measured, is changeable. Add a fact, change the outlook, and you have a new truth. Truth is a constant variable. We seek it, we find it, our viewpoint changes, and the truth changes to meet it.

William J Mayo
Ann Surgery, 1931; **94**: 799

Further reading

BOUSQUET J, HEJJAOUI A, MICHEL F-B. Specific immunotherapy in asthma. *J Allergy Clin Immunol* 1990; **86**: 292–305.

BOUSQUET J, MICHEL F-B. Immunotherapy. In: Mygind N, Naclerio RM, eds. *Allergic and Non-allergic Rhinitis. Clinical Aspects* Copenhagen: Munksgaard, 1993: 137–48.

BRINER TJ, KUO M-C, KEATING KM, ROGERS BL. Peripheral T-cell tolerance induced in naive and primed mice by subcutaneous injection of peptides from the major cat allergen *Fel d I. Proc Acad Sci USA* 1993; **90**: 7608–12.

BRUNET C, BÉDARD P-M, LAVOI A, JOBIN M, HÉBERT J. Allergic rhinitis to ragweed pollen. II. Modulation of histamine releasing factor production by specific immunotherapy. *J Allergy Clin Immunol* 1992; **89**: 87–94.

COLEMAN JW, DAVIES RJ, DURHAM SR, *et al*. Position paper on allergen immunotherapy. Report of a BSACI working party. *Clin Exp Allergy* 1993; **23**(suppl 1): 1–44.

CRETICOS PS. Immunotherapy with allergens. *JAMA* 1992; **268**: 2834–9.

DREBORG S, FREW A. Position paper: allergen standardization and skin tests. *Allergy* 1993; **48**(suppl 14): 49–54.

DURHAM SR, VARNEY V, GAGA M, *et al*. Immunotherapy and allergic inflammation. *Clin Exp Allergy* 1991; **21**(suppl 1): 206–10.

HAUGAARD L, DAHL R, JACOBSEN L. A controlled dose–response study of immunotherapy with standardized, partially purified extract of house dust mite: clinical efficacy and side effects. *J Allergy Clin Immunol* 1993; **91**: 709–22.

ILIOPOULUS O, PROUD D, ADKINSON NF, *et al*. Effects of immunotherapy on the early, late and rechallenge nasal reaction to provocation with allergen: changes in inflammatory mediators and cells. *J Allergy Clin Immunol* 1991; **87**: 855–66.

MACHIELS JJ, LEBRUN PM, JACQUEMIN MS, SAINT-REMY JMR. Significant reduction of nonspecific bronchial reactivity in patients with *Dermatophagoides pteronyssinus*-sensitive allergic asthma under therapy with allergen–antibody complexes. *Am Rev Respir Dis* 1993; **147**: 1407–12.

MAJCHEL AM, PROUD D, FRIEDHOFF L, *et al*. The nasal response to histamine challenge. Effect of the pollen season and immunotherapy. *J Allergy Clin Immunol* 1992; **90**: 85–91.

MALLING H-J. Immunotherapy in Europe. *Clin Exp Allergy* 1994; **24**: 515–21.

MALLING H-J, WEEKE B, eds. EAACI immunotherapy position paper. The recommendations of the European Academy of Allergy and Clinical Immunology. *Allergy* 1993; **48**(suppl 14): 9–36.

NORMAN PS. Modern concepts of immunotherapy. *Curr Opin Immunol* 1993; **5**: 968–73.

PLATTS-MILLS TAE. Allergen-specific treatment for asthma. *Am Rev Respir Dis* 1993; **148**: 553–5.

RAK S, BJÖRNSON A, HÅKANSON L, SÖRENSON S, VENGE P. The effect of immunotherapy on eosinophil accumulation and production of eosinophil chemotactic activity in the lungs of subjects with asthma during natural pollen exposure. *J Allergy Clin Immunol* 1991; **88**: 878–88.

REID MJ, LOCKEY RF, TURKELTAUB PC, PLATTS-MILLS TAE. Survey of fatalities from skin testing and immunotherapy 1985–1989. *J Allergy Clin Immunol* 1993; **92**: 6–15.

VAN BEVER HP, STEVENS WJ. Effect of hyposensitization upon the immediate and late asthmatic reaction and upon histamine reactivity in patients allergic to house dust mite (*Dermatophagoides pteronyssinus*). *Eur Respir J* 1992; **5**: 318–22.

VARNEY VA, GAGA M, FREW AJ, *et al*. Usefulness of immunotherapy in patients with severe summer hay fever uncontrolled by antiallergic drugs. *Br Med J* 1991; **302**: 265–9.

VARNEY VA, HAMID QA, GAGA M, *et al*. Influence of grass pollen immunotherapy on cellular infiltration and cytokine mRNA expression during allergen-induced late phase cutaneous responses. *J Clin Invest* 1993; **92**: 644–51.

Part 12 Other Allergic Lung Diseases

12.1 Allergic bronchopulmonary aspergillosis
Type I- and Type III-like reactions to bronchial saprophytes

Key points
• Patients who develop bronchopulmonary aspergillosis are often young atopics with a history of asthma.
• The asthmatic airways with mucus plugs become permanently colonized by *Aspergillus fumigatus*.
• Continuous shedding of antigen is a strong stimulus for the synthesis of IgE- and IgG-precipitating antibody.
• A combined Type I- and Type III-like reaction leads to inflammation and tissue damage (bronchiectasis and fibrosis).
• Symptoms consist of wheezing dyspnoea, productive cough and 'flu symptoms'.
• As symptoms correlate poorly to lung pathology, laboratory tests are mandatory.
• Virtually all patients have a pronounced elevation of total IgE, which closely mirrors the disease activity.
• A positive skin test is necessary but not diagnostic, and the same applies for precipitating IgG antibody.
• Untreated patients have marked blood eosinophilia.
• Microscopy of sputum reveals eosinophilia and often *Aspergillus* mycelia.
• X-ray examination shows migrating infiltrates, atelectases and proximal bronchiectases.
• The acute flare-up is associated with airway obstruction and a fall in carbon monoxide diffusion.
• Therapy, consisting of oral prednisolone, should be early and strenuous in order to prevent tissue damage.
• The patient should be followed regularly with serial IgE measurements and chest radiograms.

Aspergillus-associated diseases
The mould species, *Aspergillus fumigatus*, can cause a variety of airway diseases with distinct immunopathogenesis and clinical presentations.

1 The ubiquitous airborne *Aspergillus* spores may cause IgE-mediated *allergic asthma* in atopic subjects.
2 Non-atopic individuals can become ill when they inhale large amounts of spores; the resulting *allergic alveolitis* is largely IgG-mediated (see Chapter 12.2).
3 In some cases of chronic asthma, inhaled spores are not eliminated from the airways; they form hyphae, which multiply in the airway lumen. A combined IgE and IgG antibody response is the cause of *allergic bronchopulmonary aspergillosis*.
4 *Aspergillus fumigatus* can also colonize bronchiectatic cavities, cysts and tumours in non-atopic subjects and form an *aspergilloma*.
5 In immunodeficient patients, the moulds can become invasive and produce pneumonia, abscesses and *septicaemic aspergillosis*.

Occurrence
The prevalence of allergic bronchopulmonary aspergillosis is not known, and it may vary geographically. Almost all publications come from London and Chicago, where it has been possible to collect a sufficient number of patients for study. Apparently, the disease is rare in many parts of the world, for example the Nordic countries.

Pathogenesis
Mucus plugging of asthmatic airways can make it possible for inhaled spores of *Aspergillus fumigatus* to germinate and form mycelia. The bronchi can become permanently colonized in the case of *lung damage* resulting from previous severe asthma episodes.

The fungi do not invade the tissue but remain as *saprophytes in the airway lumen*. The continuous shedding of antigen into the tissue stimulates the production of *precipitating IgG antibody*, and atopic individuals also produce *IgE antibody*. Both types of antibody are required for the resulting inflammatory reaction that causes further damage to the bronchial wall and development of bronchiectasis.

IgE antibody and a Type I reaction make the asthma worse, contribute to the massive eosinophilia and enhance the effect of precipitating IgG antibody, probably by increasing vascular permeability. Precipitating IgG antibodies form immune complexes with the antigen, resulting in complement activation, which is largely responsible for the inflammation and tissue destruction. The immune reaction is referred to as Type III-like, as a typical Type III reaction with immune complex vasculitis does not occur.

Pathology

The affected bronchi are *bronchiectatic* and may be filled with mucus, containing *fungal elements* and *eosinophils*. The *bronchial wall is thickened* with cellular infiltration and fibrosis. The parenchyma often shows consolidation with *granulomas*, consisting of eosinophils and mononuclear cells. Although the involvement is mainly bronchial, the *alveolar wall* may be sufficiently *thickened* to produce gas diffusion problems.

Clinical characteristics

Patients who develop allergic bronchopulmonary aspergillosis: 1, have a *history of asthma*; 2, are almost always *atopic*; and 3, are often of the *younger age* group.

An acute flare-up of the disease is associated with *wheezing dyspnoea*, *productive cough*, often with expectoration of brownish plugs, 'flu symptoms', and sometimes fever. The disease may simulate recurrent infections.

Laboratory tests

When the disease is suspected, *laboratory tests are mandatory*, as the correlation between symptoms/signs and lung pathology is poor. An early diagnosis is important for the prevention of further tissue damage.

Sputum examination

Microscopy of sputum reveals eosinophilia and often, but not always, *Aspergillus* mycelia. As the organism is ubiquitous, a single positive sputum culture is not diagnostic, but repeated positive cultures are suspicious.

Blood eosinophilia

Untreated patients have *marked blood eosinophilia* with a count generally over 1000/mm³.

Skin testing

Only a minority of asthmatics with a positive skin test to *Aspergillus fumigatus* have allergic bronchopulmonary aspergillosis. When the skin test is negative, the diagnosis is very unlikely, provided a potent extract is used. Thus, a positive test is *necessary but not diagnostic*. The immediate reaction is, as a rule, followed by a late reaction, both in the skin and bronchi.

Serum immunoglobulins

Aspergillus fumigatus growing in the bronchial tree is a potent stimulus not only of specific but also of non-specific IgE. Serum IgE levels are markedly elevated, being significantly higher than in uncomplicated asthma. Virtually all patients have an *elevated total IgE*, which closely mirrors the disease activity. Serial determinations of serum IgE are of great value as a guide to therapy; a rising level is predictive of a clinical flare-up, and a stable or declining value implies remission.

The occurrence of precipitating *IgG antibody* against *Aspergillus fumigatus* can serve as a diagnostic aid.

Pulmonary function tests

The acute flare-up is associated with *reversible airway obstruction*, and, in contrast to uncomplicated asthma, with a decline in *carbon monoxide diffusion*. The latter is the best pulmonary function index of disease severity.

X-ray examination

A series of *characteristic changes* are seen; they can be *transient* or *permanent*. Migrating homogeneous shadows are a common result of parenchymal infiltrates. *Atelectasis* of a segment or a lobe or total collapse of a lung is caused by mucoid impaction. *Bronchiectasis*, which characteristically are *proximal*, account for the most important permanent change seen on the radiogram. This diagnosis can be confirmed by *CT scanning*.

Diagnostic criteria

Allergic bronchopulmonary aspergillosis should be suspected at routine examination when an atopic asthma patient has one or more of the following features: 1, a history suggesting 'recurrent airway infections'; 2, expectoration of brown plugs; 3, a positive skin test to *Aspergillus fumigatus*; 4, a high serum IgE level; 5, a high blood eosinophil count; and 6, an abnormal chest radiogram.

When the suspicion is raised, the following examinations are indicated: 1, microscopy and culture of repeated sputum samples; 2, measurement of precipitating antibody; 3, CT scanning; and 4, close follow-up of the patient.

The diagnosis is based on a *combination of symp-*

Diagnostic criteria for allergic bronchopulmonary aspergillosis
Bronchial asthma
Blood eosinophilia
Positive skin test to *Aspergillus fumigatus*
Elevated serum IgE
Precipitating antibody
History of pulmonary infiltrates
Proximal bronchiectasis

Table 12.1.1. Major diagnostic criteria for allergic bronchopulmonary aspergillosis

toms, signs and tests. The major diagnostic criteria are listed in Table 12.1.1. It has been suggested that the presence of six criteria makes the diagnosis highly likely; all seven make it certain.

Therapy

Principles

It is the aim of treatment to break the vicious circle in which the growth of fungus in the viscid secretions continues to provide antigenic material. It is, however, exceedingly difficult to clear the damaged bronchial tree, and, even when the symptoms are minimal, *early and strenuous treatment* is important.

Oral corticosteroids

Steroids are *the cornerstone of therapy*. They relieve the airway obstruction, and decrease the allergic inflammatory reaction and the production of viscid secretions, all of which lead to more effective removal of the fungi.

Steroids must be given in a large enough quantity over a sufficient period of time. A daily dose of 30–40 mg (0.5 mg/kg) prednisolone in adults is given for a few weeks in order to improve the clinical condition, stop sputum production, and clear the chest radiogram. A 3-month course of prednisolone in a lower dose with subsequent monitoring of history, serum IgE levels, and chest X-rays will suffice in most patients. Some patients, however, require prednisolone therapy indefinitely.

Other treatments

Bronchodilators will improve the asthmatic component, and *antibiotics* are indicated for bacterial infections, which are frequent complications. Inhaled steroids appear to have little effect on allergic bronchopulmonary aspergillosis. Immunotherapy with *Aspergillus* extract can deteriorate the condition and is contra-indicated.

Follow-up and prognosis

As an exacerbation of allergic bronchopulmonary aspergillosis can be associated with minimal symptoms, the patients should be followed with *serial IgE measurements and chest radiograms*.

Untreated, the patients will follow a chronic course with development of bronchiectases, fibrosis with irreversibly reduced lung function, and, in many instances, respiratory failure. With early diagnosis and proper treatment, the majority of patients will show no further functional deterioration.

As simple as that
Science is the systematic classification of experience.
George Henry Lewes

12.2 Allergic alveolitis
Type III- and Type IV-like reactions to organic dust

Key points
- Allergic alveolitis is a non-IgE mediated disease caused by inhalation of organic dust.
- The bacteria, *Micropolyspora faeni*, in hay and grain stored under damp conditions is the cause of farmer's lung.
- Exposure to mouldy organic material can cause wood worker's lung, malt worker's lung and cheese worker's lung.
- Growth of micro-organisms on an air filter in humidified hot air systems gives rise to humidifier lung.
- Proteins in dried excreta from pigeons and budgerigars are the cause of bird breeder's lung.
- Occupationally, chemicals, such as isocyanates and acid anhydrides, can cause allergic alveolitis.
- Precipitating IgG antibodies and a late response to organic dust suggest a Type III-like reaction.
- An increased number of activated CD8+ T cells, lymphocyte infiltration and granulomas indicates a role for Type IV-like reactions.
- An acute form of allergic alveolitis occurs when exposure is heavy but intermittent.
- Fever, malaise, dry cough and dyspnoea occur 4–6 hours after antigen exposure.
- A subacute form occurs when exposure is mild but continuous.
- Progressive dyspnoea, decreased exercise tolerance, productive cough, fatigue and weight loss develop insidiously.
- The chronic form, leading to pulmonary disability, occurs as the result of recurrent exposure.
- An early diagnosis is important for prevention of lung fibrosis.
- During the acute episode, the sedimentation rate is raised and there is leucocytosis.
- Precipitating antibody, as a marker of exposure, supports the diagnosis.
- Skin and inhalation tests, showing late responses, are not routine examinations.
- During an episode, the lung function is reduced, and there is hypoxaemia and a reduced diffusion capacity.
- X-ray examination shows a diffuse nodular to reticular pattern.

- A lung biopsy can be of diagnostic help showing lymphocyte infiltration, granulomas and fibrosis.
- In BAL fluid, there is an increased number and percentage of CD8+ T lymphocytes.
- Treatment consists of antigen avoidance.

Extrinsic allergic alveolitis or *hypersensitivity pneumonitis* is caused by a variety of inhaled organic materials, especially microbial products and avian proteins. It is characterized by the presence of precipitating IgG antibodies, and lymphocyte infiltration in the alveoli that may progress to fibrosis.

Aetiology
The antigens are *small airborne particles* (<5 µm), which can reach the alveoli. They occur in a wide variety of dusts mainly *of organic origin* and are products of bacteria (thermophilic actinomycetes), fungi, avian excretions and chemicals. It is likely that any organic dust of appropriate particle size can induce allergic alveolitis, and Table 12.2.1 only presents a partial list.

Thermophilic actinomycetes
The first described and probably the most frequent antigen source is *Micropolyspora faeni*. It was earlier considered to be a fungus, but it has been accepted as a bacteria because it has no nuclear membrane. It thrives well at 50–60°C, a temperature commonly reached during the decay of vegetable matter, at which it produces significant amounts of enzymes responsible for the decay process. *Micropolyspora faeni* is numerous in hay and grain stored under damp conditions. It is a common cause of allergic alveolitis among farmers: *farmer's lung*.

Thermophilic actinomycetes also grow in mouldy mushroom compost (mushroom worker's lung) and in mouldy sugar cane (bagassosis).

Other micro-organisms
Industries in which wood dust, malt, cheese and a series of other *mouldy organic materials* are handled are associated with exposure to large amounts of fungal antigens and a risk of allergic alveolitis: *wood worker's lung, malt worker's lung and cheese worker's lung*.

Humidified hot air systems in an office or factory have caused outbreaks of allergic alveolitis among the employees, and ordinary room humidifiers that generate aerosols have also been implicated. The antigen source in *humidifier lung* (humidifier fever and print-

Table 12.2.1. Examples of organic dust involved in allergic alveolitis

Antigen sources of allergic alveolitis		
Antigen source	**Exposure**	**Disease**
Thermophilic actinomycetes	Mouldy hay and grain Mushroom compost Mouldy sugar cane	Farmer's lung Mushroom worker's lung Bagassosis
Fungi	Mouldy wood chips Mouldy barley Cheese mould	Wood worker's lung Malt worker's lung Cheese worker's lung
Various micro-organisms	Contaminated water systems	Humidifier lung
Animal proteins	Avian droppings	Bird breeder's lung

Chemicals:
  Toluene diisocyanate
  Trimellitic anhydride
  Phthalic anhydride
	Paint catalyst
	Trimellitic anhydride
	Epoxy resin
		Porcelain refiner's lung
		Plastic worker's lung
		Epoxy resin worker's lung

ing worker's lung) can be bacteria, fungi, algae and amoeba, which grow on the air filters.

Avian proteins

Individuals involved in the hobby or occupation of bird handling, such as *pigeon* breeders and *budgerigar* fanciers, may develop disease as a result of inhalation of antigenic proteins from dried excreta: *bird breeder's lung* or *bird fancier's lung*.

Chemicals

Isocyanates, acid anhydrides and other chemicals used in the plastic industry may act as haptens and occasionally cause allergic alveolitis as well as occupational asthma (see Chapter 3.6).

Pathogenesis

A number of observations indicate that specific immune reactions play an important role in allergic alveolitis (Table 12.2.2). However, the nature of these immune mechanisms are far less well defined than in IgE-mediated disease.

Type I reaction

IgE antibody plays no role in the pathogenesis of allergic alveolitis, which does not occur with increased prevalence in atopic individuals. However, some persons may react with both *an early and a late*

response to organic dust, and they have coexisting *allergic asthma and allergic alveolitis*.

Type III-like reaction

When patients inhale an extract of the offending organic dust, or it is used for skin testing, *a late response* develops. In addition, virtually all patients have *precipitating IgG antibodies* in plasma.

Immune complexes can stimulate *alveolar macrophages* to produce IL-1 and TNF. Besides these pro-inflammatory *cytokines*, stimulated macrophages produce a variety of *enzymes*. These products, along with influx of *neutrophils*, contribute to early alveolar damage following acute exposure to the antigenic dust.

The significance of a Type III-like reaction in the pathogenesis of allergic alveolitis is supported by lung biopsies that sometimes reveal antigen, antibody and complement deposition. Circulating complement levels, however, are within normal range, and vasculitis does not occur.

Type IV-like reaction

A Type III-like immune reaction cannot adequately explain the pathogenesis and pathology of allergic alveolitis. There are observations to support that T-cell dependent responses, or cell-mediated immunity, are also of significance. 1, Lymphocyte transforma-

Immune reactions in allergic alveolitis		
	For	**Against**
Type III-like reaction	Late response in skin and bronchi	No vasculitis
	Late response associated with fever and leucocytosis	Normal circulating complement level
	Circulating precipitating IgG antibody in all patients	Circulating precipitating IgG antibody in 50% exposed, but non-symptomatic persons
	Deposition of antigen, antibody and complement in some lung biopsies	
Type IV-like reaction	Increased number of macrophages and activated T cells in BAL and bronchial biopsies	No delayed skin response to antigen
	Increased CD8⁺:CD4⁺ ratio	
	Formation of granulomas	

Table 12.2.2. Arguments for and against an involvement of different types of immune reactions in allergic alveolitis

tion and the production of cytokines have been detected in a significant number of patients with allergic alveolitis but not in their asymptomatic counterparts. 2, Bronchial histopathology shows *lymphocyte infiltration* and granulomas. 3, BAL studies show an increased number of *activated T cells* with a relative over-representation of *CD8⁺ cells*.

Non-antigen effects

Besides acting as antigen, organic dust has a series of other biological effects, which may contribute to disease pathology: it acts as an immunological adjuvant; it directly stimulates alveolar macrophages; it activates the complement cascade; it releases mediators from mast cells; it has enzyme activity; and it contains endotoxins.

Clinical features and diagnosis

History

In the acute form, the patient often associates exposure with symptoms, but the cause of the subacute and chronic forms is more difficult to identify. A high degree of suspicion and a detailed

environmental history are of importance for the early diagnosis.

Symptoms and signs

The *acute form* occurs when *exposure is heavy but intermittent*, for example in a pigeon breeder who occasionally cleans his or her pigeon-house. Fever, chills, malaise, chest tightness, dry cough and dyspnoea occur 4–6 hours after antigen exposure and remit spontaneously within 24 hours. The attack recurs each time the individual is exposed to the offending dust. The attacks *mimic recurrent infections* and antibiotics are often prescribed.

Examination of the patient during the attack reveals an *acutely ill, dyspnoeic* individual. Signs are often scanty; only a few râles or a fine crepitation are noted on auscultation.

Acute outbreaks of farmer's lung most frequently occur towards the end of winter following a wet summer, when farmers are handling the contaminated hay in confined areas indoors.

The *subacute form* occurs when *exposure is mild but continuous*, for example from a few pet birds kept indoors. *Progressive dyspnoea*, decreased exercise tolerance, *productive cough, fatigue* and *weight loss* develop insidiously. This is not an uncommon form of farmer's lung.

The *chronic form* with progressive shortness of breath leading to *pulmonary disability* occurs as the result of recurrent exposure. Cyanosis, clubbing and cor pulmonale develop as pulmonary fibrosis progresses.

Laboratory tests

During an acute attack, the *sedimentation rate* is raised, and there is *leucocytosis* and a generalized *elevation of serum immunoglobulins*, except for IgE which is elevated only in atopic subjects.

Precipitating antibodies

Precipitating IgG antibody to the offending organic dust antigen is found in virtually all patients, and a positive test in a symptomatic patient strongly *supports the diagnosis*. About 50% of asymptomatic persons exposed to the antigen have precipitins. Thus, a positive precipitin test without appropriate clinical findings *does not establish the diagnosis*.

Skin test

In most cases, non-irritant antigenic extracts of the organic antigens listed in Table 12.2.1 are not commercially available for skin testing. When it is performed, a positive *late skin reaction* supports the diagnosis, but, like precipitins, a positive result is merely a sign of exposure and not necessarily of disease.

Inhalation test

The diagnosis can be confirmed by controlled avoidance/exposure testing. Cautious inhalation challenge with the suspected antigen can be performed in laboratories experienced in its administration, but it is not a routine examination. An isolated *late response* is typical in sensitized patients.

Lung function tests

During an acute episode, the ventilatory capacity is reduced, showing predominantly a *restrictive* pattern with equally reduced FEV_1 and FVC, and little change in peak expiratory flow rate. There is *hypoxaemia* and a *reduced diffusion capacity*. At first the changes revert to normal, but, as fibrosis develops, the changes become irreversible.

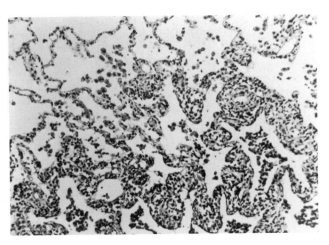

Fig. 12.2.1. Acute allergic alveolitis with lymphocyte infiltration of alveolar walls and peribronchial tissue. From Fink JN. Hypersensitivity pneumonitis. In: Middleton Jr E, Reed CE, Ellis EF, eds. *Allergy: Principles and Practice* 2nd ed. Saint Louis: The CV Mosby Company, 1983: 1085–99.

X-ray examination

In the *acute phase*, the radiogram shows a diffuse *finely nodular pattern* due to alveolar inflammation; it clears spontaneously on antigen avoidance.

In the *chronic phase*, the nodular pattern is replaced by a medium to *coarse reticular, honeycomb pattern* with parenchymal contraction and overinflation of some lung zones. These are changes of diffuse interstitial fibrosis of any origin.

Lung biopsy and bronchoalveolar lavage

Although non-specific, a biopsy may be of diagnostic help when considered together with clinical and laboratory data.

In *the acute form*, there is extensive *lymphocyte infiltration in the alveoli* and interstitial tissue (Fig. 12.2.1). Macrophages and lymphocytes also surround the epitheloid cells in some sarcoid-like granulomas. These *granulomas* may reflect a cell-mediated immune reaction of the tuberculin type.

In *the chronic form*, the most prominent feature is extensive *fibrosis*. Many alveolar spaces are obliterated and the lung architecture destroyed (Fig. 12.2.2).

In *BAL fluid*, there is an increased number and percentage of *T lymphocytes*, predominantly *CD8+ cells* (in contrast to the CD4+ cells in sarcoidosis).

Treatment

Antigen avxoidance is the cornerstone of treatment. Masks or dust filters, alteration of air conditioning systems, education of the patient and even changing

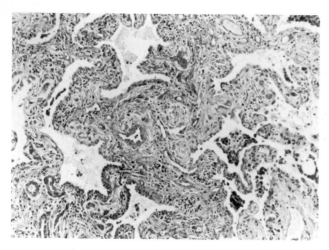

Fig. 12.2.2. Chronic allergic alveolitis with fibrosis and obliteration of many alveolar spaces. From Fink JN. Hypersensitivity pneumonitis. In: Middleton Jr E, Reed CE, Ellis EF, eds. *Allergy: Principles and Practice* 2nd ed. Saint Louis: The CV Mosby Company, 1983: 1085–99.

occupation may be necessary. *Oral corticosteroids* will abort and prevent the episodic illness, but reliance should not be placed on suppression of symptoms. As the outcome of the disease is highly dependent upon avoidance, an early diagnosis is of utmost importance.

Immunotherapy is contra-indicated in patients, having both IgE-mediated asthma and allergic alveolitis, because of the potential danger of antigen injections increasing the level of precipitating antibodies.

Non-scientific evidence
The intensity of the conviction that a hypothesis is true has no bearing on whether it is true or not.
                                                              PB Medawar

---

Further reading

DENIS MY, CORMIER J, TARDIF E. Hypersensitivity pneumonitis: whole *Micropolyspora faeni* or antigens thereof stimulate the release of proinflammatory cytokines from macrophages. *Am J Respir Cell Mol Biol* 1991; **5**: 198–203.

GREENBERGER PA, PATTERSON R. Diagnosis and management of allergic bronchopulmonary aspergillosis. *Ann Allergy* 1986; **56**: 444–9.

GREENBERGER PA, PATTERSON R. Allergic bronchopulmonary aspergillosis and the evaluation of the patient with asthma. *J Allergy Clin Immunol* 1988; **81**: 646–50.

MENDELSON EB, FISHER MR, MINTZER RA, *et al.* Roentgenographic and clinical staging of allergic bronchopulmonary aspergillosis. *Chest* 1985; **87**: 334–9.

PATTERSON R, GREENBERGER PA, HALWIG JM, LIOTTA JL, ROBERTS M. ABPA natural history and classification of early disease by serologic and roentgenographic studies. *Arch Intern Med* 1986; **146**: 916–21.

RICKETTI AJ, GREENBERGER PA, PATTERSON R. Serum IgE as an important aid in management of allergic bronchopulmonary aspergillosis. *J Allergy Clin Immunol* 1984; **74**: 68–71.

SALVAGGIO JE, MILLHOLLON B. Induction and modulation of pulmonary inflammation by organic dust: cytokines, immune complexes and 'all of those things'. *Clin Exp Allergy* 1992; **22**: 731–3.

SALVAGGIO JE, MILLHOLLON B. Allergic alveolitis: new insight into old mysteries. *Respir Med* 1993; **87**: 495–501.

SCHWARTZ HJ, GREENBERGER PA. The prevalence of allergic bronchopulmonary aspergillosis in patients with asthma, determined by serologic and radiologic criteria in patients at risk. *J Lab Clin Med* 1991; **117**: 138–43.

TRENTIN L, MARCER G, CHILOSI M, *et al.* Longitudinal study of alveolitis in hypersensitivity pneumonitis: an immunologic evaluation. *J Allergy Clin Immunol* 1988; **82**: 577–585.

Part 13 Systemic Allergic Reactions

13.1 Anaphylaxis I: mechanisms and clinical presentation
Anaphylactic and anaphylactoid reactions

Key points
- Anaphylactic reactions are usually IgE mediated.
- The causative agents are haptens or full antigens.
- Penicillin has now replaced heterologous antisera as the prime cause of anaphylactic reactions.
- Injectants are by far the most common causes, but some orally administered drugs and foods can provoke systemic reactions.
- Blood products can induce anaphylactic reactions via immune complexes and complement activation.
- Anaphylactoid reactions can be caused by radiocontrast media, dextran, morphine and muscle relaxants, which have a direct effect on mast cells.
- The generalized reactions involve respiratory, cardio-vascular and gastro-intestinal systems, and skin, singly or in combinations.
- Death is due to suffocation (laryngeal oedema and asthma) or cardiac arrest (hypotension and arrhythmias).

Anaphylactic reactions are immunologically mediated; they are acute generalized reactions often of great severity and potentially lethal. *Anaphylactoid reactions* (pseudo-allergies) are clinically similar reactions resulting from non-immune or unknown mechanisms. Otherwise, the clinical presentation and treatment of these reactions is identical. In daily routine, both are referred to as *anaphylaxis* or *anaphylactic shock*.

Patients with or without atopic disease have equal susceptibility to anaphylactic reactions, but the clinical consequences can be more serious in a patient with *asthma*, than in an otherwise healthy person. Patients taking *beta-blockers* have a significantly increased risk of severe anaphylactic reactions.

Mechanisms

IgE-mediated reactions
Human anaphylaxis is most frequently mediated through IgE antibodies (Table 13.1.1). Histamine, together with the other mast cell mediators, cause the immediate reaction, and cytokines probably augment and prolong the reaction.

Immune complex mediated reactions
The formation of immune complexes can mimic IgE-mediated anaphylaxis. This has been well demonstrated in patients with IgA deficiency; half of the cases form IgG autoantibody to IgA. An injection of *gammaglobulin*, containing IgA, in these patients will result in the formation of immune complexes consisting of host IgG and donor IgA. This activates complement resulting in the generation of the anaphylatoxins, C3a and C5a, which both degranulate mast cells and contract smooth muscles. Anaphylactic reactions to blood and other *blood products* may operate by a similar mechanism.

Direct effect on mast cells
Anaphylactoid reactions can occur as the result of release of mediators from mast cells and basophils; the pathways involved do not implicate antigen and antibody. The mechanisms are incompletely understood. In theory, an increased number of mast cells, increased cell releasability, as well as an element of increased sensitivity to mediators may all be of importance. As this type of reaction does not require prior sensitization, it may occur without previous exposure.

Presumptive abnormalities of arachidonic acid metabolism
Acetylsalicylic acid can cause asthma, angioedema

Types of anaphylactic reactions
IgE-mediated reaction   e.g. penicillin
Immune complex mediated reaction   e.g. blood products
Direct effect on mast cells   e.g. radio-contrast media
Abnormal arachidonic acid metabolism   e.g. acetylsalicylic acid

Table 13.1.1. Types of anaphylactic and anaphylactoid reactions with examples of causative agents

and an anaphylactoid reaction. The following arguments show that the reaction is mediated by a non-immunological mechanism. 1, Antibody to acetylsalicylic acid cannot be demonstrated. 2, The patients tolerate molecules that are structurally related to acetylsalicylic acid (e.g. sodium salicylate and choline salicylate). 3, They do not tolerate molecules that have biochemical activity similar to acetylsalicylic acid but are structurally unrelated. These, the *non-steroidal anti-inflammatory drugs (NSAIDs)*, inhibit the enzyme cyclo-oxygenase, which transforms arachidonic acid into prostaglandins.

Causative agents

Drugs

The list of aetiological agents, headed by drugs, is long, so the discussion is confined to those agents most frequently responsible for systemic reactions. The potency of all inducers of anaphylactic and anaphylactoid reactions is increased when given by the *parenteral route*, especially intravenously, rather than by the oral route.

The most frequent causes of anaphylaxis are *penicillin* and the synthetic penicillin derivatives. In the past, this role was played by *heterologous antisera*, used for the prophylaxis and treatment of tetanus, diphtheria, rabies, botulism and poisonous snake bites. In more recent years, anti-lymphocyte immunosuppression has become an important cause. *Peptide hormones* (insulin, ACTH and anti-diuretic hormone) and *enzymes* (streptokinase) are other causes of anaphylactic reactions.

Radiographic contrast media, opiates, anaesthetics, muscle relaxants, pentamidine and *plasma expanders* (dextran) all appear to act as direct mast cell releasing agents.

Acetylsalicylic acid and other *NSAIDs* have another non-immunological mode of action.

Human products

Blood, plasma and *immunoglobulins* can cause anaphylactic reactions by an immune complex mediated reaction, as described above. In rare cases, another homologous product, *seminal fluid*, has provoked IgE-mediated anaphylaxis during coitus.

Immunotherapy

Allergen injections frequently result in slight systemic reactions, which, in rare cases, can be severe. In unusually sensitive patients, even skin testing can result in an anaphylactic reaction.

Stinging insects

Venoms from stinging insects, especially of the *Hymenoptera* order, are relatively common causes of anaphylaxis (see Chapter 13.3).

Foods

Almost any food may cause anaphylactic reactions, but those most commonly responsible are *eggs, milk, nuts, fish* and *shellfish*.

Latex

Recently, IgE-mediated allergy to natural latex has become a prominent cause of anaphylaxis in *medical personnel* through the use of gloves. It has occurred even in *patients* due to intra-operative exposure to the surgeon's gloves (see Chapter 13.4).

Physical stimuli

A patient with *cold-induced* urticaria can experience life-threatening anaphylaxis if, for example, he or she jumps into cold water.

Patients who get pruritus and urticaria from *physical exercise* can occasionally develop vascular collapse. In some patients with this disorder, exercise following ingestion of a specific food appears to be an essential component. The mast cell plays a central role in *exercise-induced anaphylaxis*.

Idiopathic

In the rare case, anaphylaxis can occur repeatedly without any obvious reason. Mastocytosis and the carcinoid syndrome should be excluded.

Clinical manifestations

The skin, upper and lower airways, cardio-vascular system and gastro-intestinal tract may be affected singly or in combination. The severity of a systemic reaction can vary from slight itchiness and flushing to death within a few minutes. Death is either caused by suffocation (two-thirds of the cases, especially in young patients) or by cardio-vascular collapse (one-third, especially in the elderly).

Initial symptoms

The symptoms usually *start within minutes* of the injection or ingestion of the causative agent, and, in general, the earlier the symptoms occur, the more severe the clinical reaction is apt to be. The symptoms can be delayed as, for example, in the case of delayed absorption of an orally administered antigen.

The first symptom is the patient's instinctive perception that all is not well. This is soon confirmed by the occurrence of *pruritus* of the hands, feet, nose, eyes and palate, a feeling of warmth, *erythema* and faintness, and, in severe cases, *loss of consciousness*. The *pulse is rapid* and weak and the *blood pressure low*, which differentiates it from vasovagal syncope.

Skin symptoms
The initial pruritus and flushing may progress to include *urticaria* and *angioedema*, which are generally transient, lasting less than 24 hours.

Respiratory symptoms
Early stages of *laryngeal oedema* may be experienced as hoarseness, or 'a lump in the throat'. This finding is of grave importance as oedema of hypopharynx, epiglottis and larynx can quickly progress to asphyxia. Lower airway obstruction is experienced as chest tightness, noted as wheezing and can develop into severe *asthma*.

Cardio-vascular symptoms
Hypotension and shock are due to vasodilatation, with peripheral pooling of blood, and to increased vascular permeability, with *extravasation of fluid* and loss of intravascular volume. The circulatory collapse reduces coronary perfusion, which, together with *hypoxaemia*, reduces myocardial oxygenation. This may, especially in the elderly, result in *myocardial infarction*. The risk of death from anaphylaxis is considerably increased in the elderly and in patients with myocardial disease.

Gastro-intestinal symptoms
Nausea, vomiting, abdominal cramp and diarrhoea can occur but they are of less clinical importance.

Differential diagnosis
When a patient collapses after an injection, it is the physicians task to make a distinction, as quickly as possible, between a *vasovagal syncope* and an anaphylactic reaction. In the vasovagal reaction the patient is pale and sweating, the *pulse is slow* and the blood pressure maintained (low normal). There is *no pruritus* and *no skin or airway symptoms*.

The symptoms are almost immediately *relieved by recumbency*.

Hopefully not your research
The systems that fail are those that rely on the permanency of human nature, and not on its growth and development.

Oscar Wilde

Experienced doctors
Dumby: Experience is the name every one gives to their mistakes.
Cecil Graham: One shouldn't commit any.
Dumby: Life would be very dull without them.

Oscar Wilde

13.2 Anaphylaxis II: treatment

Adrenaline, oxygen and free airways

Key points

- When faced with a case of anaphylaxis, see Table 13.2.1.
- Early recognition and prompt institution of therapy is of utmost importance.
- Adrenaline is the essential drug in the treatment of anaphylaxis.
- As adrenaline has a short half-life, the injection can be repeated at 20–30-minute intervals.
- When vascular collapse is manifest, a small dose of adrenaline is given intravenously.
- Fully developed anaphylactic shock is associated with a considerable loss of intravascular fluid.
- An intravenous line is essential to ensure medication and for fluid replacement therapy.
- An H_1 antihistamine is given following the initial use of adrenaline.
- Early administration of oxygen is important.
- Oedema involving the upper airways can develop rapidly, requiring intubation or tracheotomy.
- A beta$_2$ agonist is administered early in asthma patients for prevention and treatment of broncho-constriction.
- Systemic steroids are given to prevent a secondary relapse.

Rapid action is of utmost importance (Table 13.2.1)

Anaphylaxis is a medical emergency; satisfactory treatment depends on early recognition and the prompt institution of therapy. At the first suspicion, place the patient in a *recumbent position*. Prepare an injection of adrenaline immediately.

Adrenaline

Adrenaline (epinephrine) is the *most important drug* in the treatment of anaphylaxis. As soon as anaphylaxis is recognized, it is given *intramuscularly* or sub-cutaneously in doses of 0.3–0.5 mg (0.3–0.5 ml of a 1:1000 = 0.1% = 1 mg/ml; 0.01 mg/kg body weight in children). A second dose can be given at the site of the offending injection in order to delay absorption. As adrenaline has a short half-life, the injection can be *repeated* at 20–30-minute intervals, if required and tolerated.

If vascular collapse is manifest (weak or un-obtainable pulse, and blood pressure below 60), or if upper airway obstruction is *life-threatening*, 0.3 mg adrenaline can be given *intravenously* in a running drip. The use of this route can be extremely un-pleasant for the patient and *carries a risk* of ventricular arrhythmia.

The best and safest way to administer adrenaline, in all cases of anaphylaxis, is to give it intravenously in small doses (0.1–0.3 mg), repeated at 5–10-minute intervals as required. This, in an emergency, allows the evaluation of the effect and side effects within minutes. These small doses must be given in a running drip or flushed through the vein with saline.

Oxygen

Oxygen should be administered *for hypotension and airway obstruction*, both of which cause hypoxaemia and decreased myocardial oxygenation. *Early administration* of oxygen is important for the prevention of cardiac complications.

Intravenous fluid

An *intravenous line* is essential to ensure medication and for fluid therapy. It should be inserted as quickly as possible before it is made difficult by vascular collapse. Fully developed anaphylactic shock is as-sociated with a considerable *loss of intravascular fluid* and *fluid replacement* is required.

Vasopressors

If adrenaline and intravenous fluids cannot maintain blood pressure, administer a vasopressor agent, such as dopamine, while carefully monitoring blood pres-sure and cardiac rhythm.

Antihistamines

An H_1 antihistamine is given following the initial use of adrenaline. It should be continued for 48 hours in order to prevent recurrence of circulatory shock. Concomitant use of an H_2 antihistamine can give further protection against shock.

Free airways

Upper airway obstruction

Oedema involving the epiglottis, hypopharynx and

Table 13.2.1. Treatment of anaphylaxis

Treatment of anaphylaxis
Treatment in office
Have patient *lie down* and call for assistance
Inject intramuscularly 0.5 mg *adrenaline*
Insert an *intravenous line*
Give a number of inhalations from a *beta$_2$ inhaler*
If you have time, inject an *H$_1$ antihistamine*
If the patient is still hypotensive or does not have free airways, make arrangements for transport to an intensive care unit
Treatment under transportation
Administer pure *oxygen*
Give intramuscularly 0.5 mg *adrenaline every 20–30 minutes*
If blood pressure is immeasurable, give 0.3 mg *adrenaline intravenously* (flush with saline)
If adequate ventilation cannot be maintained, insert an *oral airway* and ventilate with a compressible bag (oxygen); elevate the head of the stretcher to counteract laryngeal oedema
Be prepared to do an emergency incision in the *crico-thyroid membrane* and to insert a small ventilation tube through the incision; alternatively, puncture with large-bore needles
Treatment in intensive care unit
Do not delay *intubation*
Severe bronchospasm is treated with *intravenous beta$_2$ agonist* (salbutamol or terbutaline 250 µg, followed by 10 µg/min)
Start fluid replacement with glucose–saline and continue if necessary with a *plasma expander*
In circulatory shock, not responding to the above measures, give a *vaso-pressor* (dopamine)
Monitor respiration, blood pressure and cardiac function
Post-emergency treatment
Continue *antihistamine* treatment for 48 hours
Give *corticosteroid* in status asthmaticus doses for 48 hours
Keep the patient under *observation* for 24 hours
Thoroughly discuss *preventive measures*

larynx can occlude the airway quickly. *Adrenaline* is given in the highest tolerable dose; *H₁ antihistamines* may prevent deterioration.

A recumbent position is recommended for circulatory collapse, but when upper airway oedema is threatening, a *half-sitting position* is necessary to reduce the oedema (>20° elevation). When the epiglottis is involved, it is essential for maintenance of an open airway that the neck is kept extended while in the sitting position.

When laryngeal oedema causes considerable airway obstruction, *endotracheal intubation* must be performed. If the obstruction is too advanced to permit intubation, *crico-thyroid membrane incision* is performed with a knife. A small endotracheal tube can be inserted for short-term ventilation through the incision. Alternatively, the membrane is punctured by large-bore needles.

The administration of *pure oxygen* becomes increasingly important with the degree of ventilatory insufficiency.

Lower airways

As bronchospasm can become fulminant, treatment is started as soon as the first symptoms of bronchospasm occur and immediately in all patients with a history of asthma. It is essential, at the earliest moment, to give *serial inhalations of a beta₂ agonist* as well as intravenous beta₂ agonist.

Corticosteroids

Steroids have no place in emergency treatment as it takes 2–4 hours before they are effective. Corticosteroids in status asthmaticus doses (see Chapter 9.26) are indicated in severe cases to *prevent a secondary relapse*, which occasionally occurs within 12–24 hours.

Prevention

The life-threatening nature of anaphylaxis makes prevention the keystone of therapy. The risk of death can be minimized, but not eliminated, by the following precautions: 1, always take a careful *medical history before medication*; 2, *prefer the oral route* rather than the parenteral route; 3, require a *clear indication for intravenous drug use*; 4, *observe the patient for 30 minutes* after an allergen injection; and 5, *be prepared* to treat anaphylaxis and *have adrenaline at hand* whenever an injection is given.

Some improvement perhaps
In acute diseases, it is not quite safe to prognosticate either death or recovery.

Hippocrates

13.3 Allergy to Hymenoptera venom
Bee and wasp

Key points

- Stinging insects of the Hymenoptera order belong to two superfamilies: apids and vespids.
- Honeybees (apids) can be responsible for multiple stings when their hive is endangered (e.g. by bee keepers).
- They are not aggressive away from their hive.
- Wasp, yellow jacket and hornet (vespids) are aggressive and can sting even when unprovoked.
- There is marked cross-reactivity between venoms from wasp, yellow jacket and hornet, but bee venom is different.
- A large local reaction to a sting can be due to allergy or infection.
- A systemic reaction is always due to allergy.
- It can consist of urticaria, angioedema, asthma and cardio-vascular collapse.
- Following a serious systemic reaction, 50% will get another reaction with a subsequent sting.
- The risk of death from anaphylaxis is relatively high in the elderly and very low in children.
- The diagnosis is based on the history and allergy testing, preferably with the skin prick technique.
- Only patients with systemic reactions are tested.
- A patient who has had a severe generalized reaction should carry a syringe, preloaded with adrenaline.
- Venom immunotherapy is offered to adult patients who have had a generalized reaction with respiratory or cardio-vascular symptoms.
- A maintenance dose of 100 μg venom protein gives a 95% protection rate.
- Increased plasma level of blocking IgG antibody is probably responsible, at least in part, for the clinical efficacy.
- The duration of venom immunotherapy is 3–5 years.

Stinging insects are responsible for a vast number of trivial skin reactions, which are annoying, especially when they become infected. Occasionally, however, the reactions can be dangerous and even fatal when individuals develop an allergic reaction to the venom. This occurs with equal frequency in non-atopic and atopic subjects.

Stinging insects are by far the most important cause of allergic reactions, but biting *fire ants* are a rapidly growing problem in the southeast of USA. Their bites result in a sterile pustule and occasionally in anaphylaxis.

The Hymenoptera order

Two superfamilies of the order *Hymenoptera* cause major medical problems with their stings: *Apidae* and *Vespidae*. The insects are characterized by size, appearance, habit and venom constituent (Fig. 13.3.1).

The *honeybee* is the most important apid, while the bumblebee is a rare offender. The honeybee is amicable, it feeds its larvae pollen and honey and is not aggressive away from its hive (unless you step on it). Honeybees can be responsible for multiple stings when their hive is endangered (e.g. by bee keepers). The sting remains in the skin of the victim, along with a portion of the abdomen and venom sac of the bee, which dies following the sting.

The most important vespids are *wasp*, *yellow jacket* and *hornet* (Table 13.3.1). They use their sting to paralyse and kill insects to provide food for their larvae; they are aggressive and can sting even when unprovoked. They do not loose their sting and can sting repeatedly.

Venoms and antigens

Hymenoptera venoms are complex mixtures of pharmacologically and biochemically active substances, including enzymes (phospholipase A and hyaluronidase), peptides (melitin in honeybee venom) and biogenic amines (histamine). These substances act as *toxins*, and the proteins/peptides also act as *allergens* in sensitized persons.

There is little or no cross-reactivity between venoms from the two superfamilies, apids and vespids. Thus, although bee and wasp phosphilipase A has the same enzymatic function, they are different as antigens. There is marked *cross-reactivity* within a superfamily, especially between species within the same family. However, there can be differences between species as, for example, between the North American and the South European hornet.

Types of reaction

Local reaction

Pain, erythema and swelling, lasting for 1–2 days, are a *normal* reaction to *Hymenoptera* stings. Large reac-

Characteristics of stinging insects		
Insect type	Appearance	Habitat
Honeybee 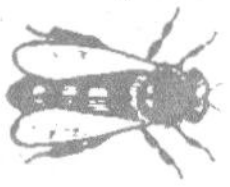	Hairy body with yellow and black markings; size 1.5 cm	Domestic hives, hollow trees or caves
Wasp 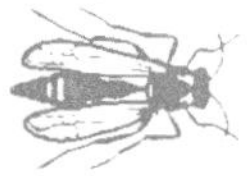	Hairless body with narrow waist, black or brown markings; size 3.0 cm	Trees, shrubs, eaves of houses
Hornet 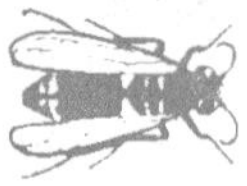	Short waist, truncated body with sparse hair, dark band under the eyes; size 2.0 cm	Oval and pear-shaped nests in trees and above ground
Yellow jacket 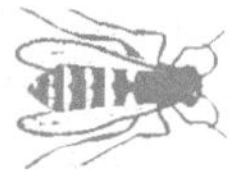	Similar to hornet with yellow markings but without dark bands under eyes; size 1.5 cm	Nests in ground and walls

Fig. 13.3.1. Characteristics of stinging insects (American nomenclature; see Table 13.3.1). From Fischer TJ, Lawlor Jr GJ. Insect allergy. In: Lawlor Jr GJ, Fisher TJ, eds. *Manual of Allergy and Immunology* Boston: Little, Brown and Company, 1981: 223–30.

tions (>10 cm) lasting for several days can occur as a result of *allergy* or *infection* (mainly vespids).

Systemic reaction

It is a major rule that any reaction remote from the sting is *allergic*. In the very rare case of multiple stings, it is possible that the remote reaction is a direct effect of the toxins; it has been estimated that 500 stings will deliver a lethal dose of venom.

The majority of reactions are mild, consisting of itching and urticaria, but a few persons get a severe and occasionally lethal anaphylactic reaction. In general, the shorter the time interval between sting and onset of symptoms, the more serious the reaction (anaphylaxis within 15 minutes; all serious reactions within 1 hour).

Three patterns of systemic reactions are recognized (but they usually occur in association): 1, generalized *urticaria* and angioedema; 2, *respiratory difficulties* with laryngeal oedema and/or asthma; and 3, *cardiovascular collapse*.

The highest incidence of *fatalities occur in middle-aged and elderly people*, probably because they have a *coexisting heart disease*. Only one-third of those who die have a history of earlier insect sting problems.

Atypical reaction

In very rare cases, an atypical reaction occurs from days to a few weeks after the sting, and it may persist over a long period of time. The reported reactions include serum sickness, vasculitis, nephrosis, neuritis and encephalopathy. The pathogenesis is unknown and immunotherapy is contra-indicated.

Natural history

About 25–50% of patients who have had a systemic reaction will get a subsequent reaction with a repeated sting. The risk is higher in adults than in children, and higher in patients who have had cardiovascular or respiratory symptoms than in those with skin symptoms only.

Bees and wasps, named in Europe and America		
Genus	Europe	America
Vespula	Wasp	Yellow jacket
Dolichovespula	Wasp	Hornet
Vespa	Hornet	European hornet
Polisters	Wasp	Wasp

Table 13.3.1. Differences in European and American nomenclature give rise to some confusion

The concentration of IgE antibodies decreases over the years and so does the risk of serious reactions, but the natural history of allergy to stinging insects, in any one patient, is *unpredictable*.

Diagnosis

History

Diagnosis of stinging insect allergy is generally self-evident. Problems arise in the identification of the causative insect. The honeybee is readily identifiable because it leaves its sting in place. Differentiation between wasp, yellow jacket and hornet is often difficult although some clues may be found if the insect is killed or the nest is near (Fig. 13.3.1).

Allergy testing

Allergy testing is performed in patients with a history of *any systemic reaction* to an insect sting, but such tests have no therapeutic value in patients with large local reactions.

A skin *prick test* is the most rapid and economic method of demonstrating venom-specific IgE antibodies. If it is negative or doubtfully positive the more sensitive intracutaneous test can be performed. A series of concentrations of venom are used for skin testing.

RAST is a good, safe substitute for skin testing and the correlation with skin tests is good.

IgE-mediated sensitivity can be demonstrated by skin testing or RAST in the large majority of those with systemic reactions and in about half the patients with a large local reaction.

Principles of avoidance

Treatment consists of avoidance, drug therapy and immunotherapy. So efficacious is modern venom injection therapy that self-treatment and the avoidance of stings have become much less important. Some guidelines on how to reduce the risk are given in Table 13.3.2. Give a copy to your patient.

Management of acute reactions

Local reactions

The sting is removed when possible. Relief of local symptoms can be obtained by pressing an *ice cube* against the sting site. Any type of *pressure* will delay absorption of venom and rapid action may prevent a progression to a more severe reaction. Folk medicine advocates application of various materials to the lesion; they may or may not be effective. An aqueous solution of aluminium sulphate (20% with 1% surfactant) denatures the injected protein and seems a better choice.

Systemic reactions

Itching and urticaria are treated with an *oral anti-*

Table 13.3.2. Patient information on how to reduce the risk of insect stings

How patients can reduce the risk of insect stings
The risk increases in summer and with outdoor activities
Be wary of outdoor eating and avoid jam, honey, sweet fruits, drinks and pickles
Always wear shoes out of doors; wear long trousers when walking in the grass or fields and gloves when gardening
Avoid bright, colourful clothing, perfumes, scented soaps and hair sprays as they attract insects
All nests or hives in the vicinity of the home should be removed – by another person
Stay away from insect feeding grounds, such as flower beds, clover fields, orchards with ripe fruit and garbage disposal areas
Have an emergency kit available at all times
Seek medical attention immediately after an emergency kit is used

histamine. A severe, generalized reaction is treated with *adrenaline* following the general rules for treatment of anaphylaxis (see Chapter 13.2). Upper airway obstruction often plays an important role in venom allergy; a *free airway* can be maintained by insertion of an oral airway, intubation or tracheotomy. Don't forget to give *oxygen* and remember that the correct position for a patient with upper airway obstruction is half-sitting, with his or her neck extended.

Self-treatment

When a patient has once experienced a severe generalized reaction, he or she should carry, and be instructed in the use of, an emergency kit. It is used immediately after a sting in patients unprotected by immunotherapy; treated patients only use the kit for a clear-cut reaction.

An *emergency kit* contains: 1, a preloaded syringe with adrenaline 1 mg/ml (sealed in nitrogen to avoid oxidation) and diluted to deliver a dose of 0.3–0.5 mg (0.01 ml/kg in children); and 2, an antihistamine tablet for immediate oral ingestion.

Venom immunotherapy

It is a dark chapter in the history of allergology that whole-body extracts, used to the satisfaction of patients and allergists for nearly 50 years, are completely ineffective. Treatment with venom extracts, on the other hand, is highly successful.

Indications

All adult patients with a *positive skin test or RAST* who have experienced a *generalized reaction with* *respiratory or cardio-vascular symptoms* should be offered immunotherapy. Untreated, they will have a 50% risk of a severe reaction at a subsequent sting. Immunotherapy can also be considered in a few patients with moderately severe systemic symptoms, who cannot avoid exposure (e.g. bakers, greengrocers, beekeepers), and when medical assistance is far away.

Allergy, causing a systemic reaction in a child, is not usually treated because fatalities are almost unknown in childhood. Patients with large local reactions are not candidates for immunotherapy as their risk of anaphylaxis is small (Table 13.3.3).

Contra-indications

Immunotherapy should not be used in patients on *beta-blocker* therapy, as the use of adrenaline can lead to unopposed alpha-receptor stimulation and may result in an overshoot in blood pressure. Immunotherapy should not be started during *pregnancy* but it may be continued when a patient on maintenance dose becomes pregnant.

Immunological changes

During venom immunotherapy, an initial increase in specific IgE antibody is followed by a slow decrease. This decrease is also seen in untreated patients who are not re-stung. Most important is the therapy-induced *increase in blocking IgG antibody*, which probably is responsible, at least in part, for the protective effect of the treatment.

Repeated stings, often occurring in beekeepers, also induces the formation of IgG antibody. This then protects those beekeepers who have developed IgE

Indication for immunotherapy	
Patients	**Indication**
Adults with a severe systemic reaction (respiratory or cardio-vascular involvement)	Yes
Adults with a moderate systemic reaction (urticaria, angioedema and mild asthma)	No/Yes*
Adults with a mild systemic reaction	No
Children with a systemic reaction	No
Patients with a large local reaction	No

Table 13.3.3. Indication for immunotherapy of patients with reactions to insect stings and a clear-cut positive allergy test. *Depends on frequency of reaction, likelihood of future exposure and access to medical service

antibody. Thus, venom-specific IgE serves as a measure of the 'state of allergy' and the venom-specific IgG as a measure of the 'state of immunity' and protection. However, measurement of IgE and IgG antibodies is not clinically useful in predicting the outcome of a sting challenge.

Therapy regimen

The goal for venom therapy is to reach a maintenance dose of *100 µg venom protein*, the equivalent of a few stings. When this dosage is reached, venom immunotherapy is highly effective, providing protection in about 95% of patients (higher protection with vespid venom than with bee venom).

The basic approach to venom immunotherapy is similar to other forms of allergen immunotherapy (see Chapter 11.5). Therapy is initiated with small doses (usually 0.01–0.1 µg) and incremental doses given until the maintenance dose is reached. There is a risk of *systemic allergic reactions*, which usually occur during the initial phase of dose increase, most often between 10 and 100 µg. Venom immunotherapy should be given only by physicians familiar with these types of extracts and in locations with all resuscitation facilities.

Duration of therapy

Studies with deliberate stings in hospital at timed intervals after discontinuation of immunotherapy indicate that venom immunotherapy can be discontinued after *3–5 years*.

On writing medical papers
Begin with an arresting sentence; close with a strong summary; in between speak simply, clearly, and always to the point; and above all be brief.

William J Mayo

13.4 Latex allergy
Gloves, condoms and balloons

Key points
- Latex is the milky sap collected by tapping the rubber tree.
- Chemicals, added to latex, can cause a Type IV reaction and contact eczema (not described in this chapter).
- Latex proteins can cause a Type I reaction with contact urticaria, airway symptoms and anaphylaxis.
- Most latex-sensitive individuals have an atopic background.
- Latex is an important cause of occupational allergy among health-care personnel.
- Contact urticaria, which arises within minutes of direct contact with gloves, is a good indicator of latex allergy.
- Pruritus alone is poorly predictive of latex allergy.
- Cornstarch powder, which absorbs latex proteins in gloves, becomes airborne and can induce symptoms in eyes, nose and bronchi.
- Patients who undergo multiple operations have a high risk of developing latex allergy.
- The group with the highest risk is children with spina bifida.
- Serious anaphylactic reactions predominantly occur during intra-abdominal surgery.
- Skin prick testing is an easy, specific and sensitive way to diagnose latex allergy, but extracts are not standardized.
- Provocation testing consists of wearing a latex glove and of handling boxes containing gloves.
- Use of non-latex gloves is necessary in sensitized health-care personnel.
- Stringent elimination of latex from the operating room is needed to protect a sensitive patient.

Type I and Type IV reactions
It has long been known that gloves of rubber can cause *contact eczema* some hours after exposure. This *Type IV reaction*, or delayed-type hypersensitivity, to *chemical additives* added to rubber can be diagnosed by *patch testing* with these chemicals.

It was not until 1979 that the first case of a *Type I reaction*, or immediate-type hypersensitivity, to *latex proteins* was described.

Since then, an increasing number of cases of local reactions to gloves, especially in health-care personnel, and of anaphylactic reactions in patients undergoing surgery, have been reported.

The frequency of latex protein allergy may have increased due to the dramatic rise in the use of gloves by medical and dental personnel for protection against HIV and hepatitis viruses.

Latex allergens

Natural rubber is obtained from the rubber tree, *Hevea braziliensis*. The milky sap of this plant, latex, contains a rubber matrix of *polyisoprene*, about 2% *protein* and water. During rubber manufacture, the polyisoprene chains are cross-linked and many *chemicals* are added (vulcanizers, accelerators, stabilizers, antioxidants). The final product contains a number of chemicals (Type IV allergy) and at least 16 different protein molecules, which are the cause of the IgE-mediated Type I reactions.

Latex allergens show *cross-reactivity* with fruit allergens. Nearly half of the latex-allergic patients report having an allergic reaction to a fruit, the most frequently mentioned being *banana*, avocado and kiwi.

Latex is a widespread product and the variety of articles containing latex is considerable. The most important are *gloves, medical equipment (catheters and tubes), condoms and balloons* (Table 13.4.1).

Latex articles causing symptoms	
Articles	**Number of patients**
Gloves	69
Sticking plaster	11
Balloons	8
Bracer	6
Condoms	5
Masks (anaesthetic or diving)	3
Stretch textiles	3
Shoes	3
Door/window isolation	2
Air mattress	1
Sailing equipment	1
Stamps	1

Table 13.4.1. List of articles, containing latex, that caused symptoms in 70 patients (64 hospital personnel) with IgE antibodies to latex. From Jaeger D, Kleinhans D, Czuppon AB, Baur X. *J Allergy Clin Immunol* 1992; **89**: 759–68

Risk factors

Atopic status and hand eczema

Most latex-sensitive patients have an atopic background, and there is a positive association between *atopic status*, defined as a positive skin test to major aero-allergens, and the risk of developing latex allergy. *Hand eczema* also predisposes to latex allergy.

Health-care personnel

Recent reports have described allergy to latex in 5–10% of *nurses* working in operating units, and in as many as 15–30% of *dental workers*. Consequently, latex is now an *important cause of occupational allergy* among health-care workers.

Patients undergoing multiple operations

Patients who undergo multiple operations or are chronically exposed to latex medical devices (catheters) have a considerable risk of developing Type I reactions. The group with the highest risk is *children with spina bifida* or severe urogenital defects. The reported incidence of latex allergy among children with spina bifida ranges from 20 to 60%. These children can get allergic symptoms from blowing-up balloons.

Rubber industry workers

Not surprisingly, workers in factories manufacturing latex gloves are at risk. A study of rubber workers showed a positive skin test to latex in 10%.

Clinical manifestations

Patients may exhibit the full range of reactions from contact urticaria to anaphylaxis (Table 13.4.2). Life-threatening reactions are typically induced by mucosal and serosal exposure, whereas cutaneous exposure leads to localized reactions. The symptoms are noted within a few minutes but the source can be difficult to identify because latex is found in more than 20000 consumer items.

Contact urticaria

Symptoms may arise from direct contact with gloves. The classical clinical picture of this Type I allergy is patchy or diffuse redness and *urticaria of the back of the hands* and fingers that stops abruptly at the wrist. The hands, however, often transfer the allergen to other parts of the body, especially the face.

Symptoms in latex-allergic patients	
Urticaria	100%
Rhinitis	51%
Conjunctivitis	44%
Dyspnoea	31%
Systemic reactions	24%
Surgery complications	6%

Table 13.4.2. Symptoms in 70 patients (64 hospital personnel) with latex allergy. From Jaeger D, Kleinhans D, Czuppon AB, Baur X. *J Allergy Clin Immunol* 1992; **89**: 759–68

When gloves induce contact urticaria, it is highly indicative of latex allergy. On the other hand, *pruritus alone is poorly predictive of latex allergy*. In a study of nurses, only 25% of those who exclusively complained of itching when wearing surgical gloves, had a positive skin prick test to latex.

Reported data suggest that only 25% of women, allergic to latex gloves, experience vaginal pruritus during or after exposure to *condoms*, but underreporting on this point is likely.

Respiratory symptoms

Cornstarch powder, used as a lubricant in medical gloves, is not, by itself, allergenic. However, it can absorb *latex proteins* and function as a carrier for latex allergens. When packages of gloves are opened, cornstarch particles become airborne, contaminating large areas. Sensitive people may experience *symptoms in eyes, nose and bronchi* within minutes. Consequently, allergic individuals may encounter difficulty in working or in undergoing treatment in environments, such as operating theatres.

Systemic manifestations

The great majority of serious reactions have occurred in patients *during surgery*. Typically, anaphylaxis is caused by contact with a surgeon's gloves during an *intra-abdominal operation*. Some patients have experienced more than one episode, as the cause of the first one has not been recognized.

Anaphylactic reactions have also occurred following *tracheal intubation*, after *insertion of a catheter*, during *gynaecologic examination* and during *barium enema examination*, as the rectal catheter has a latex cuff.

Diagnosis

Skin prick test

Prick testing is the easiest and most readily available way to diagnose latex allergy. It is highly *specific* and more *sensitive* than *in vitro* testing. It can be performed with extract both made from raw latex and from finished rubber products. However, at present, the extracts are poorly characterized and *not standardized*.

Skin testing with extracts of 19 brands of latex gloves have shown a frequency of positive reactions from 10–100% indicating that there are differences in the quantity of latex allergens eluting from different brands of gloves.

Prick test with extracts of 16 different brands of condoms have shown that four brands caused a positive reaction in 50–70% of patients allergic to latex.

Provocation test

Skin challenge can be done by placing $1\,cm^2$ pieces of latex glove material, moistened with saline, on the skin of the forearm or by *wearing a latex glove* on a dampened hand for 15 minutes. A vinyl glove can be used as negative control.

Challenge testing of the eyes and airways can consist of *handling boxes containing gloves*, or by inhalation of powder from latex gloves in a small inhalation chamber for 15 minutes.

There is a risk of eliciting systemic reactions when performing provocation tests, so they should be done only in special cases.

In vitro tests

At present, *in vitro* testing (RAST) is *less sensitive* than skin tests and provocation challenge, detecting IgE antibodies in only 50–70% of skin test positive patients.

Differential diagnosis

In patients with hand eczema, induced by latex gloves, it is often necessary to use patch testing to *rule out sensitivity to rubber chemicals*.

When allergic reactions occur during surgery, *allergy to muscle relaxants*, thiopentone, succinylcholine and other drugs used during general anaesthesia must be considered.

Prevention

Primary prevention—to avoid sensitization

People with a history of *atopic disease and eczema*, who must use gloves in their work, might be advised to use synthetic gloves instead of latex products whenever possible.

Children with spina bifida are at such high risk of sensitization that many centres recommend that latex products be avoided entirely in this group.

Encouraged by the Food and Drug Administration in the USA, the manufacturers of latex-containing medical devices are currently trying to make the protein levels in their products as low as possible.

Secondary prevention—to avoid symptoms

The principle therapeutic approach for sensitized persons, consisting of *avoiding exposure to latex*, is a method that is difficult because of the ubiquity of latex products.

A number of brands of *non-latex gloves* (plastic or vinyl) are available. The protective effect of some of these gloves has been disputed and some are unacceptable to surgeons who do not get an accurate touch.

The stringent elimination of latex from the operating room can protect the sensitive patient from an anaphylactic reaction. Health professionals should use non-latex gloves when in contact with such patients. When latex gloves are used, it is possible to diminish the allergenic material considerably by *washing the gloves*.

Avoid unanimity

Read, every day, something no one else is reading. Think, every day, something no one else is thinking. Do, every day, something no one else would be silly enough to do. It is bad for the mind to be always part of a unanimity.

Christopher Morley

Further reading

BOUSQUET J, KNANI J, VELASQUEZ G, *et al.* Evolution of sensitivity to Hymenoptera venom in 200 allergic patients followed for up to 3 years. *J Allergy Clin Immunol* 1989; **84**: 944–50.

FUCHS T, WAHL R. Immediate reactions to rubber products. *Allergy Proc* 1992; **13**: 61–6.

HAUGAARD L, NØRREGAARD O, DAHL R. In-hospital sting challenge in insect venom-allergic patients after stopping venom immunotherapy. *J Allergy Clin Immunol* 1991; **87**: 699–702.

INGALL M, GOLDMAN G, PAGE LB. Beta-blockade in stinging insect anaphylaxis. *J Am Med Wom Assoc* 1984; **251**: 1432–8.

LAGIER F, VERVLOET D, LHERMET I, POYEN D, CHARPIN D. Prevalence of latex allergy in operating room nurses. *J Allergy Clin Immunol* 1992; **90**: 319–22.

LEVY DA, CHARPIN D, PECQUET C, LEYNADIER F, VERLOET D. Allergy to latex. *Allergy* 1994; **47**: 579–87.

MÜLLER U, MOSBECH H. Immunotherapy with Hymenoptera venoms: a position paper. *Allergy* 1993; **48**(suppl 14): 37–46.

MÜLLER U, MOSBECH H, BLAAUW P, *et al.* Emergency treatment of allergic reactions to Hymenoptera stings. *Clin Exp Allergy* 1991; **21**: 281–8.

REISMAN RE. Venom hypersensitivity. *J Allergy Clin Immunol* 1994; **94**: 651–8.

TOOGOOD JH. Beta-blocker therapy and the risk of anaphylaxis. *Can Med Assoc J* 1987; **136**: 929–33.

TURJANMAA K, REUNALA T. Condoms as a source of latex allergen and cause of contact urticaria. *Contact Dermatitis* 1989; **20**: 360–4.

VALENTINE MD, SCHUBERTH KC, KAGEY-SOBOTKA A, *et al.* The value of immunotherapy with venom in children with allergy to insect stings. *N Engl J Med* 1990; **323**: 1601–3.

YUNGINGER JW. Anaphylaxis. *Ann Allergy* 1992; **69**: 87–96.

Index